ENCYCLOPEDIC HANDBOOK OF BIOMATERIALS AND BIOENGINEERING

Part B: Applications

Volume 1

ENCYCLOPEDIC HANDBOOK OF BIOMATERIALS AND BIOENGINEERING

Part B: Applications
Volume 1

edited by

Donald L. Wise
Northeastern University
Boston, Massachusetts

Debra J. Trantolo
Cambridge Scientific, Inc.
Belmont, Massachusetts

David E. Altobelli
Harvard School of Dental Medicine
Boston, Massachusetts

Michael J. Yaszemski
United States Air Force
Lackland Air Force Base, Texas

Joseph D. Gresser
Cambridge Scientific, Inc.
Belmont, Massachusetts

Edith R. Schwartz
National Institute of Standards and Technology
Gaithersburg, Maryland

MARCEL DEKKER, INC.   NEW YORK · BASEL · HONG KONG

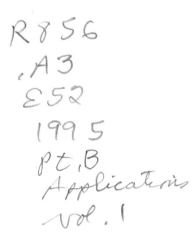

Library of Congress Cataloging-in-Publication Data

Encyclopedic handbook of biomaterials and bioengineering / edited by Donald L. Wise
... [et al.].
    p. cm.
    Contents: Pt. A., v. 1-2. Materials -- Pt. B., v. 1-2. Applications.
    ISBN 0-8247-9593-8 (v. 1 : alk. paper) — ISBN 0-8247-9594-6 (v. 2 : alk. paper)
— ISBN 0-8247-9595-4 (v. 1 : alk. paper) — ISBN 0-8247-9596-2 (v. 2 : alk. paper).
    1. Biomedical engineering -- Encyclopedias. 2. Biomedical materials--
Encyclopedias. I. Wise, Donald L. (Donald Lee)

R856.A3E52   1995
610'.28--dc20
                        95-21232
                            CIP

The publisher offers discounts on this book when ordered in bulk quantities. For more information, write to Special Sales/Professional Marketing at the address below.

This book is printed on acid-free paper.

Marcel Dekker, Inc.
270 Madison Avenue, New York, New York 10016

Current printing (last digit):
10 9 8 7 6 5 4 3

PRINTED IN THE UNITED STATES OF AMERICA

Preface

The medical device and drug industry is consistently one of the strongest performers. Materials are a key ingredient to this industry. Development of these materials is in a constant state of activity with the burdens of old materials not withstanding the tests of time and new materials needs coming to the forefront of modern applications. This handbook focuses on materials used in or on the human body — materials that define the world of "biomaterials."

The *Encyclopedic Handbook of Biomaterials and Bioengineering* covers the range of biomaterials from polymers to metals to ceramics. The depth of the field necessitated careful integration of basic science, engineering, and practical medical experience in a variety of applied disciplines. As a result, scientists, engineers, and physicians are among the chapter authors, as well as the editors. The handbook provides a detailed accounting of the state of the art in the rapidly growing biomaterials arena. Its organization reflects the diversity of the field.

The encyclopedia is a four-volume reference: Part A, "Materials," in two volumes and Part B, "Applications," in two volumes. In the Applications texts, the focus is on the actual use of the biomaterials in their applied settings. Volume 1 deals first with the general requirements in selecting a proper biomaterial for successful application, then moves to one of the original applications areas for biomaterials — orthopedics. Volume 2 focuses on biomaterials in bone cement, vascular, ophthalmic, and dental applications. Integral to all of these chapters are evaluations of the performance of the biomaterials in the projected clinical setting.

The users of this encyclopedia will represent a broad base of backgrounds ranging from the basic sciences (e.g., polymer chemistry and biochemistry) to the more applied disciplines (e.g., orthopedics and pharmaceutics). To meet varied needs, each chapter provides clear and fully detailed discussions. This in-depth coverage should also assist recent inductees to the biomaterials circle. The editors trust that this handbook conveys the intensity of this fast-moving field in an enthusiastic presentation.

The editors are grateful for the cooperation of many friends and colleagues in their support of this work. Our appreciation extends to each of the contributors for suggestions and comments as the project developed. Their interest and enthusiasm in pulling together a comprehensive reference for all our associates in the biomaterials area have been most gratifying. The editors are especially thankful to Ms. Wanda O'Connell for her patience and competence in dealing with manuscripts from more than 100 authors.

Donald L. Wise, Debra J. Trantolo, David E. Altobelli,
Michael J. Yaszemski, Joseph D. Gresser, and Edith R. Schwartz

Contents of Part B: Applications

Part II. Orthopedic Biomaterials

Part III. Metals in Orthopedics

Part IV. Bone Repair and Joint Replacement

Part V. Tissue Response and Growth

VOLUME 2

Part VI. Bone Cements

Part IX.   Ocular Applications

Part X.   Dental Applications

Contents of Part A: Materials

VOLUME 2

Part V.   Materials Based on PLGA

Part VI.   Controlled Release

Part VII.   Collagen-Based Materials

ENCYCLOPEDIC
HANDBOOK OF
BIOMATERIALS AND
BIOENGINEERING

Part B: Applications

Volume 1

I
INTRODUCTION

1

Anisotropic Biomaterials: Strategies and Developments for Bone Implants

Erich Wintermantel and Joerg Mayer
Swiss Federal Institute of Technology
Zürich, Switzerland

I. INTRODUCTION

Anisotropic biomaterials are developed in order to functionally mimic a recipient structure, i.e., bone. Anisotropy in this chapter is understood as a variation in mechanical properties depending on the geometrical orientation of tensile or compressive load application. Metals are isotropic under this definition, whereas fiber composite materials are anisotropic.

Biocompatibility is defined as surface *and* structural compatibility of an implant. Structural compatibility includes optimal load transition in an implant/materials interface. It is suggested, therefore, that anisotropic materials offer higher potential biocompatibility than metals do because mechanical properties can better be adjusted to bone.

Other properties of anisotropic, nonmetallic materials are considered: absence of metal ions in order to prevent allergic reactions, adjustability of x-ray transparency by adding contrast medium to the polymeric matrix, and full compatibility with NMR and CT diagnostic procedures.

Homoelasticity is defined as the approach in stiffness to bone. The intention is to minimize the strain mismatch between bone and implant.

II. FUNCTIONAL ELEMENTS OF CARBON FIBER REINFORCED COMPOSITES

A. The Fiber

The carbon fiber is the load-bearing element in the composite. Due to its superior strength and stiffness the fiber defines the mechanical anisotropy. Most carbon fibers are made from polymer precursor fibers such as polyacrylnitrile (PAN) or from pitch precursors. The influence of the precursor and processing conditions—i.e., carbonization and graphitization temperature or rate of drawing—on the fiber structure and the physicochemical properties has been extensively discussed[1–3]. Table 1 gives an overview of the range of achievable mechanical properties [4]. The anisotropy of the fiber itself is enhanced with increasing graphitization temperature [5].

The negative thermal expansion coefficient in the fiber axis has especially to be considered during processing, because the mismatch of thermal expansion between fiber (-10^6 m/K) and matrix (10^5 m/K) or between angle-plied fibers causes considerable internal stresses. Therefore, the orientation of the fibers in a composite has to be symmetric according to the geometric middle plane of the part.

B. Matrix

The matrix embedding the fibers guarantees the structural integrity of the fiber architecture in a composite. It has the following functions in a composite which determine the failure behavior of the composite during off-axis loading [6–10]:

- Mechanical support of the fibers if the composite is loaded by compression or shear forces
- Force transmission from fiber to fiber during crack growth or at fiber ends
- Load bearing if the composite is stressed transversally to the fiber direction
- Protection of the fiber against aggressive media

To achieve biocompatibility the matrix should expose an appropriate surface concerning surface energy, microstructure, or retention of fiber particle debris.

In the literature many matrices have been discussed, such as polysulfone [11, 12], nylon [13], epoxy resins [14–16], carbon [17], and others [18–21]. Because of the chemical long-term stability and the appropriate processing techniques, thermoplastic matrices with a special focus on polyether(ether)ketone (PEEK) are emphasized. PEEK is well characterized as bulk polymer and as matrix for carbon fibers [22, 23] considering structure and morphology [24–27], processing [28–34], mechanical properties [34–38], chemical stability [39], and biocompatibility [40–45].

Table 2 shows typical properties of the matrices used from the authors for biocompatible composites, i.e., PEEK, polyamide 12 (PA12), and polyethylmethacrylate (PEMA).

C. The Interphase

The coupling element between fiber and matrix, the so-called interface, determines most of the mechanical properties, except the elastic properties. It is responsible for the chemi-

Table 1 Mechanical Properties of Carbon Fibers

Fiber	Ultimate strength (MPa)	Young's modulus (GPa)	Elongation at break (%)	Density (g/cm^3)
Standard, AS 4 (Hercules)	3600	235	1.53	1.8
Intermediate, IM8 (Hercules)	5484	323	1.75	1.75
High-strength HS, T1000 (Toray)	7060	297	2.38	1.75
High-module HM, M50 (Toray)	2450	490	0.5	1.91

Source: Ref. 4

Table 2   Properties of Thermoplastic Matrices Used for the Described Studies

	PA 12 (Atochem)	PEEK (ICI)	PEMA (Roehm)
Tensile modulus (GPa)	1.4–1.6	3.6	1.1–1.3
Ultimate strength (MPa)	52	92	40–45
Elongation at break (%)	240	50	3–4
Melting point (°C)	178	334	–
Glass transition temp. (°C)	40–45	143	45–55
Density (g/cm³)	1.10	1.28	1.13
Crystalinity (%)	30	35	Amorphous
Water uptake at 20°C (%)	1.5	0.5	1.8 (37°C)

cal stability of the composite [46]. The definition of this coupling element is controversially discussed [46–49]. The following distinction between an interface and an interphase is illustrated in Fig. 1 for a carbon fiber reinforced semicrystalline thermoplast such as PA12 or PEEK.

Interphase: A 3-dimensional phase with physicochemical properties different from the neighboring bulk phases, i.e., matrix and fiber or other interphases. Fracture in an interphase has a cohesive morphology.

Interface: A 2-dimensional face between interphases and bulk phases. It is the surface of these phases. Fracture in an interface has an adhesive morphology.

The structure of interphases, i.e., the transcrystalline phase or the nucleation zone for spherolithes, has been extensively discussed for polyolefins and PEEK [50–52, 55, 58]. Nevertheless, the influence of such phases on mechanical properties is not clear and depends on the polymer as well as on the processing conditions [50, 51].

Closely correlated to interphases and interfaces is adhesion and wetting, which is the precondition but not the reason for good adhesion [48]. The wetting behavior is mainly determined by surface energies and processing conditions, i.e., the polymer viscosity and

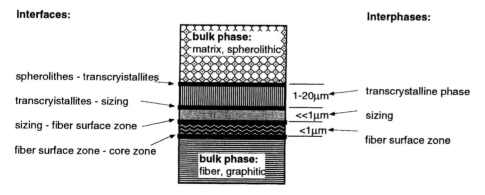

Figure 1   Location of interfaces and interphases in a carbon fiber reinforced semicrystalline thermoplast. [After Ref. 132.]

hydrostatic pressure. For adhesion, the following key factors are currently discussed [5, 48, 49, 53]:

- Mechanical interlocking by enhanced surface roughness of the fiber
- Intermolecular forces (van der Waals, dipole–dipole)
- Covalent, ionic (acid–base) and hydrogen bonds

According to Ref. 46, adhesion influences strength, fatigue resistance, and toughness, but has no significance for the elastic properties. In a typical failure sequence of an unidirectional composite, matrix fails first by transverse cracking, followed by subsequent steps, i.e., fiber–matrix debonding, tensile failure of the weakest fibers, load transfer to neighboring fibers, and crack growth with pull-out of the broken fibers [54].

Because of the higher Gibb's free energy of interphases, they are considered to be sensitive to the attack of aggressive media such as water [56, 82, 83] and body fluids. The uptake of water in an immersed composite can cause the hydrolysis of chemical bonds, debonding, and swelling. In composites, considerable reduction in compressive and off-axis strength and a reduced fatigue resistance have been observed [57]. These effects became even more relevant in short fiber reinforced composites due to the fiber discontinuity.

To improve long-term stability of composites for implant materials, fiber and matrix have frequently been tuned to an optimal interface stability [66]. On carbon fibers, reactive chemical groups have been introduced by methods such as thermal [60, 62] or anodic [53] oxidation, plasma oxidation, or polymerization treatments [61]. For the characterization of the surface properties of fiber and matrix, different methods have been used to describe the surface chemistry by x-ray photoelectron spectroscopy (XPS) [63, 64], secondary ion mass spectroscopy (SIMS) [63], Fourier transform infrared (FTIR) reflection spectrometry [65], Raman microscopy [65], and inverse gas chromatography [67]. Surface energy and the influence of adsorbed layers have been studied in Wilhelmy wetting experiments [68–71]; the surface morphology, by scanning electron microscopy (SEM) or scanning probe microscopy (SPM) [72, 73]. The accompanying figures [73] illustrate the influence of a thermal oxidative treatment at 400°–500°C for 15 min of T300 carbon fibers, which are used for the knitted fiber reinforced composites discussed in the following section. The atomic force microscopy (AFM) measurements indicated a slight increase in surface roughness as well as an obvious change of the surface morphology from parallel grooves at 400°C to a more hill-like structure (Fig. 2). The XPS measurements (Fig. 3) reveal only a slight influence of the oxidative treatment on the oxygen content (10% at 400°C, 13% at 600°C). In the carbon 1s and in the O 1s peak the high energy tail increases slightly with temperature. This indicates forced oxidation of carbon. The increasing surface energies (Fig. 4) reveal the most significant effect of this oxidative treatment.

To investigate the interaction between fiber and matrix in a microscopic scale, a sintering experiment was performed based on the solid-body wetting technique [73, 74]. PEMA powder spheres were sintered on the thermal-treated carbon fibers at 100°C. Figure 5 shows a polymer sphere of 1000 μm^3 volume after 60 min sintering at 100°C having a wetting angle of about 120°. The arrow indicates a contact area to an other fiber stressing that wetting occurs even at the submicron scale. The advancing wetting angle was measured in the SEM after 30, 60, and 90 min sintering. The sinter activity was found to increase with smaller droplets size as expected from the sinter theory and with decreasing oxidation temperature. Comparing results from the solid-body experiment with the

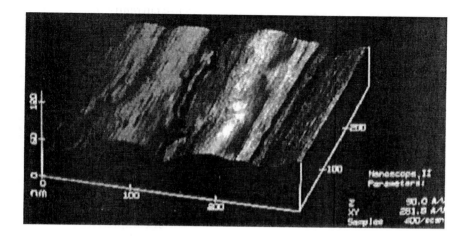

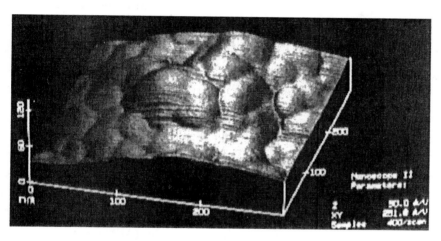

Figure 2 AFM images of the thermal oxidized T300 carbon fiber. Top: 400°C 15 min; bottom: 600°C 15 min [72].

surface energies measured, the astonishing observation is that the sinter activity is reduced for higher fiber oxidation temperatures. Explanations considered may be that, on the one hand, this interaction between fiber and matrix is controlled by the dispersive part of surface energy; on the other hand, the change of surface morphology may have had some influence as well.

D. Role of the Fiber Architecture

Fiber architecture—the arrangement of fibers in the composite—defines the thermomechanical properties of the composites. The fiber architecture itself is determined by the processing technique. Depending on the process, the fiber architecture can be built up previous to consolidation or during final shaping as it is explained in Table 3.

Well established in composite processing are lamination techniques for continuous fibers (60 vol%) and injection molding (<40 wt%). Textile preforming to net shape

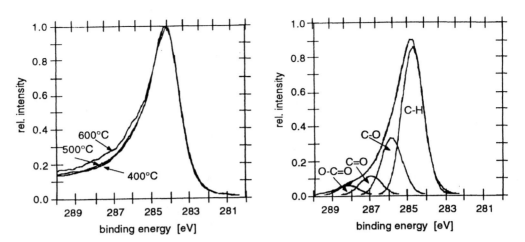

Figure 3 XPS analysis of the T300 surface after thermal oxidation for 15 min. Left: comparison of the oxidation temperatures; right: identification of fitted chemical functionalities. (Chemical shifts according to Ref. 131.)

and melt extrusion are new techniques developed for the requirements of biocompatible composites. Their application in osteosynthesis devices, i.e., plate and screw, is described in the following section [75, 76].

The goal of lamination techniques for continuous fiber reinforced composites is the optimal alignment of the fibers according to an optimization of mechanical properties. Typical fiber architectures are cross-plied layers of unidirectional laminates or woven cloths. Because of the 2-dimensional fiber orientation, these structures are used for shell constructions. The productivity of lamination techniques, i.e., filament winding or tape

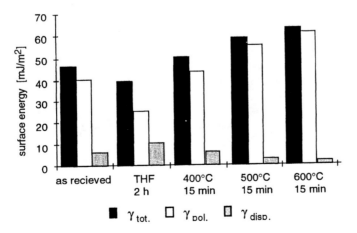

Figure 4 Surface energies of T300 fibers after 400°C, 500°C, and 600°C for 15 min. Solvents were water and ethylene glycol [73].

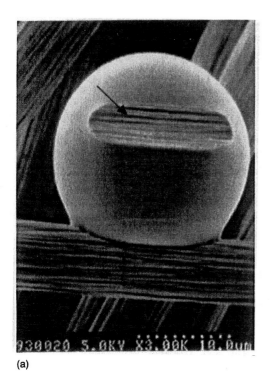

(a)

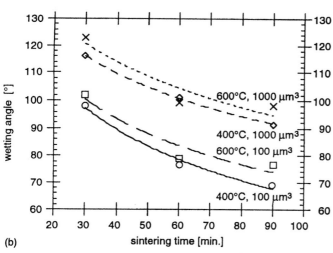

(b)

Figure 5   Solid-body wetting of PEMA powder on T300 carbon fibers. Upper: sinter conditions 100°C, 60 min [73]. Lower: sinter activity of PEMA on T300 in the solid-body wetting experiment.

Table 3 Definition of Fiber Architecture by Processing: Example of Processes

Previous to consolidation	During shaping
Lamination techniques (continuous fibers)	Injection molding (short fibers)
Textile preforming to net shape (continuous fibers)	Melt extrusion (continuous fibers)

laying, is low but at a high cost level. Disadvantages are: (1) the 2-dimensionality that restricts the application to well-defined load cases only and (2) the poor drapability due to the continuity of the aligned fibers. Three-dimensional fiber structures can be achieved using expensive techniques, i.e., 3-D weaving or braiding [77–81].

The use of injection molding techniques using short fibers is optimized to achieve suitable mechanical properties with highest productivity and lowest costs. The fiber arrangement in the mold is controlled by the melt flow. Therefore, the alignment of the fibers is more randomized even if certain preferential orientations are observed in skin zone. Disadvantages of this technique are the low fiber volume content and the fiber discontinuity, which increases the sensitivity of matrix failure during fatigue, especially in aggressive environments.

In several reviews [84–89] models are proposed for the understanding and calculation of mechanical properties from the fiber architecture as well as the common manufacturing techniques for continuous [90–92] and short fiber reinforced composites [93, 131].

III. COMPOSITES DESIGNED FOR ANISOTROPIC BIOMATERIALS, SUCH AS OSTEOSYNTHESIS DEVICES

A. Introduction

The common osteosynthesis techniques are focused on a rigid fixation of the fracture sites using plates made from stainless steel [94] or titanium alloys. To achieve primary bone healing without the formation of callus, high axial pressures are needed [95]. Isoelastic osteosynthesis is discussed as an alternative approach which includes fast mechanisms of bone healing such as callus formation [96]. Several concepts, such as the use of resorbable materials [97, 98] or reduction of plates stiffness by change of the material or of the design [110], have been discussed.

It has been found that the amount of external callus is dependent on the plate's stiffness [99]. Compared to primary bone healing, the formation of callus results in higher fracture strength of the healed bone [100, 101]. Less bone resorption underneath homoelastic plates has been observed by several authors [96, 97, 100], correlating loss of bone density with the degree of stress protection. As further reason for bone resorption, local bone necrosis due to high contact pressure of the plate, is controversially discussed [102–104]. It has been reported [105–109] that the residual strength is at its maximum before resorption by stress shielding or by necrosis takes place.

To achieve a stable homoelastic fixation, axial stiffness comparable to bone is requested [110, 111]. Bending and torsional stiffness should be higher for proper fixation of the fracture. Since 1975, numerous carbon fiber reinforced, nonresorbable composites have been studied *in vitro* and *in vivo*, using polysulfone [11, 12], nylon [13], epoxy resins [14–16], carbon [17], or other matrix systems [18–21, 112, 113]. Multistep manufacturing techniques, i.e., hot-pressing and machining techniques, were used for continuous fiber reinforced laminates. Because of the fair competitiveness of these techniques for medium-scale series, injection molding of short fiber reinforced composites has been investigated [128]. The low fiber content, and problems with reproducible fiber distribution, with fatigue behavior, and with sensitivity to environmental attack restricted the application of injection-molded plates. The possibility of hot-shaping the plate because of the discontinuity of the fibers may be an advantage for clinical application. Thermal shaping of laminated plates [112] is restricted to intra- and interlaminar shearing and intralaminar transverse flow because of the rigidity of the reinforcing carbon fibers.

Based on previous discussion, the following requirements for a homoelastic osteo-synthesis system made from anisotropic biomaterials have to be considered:

- Three-dimensional fiber orientation due to the complex load collective in an osteosynthesis
- Anisotropy for high torsional and bending stiffness combined with low axial stiffness
- X-ray transparency to allow the definition of time for the earliest possible removal
- Shaping of the plate during operation, but with minimal impact to the recipient tissue
- Costs comparable to or lower than metal plate manufacturing
- Use of screws made from composites to prevent corrosion

In the following section the results of an osteosynthesis system development are discussed. According to the concept of process-controlled anisotropic biomaterials a fiber architecture, defined previous to consolidation, is discussed for an osteosynthesis plate. A fiber architecture built up during processing is discussed for a cortical bone screw.

B. Osteosynthesis Plate, Net Shaped by a Single-Step Processing of Knitted Carbon Fiber Reinforced Thermoplastics

The net shape manufacturing technique of the 6-hole ulnar osteosynthesis plate shown in Fig. 6 uses two characteristic properties of knitted fiber structures: the drapability and the coherence which makes it possible to mold in holes by widening of single loops. The

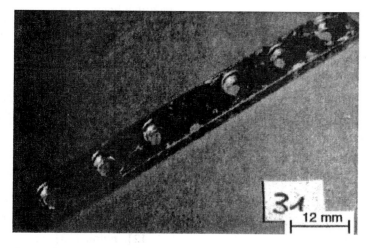

Figure 6   Six-hole ulnar osteosynthesis plate, made from knitted carbon fiber reinforced PEEK in a single-step net shape pressing technique [73].

plate is made from weft-knitted carbon fiber reinforced PEEK in a single-step net shape pressing technique [73, 74]. Knitted fibers are an unusual fiber architecture for reinforcing composite materials, and due to the curved fibers, they are claimed to have poor mechanical properties [81, 114–118]. Recent investigations [73] have shown that knitted structures have the following special features which are advantageous for anisotropic biomaterials:

- Fiber orientation is defined spatially by the geometry of the loop.
- Coherence of the knit structure guarantees fiber orientation and fiber content even during large plastic deformation.
- Drawability: due to its structure, weft knits can be drawn in wale and in course directions up to 150%.
- The unique drapability of knitted textile performs and plastic deformability of consolidated semifinished parts allow an unhampered shaping.
- Spatial interweaving of the loops hinders the formation of layer structures and excludes delamination.
- Metal-like shaping techniques such as deep-drawing or hot-stamping and waste-free net shape forming.

These aspects are discussed in the following section to give a better understanding of the behavior of complex fiber architectures and the possibilities of their application in implant materials.

1. Structure of Knitted Carbon Fiber Reinforced Composites

The carbon fiber knit investigated is characterized by its low density and by the size of the loops, as shown in Fig. 7. An optimized knitting technique is requested to knit carbon fiber with loop size of several millimeters and with minimal fiber damage [119, 120].

The weft knit has a basic periodic structure with a high symmetry having perpendicular mirror planes and screw axes (Fig. 8). As shown in Fig. 9, two stacking sequences have been assumed in the densified composite. Both indicate orthorhombic symmetry

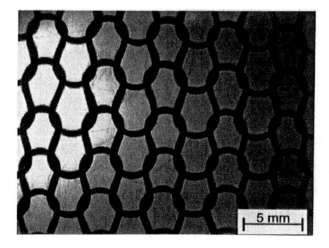

Figure 7   One layer of the circular weft knit [73].

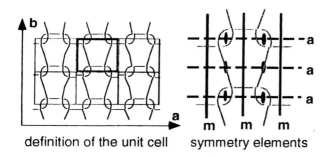

definition of the unit cell   symmetry elements

Figure 8 Definition of the unit cell of a single weft knit layer (highlighted). The size of a typical unit cell is $a = 8$ mm, $b = 6$ mm [73].

relations in the Laue group, which is the relevant one for the mechanical properties. Therefore, mechanical structure modeling based on the units cell properties is possible and, for the calculation, six independent elastic constants have to be considered. To visualize in the composite knit structure, a 100-μm copper filament has been coknitted and x-rayed after consolidation. X-ray investigations of consolidated composites indicated that both stacking sequences are present, with $a/4 + b/2$ as the most frequent.

During consolidation, knit layers interpenetrate and a 3-dimensional fiber structure is built up as shown in the cross-section in Fig. 10. A complete consolidation with fiber volume contents up to 60 vol% is possible using a knit of low area weight and high loop size.

The coherence of knit structure guarantees the fiber orientation even at high drawing ratios. Drawing induces a uniform deformation of the loops indicating a solid-body

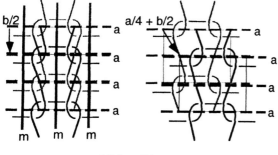

space group: triklin , P1
Laue group: orthorhombic primitive, mmm

                   b wale direction

unit cell:
$a = 8$ mm, $b = 6$ mm   c course direction

Figure 9 Symmetry in weft knits and possible stacking arrangements. The periodicity of the knit structure is a basic feature for modeling [73].

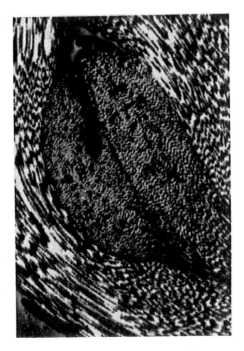

Figure 10   Cross-section in the knit plane of a knitted fiber reinforced composite [73].

deformation behavior with transverse contraction about 1. Figure 11 illustrates this observation by x-ray imaging for knits uniaxially drawn in wale and course directions. The amount of fibers aligned to the drawing direction is increased by drawing. The fibers are straightened in the drawing direction. These effects lead to the observed strain stiffening and strengthening effect shown later in Fig. 16. Drawing also enhances the anisotropy reinforcing the drawing direction. Because of the coherence, the fiber content perpendicular to the drawing direction is considerably reduced.

The analysis of the x-ray images [123] approaches the loop shape with straight, short fibers as shown in Fig. 12. Using image processing, the x-ray image is cut into single-curved fiber segments. They are analyzed according to their maximum projection and width. Both values are used to idealize the curve segment with the corresponding section of a circle, which is approximated by virtually straight short fibers. Therefore, short-fiber theories can be used for the calculation of the mechanical properties. Figures 13 and 14 illustrate the influence of drawing on the short fiber orientation and on the length distribution. It has been found [62, 121, 122] that strength properties depend on the adhesion between fiber and matrix. Based on the fiber length distribution and according to the theory of short-fiber reinforcement, a virtual critical fiber length can be introduced. If in parts of a stitch the calculated short fiber lengths become smaller than the critical fiber length, these parts do not contribute to strength. With this approach the influence of adhesion can be considered.

The orientation and ellipticity of the fiber cross-sections show the 3-dimensional fiber orientation in the composite. For the analysis of fiber cross-sections, image analysis procedures are used [123–126]. In Fig. 15 the spatial fiber orientation distribution of a

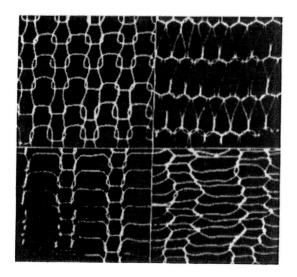

Figure 11 X-ray image of the knit structure in the composite shown for different draw ratios: undrawn (upper left), 56% drawn in wale (upper right), 20% drawn in course (lower left), and 58% in course (lower right) [73].

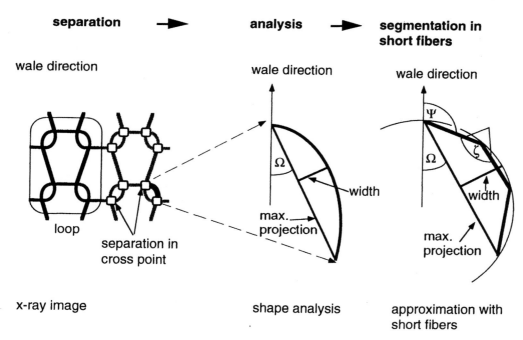

Figure 12 Analysis of the x-ray images (Fig. 11) resulting in a short fiber orientation distribution (Fig. 13) [73].

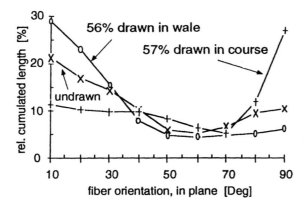

Figure 13   Influence of the drawing ratio on the fiber orientation distribution, determined by x-ray analysis [73].

knitted fiber reinforced composite is illustrated for an undrawn composite. The azimuth is the in-plane angle and the elevation is the out-of-plane angle of the analyzed fiber.

2.   *Characterization of Materials for Standard Tests*

Two different fiber–matrix systems were used in this study: HT-carbon fibers combined with polyethylmethacrylate (T300/PEMA, powder bath impregnated). The advantage of PEMA for surgical applications is its low glass transition point of approximately 65°C, which makes it possible to adapt the manufactured part to a special individual geometry by heating it up in hot water [75, 122]. HT-carbon fibers/polyether(ether)ketone (AS4/PEEK, comingled yarn) was chosen to study the highest achievable performance.

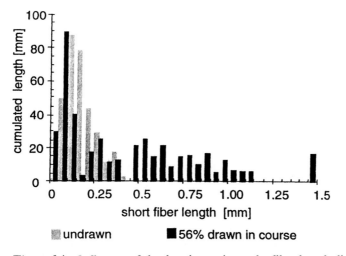

Figure 14   Influence of the drawing ratio on the fiber length distribution [73].

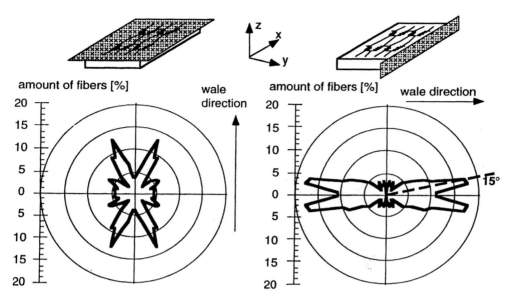

Figure 15 Spatial fiber orientation distribution in an undrawn carbon fiber reinforced thermoplastic in the knit plain and perpendicular to it [73].

To study the influences of knit structure, knit drawing, fiber matrix adhesion, and matrix properties on the mechanical properties, selected directions tested were either the wale or the course direction. Referring to DIN 29971 stress/strain behavior has been analyzed during tensile and 4-point-bending loading; interlaminar shear strength was determined in some cases [122]. Measurements were performed in a universal testing machine (Zwick 1474) with a testing speed of 0.5 mm/min.

3. General Mechanical Properties

The mechanical properties of knitted fiber reinforced composites are determined by the knit parameters, i.e., type, size and deformation of the loop. To improve mechanical properties, it is important to orient the knit layer and/or the direction of loop stretching according to the main load direction. This aligns the amount of locally straightened and load-bearing fibers to the force direction and improves strength and stiffness.

Stiffness and Static Strength.   Depending on plastic deformation during hot-forming, stiffness and strength of knits reach or even exceed the properties of 1 × 1 plain weaves referring to the direction or the main deformation (Fig. 16). These properties are anisotropic and their anisotropy can be controlled by drawing during textile preforming or plastic hot-deformation. To allow a proper comparison, all values have been recalculated for 40 vol% fibers. Here, 0° corresponds to the UD fiber direction and the weft direction of the knit; 90° or warp is the perpendicular direction. Before testing, the knits have been deformed either in the wale or the course direction and afterwards they were tested in the deformation direction and perpendicular to it. The comparison of the anisotropy between unidirectional, 1 × 1 woven and undrawn weft knit reinforced composites (Fig. 17) indicates a smoothed anisotropy for knitted structures, because the curved fiber structure

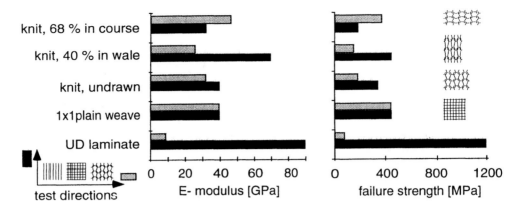

Figure 16   Comparison of the mechanical properties of 0° UD, 1 × 1 plain weave and weft knit [73].

distributes fibers homogeneously in plane and out of plane. This is also visible in the cross-section (Fig. 10).

Strain Stiffening and Strain Strengthening.   Strain stiffening and strain strengthening are characteristic properties of knitted fiber reinforced composites (Fig. 15). As illustrated in Fig. 18, Young's modulus and strength correlate with the plane fiber orientation distribution. This is shown in the linear correlation between the rate of drawing expressed by the portion of fiber length and the mechanical anisotropy shown by its portion. Fiber

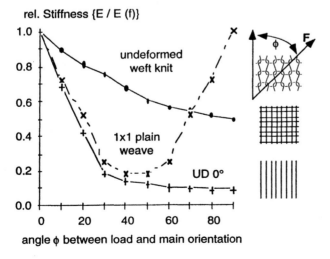

Figure 17   Comparison of the anisotropy between unidirectional, 1 × 1 woven and undrawn weft knit reinforced composites [73].

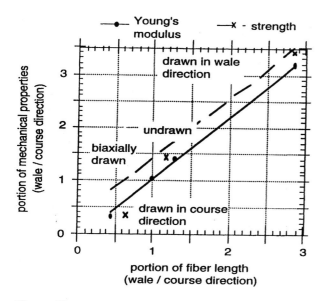

Figure 18 Influence of knit deformation on the anisotropy of the materials stiffness [73].

portions between 0°–20° and 70°–90° are taken into account. The influence of drawing on the distribution itself is shown in Fig. 19.

Failure Behavior.   Assuming good adhesion between fiber and matrix, the failure behavior is determined by the fiber orientation distribution [62]. This is illustrated in the scanning electron microscopy (SEM) image in Fig. 20, whereas the primary failure is due to fiber tensile failure of the best-oriented fiber parts.

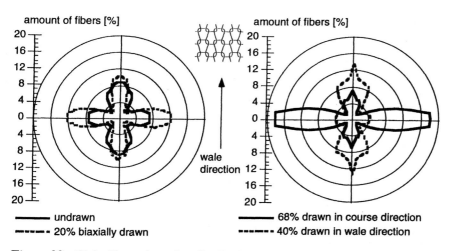

Figure 19   Plain fiber orientation distribution resulting from the short-fiber analysis of the x-ray images. The orientation of the polar diagrams is indicated according to the sketch of a knit [73].

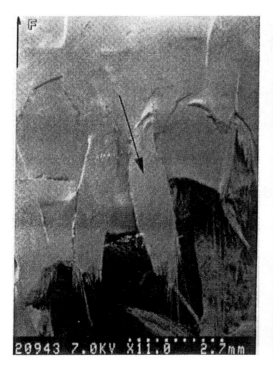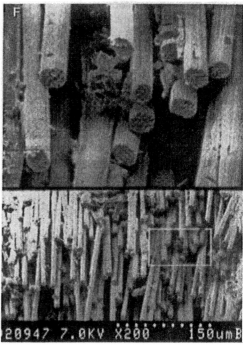

Figure 20   Failure of an undrawn knit specimen oxidized at 600°C, tested in the wale direction [73].

The improved adhesion due to the oxidative treatment influences mainly strength in wale direction and the fracture mechanisms. Based also on other experiments [61], an important feature is the critical fiber length needed for complete stress transfer. If this fiber length is short compared to the curvature of the fibers in the stitch, the stress distribution is fully determined by the fiber orientation distribution. In this case the textile properties of the knit have no influence on the mechanical properties. If the adhesion is too poor or if the loops were too small, strength and transverse contraction will be considerably influenced by the knit structure, as pointed out in Figs. 20 and 21. At 400°C, complex bending failure is observed in the contact zone of loops influenced by the textile knit structure. Insufficient adhesion between fiber and matrix is seen as the cause. This effect is visible in the splitting of the roving and in the long fiber pullout lengths. At 600°C, initial tensile fiber failure occurs within the fibers oriented to the outer force direction. Crack growth is controlled by the local fiber orientation distribution. The close-up shows the fiber-dominated crack growth, and the lower amount of fiber pull-out indicates an improved adhesion. The failure mode is elastic and microscopically comparable to a 0° UD tensile failure.

Energy release rate during crack growth in the K_i case (DCB test, area method) was measured to be twice as high for knits (PEEK-C weft knit undeformed, $G_{1c} = 4.5$ kJ/m^2) than for unidirectional reinforced composites (PEEK-C 0°, $G_{1c} = 2$ kJ/m^2). The control of fiber–matrix adhesion allows one to obtain a broad range of fracture toughness. The interwaved fiber structure of knits prevents delamination.

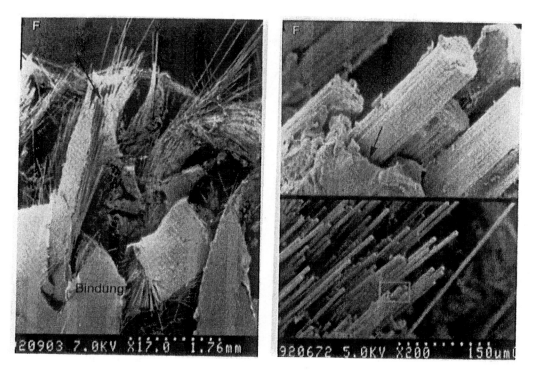

Figure 21   Failure of an undrawn knit specimen oxidized at 400°C, tested in the wale direction [73].

4.   Modeling of the Mechanical Properties

The mechanics of knits are determined by the coherence of the knitted fiber structure. The defined fiber orientation allows fundamental mechanical description of structure-properties relations as well as estimated engineering calculations [122, 123]. These relations are based on the results of different research groups [114, 115, 123]. Figure 22 compares the calculated distribution, based on the x-ray data, with the measured Young's modulus. For the calculation, a simple single-fiber approach is used [73, 114, 115]. The specimen investigated is a 13% in-wale drawn PEEK/AS4 knit composite with a fiber volume content of 40%. The calculation gives a conservative estimation.

5.   Net Shape Manufacturing of the Osteosynthesis Plate

Net shape pressing is defined as thermoinduced forming of a raw material in one production step without need of further processing. The matrix-impregnated, rolled knitting was pushed over the thorns of the form (Fig. 23). After inserting all four sidewalls, a stamp was lowered onto the knitting. Due to this process, no fibers had to be cut; the loops are distorted to a circular fiber alignment around the thorns, which has a self-reinforcing effect and the complete surface is polymer coated.

The pressing cycle for the plates containing T300/PEMA was as follows: heat-up to 190°C at a rate of 18°C/min, holding period at 190°C for 30 min, pressure 175 bar, cooling rate 10°C/min. The same cycle was applied to the AS4/PEEK composite, except

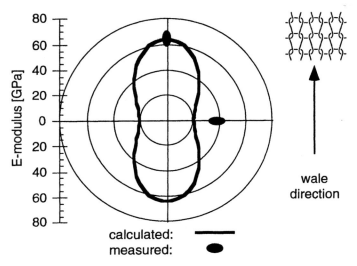

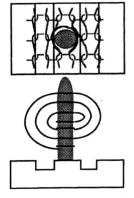

Figure 22   Comparison of the calculated Young's modulus distribution based on the x-ray analysis and a single-fiber approach [112, 113] with measured data [73].

that the holding period was at 390°C. These conditions were also used for the manufacturing of the mechanical test specimen.

Bending strength and modulus were determined by a 4-point bending test (DIN 29971, 2 mm/min) at 25°C. The support span was 97 mm and the pressure span was 41.2 mm. According to the geometry of the plate, a model for the calculation of the bending modulus and strength has been derived. The plates have been idealized as beams with two different cross-sections, a massive section and a reduced section, representing the holes [73, 75]. The fiber volume content was measured by gravimetrical and optical methods [75, 76]. The failure mechanisms were observed by SEM.

To compare net shape pressing with common lamination technologies, a laminated

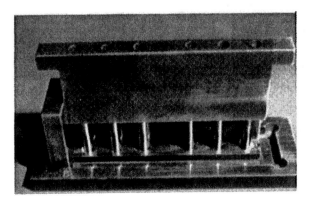

Figure 23   The net shape pressing form (left) and the stamp lowered onto the knitting (right) [73].

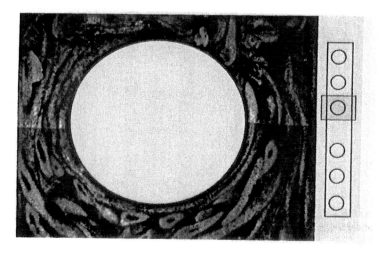

Figure 24 Cross-section of a plate as indicated. The hole-forming process induces a fiber alignment along the plate's axis [75].

osteosynthesis of identical geometry has been made from carbon-fiber reinforced PEEK laminates (APC2-AS4 from ICI). The plates had stiff outer shells and a weak core to achieve a high bending ($E_b = 107$ GPa) to axial ($E_a = 60$ GPa) stiffness ratio. The properties of these plates have been discussed in previous publications [112, 113]. A stainless steel plate (6-hole ulnar) has been used as a reference.

6. Structure and Properties of the Net Shape Osteosynthesis Plate

The cross-section shown in Fig. 24 illustrates the effect of hole forming on the fiber architecture. In the critical cross-section, a forced fiber orientation along the plates axis as well as a slightly improved fiber content can be observed. This effect results in an improvement of the mechanical properties compared to drilled plates machined from

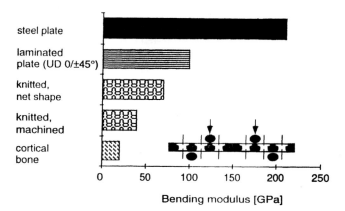

Figure 25 Bending moduli of osteosynthesis plates: made from stainless steel, UD-laminated and machined, knitted net shaped, and knitted machined (AS4/PEEK) [73].

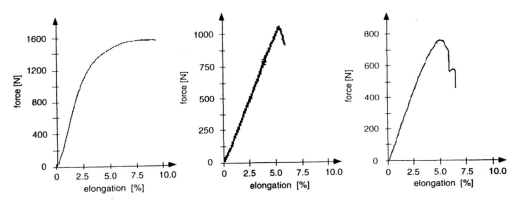

Figure 26 Comparison of the stress–strain curves for the stainless steel plate (left), the laminated plate (middle), and the net shape pressed plate (right) [73].

pressed-knitted fiber-reinforced plates [73]. Figure 25 illustrates this finding for the bending modulus of osteosynthesis plates, made from stainless steel, UD-laminated and machined, knitted net shaped and knitted machined. The Young's modulus of cortical bone is added to the figure in order to demonstrate a possible mechanical approach to homoelasticity with knit-reinforced thermoplastics.

The spatial fiber orientation around the hole as indicated in Fig. 24 induces a characteristic failure behavior for the net shape plate. Compared to the laminated plate, an improvement of damage tolerance is observed in the stress–strain curves wherein the amount of pseudoplastic failure is considerably increased (Fig. 26). These findings correlate with an increase of the damage area as illustrated in the SEM images in Fig. 27 and with the dislocation of the failure area beyond of the smallest cross-section as illustrated in Fig. 28. Primary failure occurs at the compression site: The laminated plate shows local fiber buckling of the outer 0° plies (1), with subsequent delamination (2) and compression failure of the inner 0° plies (3). In the net shape plate (PEEK-AS4), failure occurs beyond the smallest cross-section (compare to Fig. 28). The crack path is guided by fiber orientation in the loop. Primary failure is a compression failure of fibers which have been well aligned to the plates axis and are underneath the plate's surface.

An additional effect of the net shape processing is the complete coating of the plate's surface with the matrix polymer. Figure 29 shows the comparison to the drilled surface of the laminated plates, which have to be coated with a suitable polymer in an additional processing step to prevent the release of carbon fiber particles.

7. Comparison of the Homoelasticity in FEM Calculations and Strain Gauges Measurements

Three-step finite element modeling (FEM) and finite element analysis (FEA) was used to evaluate the properties of osteosynthesis plates made of anisotropic carbon fiber reinforced thermoplastics. The calculations were performed in CAEDS (I-DEAS Version 4.1) and its Integrated Finite Element Solver (IFES). The material properties were orthotropic for analysis steps 1 and 3 and isotropic for step 2. The basic setup of the FEM/FEA procedure is shown in Fig. 30 and is as follows [113]:

- *Step 1*: A 2-D model of the plate generated from parabolic thin shell elements (Fig. 31a) is used to perform a fast analysis of the deformation and the global stress distribution.

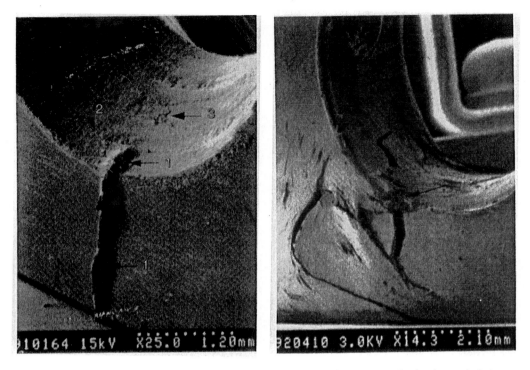

Figure 27 Comparison of the primary failure behavior of the osteosynthesis plates at their compression site. Left: laminated plate; right: net shape plate (PEEK-AS4) [73].

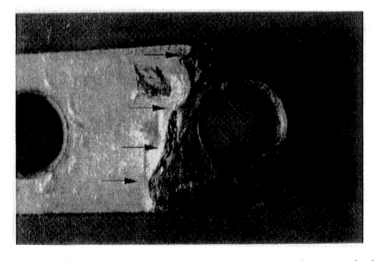

Figure 28 Tensile failure side of the net shape pressed osteosynthesis plate [73].

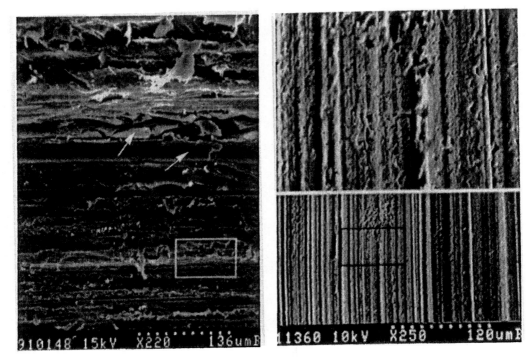

Figure 29 Comparison of the surfaces of the laminated and machined plate (left) and of the net shape pressed plate (right) [73].

- *Step 2*: A 3-D model of bone, plate, and screws generated from linear solid brick and wedge elements (Fig. 31b) is the basis for plate/bone system deformation analysis and for evaluation of the stress shielding effect. The bone is modeled as a thick walled tube. Load transfer from bone to plate is modeled with gap elements between plate and screws. The constraints of the gap elements made it possible to transmit only compression forces on the countersunk holes. Friction forces have not been consid-

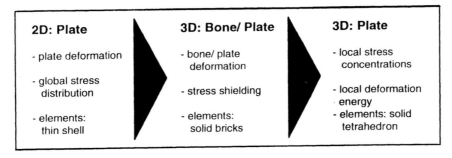

Figure 30 Schematic drawing of the proposed FEM/FEA procedure [113].

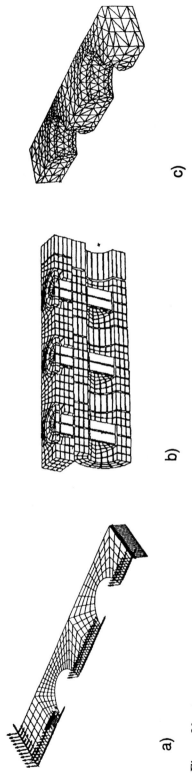

a)

b)

c)

Figure 31 (a) Example for a 2-D model for step 1 with restrains and applied bending force. (b) Part of the 3-D plate/screws/bone model with shrunken elements. (c) 3-D model of the plate for the analysis of local effects on laminates [113].

ered because the calculations have been restricted to a relaxed osteosynthesis of a reconsolidated bone. Between bone and screws, shared knots are used.

- *Step 3*: A layered model of the plate generated from parabolic tetrahedron solids (Fig. 31c) is used for the analysis of local stress concentrations with respect to the anisotropic materials behavior and the asymmetric hole geometry.

Steps 1 and 3 have been helpful in evaluating the laminate setup and the design of composite plates. The 2-D models gave a fast access to reliable deformation values varying the dimensions of the plate. The analysis of the 3-D model allowed detailed stress and strain energy analysis of the laminated plate under bending loads. The four-layered structure is considered to be a good compromise for approximating the anisotropic plate behavior with its countersunk holes. As a result, the hole design was adapted to the specific requirements of composites. However, they were not suitable for detailed study of the influence of the complex fiber structure of the knitted fiber reinforced and net-shaped plate. Therefore, the calculations have been focused on global effects such as stress shielding in model step 2. The isotropic material properties used are collected in Table 4.

The calculated strain distributions in the plate/screw/bone model have been verified in a 4-point bending test of a relaxed and reconsolidated osteosynthesis, as indicated in Fig. 32. A woven glass fiber reinforced tube ($E = 18$ GPa) has been used as a model bone and plates have been fixed on the tube with cortical steel screws.

FE calculation as well as strain gauge measurements indicate the most intensive stress protection for the steel plate (Fig. 33). The reinforcing effect of the net shape process is seen only in the strain gauge measurements. The strains around the holes are even smaller for the net shape plate although the Young's modulus of the laminate is more than 100% higher than those of the knitted plates. In the isotropic FEM calculation it is not possible to take into account the influence of local stiffening of the net shape pressed plate.

The analysis of the stress protection indicated by the dislocation of the neutral bending axis of the osteosynthesis (Fig. 34) illustrates the improvement of homoelasticity of the net shape manufactured plate. The variation of the Young's modulus along the plate axis seems to compensate the variation of the bearing cross-section. Therefore, the strain distribution in the bone becomes more homogeneous comparing an osteosynthesis using net shape plate with one using a laminated or even a steel plate.

Table 4   Isotropic Material Properties Used in the Plate/Screws/Bone FE Model

	Young's modulus (GPa)
Bone	20
Steel plate and screw	210
Laminated plate	107
Knitted net shape plate	33
Composite screw	60

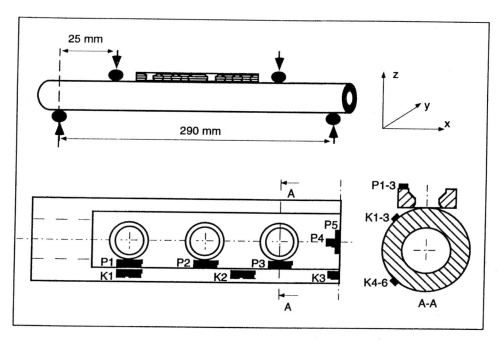

Figure 32 Four-point bending test of the osteosynthesis. The location of the strain gauges is indicated (P1-P5, K1-K6). Load applied was between 100 and 1000 N [73].

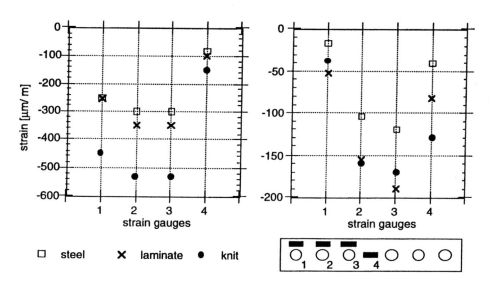

Figure 33 Comparison of the strains in the plate calculated in the FE model (left) and measured in the strain gauge measurement (right) [73].

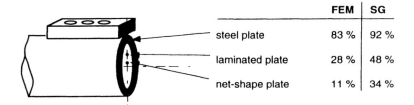

	FEM	SG
steel plate	83 %	92 %
laminated plate	28 %	48 %
net-shape plate	11 %	34 %

Figure 34 Comparison of the dislocation of the neutral bending axis measured and calculated [73].

C. Development of a Cortical Bone Screw Made with Endless Carbon Fiber Reinforced Polyether(ether)ketone (CF-PEEK) by Extrusion

1. Introduction

The development of homoelastic, anisotropic osteosynthesis systems with improved biocompatibility suggests including carbon-fiber reinforced bone plates and screws as a new implant system [123, 127]. Preliminary results have shown that short fiber reinforced bone screws, manufactured by injection molding, cannot fulfill the mechanical requirements for long bone osteosynthesis due to low volume fiber fraction, critical fiber length, and poor control of fiber orientation.

In preliminary studies, several production techniques for the fabrication of a carbon fiber reinforced bone screw were elaborated and evaluated. Based on the resulting new fabrication technique—melt extrusion—cortical bone screws were manufactured from carbon fiber reinforced polyether(ether)ketone (PEEK) and their mechanical behavior under static loads was characterized [128].

The principle of melt extrusion technique is very similar to the hot-extrusion technique used in metal working. But in contradistinction to metal working, the blanks are heated above the melting point of the matrix material prior to forming. The bone screw has a core diameter of 3 mm, a fiber volume fraction up to 62 vol%, and a matrix-coated surface. This process, which is comparable to injection molding, defines the fiber structure during processing in the liquid phase.

2. Materials and Methods

Raw Material. Round rods made from carbon fiber reinforced PEEK (APC 2/AS4 from ICI, fiber volume fraction: ~62 vol%) were used as blanks for the production of bone screws. Two types of blanks with different fiber orientations were processed:

- Type 1: blanks with pure 0° fiber orientation
- Type 2: blanks with 0°/±45° fiber orientation

Melt Extrusion Process. A blank is heated in the melt extrusion tool (Fig. 35) to forming temperature (380°–400°C) and then pressed into the mold (strain rate: 2–80 mm/s; forming force: 120 MPa) by a tool peen. While applying a dwell pressure of about 90 MPa the whole melt extrusion tool is cooled down to room temperature by a compressed air sprayer. After disassembling the extrusion tool the bone screw can be removed from the mold.

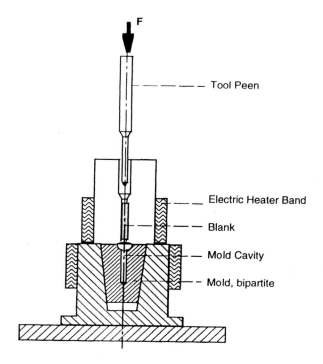

F

— — — — Tool Peen

— — Electric Heater Band

— — Blank

— Mold Cavity

— — Mold, bipartite

Figure 35 Experimental melt extrusion tool [128].

Tensile strength and Young's modulus were determined with a universal tension/ compression testing machine (Zwick 1474). Tensile strength was determined using a clamping system (Fig. 36) which provides a force induction similar to that in real application (strain rate: 1 mm/min).

For the determination of Young's modulus, specimens consisting of a screw segment (length: 6 mm) embedded in epoxy resin (Fig. 37) were subjected to a compression test. Embedding of the screw segments in epoxy resin was necessary for specimen preparation and for stabilization during compression test. The influence of this embedding on the test result was afterwards mathematically eliminated by the following algorithm:

$$ E = \frac{1}{A_{screw}} \cdot \left(P \cdot \frac{l_0}{\Delta l} - A_{epoxy} \cdot E_{epoxy} \right) $$

where

  A_{screw}: apparent cross-section of the screw*
  A_{screw}: apparent cross-section of the embedding
     P: compressive force
     Δl: longitudinal deformation
     l_0: length of the unloaded specimen

*Determined by a compression test using an equivalent specimen consisting of a screw segment made from stainless steel (same geometry).

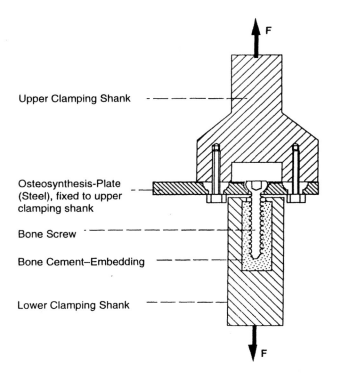

Upper Clamping Shank

Osteosynthesis-Plate
(Steel), fixed to upper
clamping shank

Bone Screw

Bone Cement–Embedding

Lower Clamping Shank

Figure 36   Test configuration for the determination of tensile strength [128].

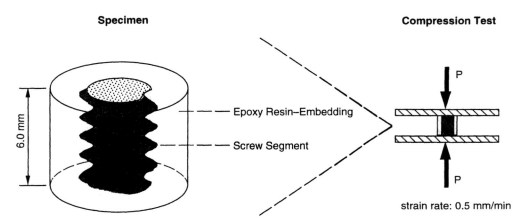

Specimen

Compression Test

6.0 mm

Epoxy Resin–Embedding

Screw Segment

strain rate: 0.5 mm/min

Figure 37   Specimen for the determination of the Young's modulus distribution along the screw axis [128].

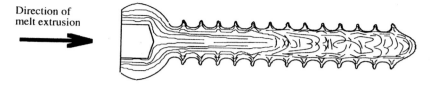

Figure 38   Fiber orientation in melt-extruded screws [128].

The ultimate torsional strain and moment were determined in accordance with ISO 6475, which describes test methods and mechanical requirements for bone screws made from stainless steel.

3.   Results

Fiber Orientation.   Figure 38 schematically shows fiber orientations in the melt-extruded bone screw, determined in ground sections. In the screw head and in the upper part of the threaded bolt, fibers are generally aligned along the screw axis. Towards the tip of the screw, fibers in the core zone become more circularly oriented. In a skin zone with an approximate thickness of 0.7 mm, fibers still follow the longitudinal profile of the thread.

Screws which were melt extruded using a blank with $0°/±45°$ fiber orientation show a significantly higher percentage of fibers with a $90°$ orientation versus screw axis than screws made from blanks with a pure $0°$ fiber orientation. Fiber layers with a $45°$ orientation in the blank seem to have a tendency to tilt during the forming process and to align parallel to the flow front.

Strain rate and forming temperature were found to have no significant influence on the fiber orientation.

Mechanical Properties.   Tensile strength of the screws shows only little dependence on the type of blank used in the melt-extrusion process. An average tensile strength of approx. 460 MPa^2 was measured (sampling size: 15 screws). Screws which were processed using a high strain rate ($≈80$ mm/s) and high forming temperature (400°C) have a slightly higher tensile strength.

The average torsional strength of screws made from type 1 blanks is 18% higher than that of the ones made from type 2 blanks (Table 5). Screws processed with a low strain rate (2 mm/s) and low forming temperature (380°C) can bear a slightly higher torsional

Table 5   Mechanical Properties of Bone Screws Made from CF/PEEK

Production technique	Fiber length	Fiber volume fraction (vol%)	Fiber orientation in the blank	Tensile strength (MPa^2)	Torsional strength (MPa^2)	Twisting angle for power failure (°)
Melt extrusion	"Endless"	62	0°	457	202	270
Melt extrusion	"Endless"	62	0°/±45°	456	171	240
Injection molding[a]	Short	15	Random	76	151	180

Source: Ref. 129
[a]Raw material: PEEK CA30 from Cellpack, Switzerland

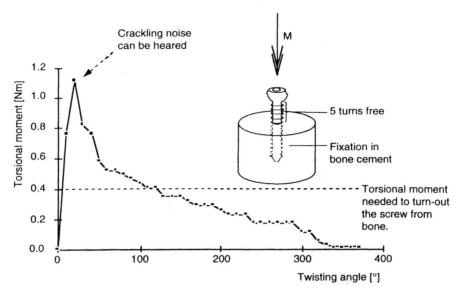

Figure 39   Typical torsion test result of a bone screw fabricated by melt extrusion [128].

moment. Initial torsion failure occurs between 30° and 60° past locking, and thereafter the residual torsional strength decreases very slowly until power failure occurs between 200° and 370° past locking (Fig. 39).

Young's modulus in axial direction of a melt-extruded bone screw does not remain constant along the screw axis. It decreases from approx. 23 GPa at the screw head to approx. 5 GPa at the tip (Fig. 40). Using a type 1 blank produces a bone screw with a slightly higher stiffness than using a type 2 blank in the melt-extrusion process.

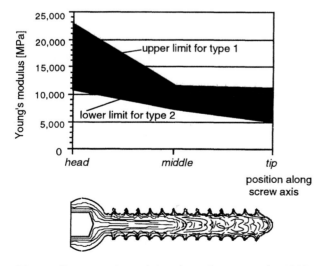

Figure 40   Young's modulus along the screw axis [128].

4. Discussion

Fabrication of a bone screw made from CF/PEEK by melt extrusion has shown that this new manufacturing technique offers an economical possibility for net shaping of endless fiber reinforced thermoplastics. Fiber orientation, as a determining factor for mechanical properties, can be controlled by fiber orientation in the blank. It was experimentally found that strain rate and forming temperature have only a very slight influence on the result of the melt-extrusion process.

Melt-extruded bone screws made from CF/PEEK attain approx. 70% of tensile strength of a conventional bone screw made from stainless steel. However, an average breaking load of 3200 N is already sufficient for osteosynthesis application. Comparable bone screws are already drawn out of the bone by stripping threads at tensile load of 800 to 1300 N [132].

ISO standard 6475 requires a maximum torsional moment of at least 4.4 Nm and a twisting angle at power failure of at least 180° for comparable bone screws made from stainless steel. It has to be mentioned, however, that these requirements have no direct correlation to the application of the screws. CF/PEEK bone screws cannot fulfill the requirements of ISO standard 6475, although breaking the screw by overturning is impossible because the thread in the bone will be stripped before failure occurs in the bone screw. However, power failure by overturning the screw would be announced by a loud crackling noise and a significant decrease in torsional stiffness. The residual strength after initial break still allows removal of the screw from the bone.

Young's modulus of bone and bone screw made from CF/PEEK are of the same order. This results in an improved stress transfer from bone to screw. Together with their insensitivity against corrosive media, CF/PEEK screws also offer an improved structural and chemical biocompatibility.

IV. CONCLUSIONS

In order to mimic natural load-transmitting structures, i.e., bone, we developed anisotropic reinforcements for osteosynthesis and for hip endoprosthesis stems (Fig. 41). The

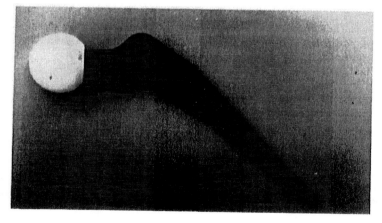

Figure 41   Hip endoprosthesis made from carbon fiber reinforced PEEK.

presented results show that it is possible to process carbon fibers and thermoplastic matrices into composites which fulfill the following requirements:

1. Optimized interface and interphase designs for long-term mechanical stability
2. Simulation of bone anisotropy with 3-dimensional reinforcement architecture due to appropriate processing
3. Preparation of cost-effective industrial manufacturing due to net shape processing.

REFERENCES

1. Donnet, J. B., and Bansal, R. C., *Carbon fibers*, 2nd ed., revised and expanded, Marcel Dekker, New York, 1990, p. 145.
2. Bennett, S. C., and Johnson, D. J., *Carbon*, *17*, 25 (1979).
3. Bascom, W. D., Fiber sizing, in *Composites* (C. A. Dostal et al., eds.), Engineered Materials Handbook, Vol. 1, ASM International, Metals Park, OH, p. 122 (1987).
4. Hughes, J. D. H., Strength and modulus of current carbon fibers, *Carbon*, *24*(5) 551–556 (1986).
5. Fitzer, E., and Heine, B., Carbon fibre manufacture and surface treatment, in *Fibre Reinforcements for Composite Materials*, (A. B. Bunsell, ed.), Elsevier, Amsterdam, 1988, pp. 74–146.
6. Maier, G., and Vetesnik, P., Matrixsteifigkeit bestimmt Druckfestigkeit von Faserverbundwerkstoffen, *Kunststoffe*, *81*, 614–616 (1991).
7. Chu, J. N., Ko, F. K., and Song, J. W., Time-dependent mechanical properties of 3-D braided graphite/PEEK composites, *SAMPE Q.*, *7*, 14–19 (1992).
8. Karger-Kocsis, J., Yuan, Q., and Czigany, T., Assignment of acoustic emission to the failure sequence and damage zone growth in glass fiber strand mat-reinforced structural nylon RIM composites, *Polym. Bull.*, *28*, 717–723 (1992).
9. Karger-Kocsis, J., and Czigany, T., Fracture behaviour of glass-fiber mat-reinforced structural nylon RIM composites studied by microscopic and acoustic emission techniques, *J. Mat. Sci.*, *38*, 2438–2448 (1993).
10. Karger-Kocsis, J., Fracture mechanical characterization and damage zone development in glass-fiber-mat reinforced thermoplastics, in *Proceedings of ICCM9*, Madrid, (A. Miravete, ed.), University of Zaragoza and Woodhead Publ., 1993, Vol. 2, pp. 275–282.
11. Claes, L., Huettner, W., and Weiss, R., Mechanical properties of carbon fibre reinforced polysulfone plates for internal fracture fixation, in *Biological and Biomechanical Performance of Biomaterials* (P. Christel, A. Meunier, and A. J. C. Lee, eds.), Elsevier, Amsterdam, 1986, pp. 81–86.
12. Huettner, W., Keuscher, G., and Nietert, M., Carbon fibre reinforced polysulfone thermoplastic composites, in *Biomaterials and Biomechanics* (P. Ducheyne, G. Van der Perre, and A. E. Aubert, eds.), Elsevier, Amsterdam, 1984, pp. 167–172.
13. Soltész, U., Hehne, H. J., and Desiderato, R., Modelluntersuchungen zum interfragmentaeren Kontakt und zur Druckverteilung bei Osteosynthesen, in *Deutsche Sektion der Internationalen Arbeitsgemeinschaft fuer Osteosynthesefragen*, DVM, 1982, pp. 6–22.
14. Bradley, J. S., Hastings, G. W., and Johnson-Nurse, C., Carbon fibre reinforced epoxy as a high strength, low modulus material for internal fixation plates, *Biomaterials*, *1*, 38–40 (1980).
15. Moyen, B., Comtet, J. J., Santini, R., Rumelhart, C., and Dumas, P., Reactions de l'os intact sous des plaques d'osteosynthese en carbone, SOFCOT reunion annuelle, Suppl. II, *Rev. Chir. Orthop.*, *68*, 83–90 (1982).
16. Tayton, K., Johnson-Nurse, C., McKibbin, B., Bradley, J., and Hastings, G. W., The use of semi-rigid carbon-fibre-reinforced plastic plates for fixation of human fractures, *J. Bone Joint Surg.*, *64-B1*, 105–111 (1982).

17. Claes, L., Kinzl, L., and Neugebaue, R., Experimentelle Untersuchung zum Einfluss des Plattenmaterials auf die Entlastung und Atrophie de Knochens unter Osteosyntheseplatten, *Biomed. Tech.*, 26(4), 66–71 (1981).

18. Hastings, G. W., Biomedical applications of CFRPs, in *Carbon Fibre and Their Composites* (E. Fitzer, ed.), Springer-Verlag, Berlin, 1983, pp. 261–271.

19. Tayton, K. J. J., The use of carbon fibre in human implants: The state of the art, *J. Med. Eng. Tech.*, 7(6), 271–272 (1983).

20. Tayton, K. J. J., and Bradley, J., How stiff should semi-rigid fixation of the human tibia be? A clue to the answer, *J. Bone Joint Surg.*, 65-B3, 312–315 (1983).

21. Woo, S. L-Y., Akeson, W. H., Levenetz, B., Coutts, R. D., Matthews, J. V., and Amiel D., Potential application of graphite fibre and methyl methacrylate resin composites as internal fixation plates, *J. Biomed. Mat. Res.*, 8, 321–338 (1974).

22. Polyetherketones, *Encyclopedia of Polymer Science and Engineering*, Wiley, New York, 1988, Vol. 12, pp. 313–320.

23. Nguyen, H. X., and Ishida, H., Poly(aryl-ether-ether-ketone) and its advanced composites: A review, *Pol. Comp.*, 8, 59–73 (1987).

24. Vautey, P., Merienne, M. C., Cottenot, C., and Favre, J. P., in *IPCM '89 Conference Proceedings*, Butterworth, Sheffield, UK, 1989, pp. 53–58.

25. Seferis, J. C., Polyetheretherketone (PEEK): Processing structure and properties studies for a matrix in high performance composites, *Pol. Comp.*, 7, 159–169 (1986).

26. Peacock, J. A., Fife, B., Nield, E., and Barlow, C. Y., A fibre–matrix interface study of some experimental EEK/carbon fibre composites, in *Composite Interfaces* (H. Ishida and J. L. Koenig, eds.), Elsevier, 1986, p. 143–148.

27. Lustinger, A., PEEK composites, processing–morphology property relationship, in *Int. Enzycl. Compos.*, 4, 156–169 (1990).

28. Scobo, J. J. R., and Nakajima, N., Strength and failure of PEEK/graphite fibre composites, *SAMPE J.*, 26, 45–50 (1990).

29. Lustinger, A., and Newatz, G. M., Interlamellar fracture and craze growth in PEEK composites under cyclic loading, *J. Comp. Mat.*, 24, 175–181 (1990).

30. Friedrich, K., Fractography and failure of unfilled and short fibre reinforced semi-crystalline thermoplastics, in *Fractography and Failure Mechanisms of Polymers and Composites* (A. C. Roulin-Moloney, ed.), Elsevier Applied Science, London, 1989, pp. 437–494.

31. Davies, P., Cantwell, W., Moulin, C., and Kausch, H. H., A study of the delamination resistance of IM6/PEEK Composites, *Comp. Sci. Tech.*, 36, 153–166 (1989).

32. Barlow, C. Y., Peacock, J. A., and Windle, A. H., Relationships between microstructures and fracture energies in carbon fibre/PEEK composites, *Composites*, 21, 383–388 (1990).

33. Ghasemi Nejhad, M. N., and Parvizi-Majidi, A., Impact behaviour and damage tolerance of woven carbon fibre reinforced thermoplastic composites, *Composites*, 21, 155–168 (1990).

34. Lustinger, A., Uralil, F. S., and Newaz, G. M., Processing and structural optimization of PEEK composites, *Pol. Comp.*, 11, 65–75 (1990).

35. Cantwell, W. J., Davies, P., and Kausch, H. H., The effect of cooling rate on deformation and fracture in IM6/PEEK composites, *Comp. Struct.*, 14, 151–171 (1990).

36. Kempe, G., Krauss, H., and Korger-Roth, G., Adhesion and welding of continuous carbon fibre reinforced polyetheretherketon (CF-PEEK, APC2), in *ECCM4*, Stuttgart, September 1990, Elsevier Applied Science, London, 1990, pp. 105–112.

37. Manson, J. A. E., and Seferis, J. C., Autoclave processing of PEEK/carbon fibre composites, *J. Thermopl. Comp. Mat.*, 2, 35–49 (1989).

38. Silvermann, E. M., and Griese, R. A., Joining methods for graphite/PEEK thermoplastic composites, *SAMPE J.*, 25, 34–38 (1989).

39. Horn, W. J., Shaikh, F. M., and Soeganto, A., Degradation of mechanical properties of advanced composites exposed to aircraft environment, *AIAA J.*, 27, 1399–1405 (1989).

40. Taylor, D., and McCormack B., The durability of materials used in orthopaedic implants, *Mat. Eng.*, *32*, 35–44 (1989).

41. Francis, D., and Williams R., Engineering thermoplastics ind reusable medical applications, *Mat. Eng.*, *105*, 21–25 (1988).

42. Turner, R. M., Swerdlow, M. S., and Bate, B., Prosthetic devices, *ICI Off. Gaz.*, 5.6.1987, 17.6.1985.

43. Wenz, L. M., Merrit, K., Brown, S. A., Moet, A., and Steffee, A. D., *In vitro* biocompatibility of polyetheretherketone and polysulfone composites, *J. Biomed. Mat. Res.*, 24, 207–215 (1990).

44. Williams, D. F., McNamara, A., and Turner, R. M., Potential of polyetherehterketone (PEEK) and carbon fibre reinforced PEEK in medical applications, *J. Mat. Sci. Lett.*, 6, 188–190 (1987).

45. Wenz, L. M., Brown, S. A., and Moet, A., Accelerated testing of a composite spine plate, *Composites*, 20, 569–574 (1989).

46. Kardos, L. J., The role of the interface of polymer composites — Some myths, mechanisms and modifications, in *Molecular Characterization of Composite Interfaces* (H. Ishida and G. Kumar, eds.), Plenum Press, New York, 1985, pp. 1–11.

47. Bascom, W. D., Interfaces in fiber reinforced composites, *Int. Enzycl. Comp. Mat.*, 2, 411–422 (1991).

48. Ryutoku, Y., Kiyotake, M., Akio, N., Yoshito, I., and Suzuki, T., *Adhesion and Bonding in Composites*, Marcel Dekker, New York, 1990, pp. 1–42, 257–332.

49. Caldwell, D. L., Interfacial analysis, *Int. Enz. Comp. Mat.*, 2, 361–375 (1991).

50. Moeginger, B., Mueller, U., and Eyerer, P., Morphological investigations of injection moulded fiber-reinforced thermoplastic polymers, *Composites*, 22, 432–436 (1991).

51. Benjamin, S., Chen, H. J. H., and Chen, E. J. H., Study of transcrystallization in polymer composites, *Mat. Res. Soc. Symp. Proc.*, 170, 117–121 (1990).

52. Peacock, J. A., Fife, B., Nield, E., and Barlow, C. Y., A fiber–matrix interface study of some experimental PEEK/carbon fiber composites, in *Composite Interfaces* (H. Ishida and L. J. Koenig, eds.), Elsevier, Amsterdam, 1986, pp. 143–149.

53. Weiss, R., Die Natur der Haftung an der Faser/Matrix-Grenzflaeche von kohlenstoffaserverstaerkten Polymerverbundkoerpern und deren Modifizierbarkeit zur Erzielung massgeschneiderter Verbundkoerpereigenschaften, Dissertation, TH University of Karlsruhe, 1984.

54. Peacock, J. A., Fife, B., Nield, E., and Crick, R. A., Examination of the morphology of aromatic polymer composite (APC-2) using an etching technique, in *Composite Interfaces* (H. Ishida and L. J. Koenig, eds.), Elsevier, Amstermdam, 1986, pp. 299–306.

55. Schoolenberg, G. E., and Rooyen, A. A., Transcrystallinity in fiber reinforced thermoplastic composites, in *Interfacial Phenomena in Composite Materials 91* (I. Verpoost and F. Jones, eds.), Butterworth Heinemann, 1991, pp. 111–114.

56. Megerdigian, C., Robinson, R., and Lehmann, S., Carbon fiber/resin matrix interphase: Effect of carbon fiber surface treatment and environmental conditioning on composite performance, *33rd Int. SAMPE Symp.*, 1989, pp. 571–582.

57. Hojo, M., Tanaka, K., Gustafson, C. G., and Hayashi, R., Fracture mechanics for delamination fatigue crack propagation of CFRP in air and in water, *Key Eng. Mat.*, *37*, 149–160 (1989).

58. Devaux, E., and Chabert, B., Particular crystalline superstructures appearing at the interface of polypropylene/glass fiber composites during a non-isothermal crystallization from the melt, in *Interfacial Phenomena in Composite Materials 91* (I. Verpoost and F. Jones, eds.), Butterworth Heinemann, 1991, pp. 115–120.

59. Ekstrand, K., Ruyter, I. E., and Wellendorf, H., Carbon/graphite fiber reinforced poly(methyl methacrylate): Properties under dry and wet conditions, *J. Biomed. Mat. Res.*, 21, 1065–1080 (1987).

60. Cziollek, J., Studien zur Beeinflussung der Verstaerkungsverhaltens von Kohlenstoffasern

durch Oberflaechenbehandlung der Fasern und durch Verwendung deines Kohlenstoff/Kohlenstoff-Skeletts als Verstaerkungskomponente, Dissertation, TH University of Karlsruhe, 1983.

61. Su, J., Tao, X., Wei, Y., Zhang, Z., and Liu, L., The continuous cold-plasma treatment of the graphite fibre surface and the mechanism of the modification of the interfacial adhesion, in *Interfaces in Polymers, Ceramic and Metal Matrix Composites* (I. Hatsuo, ed.), Elsevier, Amsterdam, 1988.

62. Mayer, J., Giorgetta, S., Koch, B., Wintermantel, E., Padscheider, J., Spescha, G., Karger-Kocsis, J., and Chuang, Y. Characterization of thermal oxidized carbon fiber surfaces by ESCA, wetting techniques and scanning probe microscopy and the interaction with polyethylenmethacrylate: Development of a biocompatible composite material, presented at Interfacial Phenomena in Composite Materials IPCM 93, Cambridge, UK, September 1993.

63. Chan, C., M., Surface analysis, *Int. Enzycl. Comp. Mat.*, (3rd ed.), *3*, 376–379 (1991).

64. Hughes, J. D. H., The carbon fiber/epoxy interface—A review, *Comp. Sci. Tech.*, *41*, 13–45 (1991).

65. Ishitani, A., Characterization of the surface and the interface of the carbon fiber, in *Molecular Characterization of Composite Interfaces* (H. Ishida and G. Kumar, eds.), Plenum Press, New York, 1985, pp. 321–331.

66. Fitzer, E., and Weiss, R., Effect of surface treatment and sizing of C-fibers on the mechanical properties of CFR thermosettings and thermoplastic polymers, *Carbon*, *25*(4), 455–467 (1987).

67. Nardin, M., Balard, H., and Papirer, E., Surface characteristics of commercial carbon fibers determined by inverse gas chromatigraphy, *Carbon*, *28*(1), 43–48 (1990).

68. Hodge, D. J., Middlemiss, B. A., and Peacock, J. A., Correlation between fiber surface and fiber matrix adhesion in carbon fiber reinforced PEEK composite, *Mat. Res. Soc. Symp. Proc.*, *170*, 327–338 (1990).

69. Donnet, J. B., Brendle, M., Dhami, T. L., and Bahl, O. P., Plasma treatment effect in the surface energy of carbon and carbon fibers, *Carbon*, *24*, 757–770 (1986).

70. Donnet, J. B., Cazeneuve, C., Schultz, J., and Shanahan, M. E. R., The surface energy of carbon fibers, in *14th Biennal Conf. Carbon: Ext. Abstr.*, June 1979, pp. 216–217.

71. Hammer, G. E., and Drzal, L. T., Graphite fiber surface analysis by x-ray photoelectron spectroscopy and polar/dispersive free energy analysis, *Appl. Surf. Sci.*, *4*, 340–355 (1980).

72. Hoffman, W. P., Hurley, W. C., Liu, P. M., and Owens, T. W., The surface topography of non-shear treated pitch and PAN carbon fibers as viewed by the STM, *J. Mater. Res.*, *6*(8), 1685–1694 (1991).

73. Mayer, J., Gestricke aus Kohlenstoffasern fuer biokompatible Verbundwerkstoffe, dargestellt an einer homoelastischen Osteosyntheseplatte, Dissertation, ETH Zuerich, 1994.

74. Mayer, J., Wintermantel, E., and Zemp, P. A., Solid-body wetting, a new method for studing the wetting behavior of thermoplastics on carbon fibers, in *Interfacial Phenomena in Composite Material '91* (I. Verpoost and F. Jones, eds.), Butterworth-Heinemann, 1991, pp. 97–100.

75. Ruffieux, K., Hintermann, M., Mayer, J., and Wintermantel, E., Enhanced local carbon fibre knitting reinforcement of isoelastic bone plates: Concept of a new implant., in *VTT Congress, Textiles and Composites '92*, Tampere, Finland, June 1992, pp. 326–332.

76. Mayer, J., Ruffieux, K., Tognini, R., and Wintermantel, E., Knitted carbon fibers, a sophisticated textile reinforcement that offers new perspectives in thermoplastic composite processing, in *Developments in the Science and Technology of Composite Materials*, ECCM6, September 1993, Bordeaux (A. R. Bunsell, A. Kelly, and A. Massiah, eds.), Woodhaed Publishing, 1993, pp. 219–224.

77. Scardino, F. An Introduction in Textile Structures and Their Behavior, in *Textile Structural Composites* (T.-W. Chou and K. F. Ko, eds.), Composites Material Series (Pipes P. B.), Elsevier, Amsterdam, 1989, pp. 1–25.

78. Planck, H., Exploiting the characteristics of textile fabrics in fiber reinforced composites, in *Proc. Verbundwerk 92, 4th Int. Conf. Reinforced Mat. Compos. Techn.* (S. Schnabel, ed.), Denat, Frankfurt, 1992, pp. 10.3–10.33.

79. Hickman, G. T., and Williams, D. J., 3-D knitted preforms for structural reaction injection molding (S.R.I.M.), in *How to Apply Advanced Composite Technology, Proc. 4th Ann. Conf. Adv. Compos.*, Sept. 1988, Dearborn MI, ASM Int., 1988, pp. 367–370.

80. Ko, F. K., and Kutz, J., Multiaxial warp knit for advanced composites, in *How to Apply Advanced Composite Technology, Proc. 4th Ann. Conf. Adv. Compos.*, Sept. 1988, Dearborn MI, ASM Int., 1988, pp. 377–384.

81. Drechsler, K., Beitrag zur Gestaltung und Berechnung von Faserverbundwerkstoffen mit dreidimensionaler Textilverstaerkung, Dissertation, University of Stuttgart, (1992).

82. Apicella, A., Environmental resistance of high-performance polymeric matrices and composites, in *International Encyclopedia of Composites* (S. E. Lee, ed.), VCH Publishers, 1990, Vol. 2, pp. 46–67.

83. Menges, G., Environmental stress cracking (ESC) and environmental stress failure (ESF), in *International Encyclopedia of Composites* (S. E. Lee, ed.), VCH Publishers, 1990, Vol. 2, pp. 67–77.

84. Talreia, R., Continuum damage mechanics, in *International Encyclopedia of Composites* (S. E. Lee, ed.), VCH Publishers, 1990, Vol. 1, pp. 483–488.

85. Chawla, K. K., Fatigue, in *International Encyclopedia of Composites* (S. E. Lee, ed.), VCH Publishers, 1990, Vol. 2, pp. 107–115.

86. Saliba, S. S., and Snide, J. A., Fractography of composite materials, in *International Encyclopedia of Composites* (S. E. Lee, ed.), VCH Publishers, 1990, Vol. 2, pp. 268–288.

87. Umar-Kitab, S. A., Laminated plate analysis using the finite element method, in *International Encyclopedia of Composites* (S. E. Lee, ed.), VCH Publishers, 1990, Vol. 3, pp. 1–10.

88. Herakovich, K. T., Lamination theory, in *International Encyclopedia of Composites* (S. E. Lee, ed.), VCH Publishers, 1990, Vol. 3, pp. 44–54.

89. Bigg, D. M., Thermoplastic matrix composites, in *International Encyclopedia of Composites* (S. E. Lee, ed.), VCH Publishers, 1991, Vol. 6, pp. 10–32.

90. Strong, A. B., Manufacturing, in *International Encyclopedia of Composites* (S. E. Lee, ed.), VCH Publishers, 1990, Vol. 3, pp. 103–126.

91. Harper, R. C., and Pugh, J. H., Thermoforming of thermoplastic matrix composites, in *International Encyclopedia of Composites* (S. E. Lee, ed.), VCH Publishers, 1991, Vol. 5, pp. 496–528.

92. Peters, S. T., Foral, R. F., and Humphrey, W. D., Filament winding, in *International Encyclopedia of Composites* (S. E. Lee, ed.), VCH Publishers, 1990, Vol. 2, pp. 167–182.

93. Advani, S. G., Molding short fiber composites, flow processing, in *International Encyclopedia of Composites* (S. E. Lee, ed.), VCH Publishers, 1990, Vol. 3, pp. 514–525.

94. Mueller, M. E., Allgoewer, M., Schneider, R., and Willenegger, H., *Manual der Osteosynthese*, Springer-Verlag, Berlin, 1977.

95. Perren, S. M., Physical and biological aspects of fracture healing with special reference to internal fixation, *Clin. Orthop. Rel. Res., 138*, 175–191 (1979).

96. McKibbin, B., The biology of fracture healing in long bones, *J. Bone Joint. Surg., 60*, 150–162 (1978).

97. Parsons, J. R., Alexander, H., Corcoran, S. J., and Weiss, A. B., *In vivo* evaluation of fibre reinforced absorbable polymer bone plates, in *Proceedings of the Second International Symposium on Internal Fixation of Fractures*, Lyon, France, September 1982, pp. 117–120.

98. Hench, L. L., and Ethridge E. C., *Biomaterials: An Interfacial Approach*, Academic Press, New York, 1982, pp. 225–252.

99. Terjesen, T., and Apalset, K., The influence of different degrees of stiffness of fixation plates on experimental bone healing, *J. Orthop. Res., 6*, 293–299 (1988).

100. Sarmiento, A., Mullis, D. L., Latta, L. L., Tarr, R. R., and Alvarez, R., A quantitative comparative analysis of fracture healing under the influence of compression plating vs. closed weight bearing treatment, *Clin. Orthop.*, *149*, 232–239 (1980).

101. Skirving, A. P., Day, R., Eng, B., McDonald, W., and McLaren, R., Carbon fibre reinforced plastic (CFRP) plates vs. stainless steel dynamic compression plates in the treatment of fractures of the tibia in dogs, *Clin. Orthop. Rel. Res.*, *224*, 117–124 (1987).

102. Stuermer, K. M., and Scholten, H. J., Periostschaedigung oder Stress-protection als Ursache der Porose im Plattenlager? Ein tierexperimenteller Rechts-Links-Versuch, *Hefte Unfallheilkunde*, *207*, 255–256 (1989).

103. Perren, S. M., Cordey, J., Rahn, B. A., Gautier, E., and Schneider, E., Early temporary porosis of bone induced by internal fixation implants. A reaction to necrosis, not to stress protection, *Clin. Orthop.*, *232*, 139–151 (1988).

104. Perren, S. M., Buchanan, J. S., and Schwab, P., Das Konzept der biologischen Osteosynthese unter Anwendung der Dynamischen Kompressionsplatte mit limitiertem Kontakt (LC-DCP): Wissenschaftliche Grundlagen, Design und Anwendung, *Injury* (suppl.), *22*(1), 1–44 (1991).

105. Hayes, W. C., Schein, S. S., Nunamaker, D. M., Heppenstall, R. B., Muller, G. W., Sampson, S., and Sapega, A., Mechanical properties of healing fractures treated with compression plate fixation, in *Proceedings of the Second International Symposium on Internal Fixation of Fractures*, Lyon, France, September 1982, pp. 81–84.

106. Liskova-Klar, M., and Uhthoff, H. K., Radiologic and histologic determination of optimal time for the removal of titanium alloy plates in beagle dogs: Results of early removal, in *Current Concepts of Internal Fixation of Fractures* (H. K. Uhthoff, ed.), Springer-Verlag, Berlin, 1980, pp. 404–410.

107. Slatis, P., Paavolainen, P., Karaharju, E., and Holmstrom, T., Structural and biomechanical changes in bone after rigid plate fixation, *Can. J. Surg.*, *23*, 247–250 (1980).

108. Braden, T. D., Brinker, W. O., Little, R. W., Jenkins, R. B., and Butler, D., Comparative biomechanical evaluation of bone healing in the dog, *J. Am. Vet. Med. Assoc.*, *163*, 65–69 (1973).

109. Noser, G. A., Brinker, W. O., Little, R. W., and Lammerding, J. J., Effect on time and strength of healing bone with bone plate fixation, *Am. Anim. Hosp. Assoc. J.*, *13*, 559–561 (1977).

110. Woo, S. L., Lothringer, K. S., Akeson, W. H., Coutts, R. D., Woo, Y. K., Simon, B. R., and Gomez, M. A., Less rigid internal fixation plates, historical perspectives and new concepts, *J. Orthop. Res.*, *1*, 431–449 (1984).

111. Woo, S. L-Y., Akeson, W. H., Simon, B. R., Gomez, M. A., and Seguchi, Y., A new approach to the design of internal fixation plates, *J. Biomed. Mat. Res.*, *17*, 427–439 (1983).

112. Mayer, J., Ruffieux, K., Koch, B., Wintermantel, E., Schulten, T., and Hatebur, A., The double die technique (DDT): Biomaterials processing for adaptable high fatigue resistance thermoplastic–carbon fiber ostheosynthesis plates, presented at the International Symposium on Biomedical Engineering in the 21st Century, Taipei, September 23–26, 1992.

113. Schaetti, T., Wintermantel, E., Meier, D., and Mayer, J., Finite element modelling (FEM) and analysis (FEA) of composite layers for an implant/bone system demonstrated in a carbon fiber/thermoplastic osteosynthesis plate, presented at IV International Symposium on Biomedical Engineering, Peniscola, Spain, September 1991.

114. Owen, M. J., Middleton, V., and Rudd, C. D., Fibre reinforcement for high volume resin transfer molding, *Comp. Manufac.*, *1*, 74–78 (1990).

115. Rudd, C. D., Owen, M. J., and Middleton, V., Mechanical properties of weft glass fibre/polyester laminates, *Comp. Sci. Tech.*, *39*, 261–277 (1990).

116. Chou, S., and Wu, C. J., A study of the physical properties of epoxy resin composites with knitted glass fiber fabrics, *J Reinforc. Plast. Compos.*, *11*, 1239–1250 (1992).

117. Ramakrishna, S., and Hull, D., Tensile behaviour of knitted carbon-fibre-fabric/epoxy laminates. Part 1: Experimental, *Comp. Sci. Techn.*, *50*, 237–247 (1994).
118. Ramakrishna, S., and Hull, D., Tensile behaviour of knitted carbon-fibre-fabric/epoxy lamninates. Part 2: Prediction of tensile properties, *Comp. Sci. Techn.*, *50*, 249–258 (1994).
119. Buck, A, Patentschrift DE 3108041 C2, 1985.
120. Vetter, S., Aktuelle R/L-Rundstrickmaschinen—Konstruktionen, *Wirkerei- und Strickerei-Technik*, *40*, 707 (1990).
121. Mayer, J., Wintermantel, E., De Angelis, F., Niedermeier, M., Buck, A., and Flemming, M., Carbon fibre knitting reinforcement (K-CF) of thermoplastics: A novel composite, presented at Euromat Cambridge UK, 1991, in *Advanced Structural Materials* (T. W. Clyne, ed.), The Institute of Materials, Cambridge, UK, 1991, pp. 18–26.
122. Mayer, J., Ha, S. W., de Haan, J., Petitmermet, M., and Wintermantel, E., Knitted carbon fibers reinforced biocompatible thermoplastics, mechanical properties and structure modelling, in *Developments in the Science and Technology of Composite Materials*, ECCM6, September 1993, Bordeaux (A. R. Bunsell, A. Kelly, and A. Massiah, eds.), Woodhaed Publishing, 1993, pp. 637–642.
123. Mayer, J., Luescher, P., and Wintermantel, E., Knitted carbon fiber reinforced thermoplastics: Structural characterization with image analysis. In *Textiles and Composites '92* (H. Meinander, ed.), VTT Symposium 133, Tampere, Finland, 1992, pp. 315–320.
124. Schwarz, P., Mueller, U., and Fritz, U., Faserorientierung bestimmt Werkstoffeigenschaften, *Kunststoffe*, *82* 239–242 (1992).
125. Toll, S., and Andersson, P. O., Microstructural characterization of injection moulded composites using image analysis, *Composites*, *22*, 298–306 (1991).
126. O'Conell, P. A., and Duckett, R. A., Measurements of fiber orientation in short-fiber-reinforced thermoplastics, *Compos. Sci. Tech.*, *42*, 329–347 (1991).
127. Williams, D. F., McNamara, A., and Turner, R. M., Potential of polyetheretherketone (PEEK) and carbon-fiber-reinforced PEEK in medical applications. *J. Mat. Sci. Lett. 6*, 188–190 (1987).
128. Loher, U., Tognini, R., Mayer, J., Koch, B., and Wintermantel, E., Development of a cortical bone screw made with endless carbon fiber reinforced polyetheretherketone (CF-PEEK) by extrusion: A new method, presented at the 7th PIMS Congress, Amsterdam, September 1993.
129. Kardos, I. J., short fibre reinforced polymeric composites: Structure–property relations, in *International Encyclopedia of Composites* (S. E. Lee, ed.), VCH Publishers, 1991, Vol. 4, pp. 130–141.
130. Carlsson, L. A., and Pipes, R. B., *Hochleistungsfaserverbundwerkstoffe*, Teubner Studienbücher Werkstoffe, Teubner, Stuttgart, 1989, pp. 11–29.
131. Drzal, L. T., Intrinsic material limitations in using interface modification to alter fiber-matrix adhesion in composite materials, *Mat. Res. Soc. Symp. Proc.*, *170*, 275–283 (1990).
132. Deger, C., Jadhav, T., and Jadav, B., Development of absorbable, ultra high strength poly (lactides), *Progress in Biomedical Polymers*, Plenum Press, S. 239–248, 1990.

2
Biomechanical Aspects of Joint and Tooth Replacements

Günther Heimke
Clemson University
Clemson, South Carolina

I. INTRODUCTION

Joint and tooth replacements belong to the group of permanent implants as compared to temporary implants like bone plates and other means of fracture fixation. Such permanent implants are intended to serve their purpose for the remaining lifetime of the patient. Presently, survival rates of up to 20 years can be realistically considered for total hip replacements and dental implants.

All these implants can be considered to consist of a functional unit, such as the crown on top of a dental implant for chewing or the articulating component of a joint replacement, and an anchoring unit for their fixation in the adjacent part of the skeleton. While the functioning portion of a dental implant can, if necessary, be replaced without an additional surgical intervention, the articulating components of a joint replacement and all anchoring portions must maintain their integrity for the whole remaining life span of the recipient.

In order to function as intended, all these replacements must transmit forces either into or from one part to another part of the skeleton. The mechanical problems resulting from this force transmission can be treated from different points of view:

1. The mechanical reliability of the implant itself
2. The response of the bony tissue to the stresses and strains created by the insertion of the implant
3. The mechanics of the interface between implant and bone

Of course, none of these viewpoints can be treated independently from the others. In every case given, the mechanical reliability depends on the dimension, the shape, and the material of the anchoring portion of the implant. The remodeling of the bony tissues concerned is largely controlled by the stresses and strains they experience (remember the occurrence of disuse atrophy), which, in turn, depend on the shape of the implant and the kind of interface. The kind of tissue at the interface is partially controlled by the implant material and strongly depends on the type of forces acting along the interface: If the forces create shear movements, a pseudarthrosis-like soft tissue layer will result, the presence of which strongly changes the stress and strain distribution inside the adjacent bony tissue as compared to the situation with direct bone contact or an intimate interlocking between implant and bone. This strong interdependence of the three points of view given above must always be kept in mind in their subsequent treatment.

II. MECHANICAL PROPERTIES OF PERMANENT IMPLANTS

In order to account for the old and general surgical requirement to sacrifice as little living tissue as possible, the anchoring portions of nearly all load-bearing implants are dimensionally confined. Thus, only high-strength materials can be considered. But all materials do interact with their environment. The materials themselves corrode and they release some components such as atoms or ions, or compounds such as monomers into the environment. These interactions are the more pronounced the higher the stresses (stress corrosion) and the higher the amplitude and the number of load changes (fatigue). In addition, the corrosion products influence the environment and (for by far most materials) are toxic to the tissues adjacent to the anchoring portions of implants. Therefore, the number of materials with just the correct combination of properties suited for permanent implants is very limited.

All major groups of solids are represented among the bone replacement materials: The oldest man-made inorganic material, ceramic, was the latest to be considered for that application; metals and plastics have been used for several decades already. The most important structural features of metallic and ceramic implant materials have been recently discussed elsewhere in much detail [1–5]. Table 1 gives a survey of the essential differences of the mechanical properties of the three types of materials.

Another viewpoint for categorizing implant materials is their degree of compatibility with living tissue, in particular bony tissue. Of course, many kinds of ratings have been suggested [6, 7]. In Table 2, a rating once given by Osborn [7] is reproduced because of its wide acceptance and simplicity, but with some modifications accounting for more recent results. The tissue reactions mentioned in column 2 of Table 2 are those essentially observed in load-free situations or during the healing period of (later to be) loaded implants. Thus, all mechanical influences which might result in movements along the interfaces and which, even in the case of fracture healing, would result in a soft tissue interlayer (a pseudarthrosis seam) are excluded [8, 9]. Table 2, therefore, mainly represents the biochemically controlled tissue responses.

The correlation between the terms mentioned in the first column of Table 2 and the summarizing description of the reactions of bony tissue around them, given in the second column, can already be regarded as an attempt to give a definition of these concepts. However, because of the importance of a correct and precise terminology, these terms are defined in more detail in Table 3.

A. Metals

Of the mechanically strong metals with a corrosion resistance sufficiently high enough to be considered for permanent implants, the stainless steels have been used in joint surgery in combination with the polymethylmethacrylate (PMMA) bone cement in the 1960s and

Table 1 Comparison of Essential Mechanical Properties of Metals, Ceramics, and Plastics (Characteristic and Simplified, Averaged Values)

Material	Elastic modulus (10^6 MPa)	Characteristic strength (MPa)	Fatigue strength (MPa)	Comments[a] (trade names)
Stainless steel	0.2	700[b]	250	—
Co–Cr–Mo alloys	0.23	500[b]	250	Old cast materials (Vitallium; Protasul 2)
	0.23	750[b]	350	Cast (Endocast; Vitallium)
	0.23	850[b]	450	Sintered (Zimmerloy)
Co–Cr–Mo–Ni alloy	0.23	950[b]	450	Forged (Protasul 10)
Titanium, commercially pure	0.11	500[b]	100	—
TiAlV- and TiAlFe alloys	0.11	950[b]	600	—
Tantalum	0.18	125[b]	—	—
Alumina-ceramics	0.38	400[c]	300	(Frialit; Biolox)
Hydroxyl-apatite	0.02	100[c]	25	
Ca-phosphate glasses	0.03	200[c]	50	(Ceravital; Bioglass)
PMMA	0.003	80[b]	20	(Palacos; Simplex)
HDPE	0.001	25[b]	10	
Cortical bone	0.020	150[b]	—	—
Cancellous bone	0.003	5[b]	—	—

[a]Averaged data, not always identical with the specifications given by the manufacturers
[b]Tensile strength values
[c]Bend strength values

Table 2 Categorization of Hard Tissue Replacement Materials According to Their Compatibility with Bony Tissue

Degree of compatibility	Characteristics of reactions of bony tissue	Materials
Biotolerant	Implants separated from adjacent bone by a soft tissue layer along most of the interface: distance osteogenesis	Stainless steels, PMMA bone cements, Co–Cr–Mo and Co–Cr–Mo–Ni alloys
Bioinert	Direct contact to bony tissue: contact osteogenesis	Alumina ceramics, zirconia ceramics, titanium, tantalum, niobium, carbon
Bioactive	Bonding to bony tissue, bonding osteogenesis	Ca-phosphate-containing glasses and glass-ceramics, hydroxyl apatite and tricalcium-phosphate ceramics, titanium(?)

Table 3 Definition of Terms Used for Rating the Degree of Compatibility of Bone Replacement Materials

Term describing degree of compatibility	Material's influence on adjacent tissue	Result
Biotolerant (distance osteogenesis)	Components of the material (e.g., ions or monomers) are leached into the surrounding tissue.	Irritation of the differentiation of precursor cells into osteoblasts; formation of a collagen-rich interlayer.
Bioinert (contact osteogenesis)	"Nothing goes into solution": leakage of ions and other matter below detectability by cells and without systemic effect. Strong and fast absorption of moleculecules from body fluids so that the surface of the implant is covered completely (coated) by the body's own matter.	No biochemical influence on cell differentiation and proliferation. No biochemical information to cells about the presence of an implant. No enzyme-controlled reactions; the implant is "camouflaged" against the host's immune system. No foreign body reactions.
Bioactive (bonding osteogenesis)	Deposition of collagen and/or hydroxyl apatite from the surrounding bone onto the surface of the implant.	Bond formation in the sense of a glueing effect (without the necessity for adding a glue).

into the '70s. However, because of their limited fatigue strength (see Table 1) and their relatively low modulus of elasticity, resulting in considerable deformations and thus, loading of the surrounding cement, their use was more and more discontinued in favor of the stiffer Cobalt-based alloys. Whether the newer high nitrogen containing material (see Table 4) will regain some of the importance of the stainless steels for permanent implants remains to be seen.

1. *Cobalt-Based Alloys*

The more corrosion resistant Co-based alloys are the most widely used implant materials in orthopedic surgery today, in particular in joint replacements in combination with PMMA bone cement. These alloys have undergone considerable improvements during about the last 20 years. While the fatigue strengths of most of the old cast versions had not been much better than those of the stainless steels, resulting in stem fractures of up to about 5% of the cases within 5 years, the newer versions offer a sufficiently high safety margin [10]. This improvement of the fatigue behavior was achieved by a reduction of the average grain size and grain size distribution by the use of either much purer raw materials (e.g., Endocast), forging (e.g., Protasul 10), sintering (e.g., Zimmerloy), or combinations of them. Now, some of these alloys have stood the test of about 20 years of clinical application and have made it possible to practically completely eliminate the occurrence of stem fracture in hip arthroplasty.

2. *Titanium and Titanium-Based Alloys*

The good compatibility observed with titanium and titanium alloy implants in bony environment and the high fatigue strength of some Ti-alloys have increased the use of these metals in reconstructive surgery during the last decade considerably. Many of the

Table 4 Composition and Mechanical Properties of Iron and Cobalt Alloys for Permanent Surgical Implants According to the ASTM Standards

Name of alloy	Main alloying elements (%)	Ultimate tensile strength (MPa)	Yield strength, 0.2% (MPa)	Number of ASTM standard
Wrought high-nitrogen strengthened stainless steel	C: 0.03 max Mn: 4–6 Cr: 20.5–23.5 Ni: 11.5–13.5 Mo: 2–3 N: 0.2–0.4	*Annealed* 690 *Cold-worked* 1035 min	380 862 min	F 1314-90
Wrought high-nickel Co-based alloy	C: 0.025 Cr: 19–21 Ni: 33–37 Mo: 9–10.5	*Cold-worked and aged* 1793 min	1586 min	F 562-84
Forgings of Co–Cr–Mo alloy	Same as for F 562	*According to F 562*		F 961-85
Cast Co–Cr–Mo alloy	Cr: 27–30 Mo: 5–7 Ni: 1 Mn: 1	655 min	450 min	F 75-87
Thermomechanically processed Co–Cr–Mo alloy	Cr: 26–30 Mo: 5–7 Ni: 1 Mn: 1	1172	827	F 799-87
Wrought high-tungsten Co-based alloy	C: 0.05–0.15 Cr: 19–21 Ni: 9–11 W: 14–16	*Annealed* 860 min	310 min	F 90-87
Wrought high-iron Co-based alloy	C: 0.05 Cr: 18–22 Mo: 3–4 W: 3–4 Ni: 15–25 Fe: 4–6	*Cold-worked and aged* 1310 min *Cold-worked and aged extrahard* 1586 min	1172 min 1310 min	F 563-88

cement-free implantable joint replacements and nearly all metal dental implants are presently made of titanium or one of its alloys. If the requirements for osseo-integration, discussed later in detail, are met, titanium implants are found in close bone contact along most of their load transmitting interfaces with essentially two different kinds of bone contact: one with a close bone contact as observed with all other bioinert materials, the other with a kind of bonding to bony tissue coming close to the definition of a bioactive material. The latter was observed around dental implants and described in detail by

Table 5 Composition and Mechanical Properties of Titanium and Titanium Alloys for Permanent Implants

Name	Main alloying elements[a] (%)	Tensile strength (MPa)	Yield strength (MPa)	Number of ASTM standard
Wrought ELI Ti6Al4V alloy	Al: 5.5–6.5 V: 3.5–4.5	*Annealed* 860 min	795 min	F 136-84
Ti6Al4V ELI forgings	Al: 5.5–6.5 V: 3.5–4.5	*Not specified*		F 620-87
Ti6Al4V alloy forgings	Al: 5.5–6.75 V: 3.5–4.5	860 min	758 min	F 1108-88
Ti3.5Al6.5Fe	Al: 3.5 Fe: 6.5	*Hot-rolled and swaged* 1234	1120	[b]
Unalloyed titanium[c]	N: 0.05 max C: 0.1 max H: 0.0125 max Fe: 0.5 max O: 0.4 max	550 min	483 min	F 67-89; values given for bars of grade 4

[a]Balance Ti
[b]Taken from Ref. 15
[c]Similar to cpTi (commercially pure titanium)

Albrektsson et al. [11] and with femoral shafts of hip replacements by Menge and colleagues [12, 13]. For the other kind of bone contact see, e.g., Stock et al. [14]. The mechanical properties of the medical-grade, commercially pure (cp) titanium and titanium alloys [15] are summarized in Table 5.

3. *Fatigue Properties*

The mechanical specifications given in Tables 4 and 5 are the tensile and the yield strength. But, of course, these are values to be taken from samples in the as-cast or as-worked (e.g., wrought or forged) condition. Thus, these specifications do not contain any informations on the fatigue properties of these materials. This is a common feature of all ASTM and other national and international standards in this field, and renders them nearly worthless for design purposes. As permanent implants have to last for the remaining life span of the patients concerned, only values describing their mechanical performance after, say realistically, about 30 years of service can be used for their design. But these data are only available, if at all, from scientific literature (for a recent summary, see Ref. 16) and, in rare cases, from the catalogues of suppliers of implant materials. The fatigue strength values given in Table 1 have been averaged from such sources.

As is discussed below, many joint replacements intended for cement-free fixation carry porous coatings along all or parts of their anchoring portions. Most of these coatings consist either of beads or of wire meshes sintered or welded onto the surfaces along which a direct, shear force resistant contact or, rather, bond to bony tissue is intended. As sintering as well as welding necessitates a reaction of both components—the bead or mesh and the substrate material—any coating process nearly inevitably results in some kind of grain growth along the contact areas. Thus, the fatigue values of such coated stems can be considerably reduced as compared to uncoated versions. The fatigue strength can additionally be impaired by crevice corrosion-like processes inside the pores and the sharp corners between the beads or wires of the meshes and the substrate's surface. Table 6 gives a comparison of the fatigue strengths of the most widely used medical-grade metals.

B. Polymers

After early attempts by Judet and Judet [17] during the 1940s to replace the articulating surfaces of femoral heads by PMMA had failed, it was not until the introduction of the so-called low-friction arthroplasty by Charnley in 1960 [18] that polymers found widespread application in bone surgery. This combination of a polyethylene acetabular socket with a metal femoral stem, both anchored in their bony bed via the PMMA bone cement, is still the most widely used kind of total joint replacement. Several hundred thousand such operations are performed per year worldwide. Therefore, an enormous amount of experiences exists for this combination. An extended follow-up study based on nearly 40,000 implants inserted between 1968 and 1978 performed in the German-speaking countries [19] resulted in much valuable information and, in particular, confirmed some observations which previously had been based on much smaller groups of patients: There is one first maximum of failures about 5 years after operation, mainly because of loosening of the femoral components due to a widening of the radiolucent seam along the PMMA/bone interface. This might mainly be due to imperfections in the operational technique and particularly in the application of the bone cement. A second increase of the failure rate was found towards the end of the 10-years observation period, and the rate continued to increase. This was mainly due to loosening of the acetabular components. To understand this trend, two influences must be considered which act in the same direction: It is now generally agreed that the combination of polyethylene with a Co–Cr–Mo femoral head results in an average wear rate of the polyethylene cup of 0.2 to 0.5 mm per year, thus reducing the thickness of the cup by 2 to 5 mm within 10 years, which is about half of its original thickness. By this reduction, of course, all fatigue phenomena, such as cold working, are enhanced [20, 21]. In addition, the stresses on the cement layer surrounding the socket are increased, making the aging processes of the PMMA more severe. Therefore, the total survival time of such cemented devices must be assumed to be limited to 15 to 20 years in the more favorable situations.

Table 7 is an attempt to summarize the standardized specifications on the mechanical performance of the most widely used polymers. However, here the same problem exists

Table 6   Comparison of Fatigue Strengths of Plain and Porous Coated Metals and Alloys for Permanent Implants

Metal or alloy	Fatigue strength (MPa)		Comments
	With plain surface	Coated	
Co-based alloys	450	Up to 234[a]	Rot. beam; $f = 167$ Hz; $N = 2 \times 10^7$
TiAl6V4	600	Up to 233[a]	Rot. beam; $f = 100$ Hz; $N = 10^7$

[a]According to Ref. 16

Table 7 Composition and Some Mechanical Properties of Plastic Materials for Permanent Orthopedic Implants

Name	Composition	Mechanically characteristic values[a] (MPA)	Standard
Acrylic bone cement (PMMA)	Polymethylmethacry-late	Cured polymer after setting: compressive strength min 70; indention max 0.14 mm	F 451-86
Ultra-high molecular weight polyethylene (UHMWPE)	Polyethylene	Tensile strength at 23 °C: ultimate 27, yield 19; hardness 60 Shore D	F 648-84

[a]For details of sample preparation and test methods, refer to the standards.

as mentioned above for the metals: No data describing the fatigue behavior of these materials are included. In addition, no information regarding the wear and tear properties is mentioned.

From all of the polymers, besides PMMA and polyethylene, silicone [poly(dimethyl-siloxane)] has found relatively widespread applications in bone surgery as artificial finger joints to restore motion to arthritic patients. With these implants, the movement of the joint is based on the deformation of the silicone in the actual joint area. This gives some additional aligning stability to the joints, but it also confines the survival rates of these replacements; i.e., if the degree of bending surpasses the limits of elasticity of these materials, an early fatigue can be caused. In addition, most of these implants are soft tissue encapsulated and, thus, separated from the bones adjacent to the joints due to their low stiffness, which can contribute to relatively early cases of loosening [22].

C. Ceramics

From the large number of ceramic materials, only a very few have been found suitable for consideration for implant purposes. These include some oxide ceramic materials, some ceramics of the calcium phosphate salts, and some calcium phosphate containing glasses and glass-ceramics. The position of these ceramics within the large family of nonmetallic, inorganic materials is shown schematically in Fig. 1. The essential structural differences of ceramics and metals have been described elsewhere in detail [1, 5]. In contrast to metals, in ceramics the ionic bond is predominant, mostly between oxygen and one or another metal ion, resulting in a strong localization of the electrical charges and rendering these materials into electrical insulators. Their ionic nature is also responsible for most of their mechanical, chemical, thermal, and electrical as well as optical properties.

1. *Oxide or Bioinert Ceramics*

Oxide ceramics are mostly single-phase materials, essentially free from silicates. They are composed of the oxides of the least noble metals, the metals with the highest energies of oxide formation. Thus, they have a high chemical stability and already have been used in chemical engineering in highly corrosive and abrasive environments for more than half a century.

Alumina Ceramics.   The prototype of the oxide ceramics, aluminum oxide-, alumina-, Al_2O_3-, or corundum-ceramic is the most widely used ceramic material for permanent

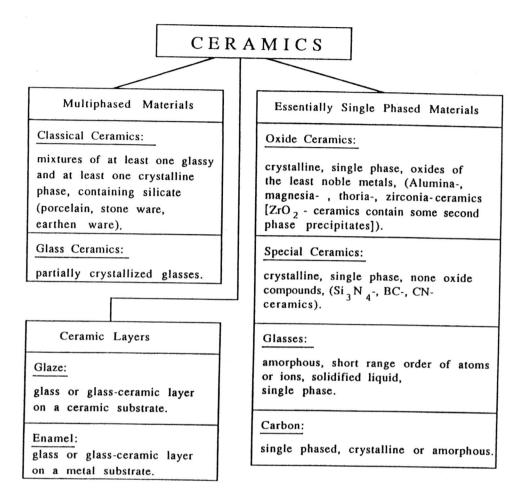

Figure 1 Ceramic materials grouped into single- and multiphased materials. All "classical" ceramics are multiphased and always contain some kind of clay allowing for the typical ceramic manufacturing techniques based on the plasticity of clays. The production techniques of the oxide and special ceramics are similar to the manufacturing processes of powder metallurgy. About 30 μm to several 100 μm thick flame- or plasma-sprayed ceramic layers have essentially the same properties as bulk materials of the same composition.

surgical implants. Corundum is the colorless version of sapphire and ruby. It is the most stable phase in the Al/O system, with a melting temperature of 2050°C. In general ceramic terminology, all ceramics having an Al_2O_3 content above about 85% are called alumina-ceramics. However, it was soon realized that ceramics with an alumina content of at least 99.5% were needed to meet the requirements of medical applications [23]. The specifications of this first generation of medical-grade alumina-ceramic are given in the first column of Table 8.

Most of the alumina-ceramic implants introduced into clinical trials and applications during the 1970s met these requirements. They became the base of many national stan-

Table 8   Properties of Medical-Grade Alumina-Ceramics According to International and Some National Standards, and of Some Commercially Available Materials with an Increased Safety Margin

Property	Unit	Ceramic according to ASTM F603-83, DIN 58 8353, ISO 6474	FRIALIT-, BIOLOX- bioceramics
Density	g/cm^3	≥ 3.9	≥ 3.98
Alumina content	%	≥ 99.5	≥ 99.9
SiO_2 and alkaline metal oxides	%	≤ 0.1	≤ 0.05
Microstructure, average grain size	μm	≤ 7	≤ 2.5
Microhardness	MPa	23,000	23,000
Compressive strength	MPa	4,000	4,000
Bend strength	MPa	≥ 400	≥ 450
Young's modulus	MPa	380,000	380,000
Impact strength	cm MPa	≥ 40	≥ 40
Wear resistance	mm^3/h	0.01	0.001
Corrosion resistance	$mg/m^2/day$	≤ 0.1	≤ 0.1

dards and the ISO standard for these materials. Detailed follow-up studies and examinations of retrieved implants [24, 25], together with some observations of an unexpected influence of minor CaO contaminations on the fatigue behaviour [26], however, clearly indicated the necessity for a further increase of the safety margin. The results of these efforts are expressed in the second data column of Table 8. Many details of this increase of mechanical properties and of the possibilities for reliable life time predictions based on the crack propagation theories developed during the 1970s are available elsewhere [27].

After an early mentioning of this material for "panoptical and medical purposes" [28], as far back as 1933, this ceramic was again recommended for implants and medical instruments in a patent application filed in the mid-1960s [29]. But it was not until the end of that decade that scientifically sufficiently detailed studies became available [30, 31]. Boutin immediately commenced clinical trials and, thus, was the first to insert a hip prosthesis containing an alumina-ceramic component into humans [32, 33]. Simultaneously, in very detailed compatibility studies, test pieces were placed in the bony tissue under nearly load-free conditions. Their results confirmed the high degree of tissue compatibility [34] of this material and the adequacy of the definition of the term "bioinert" mentioned in Table 3. The essential observation was that the recovery and restructuring of the bony tissue adjacent to such a bioinert implant exactly follows the same sequence of reactions characteristic of fracture healing. In addition, the tissue responses to alumina-ceramic wear particles and the cancerogeneity of this material were tested [35, 36].

The statement in the definition of the term "bioinert" in Table 3, "leakage of ions or other matter from the implant into the surrounding tissue below detectability by the cells . . . " needs an additional comment for one type of cell, in view of a more recent observation [37]: No increase in Al ion concentration was found in a protein-free saline solution even after 12 months; in a protein-containing tissue culture media, however, an increase of the Al ion concentration was observed as early as 2 weeks after immersion. The increase in the diameters of the prikaraya of neurons typically observed after their explantation under control conditions was inhibited or stopped in the presence of aluminum oxide ceramic material. But the bioelectric properties of the small neurons were unchanged after exposure to alumina-ceramic when compared with those grown under control conditions. Furthermore, even Al ion concentrations 100 times higher than those found in media exposed to this ceramic material had no effect on the bioelectric properties of sensory spinal ganglion cells. Such high concentrations, however, depressed the spontaneous bioelectric activities of some CA3 neuronal pools in hippocampal sections. It is concluded from the latter findings that micromolar concentrations of Al ions hardly affect the membrane properties of neurons but possibly exert effects on the metabolism or the release of specific transmitters. Clinically, however, a return of sensory activity was measured for alumina-ceramic dental implants starting about 2 years after implantation [38]. In animals the presence of nerve fibers was demonstrated histologically in the contact zone around such implants [39].

Because of their particular kind of property combination, ceramics have recently entered fields of engineering in which, in most cases, no experience in using this kind of hard and brittle material existed. This necessitated some kind of learning period and, nearly inevitably, led to some initial problems. The introduction of ceramics into medical technology was and, obviously, is no exception. Thus, while the handling of the medical-grade metals, mentioned above, does not require particular instructions, the rapid expansion, in particular in the use of ceramic balls in total hip arthroplasty, necessitates some warning comments. Their number is increasing rapidly due to the extremely low wear rates in their articulation against the same ceramic [23, 40, 41] and against polyethylene sockets where the wear rate is reduced by a factor of about 2 as compared to the Co–Cr–Mo alloys [42, 43]. These balls are fixed to the tapered necks of the metal shafts of the femoral components via conical holes. More than 1.2 million of them have been implanted since their introduction in 1974 [44]. The oldest have, subsequently, stood the test of nearly 20 years of continuous application, and their use now ranges to more than 150,000 annually.

The teams who had developed and introduced this composite system into orthopedic surgery had tried everything possible to pass on their know-how gained during the initial clinical trial period, in order to help others to avoid any of the early problems [24, 25, 45]. Occasionally, however, one or another of the safety precautions appears to have lost attention. Particular care must be taken if metal components are to be fitted with a taper in shops that are not, or not yet, properly instructed and equipped with the necessary high-precision tools and testing instruments. But also in long-term clinical routine as well as with teams newly adopting this low-wear system, not all safety features might consistently be observed.

Standards and government regulations may help to provide conditions necessary for the safety of the components concerned, but they are not sufficient as some safety-relevant handling details of these systems are completely confined to the operating room. However, even specifications for the surface roughness of the conical surfaces presently under discussion for worldwide standardization appear to need some modifications in order to provide for the required safety margins.

The design features of the most widely used conical fixation of the ceramic ball to the tapered metal stem can best be discussed using the schematic presentation in Fig. 2. Most of the details of this design resulted from extended experimental, theoretical, finite element, and optical stress analysis studies by different research teams [34, 46–48]. The

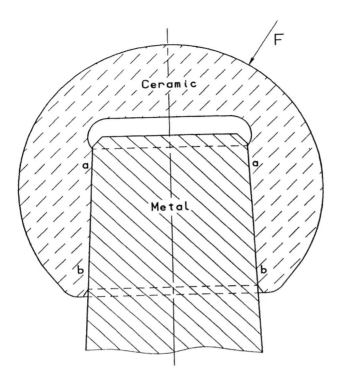

Figure 2   Cross-section of a ceramic ball joined to a metal stem via a conical sleeve. a and b indicate the inner and the outer portion of the interface between the conical hole inside the ceramic ball and the tapered neck of the metal stem respectively. F indicates the direction of the resulting force acting in the physiological situation.

results of clinical follow-up studies of these devices and the experiences in their manufacture led to the specifications presently under discussion for standardization; these are shown in Table 9.

The perfect matching of the inner, metal taper and the outer, ceramic cone as shown in Fig. 2 cannot be maintained in manufacturing, of course. Unavoidable machining tolerances will result in deviations from roundness, straightness of the dip lines, and cone

Table 9   Specification for the 12/14 Metal Taper (also Called "Eurocone") with Two Types Suggested for Standardization

Parameter	Type I	Type II
Cone angle variation	Between 5°37.5′ and 5°42.5′ for both types[a]	
Roundness deviation	<8 μm	<15 μm
Straightness deviation	<3 μm	<12 μm
Roughness, R_z	6–20 μm	60–90 μm

[a]5°37.5′ is the lowest value according to FDA requirements.

angle. In order to study the relative importance of these deviations on the load-bearing capacity, all three parameters should be treated separately. However, the preparation of test specimens also requires tolerances; thus, their effects will always overlap and a relatively large scatter of values must be expected.

If the roundness deviations are described as a change of the cross-section from circular to elliptical, the orientation of the long axis of this ellipsoid to the plain of the femoral shaft also needs to be considered. In studies disregarding this orientational effect, a marked decrease in load-bearing capacity was observed for roundness deviations exceeding 8 μm for metal tapers with a roughness below $R_z = 20$ μm.

Figure 3 shows the influence of the straightness deviations on the load-bearing capacity and indicates that the FDA requirement of 46 kN can be maintained if the deviation is kept smaller than 3 μm.

In Fig. 4 a general increase of the load-bearing capacity with decreasing absolute values of the angle deviation can be seen. The lower level of the values on the right-hand side clearly demonstrate the dangers of too large angles of the metal taper because of a shift of the contact area to the opening end of the ceramic cone, as marked with the letters b in Fig. 2. The generally lower values for the load-bearing capacities (below 20 kN) in Fig. 4 as compared to the level shown in Fig. 3 (up to more than 50 kN) result from the difference in the application of the forces to the ceramic balls: The arrangement with a ring-shaped loading zone according to ISO 7206-5 always yields markedly higher fracture loads than the load transmission via a ceramic plate (as was used in Fig. 4) or against a ceramic and even a polyethylene socket.

Besides deviations from the ideal shape, unavoidable surface undulations such as turning or grinding grooves must be considered. In addition, as all contaminations, e.g., particles and lubricants, will have the most detrimental effect on absolutely flat surfaces,

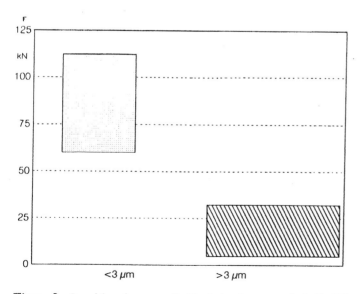

Figure 3 Load-bearing capacity F of alumina-ceramic balls (28 mm diameter) on standard 12/14 tapers of TiAl6V4 stems as a function of two artificial deviations *D* from the straightness of the dip lines. Test conditions according to ISO 7206-5.

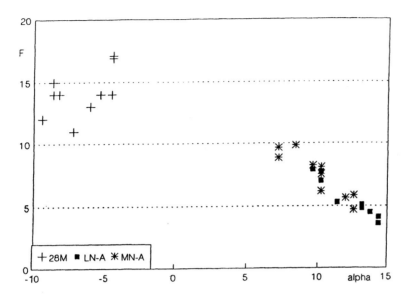

Figure 4   Load-bearing capacity F of alumina-ceramic balls (axial load) versus differences of angles of the ceramic cone and metal taper (alpha in minutes). (Crosses: values measured with 28-mm balls and medium neck length against ceramic plates; stars: values measured with 32-mm balls and medium; and squares: long neck lengths against polyethylene.) (From Andrisano et al., Ref. 91.)

a minimum surface roughness must be provided. There is still another requirement not yet accounted for in the standards presently under discussion: In order to reliably exclude all frictional movements along the interface, it is necessary to achieve some kind of cold welding at least along parts of the interface. This cannot be achieved if the required roughness consists of isolated holes or grooves extending into an otherwise plain surface. Only a roughness providing for a sufficient number of relatively sharp peaks can yield the high stresses necessary for cold flow and the formation of a sufficient number of oxygen bridges.

This latter requirement demands particular attention in the interoperational handling of these devices: Any kind of body fluid or tissue remaining along the interface during the final joining of the two components will severely impair the safety of the whole device.

There has always been, and still is, the temptation to ask a workshop, not yet completely instructed and equipped, to machine a cone onto a metal stem, which might be regarded as optimal in one or another clinic for particular indications but which is not supplied routinely by the supplier of ceramic balls. The following two examples demonstrate the necessity for additional attention to not always obvious deviations:

The taper shown in Fig. 5 meets the angle (with 5° 40′ 26″), the roundness (with deviations up to 2.3 μm), and along most of its surface the roughness specification (with $R_t = 6.37$ μm) of Table 9, but misses the straightness requirement (with 3.34 μm). Further on, there is a shiny area inside of which the roughness is reduced, probably caused by an additional touch with the grinding tool.

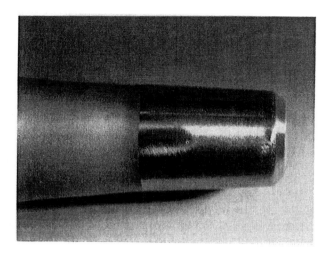

Figure 5   Taper with a shiny area.

Figure 6 gives an example of a particularly dangerous deviation. While the roundness and straightness requirements are met, the roughness of $R_t = 3.65$ μm is much too small. But the most dramatic deviation is a generally too short taper resulting in the furrow to be seen in the sand-blasted area below the taper. This is caused by the rim at the entrance of the conical hole of the ceramic ball contacting this metal portion. If this had happened in a clinical case, the metal taper would not penetrate into the ceramic cone completely

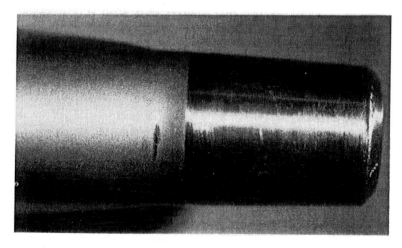

Figure 6   Cone with furrow on the lateral side of the sand-blasted area.

but would remain loose, and would soon start to grind away the metal, ending in catastrophic failure.

ZrO_2, SiC-, Si_3N_4-, and Sialon-Ceramics.   Other mechanically strong and highly corrosion resistant ceramics have also been considered for implant purposes. Table 10 summarizes their main mechanical characteristics. During the 1970s the mechanical strength of some zirconia-ceramics could be increased considerably [49], even surpassing the bend strength of the medical-grade alumina-ceramic mentioned in Table 8. Short-term compatibility studies in soft tissue of some modifications of these high-strength ZrO_2-ceramics showed relatively favorable tissue responses [50]. The high strength of these ceramics, however, is based on the presence of carefully controlled tetragonal precipitates in a cubic matrix. Because of a considerably reduced corrosion resistance of the tetragonal phase [51], a marked fatigue must be expected in body environment. This selective solubility (of the tetragonal precipitates) might also be one of the reasons for the less favorable wear behavior of zirconia-ceramic balls as compared to alumina-ceramic balls observed and described in Ref. 43. The fact that the raw materials from which the zirconia is derived are always accompanied by at least some tenth of a percent of urania and thoria renders most zirconia-ceramics radioactive, usually just to the legal limit for implant purposes [52]. Thus, only zirconia-ceramics made from raw materials from which all radioactive contaminations have been removed carefully can be considered for medical applications.

Some special, nonoxide ceramics such as silicon-carbide and silicon-nitride had also been considered for medical applications but were found without advantages or even inferior in their body compatibility to alumina-ceramic [53]. The same is true for some mixtures of special silicon-nitride-ceramics with oxide ceramics, the so-called Sialon-ceramics (*si*licate *al*uminum *o*xide and *n*itride ceramics) [54].

Carbon.   Different versions of solid carbon have also been considered again and again as bone substitutes (for a summary, see Ref. 55). For high load bearing applications carbon fiber reinforced carbons were developed in an attempt to combine high strength with a low Young's modulus in order to realize a so-called isoelastic prosthesis together with graphite surfaces reacted with nitrogen to form highly wear resistant layers along the articulating areas [56]. But the results of the first clinical trial were discouraging. Whether this was due to the implant design, a femoral cup with a central pin, or really attributable to the materials was never resolved.

Table 10   Mechanical Properties of Some ZrO_2-, SiC-, and Si_3N_4-Ceramics

Kind of ceramic	Density (g/cm^3)	Porosity (%)	Young's modulus (GPa)	Bend strength (MPa)	Comment
ZrO_2	6	<0.1	210	Up to 1000	a
SiC	3.15	<2	400	400	Sintered
SiC	3.2	0	420	550	Hot-pressed
Si_3N_4	3.3	<2	310	500	Sintered
Si_3N_4	3.2	0	320	760	Hot-pressed

[a]All values strongly depend on kind and amount of the stabilizing dopant and on the kind of heat treatment.

2. Ca-Phosphate and Bioactive Ceramics

Since the discovery of the ability of the formation of some kind of a direct, mechanically strong bond to living bony tissue in the late 1960s, particular interest has been focused on these ceramics. The term "bioactivity" was soon coined for this kind of material. There are two kinds of bioactive ceramics: an essentially silicate-free, sintered ceramic approaching the composition of the mineral phase of bone, and a silicate glass or glass-ceramic containing CaO and P_2O_5 in about the ratio in which it is present in bone.

Sintered Ca-Phosphate Materials. These more or less closely resemble the mineral phase of bone like hydroxylapatite- [$Ca_5(PO_4)_3OH$] (HA) and tricalcium phosphate-[$Ca_3(PO_4)_6$] (TCP) ceramic [57, 58]. The crystal lattices of these materials are relatively complicated and allow for many other ions to enter. This is the major reason for the problem of reproducability encountered with these materials. With some reasonable degree of approximation, the TCP-ceramic can be regarded as the dehydrated version of the HA material. The essential feature of the fascinating bonding to bony tissue phenomenon of these materials is the deposition of a layer of tiny hydroxylapatite particles by the body onto the implant surface from which the bond formation then continues. As was already shown in Table 1, the mechanical strength of these ceramics is low, so that they cannot directly be used for load-bearing applications. All attempts to compensate this mechanical handicap by coating these ceramics onto mechanically strong substrates such as alloyed Ti or Co femoral stems must consider their high-fatigue behavior caused by their at least slight solubility in the body environment inherently associated with their bioactivity [59].

Ca-Phosphate-Containing Glasses and Glass-Ceramics. The other materials with bone-bonding ability are the Ca-phosphate-containing glasses and glass-ceramics [60]. Their bond formation is different from the one observed with the bioactive ceramics: detailed studies (for a survey, see Hench and Ethridge, Ref. 61) revealed a gel-like, silicate-rich interlayer from which most of the Ca and phosphate ions had leached out. This interlayer was assumed to act as some kind of a diffusion barrier preventing this leaching process to continue. On top of this gel-like layer the composition soon reached the values of normal bony tissue. The bonds thus formed were found to have a mechanical strength higher than either of the adjacent materials if the interfaces had been kept unloaded or under pure compression during the implantation period. However, clinical study with dental implants made of a variation of the original material with a somewhat reduced solubility [62] indicated that this gel-like layer does not prevent the destruction of the material if loaded by sheer forces [63]. This same leaching phenomenon had also been found with Bioglas coatings on alumina-ceramic components of experimental hip replacements [64, 65]. Thus, at present and until the newly developed apatite–wollastonite-containing glass-ceramics [66] have been shown to reliably maintain their integrity in body environment, there does not seem to be much hope of using the bone-bonding ability of the bioactive glasses for improving the fixation of load-bearing implants. A new aspect might be resulting from the recently discovered process for creating an apatite layer on nearly all materials [67].

III. MECHANICAL ASPECTS OF IMPLANT FIXATION

The ideal fixation of a bone substitute would be identical to or approach as closely as possible the integration of vital bone as realized in fracture healing or, for example, in the microsurgical osteomyocutaneous flap grafting technique [68]. In these cases the transplant is completely osseo and functionally integrated [69], and all (former) interfaces will be able to transmit tensional, compressional, and shear forces. Any alloplastic material can only be expected to come close to this fixation mode, hardly ever surpassing it.

There are three major groups of influences from which deviations of the interface reactions of bony tissue adjacent to an implant, as compared to the sequence of reactions during fracture healing, must be considered: mechanical, chemical, and biological or biochemical.

The main mechanical requirement for undisturbed fracture healing is motionlessness along the fracture site. The successes of pressure osteotonies indicate that there is no general requirement for the absence of forces. Only those forces are to be excluded which would cause relative movements along the interface. Thus, forces or components of forces oriented parallel to the surface of the fracture (shear forces) must be excluded or kept small enough. If this requirement is not met and a fracture site is not sufficiently stabilized, fracture healing will be prevented and a soft tissue layer will be formed along the surface of the fracture. This soft tissue layer is composed essentially of relatively dense, cell-depleting layers of collagen fibers preferably oriented parallel to the surface. Later, the formation of a layer of densified bone resembling a lamella of cortical bone between the soft tissue and the underlaying bone can be observed. This soft tissue layer is called a "pseudarthrosis seam." Clinically, of course, this is the nonunion situation.

According to this consideration, summarized in Table 11, the most favorable implant material would allow for a sequence of reactions in the adjacent bony tissue exactly matching fracture healing. This, however, can only be expected if all other possible influences, besides mechanical ones, can also be excluded. These other influences might be chemical, by some matter being released from the implant disturbing or even prevent-

Table 11   Survey of the Sequence of Interface Reactions of Bony Tissue

Cause	Reaction
Trauma or surgical intervention	Bleeding, stimulation of immune system by cell and other debris. Thus activated cells start to remove remainders of disrupted tissues and cells.
Insertion of implant	Nutrition of tissue layer in contact with implant is severely reduced (one half space is no longer contributing) and openings of blood vessels are blocked by clotting, resulting in predominate osteoclastic activity. Surface layer of tissue loses much of its mechanical strength.
Motionlessness at interface and absence of chemical influences	Osteoblastic activity increases, first at contact of bony tissue to implant surface where softened interlayer was thinnest (in most cases, at corners and edges).
Blood clot formation in spaces between implant surface and tissue, and inside surface undulations such as lacunae or pores	If dimensions of clot are small enough, either osteoblasts or their precursor cells migrate into the clot along the fibrinogen fibers and start bone formation.
Load application	Along pressure-loaded interfaces: further bone deposition until surface area has become large enough for pressure to reach optimum of Wolff's law. Along interfaces with shear motion: formation of a pseudarthrosis seam.

ing one or several of the steps of cell differentiation and activity. Or they might be more biological; the implant surface can cause the body's immune system to stimulate processes which would suppress one or several of the reactions necessary for the complete restoration of the interface.

Using the rating of implant materials given in Table 2, the concept of bioinert materials appears to include the possibility of an interfacial bone remodeling closely resembling fracture healing. This was confirmed for the dense alumina-ceramic for load-free situations and for mainly pressure-loaded interfaces [39, 70, 71]. This statement is based on observations with light microscopy in which osteocytes can be seen in the immediate vicinity of the alumina-ceramic surface extending their plasmatic protuberances into the crystalline surface irregularities of the otherwise dense material [72–74]. Along interfaces which could not be prevented from shear movements during the first weeks after implantation — the healing period — the formation of a pseudarthrosis seam was seen as in nonunion cases [75].

This purely mechanical (stress and strain field controlled) influence on bone remodeling must also be remembered in testing implant materials for their degree of compatibility. If tested by insertion into bony tissue, the results can be obscured completely if the load situation prevailing during implantation at the site of the histological inspection is not noted and taken into consideration. At sites along which shear movements occurred, a pseudarthrosis seam will be seen, and at sites of motionlessness, a direct bone contact will develop along a bioinert material. Thus, as far as the interfacial tissue reactions are essentially mechanically controlled and, therefore, rather material independent, reports on tissue responses to implant materials disregarding the loading situation at the point of inspection during the test are rather worthless [8, 9, 76].

Basically, because of their ability to form a mechanically stable bond to bony tissue, the bioactive materials appear to allow for reactions of the surrounding bony tissue still further resembling the processes of fracture healing. As, however, the gel-like layer formed on the surfaces of the bioactive glasses and glass-ceramics is not stable against shear forces, these materials have not yet found large-scale applications as anchoring means of load-bearing implants. The bond between hydroxylapatite ceramics and bony tissue has been shown to withstand long-term shear loadings [77], but their low mechanical strength and the high fatigue of these materials does not allow their application as anchoring means of load-bearing, permanent implants. For the same reason, coatings of these ceramics onto high-strength substrate materials appear justified only on those implants which do carry other means of load transfer such as pores, lacunae, grooves, or threads in addition.

The previously discussed comparison between the healing processes along a fracture site and the remodeling of bony tissue facing an implant results in some shape requirements for the anchoring portions of load-transmitting bone replacements. The consequences of the essential condition of permanent motionlessness along the interface are schematically shown in Fig. 7 and detailed in its legend. If the interfacial motion during the healing phase can be kept small enough, a close bone contact can also be achieved and maintained even along essentially shear-loaded cylindrical portions of implants by interlocking via ingrowth of bony tissue into grooves or lacunae making use of the so called "load–line–shadow effect" [78–80]. The validity of this concept and its consequences for the anchorage of implants have been demonstrated for a total hip replacement system [24, 25, 81] and a particular type of dental implant by clinical mobility measurements [82, 83], histologically [84, 85], and by the results of follow-up evalua-

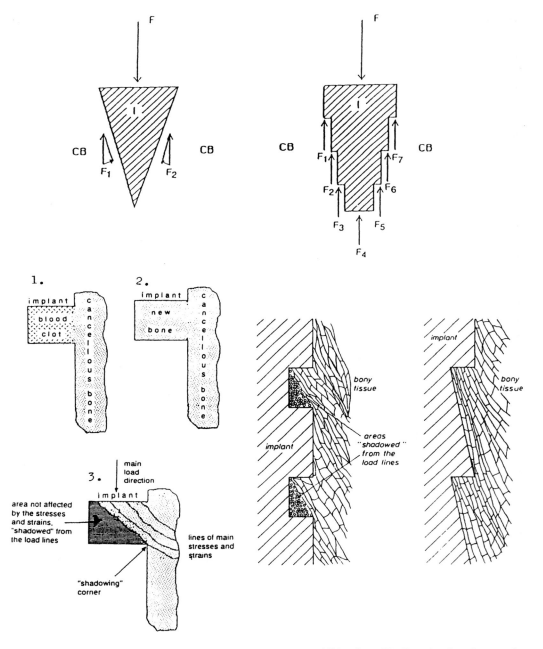

Figure 7 The interfacial mechanical conditions around a stiff implant (I). Top: implant in cancellous bone (CB) under the influence of intermittent force (F), equilibrated by the forces ($F_1 \ldots F_n$). Left: along an essentially wedge-shaped implant, large shear forces along the whole interface inevitably result in shear movements as long as there is no interfacial bonding. Right: the surfaces of the "steps" facing into the bone are met by the forces perpendicularly (are pressure loaded only), thus, remaining essentially at rest. Bottom left group (the "load–line–shadow effect"), from top to bottom: 1, implant with one lacuna press-fitted into cancellous bone shortly after implantation, lacuna filled by blood clot; 2, after the healing period, lacuna homogeneously filled with bony tissue; 3, some time after load application, area "shadowed" from load lines shows disuse atrophy. Bottom right row: the application of this phenomenon to achieve close bone contact along essentially shear-loaded interfaces by "interlocking."

tions [86, 87]. The presence or absence of interfacial motions can also be regarded as being controlled by the stress and strain field created by the insertion of an implant in the adjacent bone.

The application of these considerations for the analysis of the failure modes of the two most widely used types of load-bearing, permanent implants — total hip replacements and dental implants — allows for some summarizing judgment and suggestions for further improvements of the presently already high success rates.

IV. SOME FINAL REMARKS

From the presently available materials for bone, joint, and tooth replacements, titanium alloys appear to be the best-suited material for the anchoring portions of these devices for cement-free applications. For cemented implants, the use of the high-strength (low grain size) Co-based alloys has the advantage of higher elastic moduli, and, thus, smaller deformations and reduced fatigue of the surrounding cement mantle [88]. For the socket components of total hip replacements, a cemented polyethylene cup in combination with an alumina-ceramic ball appears the best solution from the friction and wear point of view, while the higher stresses within the polyethylene linings in the so-called metal-backed acetabular cups result in markedly increased amounts of polyethylene wear particles [88]. From the list of materials, the titanium and cobalt alloys have stood the test of several decades of clinical application. The PMMA bone cements have also stood the test of several decades of continuous application if combined with sufficiently stiff metal components. From the two most favorable partners of the articulating materials, it might be useful to further increase the safety margin of the ceramic and its joining to the metal stem. What definitely needs to be looked into is the fatigue and wear behavior of the polyethylene.

The formation of essentially similarly stable bony structures around long-term successful cemented stems, a particular type of titanium stem [89], and around dental implants [90] can be regarded as evidencing the ability of the bony tissues concerned to remodel into bony structures that allow reliable stabilization of the implants in their position and simultaneously allow maintenance of all other functionally necessary features such as blood supply and nerve and muscle activities, provided the implants carry load-transmitting structures allowing for the right amount of load transfer at the right location — in other words, the physiologically correct interface mechanics. However, the still remaining failure rates, in the order of 2% to 5% after about 10 years and more than 10% after 15 years, in the best clinics clearly demand further improvements.

ACKNOWLEDGMENTS

Thanks are due to P. D. Dr. G. Willmann and Dr. H. Richter, Plochingen, Germany, for providing some of the experimental data mentioned in the section on alumina-ceramics and for helpful discussions.

REFERENCES

1. Heimke, G., Structural characteristics of metals and ceramics, in *Metal and Ceramic Biomaterials*, Vol. 1 (P. Ducheyne and G. W. Hastings, eds.), CRC Press, Boca Raton, FL, 1984, pp. 7–61.

2. Pilliar, R. M., Manufacturing processes of metals: the processing and properties of metal implants, Ref. 1, pp. 79–90.
3. Keller, J. C., and Lautenschlager, E. P., Metals and alloys, in *Handbook of Biomaterials Evaluation* (A. F. von Recum, ed.), Macmillan, New York, 1986, pp. 3–23.
4. Leininger, R. I., and Bigg, D. M., Polymers, Ref. 3, pp. 24–37.
5. Heimke, G., Ceramics, Ref. 3, pp. 38–54.
6. Heimke, G., and Griss, P., Tissue interactions to bone replacement materials, in *Bioceramics of Calcium Phosphate* (K. de Groot, ed.), CRC Press, Boca Raton, FL, 1983, pp. 79–97.
7. Osborn, J. F., in *Fortschritte der Kiefer- und Gesichtschirurgie XXVIII* (Pfeifer and Schwenzer, eds.), Thieme Verlag, Stuttgart, May 1983.
8. Heimke, G., Griss, P., Jentschura, G., and Werner, E., Die Aussagefähigkeit histologischer Befunde zur Beurteilung von Knochenersatzwerkstoffen, *Arch. Orthop. Traumat. Surg.*, *91*, 267–276 (1978).
9. Heimke, G., Griss, P., Werner, E., and Jentschura, G., The effects of mechanical factors on biocompatibility tests, *J. Biomed. Eng.*, *3*, 209–213 (1981).
10. Semitsch, M., and H. G. Willert, Metallic materials for artificial hip joints, in *Encyclopedia of Medical Devices and Instrumentation* (J. G. Webster, ed.), Wiley, New York, 1988, pp. 137–149.
11. Albrektsson, T., Branemark, P. I., Hansson, H. A., and Lindstrom, J., Osseointegrated titanium implants, *Acta Orthop. Scand.*, *52*, 155–163 (1981).
12. Menge, M., Klinische Erfahrungen mit dem System Zweymüller-Endler: Analyse der Folgebeschwerden, in *Aktueller Stand der zementfreien Hüftendoprothetik* (B. Maaz and M. Menge, eds.), Georg Thieme Verlag, Stuttgart, 1985, pp. 44–50.
13. Lintner, F., Zweymüller, K., and Brand, G., Die knöcherne Reaktion auf zementfrei implantierte Titaniumschäfte, Ref. 12, pp. 33–43.
14. Stock, D., Gottstein, J., Griss, P., Winter, M., Heimke, G., and Büsing, C. M., Experimentelle Ergebnisse an Stufenschäften aus Titan für Hüftendoprothesen, *Z. Orthop.*, *121*, 640–645 (1983).
15. Breme, J., and Schmid, H-J., Criteria for the bioinertness of metals for osseo-integrated implants, in *Osseo-Integrated Implants*, Vol. 1, *Basics, Materials, and Joint Replacements* (G. Heimke, ed.), CRC Press, Boca Raton, FL, 1990, pp. 31–80.
16. Kohn, D. H., and Ducheyne, P., Materials for bone and joint replacements, in *Material Science and Technology*, Vol. 14, *Medical and Dental Materials* (D. F. Williams, ed.), VCH, Weinheim, 1992, pp. 29–109.
17. Judet, J., and Judet, R., The use of an artificial femoral head for arthroplasty of the hip joint, *J. Bone Joint Surg.*, *32B*, 166–170 (1950).
18. Charnley, J., Follacci, F. M., and Hamond, B. T., The long term results of low-friction arthroplasty of the hip as a primary invention, *J. Bone Joint Surg.*, *B*, *54*, 61–66 (1972).
19. Griss, P., Hackenbroch, M. H., Jäger, M., Preussner, B., Schäfer, Th., Seebauer, R., van Eimeren, W., and Winkler, W., Ten year results of total hip replacement. A retrospective multicenter study based on a ten percent random sample of 39,000 total hip replacements after ten years of observation, in *Aktuelle Probleme in Chirurgie und Orthopädie*, Vol. 21, H. Huber Verlag, Bern, 1982.
20. Eyerer, P., Property changes of UHMWPE during implantation—First hints for the development of an alternative polyethylene, in *ANTEC 85*, 43rd Annual Technical Conference, Washington, DC, 1985, p. 62.
21. Eyerer, P., and Ke, Y. C., Property changes of UHMWPE hip cup endoprostheses during implantation, *J. Biomed. Mater. Res.*, *18*, 1137–1142 (1984).
22. Swanson, A. B., de Goot Swanon, G., and Frisch, E. E., Flexible (silicone) implant arthroplasty in small joints of extremeties: Concepts, physical and biological considerations, experimental and clinical results, in *Biomaterials in Reconstructive Surgery* (L. R. Rubin, ed.), C.V. Mosby, St. Louis, 1983, pp. 595–599.

23. Griss, P., v. Andrian-Werburg, H., Krempien, B., and Heimke, G., Biological activity and histocompatibility of dense Al₂O₃/MgO ceramic implants in rats, *J. Biomed. Mater. Res. Symp.*, *4*, 453–462 (1973).

24. Griss, P., and Heimke, G., Five years experience with ceramic–metal–composite hip endoprostheses. I. Clinical evaluation, *Arch. Orthop. Traumatol. Surg.*, *98*, 157–164 (1981).

25. Heimke, G., and Griss, P., Five years experience with ceramic–metal–composite hip endoprostheses. II. Mechanical evaluations and improvements, *Arch. Orthop. Traumatol. Surg.*, *98*, 165–171 (1981).

26. Österholm, H. H., and Day, D. E., Calcium migration in dense alumina aged in water and physiological media, *Ceramic Bull.*, *60*, 955–959 (1981).

27. Soltész, U., Strength characterization of alumina bioceramics according to the new ISO draft, in *Bioceramics*, Vol. 2 (G. Heimke, ed.), German Ceramic Society, Cologne, 1990, pp. 160–171.

28. Rock, M., Künstliche Ersatzteile für das Innere und Äussere des menschlichen und tierischen Körpers, German Patent 583,589, 1933.

29. Sandhaus, S., Bone implants and drills and taps for bone surgery, British Patent 1083769, 1967.

30. Hulbert, S. F., Talbert, C. D., and Klawitter, J. J., Investigation into the potential of ceramic materials as permanently implantable skeletal prostheses, in *Biomaterials* (A. M. Bement, ed.), University of Washington Press, Seattle, 1971, pp. 3–77.

31. Hentrich, R. L., Graves, G. A., Stein, H. G., and Bajpai, P. K., An evaluation of inert and resordable ceramics for future clinical orthopedic applications, *J. Biomed. Mater. Res.*, *5*, 25 (1971).

32. Boutin, P., L'alumine et son utilisation en chirurgie de la hanche (étude experimentale), *Presse med.*, *79*, 14 (1971).

33. Boutin, P., Arthroplastie de la hanche par prothese en alumine fritté. Etude experimentale et premieres applications cliniques, *Rev. Chir. Orthop.*, *58*, 229–246 (1972).

34. Griss, P., Heimke, G., v. Andrian-Werburg, H., Krempien, B., Reipa, H., Lauterbach, J., and Hartung, H. J., Morphological and biomechanical aspects of Al₂O₃ ceramic joint replacements: Experimental results and design considerations for human endoprostheses, *J. Biomed. Mater. Res. Symp.*, *6*, 177–188 (1975).

35. Griss, P., Krempien, B., v. Andrian-Werburg, H., Heimke, G., and Fleiner, R., Experimental study of the tissue compatibility of oxide ceramic (Al₂O₃) wear particles, *Arch. Orthop. Unfall-Chir.*, *76*, 270–279 (1973).

36. Griss, P., Werner, E., Buchinger, R., Büsing, C. M., and Heimke, G., Zur Frage der unspezifischen Sarkomentstehung um Al₂O₃-keramische Implantate, *Arch. orthop. Unfall-Chir.*, *90*, 29–40 (1977).

37. Bingmann, D., Tetsch, P., and Bertram, H. P., Aluminiumoxidkeramik in der Nervenzellkultur, *Z. Zahnärztl. Implantol.*, *4*, 4–9 (1988).

38. Lukas, D., Meyle, J., Mühlbrad, L., and Schulte, W., Die Tastsensibilität Tübinger Sofortimplantate, *Dtsch. Zahnärztl. Z.*, *35*, 334–338 (1980).

39. d'Hoedt, B., and Büsing, C. M., Die Einheilung von Al₂O₃-Keramik am Beispiel des Tübiner Implantates (Frialit): Histologische und röntgenologische Ergebnisse, *Fortschr. Zahnärztl. Implantol.*, *1*, 150–161 (1985).

40. Mittelmeier, H., Zementlose Verankerung von Endoprothesen nach dem Tragrippenprinzip, *Z. Orthop.*, *112*, 27–33 (1974).

41. Dörre, E., and Dawihl, W., Ceramic hip endoprostheses, in *Mechanical Properties of Biomaterials* (G. W. Hastings and D. F. Williams, eds.), Wiley, Chichester, UK, 1980, pp. 113–127.

42. Semlitsch, M., Lehmann, M., Weber, H., Dörre, E., and Willert, H. G., New prospects for a prolonged functional life span of artificial hip joints by using the material combination polyethylene/aluminum oxide ceramic/metal, *J. Biomed. Mater. Res.*, *11*, 537–542 (1977).

43. Streicher, R. M., Semlitsch, M., and Schön, R., Ceramic surfaces as wear partners for

polyethylene, in *Bioceramics*, Vol. 4 (W. Bonfield, G. W. Hastings, and K. E. Tanner, eds.), Butterworth–Heinemann, 1991, pp. 9–16.

44. Willmann, G. (Plochingen), Personal communication (1993).

45. Mittelmeier, H., 4 Jahre Erfahrungen mit Autophor-Keramik-Hüftprothesen, *Med. Orthop. Tech.* (MOT), *100*, 19–26 (1980).

46. Heimke, G., Griss, P., Jentschura, G., and Werner, E., Mechanical testing of ceramic materials and components for bone and joint replacements, in *Mechanical Properties of Biomaterials* (G. W. Hastings and D. F. Williams, eds.), Wiley, Chichester, UK, 1980, pp. 129–145.

47. Siedelmann, U., Richter, H., and Soltesz, U., On the structural safety of ceramic hip joint heads, in *Biomaterials 1980* (G. D. Winter, D. F. Gibbons, and H. Plenk, eds.), Wiley, Chichester, UK, 1980, pp. 213–218.

48. Soltesz, U., and Heimke, G., Stress analysis in ceramic hip joint heads of various shape and fitting, in *Biomechanics: Principles and Applications* (R. Huiskes, D. van Campon, and J. de Wijn, eds.), Martinus Nijhoff, The Hague, 1982, pp. 283–290.

49. Claussen, N., Umwandlungsverstärkte keramische Werkstoffe, *Z. Werkstofftech.*, *13*, 138–145 (1982).

50. Garvie, R. C., Urbani, C., Kennedy, D. R., and NcNeuer, J. C., Biocompatibility of magnesia partially stabilized zirconia (Mg-PSZ) ceramics, *J. Mater. Sci.*, *19*, 3224–3229 (1984).

51. Nakajima, K., Kobayashi, K., and Murata, Y., Phase stability of Y-PSZ in aqueous solutions, in *Advances in Ceramics*, Vol. 12, *Science and Technology of Zirconia II* (N. Claussen, M. Rühle, and A. H. Heier, eds.), American Ceramic Society, Columbus, OH, 1984, pp. 339–345.

52. Cieur, S., Heindl, R., and Robert, A., Radioactivity of a femoral head of zirconia ceramics, in *Bioceramics*, Vol. 3 (S. F. Hulbert, ed.), Rose-Hulman Institute of Technology, Terre Haut, IN, 1992, pp. 367–371.

53. Griss, P., Werner, E., and Heimke, G., Alumina ceramic, bioglass, and silicon nitride: A comparative biocompatibility study, in *Mechanical Properties of Biomaterials* (G. W. Hastings and D. F. Williams, eds.), Wiley, Chichester, UK, 1980, pp. 217–226.

54. Clark, I. E., Philips, McKellup, H. A., Moreland, J., and Amstutz, H. C., Sialon ceramic—A candidate material for total joint replacements, Ref. 53, p. 155.

55. Haubold, A. D., Shim, H. S., and Bokros, J. C., Carbon in medical devices, in *Biocompatibility of Clinical Implant Materials*, Vol. 2 (D. F. Williams, ed.), CRC Press, Boca Raton, FL, 1981, pp. 3–19.

56. Bruckmann, H., Maurer, H. J., Hüttinger, K. J., Rettig, H., and Weber, U., New carbon materials for joint prostheses, in *Biomaterials 1980* (D. D. Winter, D. F. Gibbons, and H. Plenck, eds.), Wiley, Chichester, UK, 1982, pp. 27–38.

57. Jarchow, M., Calcium phosphate as a hard tissue prosthetics, *Clin. Orthop. Relat. Res.*, *157*, 259–278 (1981).

58. de Groot, K., ed., *Bioceramics of Calcium Phosphate*, CRC Press, Boca Raton, FL, 1983.

59. Bauer, G., Biochemical aspects of osseo-integration, in *Osseo-Integrated Implants*, Vol. 1, *Basics, Materials, and Joint Replacements* (G. Heimke, ed.), CRC Press, Boca Raton, FL, 1990, pp. 81–97.

60. Hench, L. L., Splinter, R. J., Allen, W. C., and Greenlee, T. K., Bonding mechanism at the interface of ceramic prosthetic materials, *J. Biomed. Mater. Res. Symp.*, *2*, 117–141 (1971).

61. Hench, L. L., and Ethridge, E. C., *Biomaterials: An Interfacial Approach*, Academic Press, New York, 1982.

62. Bunte, M., Strunz, V., Gross, U., Brömer, H., and Deutscher, K., Vergleichende Untersuchungen über die Haftung verschiedener Implantatmaterialien im Knochen, *Dtsch. Zahnärztl. Z.*, *32*, 825–830 (1977).

63. Strunz, V., Paper presented at the 107th Annual Meeting of Deutsche Ges. für Zahn-, Mund-, und Kieferchirurgie, Garmisch–Partenkirchen, Germany, September 23–25, 1982.

64. Griss, P., Werner, E., Heimke, G., and Buchinger, R., Vergleichende experimentelle Untersu-

chungen an Bioglas (L. L. Hench), Al₂O₃-Keramik und mit Bioglas beschichteter Al₂O₃-Keramik. I. Ergebnisse mit unbelasteten Implantaten, *Arch. Orthop. Unfall-Chir.*, *90*, 15–27 (1977).

65. Griss, P., Werner, E., Heimke, G., and Raute-Kreinsen, U., Vergleichende experimentelle Untersuchungen an Al₂O₃-Keramik und mit mod. Bioglas (L. L. Hench) beschichteter Al₂O₃-Keramik: Ergebnisse mit belasteten Implantaten, *Arch. Orthop. Traumat. Surg.*, *92*, 199–210 (1978).

66. Kokubo, T., Ito, S., Sigematsu, M., Sakka, S., and Yamamuro, T., Fatigue and lifetime of bioactive glassceramic A-W containing apatite and wollastonite, *J. Mater. Sci.*, *22*, 4067–4070 (1987).

67. Abe, Y., Kokubo, T., and Yamamuro, T., Apatite coating on ceramics, metals, and polymers utilizing a biological process, *J. Mater. Sci., Mater. Med.*, *1*, 233–238 (1990).

68. Riediger, D., d'Hoedt, B., and Pielsticker, W., Wiederherstellung der Kaufunktion durch enossale Implantate nach der Beckenkammtransplantation mit mikrochirurgischem Gefässanschluss, *Dtsch. Z. Mund Kiefer Gesichts Chir.*, *10*, 102–110 (1986).

69. Riediger, D., Büsing, C. M., d'Hoedt, B., and Pielsticker, W., Knochentransplantat mit mikrovaskulärem Anschluss als Implantatbett für enossale Implantate, *Dtsch. Zahnärztl. Z.*, *41*, 989–998 (1986).

70. Griss, P., Krempien, B., v. Andrian-Werburg, H. Frhr., and Heimke, G., Experimental analysis of ceramic–tissue interactions: A morphological, fluorescenceoptical, and radiographic study on dense alumina oxide ceramic in various experimental animals, *J. Biomed. Mater. Res. Symp.*, No. 5 (Part 1), 39–48 (1974).

71. Griss, P., Heimke, G., Krempien, B., Silber, R., Haehner, K., and Merkle, B., Erste Erfahrungen mit der Keramik–Metallverbundprothese, *Med. Orthop. Techn. (MOT)*, *95*, 159–162 (1975).

72. Griss, P., and Heimke, G., Biocompatibility of high density alumina and its application in orthopedic surgery, in *Biocompatiblity of Clinical Implant Materials* (D. F. Williams, ed.), CRC Press, Boca Raton, FL, 1981, pp. 155–198.

73. Büsing, C. M., and d'Hoedt, B., Die Knochanlagerung an das Tüberinger Implantat beim Menschen, *Dtsch. Zahnärztl. Z.*, *36*, 563–566 (1981).

74. Schulte, W., Das enossale Tübinger Implantat aus Al₂O₃ (Frialit): Der Entwicklungsstand nach 6 Jahren, *Zahnärztl. Mitt.*, *71* (19–20) (1981).

75. Krempien, B., Griss, P., Heimke, G., v. Andrian-Werburg, H., Hartung, H. J., Reipa, S., and Lauterbach, H. J., Remodelling dynamics of cortical bone under the influence of ceramic implants in sheep, *Acta orthop. Belg.*, *40*, 624–638 (1974).

76. Soltesz, U., Siegele, D., and Baudendiestel, E., Might biomechanical effects influence biocompatibility tests in bone? in *Clinical Implant Materials* (G. Heimke, U. Soltesz, and A. J. C. Lee, eds.), Elsevier, Amsterdam, 1990, pp. 657–662.

77. Putter, C. de, Groot, K. de, and Sillevis-Smitt, P. A. E., Implants of dense hydroxylapatite in prosthetic dentistry, in *Clinical Application of Biomaterials* (A. J. C. Lee, T. Albrektsson, and P.-I. Branemark, eds.), Wiley, Chichester, UK, 1982, pp. 125–130.

78. Büsing, C. M., Heimke, G., Schulte, W., and Linn, W., Gibt es ein Lastschatten-Phänomen? Biomechanische Aspekte bei Zahnimplantaten aus Al₂O₃-Keramik, *Pathologe*, *1*, 61 (1979).

79. Heimke, G., Schulte, W., Griss, P., Jentschura, G., and Büsing, C. M., Possibilities and limitations for the fixation of alumina bone, joint, and tooth replacements: Some general considerations. *cfi/Ber. DKG*, *60*, 2–6 (1983).

80. Heimke, G., Schulte, W., d'Hoedt. B., Griss, P., Büsing, C. M., and Stock, D., The influence of fine surface structures on the osseo-integration of implants, *Int. J Artif. Organs*, *5*, 207–212 (1982).

81. Stock, D., and Geissler, M., The FRIALIT total hip system — Design considerations and clinical results, in *Osseo-Integrated Implants*, Vol. 1, *Basics, Materials, and Joint Replacements* (G. Heimke, ed.), CRC Press, Boca Raton, FL, 1990, pp. 127–151.

82. Scholz, F., Bewegungsverhalten bei Stossanregung des Tübinger Implantates im Vergleich zum natürlichen Zahn, *Dtsch. Zahnärztl. Z.*, *36*, 567–570 (1981).

83. Ney, Th., Die vertikale Beweglichkeit des Tübinger Implantates im Vergleich zum natürlichen Zahn, *Z. Zahnärztl. Implantol.*, *2*, S21–S25 (1986).

84. Büsing, C. M., d'Hoedt, B., Schulte, W. and Heimke, G., Morphological demonstration of direct deposition of bone on human aluminum oxide ceramic implants, *Biomaterials*, *4*, 125–127 (1983).

85. Bruschi, G. B., and Scipioni, A., Alveolar augmentation: New applications for implants, in *Osseo-Integrated Implants*, Vol. 2, *Implants in Oral and ENT Surgery* (G. Heimke, ed.), CRC Press, Boca Raton, FL, 1990, pp. 35–61.

86. d'Hoedt, B., and Lukas, D., Statistische Ergebnisse des Tübinger Implantates, *Dtsch. Zahnärztl. Z.*, *36*, 551–562 (1981).

87. d'Hoedt, B., 10 Jahre Tübinger Implantat aus Frialit: Eine Zwischenauswertung der Implantatdatei, *Z. Zahnärztl. Implantol.*, *2*, S6–S10 (1986).

88. Heimke, G., Orthopaedic reconstruction: Taking the right approach, *Adv. Mater.*, *4*, 676–679 (1992).

89. Heimke, G., Disuse atrophy and adaptive remodeling in the implant-carrying proximal femur, *Semin. Arthroplasty*, *4*, 261–276 (1993).

90. Heimke, G., Die Arten der Implantatverankerung, in *GOI Jahrbuch*, Quintessenz, Berlin, 1992, pp. 57–71.

91. Andrisano, A. O., Dragoni, E., and Strozzi, A., Axissymmetric mechanical analysis of ceramic heads for total hip replacements, *Proc. Instn. Mech. Engr.*, *204*, 157–167 (1990).

3
General Requirements for a Successful Orthopedic Implant

Thomas D. McGee and Curtis E. Olson
Iowa State University
Ames, Iowa

I. INTRODUCTION

When viewed from an engineering perspective the human skeleton is a marvelous engineering structure. For the long bones, for example, the cartilage-covered epiphyseal surfaces of articulating joints cannot carry heavy stresses [1]. So the joints are enlarged to reduce that stress and provide smooth articulating surfaces with extremely low friction. These bearings are supported by a thin layer of dense bone supported by trabecular bone, with the trabecular bone aligned in accordance with Wolff's law to convey the low-stress bearing forces to the dense, high-stress cortical bone of the diaphysis [2]. This remarkable structure is even more remarkable because, during growth, the dense ring of diaphysis bone just below the growth plate is continuously elongated, with cartilage calcifying below the growth plate and chondrocytes building cartilage above, all without loss of strength as the process operates to elongate the bones [3]. In this process the cell differentiation, and the vascularization and ossification mechanisms, operate continuously to produce the dense bone of the diaphysis, and still maintain the large-area bearing surfaces. The stiffness of the diaphysis, with its dense cortical bone forming a tube, is much greater than that of a solid rod of the same mass. The exterior of the epiphysis is a structural membrane. From a mechanical point of view this is an example of a marvelous engineering structure.

The physiological process mentioned above can also be approached from an engineering point of view. We see that, in each part of the structure there is a supply of cells, nutrients, enzymes, and chemicals to provide for growth, repair, and remodeling. Using the long bone joint as an example, we see that provision for cellular activity is essential for both growth, repair, and remodeling. For growth to take place there must be a steady supply of the necessary nutrients. Mechanisms for controlling that supply are extraordinarily complex [4]. For example, at the growth ring, formation of cartilage is inhibited by its own growth, causing differentiation of chondrocytes into osteoblasts. The

69

perichondrium becomes a periosteum. The chondrocytes hypertrophy and die, producing a collagenous matrix containing cavities left by the empty chondrocyte lacunae. Osteoblasts line the cartiledge and synthesize osteoid. The cartiledge begins to calcify. This mineralization reduces diffusion of nutrients and the osseous tissue contracts, producing dense osseous tissue of smaller diameter, that of the diaphysis. The mechanisms are not understood. For example, the mechanism of precipitation of hydroxyapatite is unknown [5]. Transport of calcium and phosphate ions proceed separately. Nucleation may take place homogeneously in matrix vesicles, or heterogeneously at collagen fibril voids [6]. Regardless of the mechanisms and the complexities, however, this can be considered analogous to an engineering system, something like the logistics of battle support. The necessary nutrients, mechanisms, and other factors must be provided in a timely manner for the tissue to remain healthy and strong. This can include electrical transport, the effects of stress, and many other factors. In order to have a successful prosthesis, then, we must consider all aspects of skeletal engineering. Unfortunately this has not been done. This chapter explains some of the problems using our existing research and gives an example of an attempt to consider the whole engineering analysis to establish the general requirements for successful orthopedic implants.

It is not the intent of this chapter to disparage in any way the tremendous success already achieved by current orthopedic implants such as total hip replacement. Rather this analysis is intended to call attention to possible improvements by employing a biomedical engineering approach.

II. THE PRESENT STATE OF THE ART

Orthopedic research can be divided into two areas, clinical and academic. Clinical research includes the improvements and modifications of existing prostheses and surgical procedures to improve patient care. Outstanding surgeons often work with prosthesis manufacturers to modify the existing practice in attempts to improve the performance [7]. Recently this has included the introduction of beads, mesh, and other structures on the surface of metallic implants to provide for tissue ingrowth and assist in stabilization [8]. Unfortunately a roughened implant can also cause tissue irritation and lead to failure. New ideas, such as the substitution of pure titanium for the 6Al4V alloy, have been tested in the clinic. In the dental area, for example, two tooth-root prostheses made of carbon have been introduced into clinical practice and subsequently withdrawn because of failure [9,10]. Thus the industry often is doing its research in the clinic.

Academic research is conducted through government laboratories, private laboratories, and academia. Here the research is highly specialized. Each individual specialty is dominated by the theory and practice of that specialty. For example, new materials are often evaluated on the basis of specific cellular responses to those materials regardless of whether the material is successful [11]. For example, carbon/teflon mesh has been tested as an orthopedic material despite the fact that it is easily crushed in one's fingers [12]. Also, only after other countries adopted the idea of osseous integration was the Branemark titanium implant for tooth roots accepted here. Before that time osseous integration was not considered grounds for acceptance.

The special nature of academic research has been allowed to dictate the research results. For example, bone and tissue interactions are often modeled by finite element methods to determine stress distributions in the prosthesis and in the bone [13]. But bone is complex. Almost all of these efforts have modeled bone as a continuum. In fact, bone is not isotropic and not homogeneous. Even today most finite element analyses are conducted assuming cortical bone has one set of homogeneous properties and cancellous bone has another set of homogeneous properties [14]. Actual bone varies tremendously, and the structure of the bone must be considered. When this is not done the results may be wrong and misleading. An even more serious criticism of this research is that the bone changes in response to the prosthesis. Where stresses are very high, bone is resorbed, distributing the stress and changing the geometry. This is not modeled, so the model is inaccurate as soon as the implant is in place.

The political desires of research funding also strongly affect academic research. There is a large funded effort to study orthopedic materials *in vitro*, to avoid *in vivo* studies. Programs in cell attachment and other areas are funded despite the fact that the correlation of *in vivo* with *in vitro* has not been established [15].

The research method of academia is to divide and conquer; to study one variable while keeping all others constant. This advances fundamental knowledge but does not consider the interaction of various factors. Real orthopedic implants require the simultaneous application of chemistry, basic biological science, physiology, anatomy, materials science, stress analysis, and systems analysis. The bottom line is successful orthopedic performance. This requires synthesis from all pertinent areas, identification of the important and the trivial factors, experimentation, and decision making. This is the essence of engineering design. This chapter, then, is offered as an example of biomedical engineering in its broadest sense applied to the problems of successful orthopedic implants.

III. THE GENERAL REQUIREMENTS FOR A SUCCESSFUL IMPLANT

There are at least five general requirements for a successful implant. These include tissue compatibility; sufficient strength and wear resistance for the application, including a low coefficient of friction where total joints are replaced; an adequate surgical procedure; provision for transfer of loads from the prosthesis to the tissue; and provision for the tissue to remodel, bond to, and support the tissue. Each of these is discussed separately.

A. Tissue Compatibility

Tissue response is critical to the success of an implant. It is the tissue response that determines the life of the implant because the hard tissue is continuously remodeling. Only if the tissue continues to support the implant can it be successful. The tissue response depends, in part, on the material from which it is made.

There are three classes of materials: metals, organic materials, and ceramics. The wrong material invokes classical tissue responses. This includes inflammation, the presence of macrophages, a fluid-filled capsule, and resorption of surrounding tissue [16]. Most materials in all three classes invoke this response if they have any solubility in the tissue fluids. This puts serious limitations on the materials that can be considered. All the structural components of existing prostheses are selected to be bioinert [17]. These have minimum solubility. Metals such as titanium, 316-L stainless steel, 6Al4V titanium, and cobalt–chrome alloys all are inert; although, especially in wear situations, some solubility and tissue reaction does occur. The organic polymers such as very high molecular weight (VHMW) polyethylene also are chosen for their minimum tissue response. Ceramic components such as alumina and zirconia are also bioinert. As such, all the inert materials are foreign bodies and are walled off by a thin fibrous capsule. The better materials have thinner capsules. However there is not a direct bond of osseous tissue to the implant. Such implants are only successful if the remaining tissue continues to support it. This will be time dependent because any movement of the prosthesis will increase the thickness of the fibrous capsule, leading to more movement and progressive failure. The undesirable effects of electrochemical cells for electronic conductors such as metals and the degeneration of organics such as methacrylates and polyethylene would make the ceramic materials more attractive. Many ceramic compounds are highly insoluble and inert in a physiological environment, and most are electrical insulators. However, the ceramics are brittle. This limitation is discussed later.

Materials that are not inert but are not walled off by a foreign-body capsule have especially desirable tissue response. The only known materials of this nature are calcium phosphates. The ions released by the calcium phosphates, Ca^{2+} and $(PO_4)^{-3}$ are also present in bone. The natural mineral in bone is hydroxyapatite, $Ca_{10}(PO_4)_6(OH)_2$, which contains water. Ceramic processes that require firing at high temperatures remove all or part of the water in hydroxyapatite. The residue may be oxyapatite of the same crystalline structure, or it may disproportionate into $Ca_3(PO_4)_2$ and $Ca_2P_2O_7$. Both are only slightly soluble and hydrolyze on the surface to hydroxyapatite. The tissue response for calcium-to-phosphorous ratios between 1.5 [$Ca_3(PO_4)^2$] and 1.67 [hydroxyapatite] is known to be extremely compatible with hard tissue. Their performance is often called *osteoconductive* to distinguish it from *osteoinductive*, the latter being the production of osseous tissue in soft tissue sites. The lack of a fibrous capsule and the ability of bone to bond to the calcium phosphates makes them very interesting for prosthesis applications. Tissue response is critical, and if calcium phosphates can be used to achieve a bond between the implant and the hard tissue, they make long life a possibility. It is the tissue life that is so important. Therefore, to obtain improvement in tissue response to the current metals and alloys, the use of calcium phosphates is the only choice known at the present time.

B. Strength and Wear Resistance

1. General Considerations

The contact of the tissue with an implant should not cause wear. Wear occurs at the articulating joints, where movement is mandatory. For most applications, then, strength is a critical element. Much research has been conducted on the strength of metal and plastic prosthesis materials. Because there are so few suitable metals that have reasonable tissue compatibility, the properties and the manipulation of the properties are well known [18]. Within the limitations of the properties, the geometry of the prosthesis must be selected to provide suitable strength.

There are two obvious strength limitations. One is that the strength of the implant must be sufficient to support the loads applied to it. The other is that the implant should be at least as strong as the bone. Load-bearing orthopedic implants often are anchored in dense bone so the latter limitation requires a minimum tensile strength of about 140 MPa to match the strength of the bone [19]. Within this limitation, because bone geometrics support the load, it should be possible to design implants that also will support the load.

Metals have much higher strength and higher modulus of elasticity than bone. This makes manipulation of the geometry to support the load relatively easy. However, the high modulus of elasticity can cause stress concentration in the presence of shear stresses. (A simple compressive stress does not cause stress concentration if the Poisson component of the strain can be accommodated.) Where "stress shielding" has been identified as a failure mode (plates and femoral components), the interface is in shear. This experience tells us that the implant design is best if shear situations are minimized. However, because requirements for tissue compatibility favor calcium phosphate ceramics, we need to examine them carefully. Calcium phosphates are not hard; they would not be used for articulatory bearing surfaces. Hard, inert ceramics have superior wear resistance. Metal on polyethylene wears 50 mm^3 per year, but polycrystalline alumina on polycrystalline alumina wears only 0.01 to 0.02 mm^3 per year, a factor of 1/2000 to 1/5000 better [20]. Obviously, if wear is important, ceramic materials have great prospects. For this discussion we avoid the wear problem by considering a more simple kind of prosthesis.

2. Strength of Calcium Phosphate Ceramics

Two calcium phosphates—tricalcium phosphate, $Ca_3(PO_4)_2$; and hydroxyapatite $Ca_{10}(PO_4)_6(OH)_2$—have been extensively studied for tissue compatibility [21]. Because of their excellent tissue response they are now being used in granular and block form for orthopedic repair. Current practice is to use them primarily as fillers for periodontal or bone cavities. Successful use in load-bearing situations has not been reported. Fatigue failure occurs even when prestressed, dense hydroxyapatite is used [22]. This is to be expected because of the brittle nature of calcium phosphates. This is also true of various bioglasses and glass ceramics that react with tissue because the very fact of reactivity introduces weakness. Thus calcium phosphates, by themselves and in bioglasses, can be expected to fail under functional loads.

Calcium phosphate coatings, plasma-sprayed on the surface of metals or ceramics, have similar weakness. Although wound healing may be enhanced by the presence of calcium phosphates, the bond between the calcium phosphate and the substrate is only mechanical. Thick coatings fracture off spontaneously, so only a few microns can be applied, typically 20–40 μm. This is easily removed by the tissue. Osteoclasts dissolve readily both tricalcium phosphate and hydroxyapatite. Before proposing a solution to this problem, let us consider the reasons for the weakness.

In common with almost all ceramics the calcium phosphates are brittle materials. They have no ductile or plastic deformation mechanisms. So the presence of a surface flaw causes severe stress concentration that cannot be relieved by plastic or ductile flow. The strength, then, depends upon the flaw distribution in the material. It is different for each source of material, depending on the manufacturing process. The calcium phosphates are never completely dense. They have some porosity. This reduces the strength (Fig. 1) [23]. When large pores are introduced deliberately to enhance tissue ingrowth, they seriously weaken the material. The pores serve as flaws. Although their shape is important, the strength is inversely proportional to the square root of the pore size. Even small pores cause weakness. If a calcium phosphate implant, or a bioglass implant, is modified by host dissolution, then the strength is reduced because flaws are introduced. This is a fatal limitation for such materials in load-bearing applications [24].

Ceramic materials fail in tension because of the effect of the flaws. Typically they are 10 times stronger in compression than in tension. And when stressed to the ultimate in compression, they fail in shear. Obviously, loading them in compression, and prestressing them in compression, will help prevent failure.

Many attempts have been made to produce flaw-free ceramics. The best polycrystalline alumina hip components are the state of the art in obtaining high strength. And their insolubility helps preserve that strength. Unfortunately, the calcium phosphate ceramics

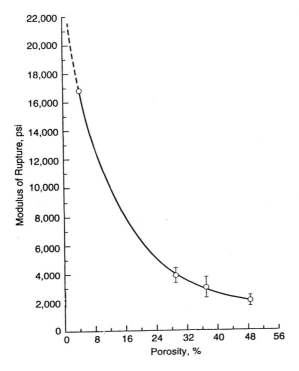

Figure 1   The effect of porosity on the strength of a fluorapatite ceramic.

cannot be made strong and retain that strength because of their most valuable feature, their solubility in the host. Some other way must be found, then, to take advantage of the biocompatibility of the calcium phosphates. This is considered in a later section. Obviously, implants should never be attempted until after testing them in the host environment.

C.   Surgical Procedure

The surgical procedure used to place an orthopedic implant is critical to the success. Recently computer controlled machinery has been used in the operating room to improve the placement and alignment of prostheses. Of course, aseptic methods are required. Yet it is obvious that the skill and knowledge of the surgeon is critical to the success of the implant. The surgeon's skill in maintaining sterility, sectioning, alignment, torquing screws, and many other factors determines whether the implant has the possibility of success.

D.   Provision for Transfer of Loads from the Prosthesis to the Tissue

Each type of implant must replace a functional orthopedic component. For that to occur, the loads imposed on the component must be known. In the case of a joint replacement the kinematics of the joint must also be known. Such loads are always dynamic. They may be suddenly applied and have a higher value than the static load. Many studies have been conducted on the kinematics and loads of the human skeleton. So the basic information is available. The difficult task is to devise a geometry for the implant that allows for load transfer to the tissue in such a way that the tissue will respond and support the prosthesis. Every application is different. The replacement of a section of a long bone is used here to discuss the principles involved. We will consider a "bone bridge" replacement of a section of a dog's femur.

The diaphysis of the femur of a dog is in the shape of a tube, slightly curved. The cortical bone of the tube is thin. The forces imposed on the tube are compressive, bending, tension, and rotation. Because of the offset neck of the femur, important bending forces put the tube in tension laterally and in compression medially. A prosthesis put into place must withstand these forces; but, more importantly, the bond of the tissue to the implant must also be strong enough to withstand these forces. The structure of the tissue implant interface must be adjusted to achieve this. When no implant is in place the continuous remodeling of mature bone, which is known to be stress regulated, maintains the tube shape and thickness. Any implant, then, should produce the same field of stresses as the natural bone. This dictates the nature of the contact between the bone and the implant. The resolved area of contact for the implant should be the same as the area would be if bone were present instead of the implant. The structure of the implant in contact with the bone should encourage bone bonding.

E. Provision for Tissue Remodeling

Once an implant is in place the natural physiological response of wound healing, callus formation, and remodeling must take place for the implant to be successful. This means that the geometry of the implant should not interfere with the transport processes and cellular responses required for repair. Most current implants are placed without regard for this principle. Crushing or drilling of cancellous bone through stem placement, and removal of important supply routes, often occurs.

The blood supply for cortical bone in the diaphysis is supplied by the medulla and the surrounding muscle. Bone repair is more rapid endosteally than periosteally. This means that the implant must also be a tube, so that the medulla can regenerate to supply blood and fluids to the wound-healing site. Then both the external and internal processes can operate normally.

IV. DESIGN OF AN IMPLANT TO SATISFY THE REQUIREMENTS

Based on the above considerations the details of the design can now be specified using a bone bridge as an example. These requirements are:

1. The chemistry of the host reactions must be dominated by a calcium phosphate ceramic.
2. The implant should have a tensile strength at least as strong as the cortical bone it contacts. The strength should not depreciate in the host atmosphere.
3. The surgical procedure should be appropriate to the implant site, aseptic, and without unnecessary trauma to the tissue.
4. The design of the implant should provide stress levels normal to the bone and allow

for tensile, compressive, bending, and torsional loads. Shear stresses at the interface should be minimized.

5. The implant should not interfere with the normal internal and external processes associated with wound healing, recovery, and remodeling.

A. The Material Design

1. Design Considerations

An obvious approach to utilizing calcium phosphates, where they do not have the required strength, is to incorporate them into a composite. Combinations with plastics, metals, and ceramics were considered. Composites based on plastics were rejected because it was difficult to expose the calcium phosphate when embedded in plastics. The limited rigidity was also a detriment. Composites based upon carbon were rejected for the same reasons, although fiber reinforcement was a desirable possibility. Composites based on metals were rejected because of reactions with the metals, including phosphorous embrittlement. High-temperature processing of metals alters the physical properties and requires reducing atmospheres, whereas the phosphates require oxidizing atmospheres. Therefore ceramic–ceramic composites appear to be more promising.

Not many ceramic materials have no reaction with calcium phosphates at processing temperatures (up to 1500°C). Based on physical chemistry and crystallographic considerations, magnesium aluminate spinel ($MgAl_2O_4$) was selected as a suitable second phase to use with a calcium phosphate [25,26]. The ionic size of Mg is too small for extensive solid solution in calcium phosphates. The aluminum ion is too large to proxy for phosphorous. Spinel is an extremely stable compound, as are tricalcium phosphate and calcium pyrophosphate. Spinel is known to be an excellent, inert ceramic in its tissue response. If the calcium phosphate is to control tissue response, it must be distributed on a very fine scale. If it is not to cause large flaws, it also must be very fine grained. The calcium phosphate should not be easily leached away, so the calcium phosphate phase should be interconnected, not isolated. For this to occur the calcium phosphate phase should be at least 25 vol%. Fifty percent would be better.

2. Experimental

Commercial tricalcium phosphate and commercial spinels were ball-milled together in water and an organic binder for 24 to produce a fine-grained mixture. They were filtered and dried to produce a cake. The cake was broken up and sieved to a free-flowing powder. The powder was pressed in a cylindrical mold at 4000 psi and isostatically pressed at 25,000 psi. An axial hole was drilled and the tube was carved by hand to the desired geometry. Bars and pellets were also produced for property measurements.

Twenty bars were tested for cross-breaking strength to determine their tensile strength. One half of each bar was tested after implanting them in the backs of dogs for 10 months. The other half was tested for comparison after the same time period. There was no statistical difference, indicating that the composite had enduring strength. This is logical because the calcium phosphate phase had the largest grain size and was the large flaw in the composite. The structure is like that of a sponge. The skeleton of the sponge is the inert spinel. The holes in the sponge are filled with calcium phosphate. The composite is called an *osteoceramic*.

Numerous tests of the osteoceramic show that bone bonds to it in the same way it does to tricalcium phosphate and hydroxyapatite. This satisfies the material requirements.

B.   The Implant Design

The basic tubular shape was adopted to provide for normal healing. The wall thickness was the same as the cortical bone, so that the compressive stresses delivered to it would be the same as if the bone were continuous. (Several specimens were provided so that the surgeon could choose the appropriate one.) Tensile and torsional forces were accommodated by forming the end of the tube with dove-tailed recesses so that bone could grow into the recess. After the recesses were filled the bone could not be withdrawn, providing tensile force accommodation. Torsional stresses were also accommodated by the bone grown into the recesses. After the recesses were filled bending stresses also could be accommodated. However, it is critical that the bone maintain the bond with the implant. This was encouraged by a series of axial grooves on the outside of the implant, with radial holes conducting blood from the medulla to the grooves (Fig. 2). The net result looks like a splined tube. It can accommodate tensile, compressive, bending, and torsional loads. It does not interfere with wound healing, callus formation, and remodeling. This satisfies the physical design requirements.

C.   The Surgical Procedure

Anesthesia was induced with intravenous thiamylal sodium (17.5 mg/kg) and maintained with 1–3% halothane gas. Cephalothin sodium was administered pre and post surgical procedure as an antibiotic (20 mg/kg). The rear quarter of the dog was clipped and prepped using alternately Betadine and 95% alcohol. A 5-min sterile scrub with Betadine was performed following the initial preparation. The ECG was monitored. The leg was draped using aseptic technique and covered with a sterile stockingette.

A skin incision was made along the cranial border of the biceps femoris muscle from the level of the greater trochanter to the proximal patella. The skin was sewn to the stockinette using 2/0 monofilament nylon. Electrocautery was used to help provide hemostasis. The skin margins were retracted and the fascia lata was incised along the cranial border of the biceps femoris muscle. The biceps femoris was retracted caudally and the

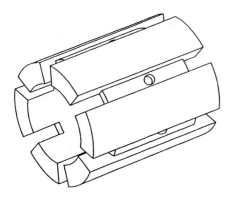

Figure 2   Geometry of the diaphysis implant.

vastus laterus muscle was retracted cranially to expose the shaft of the femur. An 8-hole 316L stainless steel compression plate was contoured to the lateral aspect at the center of the femur for later use. A section of the adductor muscles, which insert on the caudal aspect of the femur, was elevated at middiaphysis. The vastus intermedius was retracted from the cranial aspect of the femur at the same level. Two transverse osteotomies were then made with an oscillating saw (Fig. 3a). Each was approximately 12 mm from the midshaft. The diameter and the length of the osteotomy were measured, and an implant was selected of the same length and cortex thickness.

The implant was secured to the contoured plate with Kirschner wire (Fig. 3b and 3c). The plate was clamped to the lateral aspect of the femur to oppose the proximal and distal osteotomy sites to the ends of the implant. Three 3.5-mm cortical screws were placed on each side of the implant. The first screws on each side were aligned with a guide to produce compression of the bone to the implant. The area was irrigated with saline. The facia latera was closed with 0 monofilament polyglyconite sutures. The subcutaneous fat and fascia were closed with 2/0 monofilament nylon sutures. The skin was apposed with 4/0 surgical steel sutures. Cefadroxil (10 mg/kg per dose) was given twice a day for 6 days. The steel sutures were removed after 10 days.

V.   RESULTS

This procedure produced an implant that was in compression at the ends, the bone plate taking the tension forces in bending and pulling (Fig. 4). After wound healing took place

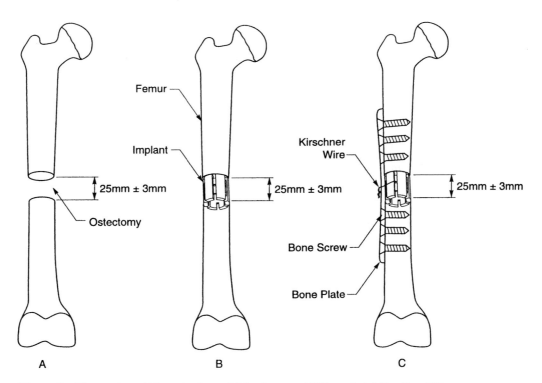

Figure 3   Illustration of the osteotomy (A), placement (B), and stabilization (C).

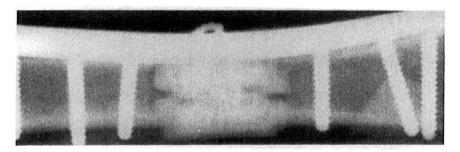

Figure 4   Radiograph of the stabilized implant, postop.

the bone began to attach to the implant. The bone plate provides a resistance to bending loads. The edges of the bone plate, held tightly against the periosteum by the bone screws, cut through the periosteum and interfered with the external blood flow at that location, producing a weaker bone under the bone plate. The bone plate and the bone screws are walled off by the foreign-body capsule in such a way that movement becomes possible with time. The compressive and tensile loads gradually shift to the implant as the tissue responds to the stress stimulus, gradually taking more of the load. This can be observed radiographically as the bone fills the dovetail recesses and the longitudinal recesses (Fig. 5). After about 1 year the bone plate was removed in a second surgical procedure (Fig. 6). Enough stress had been transferred to the implant so that the bone plate was no longer

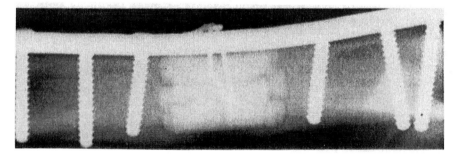

Figure 5   Radiograph of the implant at 2 months.

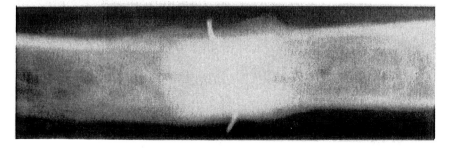

Figure 6   Radiograph of the implant immediately after bone plate removal, 13 months.

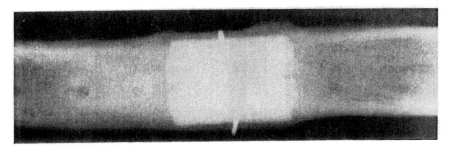

Figure 7   Radiograph of the implant 4 months after bone plate removal (total 17 months).

necessary. The weak area under the plate was sufficiently local that fracture did not occur. The bone continued to remodel over 4 months (Fig. 7). Two years after removal of the bone plate the dog was active, continuing to stress the implant normally without evidence of pain or gait variations. No further changes in remodeling occurred although it is believed the longitudinal recesses are completely filled with bone (Fig. 8).

VI.   CONCLUSION

An orthopedic bone bridge has been designed in accordance with engineering design requirements to become a functional part of a living orthopedic system. By adhering to the requirements for (1) tissue compatibility, (2) strength, (3) surgical procedure, (4) load transfer to the living tissue, and (5) tissue remodeling, the bone bridge was made functional. It was necessary to control the tissue reaction to make the tissue form an enduring attachment. No previous implant has achieved this result. This is a successful orthopedic implant.

Existing implants violate some of the principles presented here. It should be very interesting to modify existing practice to conform to these engineering principles, to determine if they can be successfully applied to more complex systems.

ACKNOWLEDGMENTS

This research could not have been conducted without the outstanding surgical skills of two veterinary surgeons, Dr. William Hoefle and Dr. Ray Kudej. Many graduate students participated in the various experiments necessary to develop the bone bridges. These

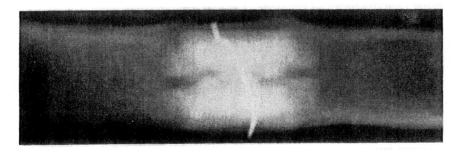

Figure 8   Radiograph of the implants 14 months after bone plate removal (total 27 months).

include Mr. Curtis Olson, who did the bone bridge research reported here, assisted by an undergraduate student, Mr. Mark Quillin. Other graduate students include Denginu Aksaci, Catherine Tweden, Ann Graves, Catherine McMahon, and Gabriele Niederauer. Important, necessary, support was provided by faculty in departments of radiology, pathology, and physiology of the ISU College of Veterinary Medicine.

REFERENCES

1. Mow, V.C., Roth, V., and Armstrong, C.G., Biomechanics of joint cartilage, in *Basic Biomechanics of the Skeletal System* (Frankel, V.H., and Nordin, M., eds.), Lea and Febiger, Philadelphia, 1980.
2. Wolff, J.L., *Das Gesetz der Transformation of Knochen*, A. Hirschwald, Berlin 1892.
3. Cowin, S.C., VanBurshirk, W.C., and Ashman, R.B., Properties of bone in *Handbook of Bioengineering* (Skalak, R., and Chien, S., eds.), McGraw-Hill, New York, 1982.
4. Bouvier, M., The biology and composition of bone, in *Bone Mechanics* (Cowin, S.C., ed.), CRC Press, Boca Raton, FL, 1989.
5. Hargest, T.E., Gay, C.V., Scharer, H., and Wasserman, A.J., Vertical distribution of cells and matrix of epiphyseal grow plate cartilage determined by quantitative electron probe analysis, *J. Histochem. Cytochem., 4(33)*, 275, 1985.
6. Glimcher, M.J., Composition, structure and organization of bone and other mineralized tissues and the mechanism of calcification, in *Handbook of Physiology*, Vol. 7, American Physiology Society, Washington, DC, 1976.
7. von Recum, A.F. (ed.), *Handbook of Biomaterials Evaluation*, Macmillan, New York, 1986.
8. Ducheyne, P., Martens, M., Aernocedt, E., Mulier, J., and DeMeester, P., Skeletal fixation by metal fiber coating of the implant, *Acta Orthop.* (Bel) *40*, 799, 1974.
9. Grenoble, D.E., and Voss, D., Materials and designs for implant dentistry, *Biomed. Mater. Devices Artif. Organs, 4*, 133, 1976.
10. Bokros, J.C., Carbon biomedical devices, *Carbons, 15*, 355, 1977.
11. Kay, J.F., Bioactive surface coatings for hard tissue biomaterials, *Handbook of Bioactive Ceramics*, Vol. 2 (Yamamuro, T., Hench, L.L., and Wilson, J., eds.), CRC Press, Boca Raton, FL, 1990.
12. Spector, M., Harmon, S.L., and Kreutner, A., Characteristics of tissue ingrowth into Proplast and porous polyethylene implants in bone, *J. Biomed. Mater. Res., 13*, 672, 1979.
13. Brunsky, J.B., Implants: Biomaterials and biomechanics, *J. Cal. Dent. Assoc., 16*, 66, 1988.
14. Brunsky, J.B., Biomechanical factors affecting the bone dental implant interface, *Clin. Mater., 10*, 153, 1992.
15. Didisheim, P., Dewanjee, M.K., Kaye, M.P., et al., Nonpredictability of long-term *in vivo* response from short-term *in vitro* or *ex vitro* blood–material interactions, *Trans. Am. Soc. Artif. Intern. Org., 30*, 370, 1984.
16. Hulbert, S.F., Levine, S.N., and Moyle, D.D., *Prosthesis and Tissue: The Interfacial Problems*, Wiley, New York, 1974.
17. Park, J.B., and Lakes, R.S., Tissue response to implants, in *Biomaterials: An Introduction*, 2nd ed., Plenum Press, New York, 1992, Chap. 10.
18. Ref. 17, Chap. 5.
19. Yamada, H., in *Strength of Biological Materials* (Evans, F.G., ed.), Williams & Wilkins, Baltimore, 1970.
20. Clark, C., Dorlot, J.M., Graham, J., Levine, D.J., Oonishi, H., Rieu, J., Rigney, D., Schwartz, G., Sedel, L., Toni, A., and Zitelli, J., Biomechanical stability and design, wear, *Ann. NY Acad. Sci., 23*, 292–296, 1988.
21. deGroot, K. (ed.), *Bioceramics of Calcium Phosphate*, CRC Press, Boca Raton, FL, 1983.
22. deGroot, K., Dental implants, in *Bioceramics of Calcium Phosphates* (deGroot, K., ed.), CRC Press, Boca Raton, FL, 1983.

23. Aksaci, D., Evaluation of a fluorapatite–spinel ceramic as a bone implant, Ph.D. Thesis, Iowa State University, 1981.
24. Park, J.B., and Lakes, R.S., Hard tissue replacement, II, in *Biomaterials: An Introduction*, 2nd ed., Plenum Press, New York, 1992, Chap. 11.
25. Janikowski, T., and McGee, T.D., Tooth roots for permanent implantation, *Proc. Iowa Acad. Sci., 76*, 1969, p. 113.
26. McGee, T.D., and Wood, J.L., Calcium phosphate osteoceramics, *J. Biomed. Mater. Res. Symposium, 5*(Pt. I), 137, 1974.

4

Structure–Property Relations of Biomaterials for Hard Tissue Replacement

David H. Kohn
University of Michigan
Ann Arbor, Michigan

1. INTRODUCTION

Total joint replacements have improved the quality of life for people with debilitating diseases such as osteo- and rheumatoid arthritis, avascular necrosis, and bone cancer. From an engineering standpoint, the function of an implant is to provide as physiologic a stress as possible to the remaining tissue so that the integrity and functionality of the tissue and biomaterials are maintained over a lengthy (i.e., >10 years) service life. Materials suited for joint replacements are those that are well tolerated by the body and can withstand cyclic loading in an aggressive environment.

An objective of implant development is often to improve interfacial bonding and stress transfer among the various components, within the constraints of material selection and design. Interfacial integrity depends upon a combination of factors, including stress levels and stress distribution, tissue modeling and remodeling, tissue reaction to the implant materials, trauma at surgery, and relative motion between the bone and implant [1–8]. The design, development, and analysis of implants is therefore interdisciplinary, involving materials, mechanical, chemical, surface science, environmental, and biological parameters. Adding to the complexity is that each of these parameters cannot be treated as a separate design parameter, but rather as an integrated set of sometimes competing parameters (Fig. 1). Interrelated factors necessary for the success of total joint prostheses are:

1. Mechanical properties of implant materials, grouting agents, or coatings [9–14].
2. Mechanisms of tissue attachment to the implant [15–17].
3. Surface state of implant materials and/or coatings [16,18,19].
4. Adhesion of any grouting agents or coatings to the substrate [20–22].
5. Size, shape, and distribution of any surface porosity [7,23–25].
6. Viability and mechanical properties of the surrounding tissue [3,7,8].

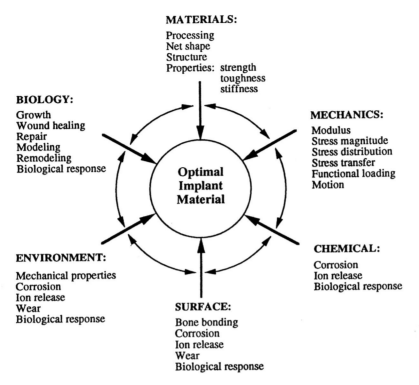

MATERIALS:

Processing
Net shape
Structure
Properties: strength
toughness
stiffness

BIOLOGY:

Growth
Wound healing
Repair
Modeling
Remodeling
Biological response

MECHANICS:

Modulus
Stress magnitude
Stress distribution
Stress transfer
Functional loading
Motion

**Optimal
Implant
Material**

CHEMICAL:

Corrosion
Ion release
Biological response

ENVIRONMENT:

Mechanical properties
Corrosion
Ion release
Wear
Biological response

SURFACE:

Bone bonding
Corrosion
Ion release
Wear
Biological response

Figure 1 Schematic of interdependent engineering factors affecting the success of total joint replacements. (From Ref. 63.)

7. Initial stability and stimulation of tissue apposition/ingrowth [2,17,26–28].
8. Elastic properties of implants, grouting agents, coating, and tissues [4,6,17,29–32].
9. Type of loading and effect of such loading [25,29,30,33].
10. Implant design [34].
11. Biological response of the materials [5,35].
12. Considerations for revision surgery, should it become necessary [4].

A. Materials Used in Bone and Joint Replacement

Because of the complexities involved in replacing joints, no one material or class of materials is sufficiently versatile. Implant systems require multiple materials to perform a variety of simultaneous functions, such as load bearing, articulation, and grouting. All classes of materials — metals, ceramics, polymers, and composites — are therefore used, many times in combination with one another (Table 1). This chapter focuses on some current problems in joint replacement and materials engineering concepts used to evaluate and potentially solve these problems. The focus is with respect to the synergy between processing, composition, structure, and properties of metals, ceramics, polymers, and composites; and how understanding this synergy helps us better understand and solve clinical problems.

Table 1   Biomaterials Used in Total Joint Replacement

Material	Application
Metals	
Stainless Steels	Femoral stems, heads
316L	
Cobalt-based alloys	Porous coatings, femoral stems, heads, tibial and femoral components
Cast Co-Cr-Mo	
Wrought Co-Ni-Cr-Mo	
Wrought Co-Cr-W-Ni	
Titanium-based materials	
CP Ti	Porous coatings, second phase in ceramic and PMMA composites
Ti-6Al-4V	Femoral stems, heads, tibial and femoral components, porous coatings
Ti-5Al-2.5Fe	Femoral stems, heads
Ti-Al-Nb	Femoral stems, heads
Ceramics	
Bioinert	
Carbon	Coatings on metallic femoral stems, second phase in composites and bone cement
Alumina	Femoral stems, heads, acetabular cups
Zirconia	Femoral heads, acetabular cups
Bioactive	
Calcium phosphates	Coatings on metallic and ceramic femoral stems, scaffold materials, second phase in PMMA and UHMWPE composites
Bioglasses	Coatings on metallic and ceramic femoral stems
Polymers	
PMMA	Bone cement
UHMWPE/HDPE	Acetabular cups, tibial and patellar components, porous coatings on metallic femoral stems
Polysulfone	Femoral stems, porous coatings on metallic femoral stems
PTFE	Femoral stems, porous coatings on metallic femoral stems
Composites	Femoral stems
Polymer-based	
Polysulfone-carbon	
Polycarbonate-carbon	
Polysulfone-Kevlar	
Polycarbonate-Kevlar	
Ceramic-based	
Carbon-carbon	

1. Implant Systems

Total joint replacements are typically classified according to the mechanism of implant/ tissue fixation. In general, implants are either cemented or cementless, referring to whether an implant is stabilized with a grouting agent or by direct contact between the tissues and the implant surface.

A cemented total hip replacement system, depicted schematically in Fig. 2, typically consists of a metallic femoral stem (stainless steel, cobalt–chromium alloy, or titanium alloy) fixed inside the medullary canal of a femur with a polymeric (polymethylmethacrylate — PMMA) bone cement. The metallic femoral head articulates in a polymeric (ultrahigh molecular weight polyethylene — UHMWPE) acetabular cup, which is also fixed in place with PMMA. Stress transfer from the pelvis to the femur is a function of the materials used and of the interfaces between the various materials and between the tissues and materials.

The long-term (i.e., >10 years) clinical results of cemented total joint replacements have been excellent in elderly (>65 years), sedentary populations, with rates of loosening and revision rates being only 1–2% per year [36].

Cementless fixation is achieved by establishing an interference fit between the implant and tissue. An inherent difference between cemented and cementless implant systems lies in the time necessary to achieve stability of the prosthesis. With a cemented implant system, fixation is achieved almost immediately postoperatively, whereas with a cementless system, tissue integration must occur before the prosthesis may be loaded. Thus, one design approach for cementless implants is to minimize the time necessary for tissue integration and maximize interfacial stability.

Ideally, for prostheses dependent upon direct tissue apposition, the materials used should elicit the formation of normal tissue at the surface and establish a continuous

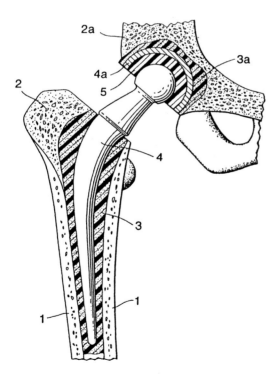

Figure 2   Schematic of the components of a cemented total joint replacement: (1) cortical bone, (2, 2a) trabecular bone, (3, 3a) bone cement, (4) metallic femoral prosthesis, (4a) metal backing of acetabular cup, (5) polyethylene acetabular cup. (From Ref. 178, with permission.)

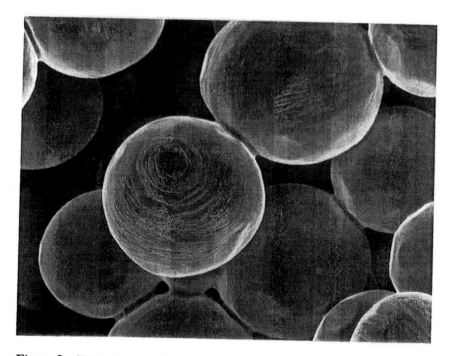

Figure 3 SEM of porous titanium surface made from powder microspheres approximately 300 μm in diameter (160×). (From Ref. 63.)

interface capable of supporting service loads over time [37]. Factors affecting the development of this interface include the bulk and surface properties of the material, interfacial motion, and tissue reaction [38].

Cementless fixation may take one of three forms: surface-textured materials, porous-coated materials, or surface-active materials. With surface-textured materials, there is bone apposition onto the surface of a grooved or textured metal [39] or polymer [40,41] surface. Surface-active materials lead to fixation through a chemical reaction between tissues and a bioactive implant surface [17,42].

The most prominent method of cementless fixation is bone ingrowth into the pores of a porous or porous-coated material. Porous coatings have been fabricated from: *polymers*—proplast [40], polysulfone [41], polyethylene [23], and PMMA [43]; *ceramics*—cerosium [44] and calcium aluminate [7]; and *metals*—stainless steel [45], cobalt-based alloys [46,47] and titanium-based alloys [15,31]. Porous metal coatings are made from powdered spheres [47], fibers [15], wires [31], or other porous structures [48], which are mechanically or chemically bonded onto a dense metal substrate to produce an inhomogeneous, porous surface geometry (Fig. 3).

B. Generalized Problems with Implant Fixation and Outline of Chapter Contents

Because of the success of joint replacement surgery in the elderly, the number of primary total joint replacements performed each year has more than doubled since 1970 [49]. The success of joint prostheses has also prompted the use of prostheses in younger (i.e., < 50 years) and more active patients, who aside from the ailments prompting the need for joint replacement, are generally healthy otherwise. Cemented total joint replacement surgery has been less successful in younger patients. Rates of radiographic failure as high as 57% after only 5 years have been reported for patients younger than 30 years of age [50].

The increasing number of prostheses implanted and the addition of the younger patient population necessitates better long-term prosthetic fixation. This need is supported by the fact that the number of revision surgeries performed is increasing at twice the rate of primary surgeries [49]. Additionally, rates of implant loosening are higher following revision joint replacement than they are following primary joint replacement [51]. Incidences of femoral loosening as high as 44% have been reported after only 4.5 years [51].

There are few long-term clinical studies on porous-coated prostheses, and whether cementless fixation will serve the long-term needs of patients better than cemented fixation is still to be determined. Because of the intimate biological contact and means of fixation, bone loss is a serious complication with cementless implants [52]. Implant failure due to bone loss may manifest itself through loss of interfacial integrity, focal loss of bone, fracture, and pain.

In general, failure of prosthetic systems may arise due to material failure of the prosthesis [53,54], the cement [55,56], or the polyethylene [57]; bone remodeling due to stress shielding [58]; corrosion [59]; and wear or other particulate debris leading to material failure or osteolysis [60–62].

In this chapter, we first summarize some of the current problems with biomaterials for hard tissue replacement: (1) biologically mediated bone loss, due to particulate debris; (2) material failure; and (3) systemic or remote-site effects. Loss of fixation due to mechanical reasons is well documented; it is summarized above and discussed in detail elsewhere [1,3,4,49,56,58,63]. Next, using a materials engineering approach of relating material processing, composition, structure, and properties, we discuss biomaterial properties and some current technologies important to understanding and solving these clinical problems. Regarding the four problems mentioned above, we focus on: (1) mechanisms of wear and surface treatment techniques; (2) metallurgical advances and nondestructive testing techniques; (3) corrosion and surface analysis techniques; and (4) improvements in fixation with advances in cements, ceramics, and composites.

II.   CURRENT PROBLEMS WITH IMPLANTS

A.   Biologically Mediated Bone Resorption—Particulate Debris

A primary problem with joint replacements is the stimulation of bone resorption by wear products. Osteolysis manifests itself as either focal lesions or cortical thinning and occurs in both cortical and trabecular bone, adjacent to both femoral and acetabular components [60,62–66]. Osteolysis has been associated with loose [67,68] and stable [62,65] cemented femoral components; loose cemented acetabular components [67] and loose and well-fixed cementless acetabular components [69].

Observations of membranous tissue adjacent to both loose and stable prostheses have shown these tissues to be infiltrated with histiocytes, foreign-body giant cells, macrophages, lymphocytes, and granulation tissue. Tissues may be laden, both intra- and extracellularly, with granules of PMMA, polyethylene, and metal wear debris of varying quantity and ranging in size from submicron to over 50 μm [60,70–72]. It is generally hypothesized that wear products stimulate macrophage activity, phagocytosis and secretion of various cytokines and intercellular mediators, which trigger osteoclastic bone resorption [60,70–72]. Since a variety of particulate materials (polyethylene, PMMA, cobalt and titanium-based alloys, calcium phosphate ceramics, and bone) and a variety of cytokines (prosthaglandin E_2, interleukins-1 and -6, tumor necrosis factor, and collagenase) can exist in the membranous tissue, dose–response relations between specific materials and cytokines are unknown, as are any possible synergistic effects and transport mechanisms.

Observation of particulate debris under polarized light and concomitant Fourier transform infrared spectroscopy (FTIR) analyses indicate that most of these particles are birefringent. This fact, along with morphological assessments, indicates that the particles are polyethylene [66]. Electron microprobe analyses reveal the existence of titanium, aluminum, and vanadium, suggesting the presence of submicron metal particles also, and more quantitative microscopic methods show submicron polyethylene, titanium alloy, pure titanium, and bone particles [73].

In addition to wear of polyethylene, *in vivo* wear of the metallic components of total joint prostheses has also been reported [61]. The cause of failure of these prostheses was speculated to be metallosis, secondary to wear and fretting of the femoral head. Fretting and corrosion at Morse taper junctions may generate particulate debris and may also be regions of fatigue initiation [53,59].

Current thought is that polyethylene debris are the main degradation products triggering bone resorption [52,60,72]. Much of this thought is based on the fact that lytic lesions are found in both well-fixed and loose [63,65] cementless femoral components. However, there may be a synergistic cascade involving the interaction of multiple materials particles and mechanical factors and more research is needed.

B. Fatigue Fracture

In the 1970s there were many fatigue fractures of cemented prostheses [54,74]. Today, however, metallurgical fatigue of cemented joint replacements has largely been eliminated through better surgical and cementing techniques, patient selection, implant design, and metallurgical advancements. The use of higher-strength wrought cobalt- and titanium-based alloys, compared to previously used annealed stainless steel and cast cobalt–chromium was important in reducing cemented prosthesis fractures.

Advances in metallurgy that helped reduce fatigue fracture in cemented prostheses are now compromised in coated implants. In porous-coated cobalt–chromium alloys, for example, the microstructure and mechanical properties are similar or sometimes inferior to those of a cast alloy, with coarse grains, carbides, interdendritic shrinkage, gas porosity, and inclusions present [75]. In porous-coated titanium, the 75% reduction in fatigue strength compared to uncoated titanium is due solely to the notch effect of the coating [10]. However, as with cobalt-based implants, even non-coated regions exhibit reduced properties because of sintering [9,10,12,76]. Metallurgical concepts associated with sintering and mechanical properties are discussed in Section III.

Fatigue fractures of porous coated prostheses are now occurring [53,77–79]. Studies have also noted regions of coatings becoming detached [80,81], but more typically this was only a secondary observation. Fatigue failures that do occur generally do so after only a few years of service [53]. These fatigue failures are due in part to some of the microstructural and geometric consequences of metallurgical processing mentioned above, which are expanded upon in Section III.

C. Remote-Site and Systemic Effects

With improved implants, the use of implants in younger patients, the greater surface area of some cementless devices, and patients living longer, the chances of systemic and remote-site effects are more likely. Determining these effects is difficult, however, since many systemic effects are not specific and may occur normally in other populations [52,82]. However, the consequences of some systemic effects may be severe enough to warrant study, even in the absence of compelling current clinical need [52,83]. The occurrence of systemic effects is recognized and, for some biomaterials, linkages between biomaterial moiety and biological response have been demonstrated *in vitro*, in animal models or in humans. The release and transportation of biomaterial degradation products in particulate and ionic forms are well demonstrated [83–85]. Implant materials may corrode and/or wear, leading to the generation of particulate debris, which may, in turn, elicit both local and systemic biological responses. These biological reactions are grouped into four categories: metabolic, bacteriological, immunological, and neoplastic [35]. Minimizing mechanical and chemical breakdown of biomaterials is therefore an important goal.

Although metals exhibit high strength and toughness, properties needed in an implant, they are more susceptible to electrochemical degradation than ceramics or polymers. Therefore, a fundamental criterion for choosing a metallic implant material is that the biological response it elicits is minimal. Because of the combined mechanical and environmental demands, the metals used in bone and joint reconstruction have been limited to three classes: stainless steels (iron-based), cobalt-based alloys, and titanium-based materials. Each of these materials is well tolerated by the body because of its passive oxide layer. Most metals have specific biological roles and are therefore essential. However, larger amounts of metals usually cannot be tolerated. The main elemental constituents, as well as the minor alloying constituents, of these metals can be tolerated by the body in trace amounts.

Many metallic ions released from implants, particularly nickel, chromium, and cobalt ions, can elicit delayed hypersensitivity reactions [86]. Although most reactions occur in previously sensitized patients, the higher rate of release in patients with loose implants may sensitize some previously unsensitized patients [86]. Metallic ions may also burden the immune system. Immune responses to titanium [87] and PMMA [88] have also recently been reported. Metallic species released from implants, such as nickel, chromium, and cobalt, are also known carcinogens [35]. Although very small in number and with no definitive linkage established, there are known cases of tumors in the region of total joint replacements [89–91]. Although small in number, the magnitude of these consequences alone warrants the study of biomaterial degradation products [52,83].

III. MATERIALS SCIENCE PRINCIPLES ASSOCIATED WITH CLINICAL PROBLEMS

A. Particulate Material Formation: Wear and Gross Corrosion Resistance

Particulate debris from metals (i.e., particles resulting from gross corrosion, wear debris, or loose particles), PMMA (wear debris), polyethylene (wear debris), ceramic (debonded hydroxyapatite), and bone may be generated by both chemical and mechanical means. Frequently, electrochemical breakdown is enhanced by mechanical processes such as wear, and the two processes are coupled. The importance of minimizing such debris is underscored by recent symposia [92,93].

1. Metallic Wear and Corrosion

Cobalt and chromium can release large amounts of dissolution products during repassivation due to solution supersaturation at the metal surface. Titanium repassivates almost instantaneously through surface-controlled oxidation kinetics. Titanium release that occurs is a result of chemical dissolution of titanium oxide [94].

In addition to the release of particulate debris from corrosion, mechanical factors such as wear, fretting, and fatigue can generate debris. The abrasion resistance of titanium-based materials is lower than that of other materials [95]. The mechanism of titanium wear is believed to be a spalling of the titanium oxide in which needle-like particles are generated.

In studying wear, not only must the individual materials be considered, but also the environment, in terms of solution, pH, proteins, metallic dissolution products, and particulate materials. In this regard, titanium has demonstrated inferior wear qualities in the presence of PMMA and metallic debris [95,96].

2. Polyethylene

The properties of polyethylene are related to the rigidity of the molecular chains and degree of crystallinity. As chain rigidity increases, melting point, tensile strength, resistance to degradation, and glass transition temperature all increase. As the crystalline/amorphous ratio increases, stiffness, yield strength, and softening point increase, while crack resistance and low-temperature brittleness are reduced [86]. In general, tensile and impact strength increase with molecular weight.

Although polyethylene acetabular and patella components do fracture [97], creep and wear are the most important properties. Adhesive wear, two-body abrasive wear and three-body wear are the most important wear mechanisms. Fatigue and environmental cracking have also been noted as secondary or possibly resultant factors [98]. The factors affecting these mechanical failure modes are most likely component orientation, direction of loading, and the resultant contact stresses.

In vitro studies on a wear simulator [95,96] show that polyethylene wear against the commonly used implant metals is low (0.4–0.9 μm/year). This wear rate is independent of the metal and does not change upon irradiation of the polyethylene. Wear is also low against fully dense ceramics, such as alumina and graphite (0.2–0.5 μm/year). Roughening of the metal or ceramic surfaces increases polyethylene wear [95,99]. Wear rate tends to be inversely proportional to molecular weight, but this relationship may be due to differences in material processing rather than molecular weight per se [100]. The size distribution of wear particles tends to be bimodal, with peaks at 1 μm and 0.1–1.0 mm. The larger particles are associated with higher wear rates [100]. Wear is dominated by contact stresses, underscoring the importance of implant design and alignment.

The friction and wear characteristics of polyethylene reported in the literature show a wide scatter, due in part to variations in contact load, contact area, velocity, and lubricant. Polyethylene wear is strongly dependent on the lubricant used, with the wear rate in distilled water being an order of magnitude less than the wear rate in serum and 2 orders of magnitude less than the wear rate in saline [99].

In vivo wear rates are 0.05–0.5 mm/year [101], compared to maximum rates of approximately 1 μm/year determined on wear simulators. The combined effect of environmentally assisted three-body wear between polyethylene, metal, and PMMA particles; creep; fatigue; and fretting *in vivo* may account for the differences between *in vivo* and *in vitro* wear rates.

Retrieval analyses of worn components indicate regions of loose polyethylene material. This surface delamination is thought to originate from material inhomogeneities or as a result of structural or chemical differences between the bulk and surface of the polyethylene [102]. Infrared spectroscopy shows that gamma-irradiation affects different crystalline bands differently but has no effect on crystallinity below 100 μm in depth. However, following gamma-irradiation, oxidation is apparent at depths of up to 1 mm, with oxidation increasing with dose [103]. Characterization of UHMWPE acetabular cups run on a joint simulator reveals oxidative degradation and crosslinking. Higher oxidative chain scission and a reduction in molecular weight occurs at the component surfaces, while greater crosslinking exists in the interior [104].

Retrieval analyses of polyethylene total knee components have shown reduced molecular weights and surface degradation adjacent to load-bearing surfaces and indicated that damaged areas tended to be oxidized [104]. Higher levels of oxidation have also been observed in areas of subsurface damage. Other retrieval and contact stress analyses reveal that peak shear stresses occur in subsurface regions, and that modes of subsurface damage include creep, fatigue, delamination, pitting, abrasion, burnishing, and oxidation [57,105]. Therefore, there appears to be a synergy among maximum shear stress, oxidation, and chemical reactions, all relating to failure of polyethylene implant materials.

3. Polyethylene Modifications

Attempts have been made to improve the properties (primarily strength, wear, and creep resistance) of polyethylene through fiber reinforcement [106], modified gamma-radiation [107], and increased crystallinity [108].

The addition of carbon fibers increases tensile, compressive and fatigue strength, bending stiffness, and creep resistance of polyethylene [106], but fatigue crack propagation rates increase [11] and wear rates of carbon fiber reinforced polyethylene (CFRPE) can be almost an order of magnitude greater than conventional polyethylene [95]. Numerical analyses indicate that contact stresses in CFRPE tibial components may be as much as 40% greater higher than in conventional polyethylene components [105].

Oxidation inhibits crosslinking of polyethylene. Although shorter segments are more mobile, can lead to crystallization, and improve static mechanical properties, the loss in toughness reduces wear resistance [107]. By excluding oxygen during ionizing radiation sterilization, crosslinking is promoted, potentially leading to a more wear- and creep-resistant polymer [107].

A higher-crystalline polyethylene (enhanced UHMWPE) has been developed through conversion of conventional UHMWPE [108]. Preliminary studies indicate that the yield strength of enhanced UHMWPE is double that of conventional UHMWPE, that creep resistance is doubled at 7 MPa, and hardness, crack growth resistance, and oxidation resistance are greater. These improvements in properties may be attributed to the greater and more controlled crystalline morphology. It is unclear whether wear resistance, the most important property, improves.

4. Advanced Ceramics

Alumina. High-density polycrystalline alumina is used for femoral stems, femoral heads, and acetabular components [109–111]. The attributes of alumina are its chemical stability, biological inertness, hardness, friction, and wear properties.

The amount of wear with an alumina–alumina combination can be 10 times less than with a metal–polyethylene system. However, the polyethylene wear rate is similar whether the countermaterial is a metal or ceramic [95]. The coefficient of friction of both alumina–alumina and alumina–polyethylene is less than that of metal–polyethylene, because of alumina's low surface roughness and wettability [111].

The physical and mechanical properties (Table 2) of α-alumina are a function of purity, grain size, grain size distribution, porosity, and inclusions [111]. For example, increasing the grain size from 4 μm to 7μm reduces the strength by approximately 20% [112]. With advanced ceramics technology, it is now possible to produce alumina with a grain size of 1 μm and a small size distribution, material characteristics known to strengthen the material (Fig. 4).

Alumina has a reduced fatigue strength in an aqueous environment, due to subcritical crack growth [113]. As with other mechanical properties, threshold stresses for subcritical crack growth are a function of processing and purity. Thermal cycling can lead to locally high residual stresses at pores, inclusions, and grain boundary triple points, which can lead to microcrack nucleation [111].

The major limitation of alumina is that it possesses relatively low tensile and bending strengths and fracture toughness, and as a consequence, is sensitive to stress concentrations and overloading. Alumina can be damaged by a fatigue-like failure process, caused by fatigue, impact, or overload [114]. Elevated contact and shear stresses, which lead to subsurface damage accumulation at microstructural defects and grain boundaries, may initiate failure [114]. These local stresses can also lead to grain excavation and third-body wear [115], mechanisms that can be attributed to the anisotropy of alumina [111].

Zirconia. Yttrium oxide partially stabilized zirconia (YPSZ) is another alternative to metal and polyethylene articulating components [116]. This ceramic is tougher than alumina since it can be transformation toughened. At room temperature, zirconia has a monoclinic crystal symmetry. Upon heating, it transforms to a tetragonal phase at approximately 1000–1100°C and then to a cubic phase at approximately 2000°C. A partially reversible volumetric shrinkage occurs during the monoclinic to tetragonal transformation. The volumetric changes resulting from the phase transformations can lead to residual stresses and cracking. Yttrium oxide (Y_2O_3) stabilizes the tetragonal phase so that, upon cooling, the tetragonal crystals can be maintained in a metastable state and not transform back to a monoclinic structure. The normal tetragonal-to-monoclinic

Table 2   Physical and Mechanical Properties of Bioinert Ceramics

Material	Porosity (%)	Density (mg/m³)	Young's modulus (GPa)	Compressive strength (MPa)	Tensile strength (MPa)	Flexural strength (MPa)
Al_2O_3	0	3.93–3.95	380–400	4000–5000	350	400–560
	25	2.8–3.0	150	500	—	70
	35	—	—	200	—	55
	50–75	—	—	80	—	6–11.4
ZrO_2, stabilized	0	4.9–5.6	150–190	1750	—	150–700
	1.5	5.8	210–240	—	—	280–450
	5	—	150–200	—	—	50–500
	28	3.9–4.1	—	<400	—	50–65

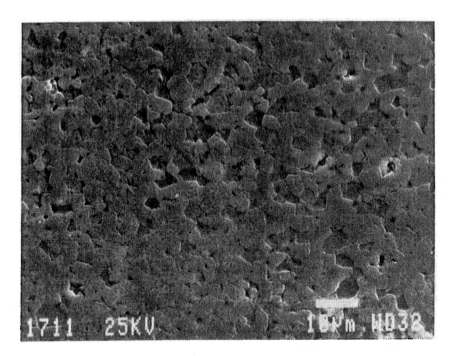

Figure 4   Microstructure of high-purity alumina, having grain sizes less than 5 μm (1000×). (From Ref. 111, Boutin et al., *J. Biomed. Mater. Res., 22*, 1203–1232, Copyright © 1988. Reprinted by permission of John Wiley and Sons, Inc.)

transformation and volume change is also prevented by neighboring grains inducing compressive stresses on one another [116].

Table 2 also lists some properties of YPSZ. The modulus is half that of alumina, while the bending strength and fracture toughness are 2–3 and 2 times greater, respectively. The increased mechanical properties may allow for smaller-diameter femoral heads to be used, compared to alumina. The wear rate of YPSZ on UHMWPE is 50% less than the wear rate of alumina on UHMWPE [117]. The wear resistance is a function of the fine grain size, lack of surface roughness, and residual compressive stresses induced by the transformation back to a monoclinic system.

5. Surface Modifications and Surface Characterization

Surface modifications aimed at reducing wear, such as ultrapassivated titanium oxide layers [118], nitriding [119], ion implantation [120], and oxygen diffusion hardening [121] have typically focussed on modifying the surface of the material wearing against polyethylene, rather than modifying the polymer itself.

Wear of Ti–6Al–4V against UHMWPE is reduced by ion implantation [96]. Ion implantation also reduces metallic wear in the presence of PMMA particles. However, with titanium third-body particles, there is still severe wear. It is therefore imperative to eliminate metallic wear debris, such as that generated from loose porous coating particles, screws, stem–bone abrasion, and fretting at Morse taper junctions. It should be noted that the depth of the ion implanted layer is only approximately 0.5 μm. *In vitro* tests of femoral heads in a wear simulator show that after only 1 million cycles (~ 6–12 months of service) the thickness of the ion implanted layer halved [96]. Thus, ion implantation may not reduce the incidence of late loosening due to particulate debris. Titanium nitride coatings may also reduce wear [119]. However, coatings can spall off and, like ion implantation, seem to have a limited life. Oxygen diffusion hardening results in a greater depth of hardening, potentially leading to greater wear resistance [121].

In vitro and *in vivo* corrosion and wear studies have been largely observational. Improvement in implant tribology will result from understanding the mechanisms governing corrosion and wear. Reaching this understanding will require analyses of implant material surfaces. The role of surface analysis in implantology, therefore, is to characterize the materials, determine the structural and composition changes occurring during processing, identify biologically induced surface reactions, and analyze the effects of the environment on the interfaces [122].

The surface of a material is almost always different in chemical composition and morphology than the bulk material. These differences arise from the molecular arrangement at the surface, surface reactions, and contamination [123]. Surface composition, binding state, and morphology are all important in the analysis of implant surfaces and implant/tissue interfaces.

The chemistry of metal implant–tissue interfaces is determined primarily by the properties of the metal oxide. Metal oxides dictate cell and protein binding at the implant surface. Surface oxides are continually altered by the in-diffusion of oxygen, hydroxide formation, and the out-diffusion of metal ions. Thus multiple oxide stoichiometries exist [18]. The dissolution kinetics of titanium oxide follow a dual logarithmic model, while oxide growth kinetics are logarithmic [18]. Although the properties of metals and their oxides are different [124], adsorption and desorption phenomena can still be influenced by properties of the underlying metal [125].

Surface potentials may also affect osseointegration. For example, it is postulated that oxides with high dielectric constants inhibit certain cell movement to an implant surface [16]. It is therefore suggested that the positive biological response to titanium is due to its high dielectric constant.

Methods of surface characterization important in defining the nature of implant surfaces and implant–tissue interfaces have been summarized in detail [123] (Table 3). These techniques will increase in importance as biomaterialists develop new materials and must characterize all of the parameters necessary to fully describe an implant surface. It should be noted that there may not be a singularly optimal surface for all types of cells and functions.

B. Physical and Mechanical Properties of Porous Metals

Due to the long service life requirements $[N = O(10^7)]$ of implants, the most critical mechanical property is high-cycle fatigue strength. The majority (80–90%) of a smooth material's high-cycle fatigue life is spent initiating a fatigue crack. Thus, factors inhibiting crack nucleation produce good high-cycle fatigue strength.

1. Physical Properties of Porous Metals

Porous-coated Co-Cr-Mo alloys are made by sintering powdered Co-Cr-Mo microspheres, approximately 100–300 μm in diameter, onto a Co-Cr-Mo substrate at 1200–1300°C for 1–3 h. Since these temperatures are above the eutectic point [126], local

Table 3   Surface Science Techniques of Use in Biomaterials Characterization

Morphological techniques
    Light microscopy
    Scanning electron microscopy (SEM)
    Energy dispersive x-ray analysis (EDXA)
    Transmission electron microscopy (TEM)
    Profilometry
    Scanning tunneling microscopy (STM)
    Tunneling spectroscopy
    Atomic force microscopy (AFM)
Diffraction techniques
    X-ray diffraction
    Electron diffraction
    Low-energy electron diffraction (LEED)
Thermodynamic analyses
    Wettability (contact angles)
    Absorption/adsorption/desorption
Electron spectroscopies
    Auger electron spectroscopy (AES)
    Electron spectroscopy for chemical analysis (ESCA)
Ion spectroscopies
    Ion-scattering spectroscopy (ISS)
    Secondary ion mass spectroscopy (SIMS)
    Rutherford backscattering spectroscopy (RBS)
    Surface extended x-ray absorption fine structure (SEXAFS)
Vibrational spectroscopies
    Infrared spectroscopy (IR)
    Electron energy loss spectroscopy (EELS)

melting accelerates particle bonding. Processing at these temperatures results in the formation of eutectic phases and grain boundary carbides.

To produce sufficient energy to bond titanium coatings to substrates, temperatures in the range of $1200°$–$1400°$C are usually necessary [75]. At these temperatures, bonding of titanium and its alloys occurs by solid-state diffusion. Temperatures in the $1200°$–$1400°$C range are above the β-transition temperature of Ti–6Al–4V, leading to a coarse ($\alpha + \beta$) lamellar microstructure (Fig. 5a). Additional effects of high-temperature sintering are thermal etching and surface pitting (Fig. 5b). These microstructural and surface phenomena contribute to a generalized loss in fatigue strength. Fiber or wire mesh coatings may be bonded to a substrate by pressure sintering, a technique that utilizes a combination of temperature and pressure to provide the necessary energy for diffusion and sintering. The use of pressure as an activator allows for lower sintering temperatures in comparison to conventional sintering. Therefore, Ti–6Al–4V can be sintered at temperatures below the $(\alpha + \beta) \rightarrow \beta$ transition temperature, allowing the retention of an equiaxed microstructure [31].

2. Mechanical Properties
Cobalt–Chromium Alloys.   The mechanical properties of cobalt-based alloys are well documented [127]. The high ultimate and fatigue strengths make this alloy a prime alloy

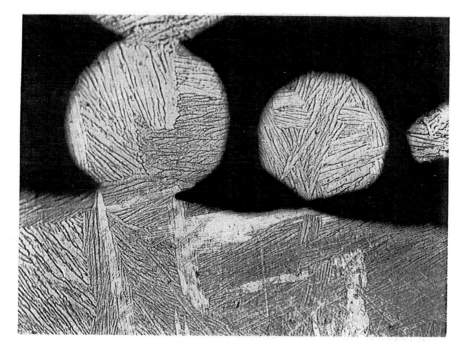

(a)

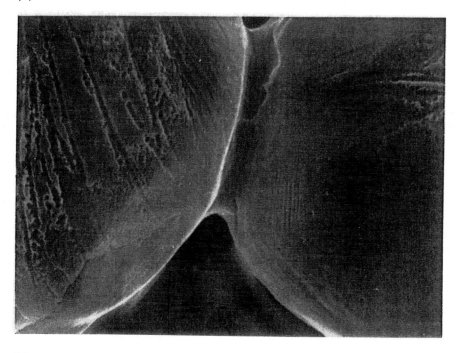

(b)

Figure 5   (a) Microstructure of porous-coated lamellar Ti–6Al–4V (200×). Sintering above the
β-transus results in a lamellar microstructure. (b) SEM of β-sintered, commercially pure titanium
microspheres, showing thermal etching and surface pitting (640×). (From Kohn and Ducheyne,
Ref. 10.)

system for use in joint reconstruction. The coarse grain size and interdendritic carbide and σ-phases present in cast Co–Cr–Mo limit the strength and ductility of the as-cast alloy [14,127]. Therefore, cast Co–Cr–Mo implants are usually solution annealed, a treatment that can result in increased yield strength and ductility, if the treatment and chemical composition are well controlled. Prolonged annealing however results in complete carbide dissolution and a decrease in fatigue strength [14]. In general, the yield and fatigue strengths of Co–Cr alloys are controlled by the ability of the solute atoms C, Cr, and Mo to inhibit dislocation motion [14].

The effect of microstructure on the fatigue strength of Co–Cr alloys is not as well defined as the effect on tensile strength. There is only a minimal difference in the median fatigue lives of cast vs. cast and solution-treated alloys [128], and solution annealing produces only a slight increase in high-cycle fatigue strength [129].

Hot isostatic pressing (HIP-ing) increases the fatigue strength of cast alloys by reducing porosity and eliminating grain boundary carbides [129]. The use of this technique is important, since a contributing factor to *in vivo* failure of Co–Cr–Mo femoral stems is fatigue crack initiation at casting defects [74].

The mechanical properties of wrought Co–Cr–Mo are superior to those of both the cast and the cast and solution-treated alloy because of the finer grain size and more homogeneous microstructure [130].

Ti–6Al–4V.   The high-cycle fatigue strength of Ti–6Al–4V has been studied extensively [9,10,131–136]. In general, mechanical properties of (α + β) titanium alloys are dictated by the amount, size, shape, and morphology of the α-phase and density of α/β interfaces [132,134,135].

Microstructures with a small ($<$20 μm) α-grain size, a well-dispersed β-phase and a small α/β interface area, such as equiaxed microstructures, resist fatigue crack initiation best and have the best high-cycle fatigue strength ($\sim$500–700 MPa) [9,132,134]. This is because a small α-grain size decreases the available reversible slip length. Minimizing the volume fraction of the β-phase decreases the length and density of α/β interfaces, locations where fatigue cracks initiate preferentially.

Lamellar microstructures, which have a greater α/β surface area and more oriented colonies, have lower fatigue strengths ($\sim$300–500 MPa) than equiaxed microstructures. In lamellar microstructures, slip is easily transmitted from one plate to another, because of the crystallographic relation between the α and β phases. The increased slip length causes a strain intensification and therefore lower resistance to fatigue crack initiation and a lower fatigue strength.

Mechanisms governing fatigue crack propagation in Ti–6Al–4V are different from those governing fatigue crack initiation. Microstructures with large grains and large α/β interfacial areas, such as lamellar microstructures, have lower fatigue crack propagation rates and higher threshold stress intensities (ΔK_{th}) than fine-grained microstructures [133–136]. Therefore, there are conflicting microstructural requirements for enhancing fatigue crack initiation and propagation resistance. The lower crack propagation rates in lamellar structures are due to larger slip lengths and more inhomogeneous slip, which improve slip reversibility at the crack tip and provide a mechanism for a fatigue crack to change its path [135].

Traditional fatigue crack propagation tests have focused on macroscopic propagation (i.e., crack length, a = 100–1000 μm). Only recently has microcrack (i.e., a = 10–100 μm) propagation been studied [136,137]. Microcracks grow at higher ΔK values for fine-grained microstructures than for coarse-grained microstructures [136,137]. The microstructural effects on microcrack and macrocrack propagation are opposite to one another. This is thought to be due to the fact that the more tortuous crack front needed to inhibit propagation has not yet formed during microcrack propagation [137]. The importance of short fatigue crack propagation of titanium alloys is brought out in the next section, as this is the governing stage of fatigue for porous-coated Ti–6Al–4V [10].

3. Fatigue of Porous-Coated Metals

The microstructural and geometric changes brought about by the deposition of a porous surface layer onto a substrate metal reduce the high-cycle fatigue strength of porous-coated titanium and cobalt–chromium alloy total joint replacements by approximately 75% compared to uncoated total joint replacements [12,76,138,213] (Table 4).

The high-cycle fatigue strength of porous-coated Co–Cr–Mo ranges between 180 and 235 MPA [14,75,138]. The same sinter-annealing treatment applied to uncoated specimens leads to similarly low fatigue strengths [75,138]. The high-temperature (1200–1300°C) sintering required to bond the coating to the substrate results in substrate porosity and the formation of eutectic phases. The physical metallurgy of these high-temperature microstructures is similar to that of cast structures. The reduction in fatigue strength of Co–Cr–Mo can be attributed for the most part to sintering. Postsintering treatments sufficient to refine cast structures and improve mechanical properties are therefore applicable to porous coated Co–Cr–Mo alloy [14,129,138].

The reduced fatigue strength of porous-coated titanium alloys is attributed to a combination of three factors: (1) stress concentrations at the porous coating/substrate interface and within the porous coating: local stresses can be as high as six times the nominally applied stress [30,139]; (2) changes in microstructure due to sintering treatments: the resulting lamellar microstructures have a high-cycle fatigue strength approximately 20–40% lower than the fatigue strength of wrought, equiaxed Ti–6Al–4V [10,12,76,136]; and (3) surface contamination from oxygen, hydrogen, and nitrogen, and thermal etching, from sintering [76].

4. Thermochemical Material Treatments

Novel thermochemical treatments using hydrogen as a temporary alloying element can significantly refine post-sinter annealed [9,10,140] or post-cast [141–143] titanium microstructures. These treatments break up the continuous grain boundary α-phase (GBα) and colony structure of lamellar microstructures, producing a homogeneous microstructure consisting of refined α-grains in a matrix of discontinuous β. These changes in microstructural morphology result in significant increases in yield strength (975–1120 MPa), ultimate strength (1025–1150 MPa), and fatigue strength (645–670 MPa) compared to respective values for lamellar (902,994,497 MPa) and equiaxed microstructures (914,1000,590 MPa) [9]. The static and dynamic strengths of hydrogen-alloyed titanium are therefore superior to strengths attainable via other thermal cycling techniques. The fatigue strength of hydrogen-alloyed microstructures increases with decreasing α-grain size; however, unlike fine-grained equiaxed structures, ductility is reduced [9,141]. Fatigue crack growth rates in hydrogen-alloyed structures are higher than in lamellar structures.

Treatment of porous-coated Ti–6Al–4V with hydrogen does not improve fatigue strength [10] and, in general, fatigue strength of porous-coated Ti–6Al–4V is independent of microstructure. The notch effect of the surface porosity does not allow the material to take advantage of the superior fatigue crack initiation resistance of a refined α-grain size. Thus, sinternecks act as initiated microcracks and fatigue of porous coated Ti–6Al–4V is propagation controlled [10].

Table 4   Fatigue Strengths of Porous-Coated Metals Tested in Reversed Bending ($R = -1$)

Author(s)	Treatment	σ_{fat}(MPa)	Testing parameters
	Co–Cr–Mo		
Georgette and Davidson [138]	As cast	267	$N = 2 \times 10^7$; 167 Hz
	Sintered + HT[a]	177	
	Sintered + HIP-ed + HT	255	
	Porous coated:	193	
	Sintered + HT		
	Sintered + HIP-ed + HT	234	
	Ti–6Al–4V		
Yue et al. [76]	Wrought	625	$N = 10^7$; 50 Hz
	β-Sintered	500	
	β-Sintered/porous coated	200	
Cook et al. [12]	Wrought	617	$N = 5 \times 10^7$; 167 Hz
	β-Sintered	377	
	β-Sintered/porous coated	138	
Cook et al. [213]	Wrought	668	$N = 5 \times 10^7$; 167 Hz
	β-Sintered	394	
	β-Sintered + BAA-1[b]	488	
	β-Sintered + BAA-2[b]	494	
	Porous coated:	140	
	β-Sintered		
	β-Sintered + BAA-1	161	
	β-Sintered + BAA-2	162	
Kohn and Ducheyne [9,10]	Wrought	590	$N = 10^7$; 100 Hz
	β-Sintered	497	
	β-Sintered + HAT-1[c]	669	
	β-Sintered + HAT-3[c]	643	
	β-Sintered + BAA-3[b]	538	
	Porous coated:	218	
	β-Sintered		
	β-Sintered + HAT-3	177	
	β-Sintered + BAA-3	233	

[a]Proprietary post-sintering heat treatment
[b]BAA = post-sintering β-annealing and aging treatments: BAA-1: 1250°C–2h–slow cool; BAA-2: 1250°C–2h–slow cool/Ar cool/($\alpha + \beta$) anneal–4h–Ar cool; BAA-3: 1030°C–20 min–Ar quench/540°C–4h–Ar quench
[c]HAT = post-sintering hydrogen–alloying treatments: HAT-1: 850°C–0.5 h in H_2/650°C–16 h in vac; HAT-3: 850°C–0.5 h in H_2/590°C–4 h in Ar/775°C–4 h in vac

High-cycle fatigue strength as a function of microstructure and interfacial geometry is depicted schematically in Fig. 6. As stress concentration increases, the controlling stage of fatigue changes from fatigue crack initiation, to short fatigue crack propagation, to long fatigue crack propagation. Similarly, as the governing stage of fatigue changes, the microstructure which maximizes the resistance to damage accumulation during that particular stage also changes. If there is no stress concentration (i.e., $K_t = \sigma_{max}/\sigma_{nominal} = 1$), fatigue crack initiation is the governing stage of fatigue, and microstructures with

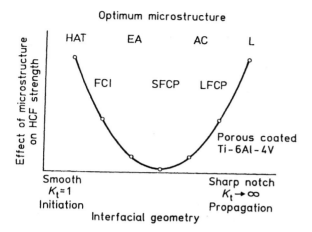

Figure 6 Schematic of Ti–6Al–4V fatigue strength and governing stages of fatigue (FCI = fatigue crack initiation, SFCP = short crack propagation, LFCP = long fatigue crack propagation) as functions of microstructure (HAT = hydrogen alloy treated, EA = equiaxed, AC = acicular, L = lamellar) and interfacial geometry. (From Kohn and Ducheyne, Ref. 10.)

small grains (equiaxed and hydrogen alloy treated microstructures) possess the greatest high-cycle fatigue strength. At high stress concentrations ($K_t > 3.5$), fatigue is governed by long crack propagation, and coarse lamellar microstructures possess the greatest high-cycle fatigue strength [144]. However, at intermediate stress concentrations, such as the stress concentrations at sinternecks [30,139], fatigue strength is independent of microstructure. Since the fatigue life of a material with stress concentrations of this magnitude is equally dependent on the different phases of fatigue, the beneficial and detrimental attributes of different microstructures are equalized. Current porous coatings, which affect fatigue strength in the same manner as notches do, lie in the crack growth region of Fig. 6. Only upon reducing the stress concentrations at the porous coating/substrate interface will the merits of post-sintering treatments on porous-coated Ti–6Al–4V be achieved.

5. Detection of Incipient Damage

As a result of the stress intensifications in porous-coated materials, crack initiation is no longer a valid determinant of fatigue life. Therefore, a technique of detecting incipient failure and distinguishing between fatigue crack initiation and propagation must be utilized to study fatigue. In implementing such a technique with porous-coated Ti–6Al–4V, several unique material qualities must be considered: the complex surface geometry; the potential for simultaneous crack nucleation at multiple, unknown sites; and irregular crack contours. The ability to detect multiple cracks is particularly important in the study of porous materials, since crack nucleation occurs at multiple sites simultaneously [20,21,80].

Acoustic emission (AE) is currently the most sensitive method of monitoring these potential fatigue phenomena, in real-time [145]. AE can detect incipient flaw sizes of 10 μm in Ti–6Al–4V [20,146], monitor cumulative damage, and distinguish different microstructural failure mechanisms [21,145,147]. Based on AE data that was verified optically, fatigue of porous-coated Ti–6Al–4V is governed by a sequential, multimode fracture process of: transverse fracture in the coating, sphere–sphere and sphere–substrate debonding, substrate fatigue crack initiation, and slow and rapid substrate fatigue crack propagation. These modes of fatigue failure are analogous to modes of failure observed in composites (i.e., matrix fracture, fiber fracture, and fiber–matrix delamination). Because of the discontinuity of the porous coating, these stages of fracture occur in a discontinuous fashion. As a result, the AE generated is intermittent and the onset of each mode of fracture can be detected by increases in AE event rate. AE therefore offers two distinct advantages over conventional optical and microscopic methods of analyzing fatigue cracks—it is more sensitive and it can determine the time history of damage progression.

Acoustic emission event amplitudes may be related to microstructural failure mechanisms. For example, in titanium alloy, transgranular cracking, fatigue striations, and void coalescence are characterized, respectively, by AE signals of 70, 80, and 100 dB [21,147]. There is not a uniqueness between signal amplitude and failure mechanisms though. In other words, given a failure mechanism, it is possible to predict an associated signal parameter. However, given a signal, it is not possible to predict the associated failure mechanism. We have therefore been analyzing the frequency characteristics of AE signals to produce such a 1:1 correspondence and also expanding our work to include other composites and bone [145].

C. Electrochemical Properties

Even though most biomaterials in clinical use are reasonably inert and well tolerated in bulk form, there is still release and transportation of biomaterial degradation products in particulate and ionic forms. Based on knowledge of electrochemical behavior, metals can be selected for implantation for which gross corrosion is unlikely, and even impossible. All currently used implant metals are in their passive state under typical physiological conditions. With the exception of some stainless steels, breakdown of passivity should not occur. In this section, the basis for the corrosion resistance of currently used implant metals is explained.

Cobalt–chromium alloys are highly corrosion resistant, because of their passive chromium oxide layer. The inhomogeneous microstructure of cast Co–Cr–Mo makes it more susceptible to corrosion than the forged alloy [130], presumably due to the presence of chromium-depleted dendritic regions acting as the more anodic sites in a galvanic reaction. Wrought Co–Cr–Mo has a lower carbon content than cast Co–Cr–Mo and, as a result, a lower corrosion resistance when tested in physiologic solution [130]. However, the rest potentials of both alloy types are well below the breakdown potential. Furthermore, the breakdown potential exceeds the potential of the oxygen reduction reaction [86,148].

Both titanium and Ti-6Al-4V possess excellent corrosion resistance for a full range of oxide states and pH levels. The corrosion resistance of titanium-based alloys is due to the extremely coherent oxide layer. The resultant low dissolution rate and near chemical inertness of titanium dissolution products allow bone to thrive and osseointegrate with titanium [86,149].

It must be emphasized that even in their passive condition, metals are not inert and there is a passive dissolution from the metal [5,18,86,149]. Linked to the issue of electrochemical behavior (as well as wear) are six questions that must be addressed [150–152]: (1) What material is released? (2) How much material is released? (3) What subsequent reactions do the release products get involved in? (4) What percentage of the release products is excreted and what percentage is retained? (5) Of the percentage that is retained, where does it accumulate? (6) What biological response(s) will result from the retained fraction?

Focusing on the major alloying elements in cobalt-based materials, Co and Ni ions bind to serum albumin, and Cr^{6+} binds to red blood cells [151]. Chemical analyses of urine from animals subjected to metal salts indicated that most Co and Ni are rapidly excreted, while less than 50% of the Cr is excreted, and this occurs at a slower rate than Co or Ni excretion [152,153]. Organ levels of Co and Ni are not significantly elevated, whereas they are for Cr.

Implantation of Co–Cr–Mo microspheres subcutaneously in rats revealed dose related elevations in serum Co and Cr, with peak concentrations achieved three days after implantation [150]. Scaling for the implant surface area to animal body weight ratio (300×), the Co and Cr elevations were 20× and 12×, respectively. The form of the released chromium is Cr^{6+}, a more biologically active form of Cr than Cr^{3+} [154].

Titanium is preferentially accumulated locally, with elevated levels of Ti in adjacent soft tissue and bone [155]. Serum proteins increase the release rate kinetics of titanium compared to solutions containing only serum electrolytes [18]. Dependent on the specific physical and chemical characteristics of the material surface, HA coatings may or may not reduce the titanium dissolution rate from porous coated Ti–6Al–4V [156].

Serum and urine analyses of patients with total joint replacements have also indicated a dose–response relationship [84]. In another study [83], patients with loose porous-coated titanium total hip replacements had double the serum concentration of titanium compared to patients with well-fixed implants. Patients with well-fixed implants had levels of serum titanium similar to those of persons without any prosthesis. No differences in serum aluminum and vanadium or in urine concentrations of any of the three elements were found between any groups. It should be noted that this study was conducted at only one time point, but questions of systemic and remote-site effects are better answered by determining the time history of elemental release and transport.

D. Advances in Fixation

1. Bone Cement

Polymethylmethacrylate (PMMA) is a widely used industrial acrylic and has had a long history as a dental cement. The properties of PMMA are well documented and have been reviewed in depth [63,157,158]. The focus of this review is on developments aimed at improving the properties of bone cements.

Porosity Reduction.   Flaws are introduced into PMMA by air entrapment during mixing and by expanding monomer vapors during polymerization. Pressurization, vacuum mixing, and centrifugation reduce porosity, with a concomitant effect on mechanical behavior [159–161]. In one study, for example, tensile strength, tensile strain and fatigue life at 5000 $\mu\epsilon$ micro strain (10^{-6}) were increased by 24%, 54% and 136%, respectively, while setting time, peak temperature, and modulus did not change [161]. Centrifugation also increases fatigue life for a range of low-cycle strain amplitudes (1000–10,000 $\mu\epsilon$) [162]. Estimates of fatigue limits for uncentrifuged and centrifuged cements at these strain levels are 3.5 and 4 MPa, respectively [158]. Thus, there is not a substantial increase in high-cycle fatigue strength following centrifugation. At lower stresses, the effect of centrifugation is minimized since fatigue failure is dictated by the micromechanics of the specimen surface [163]. As samples with notches of increasing initial stress intensity are tested, the effect of porosity reduction is minimized [163].

It is hypothesized that material imperfections at the bone–cement interface, created as a result of cement interdigitation, act as crack initiation sites [164]. Therefore, crack propagation governs fatigue of PMMA *in vivo* and fracture toughness and fatigue crack growth rate are the most important properties. Centrifugation does not effect these properties [164].

It is necessary to determine the critical flaw size and stress intensity at which the governing stage of fatigue changes from initiation to propagation. An analysis similar to that performed for porous metals (Fig. 6) is in order. Eliminating porosity completely may not maximize strength either, as there may be a critical void size and fraction below which crack blunting is less likely to occur.

PMMA Composites.   Reinforcing agents are frequently used to increase the tensile load bearing capacity of brittle materials like bone cement. Wires, fibers, and particles made of carbon and graphite [165–168], aramid [168–170], stainless steel [171,172], titanium [173,174], glass [175], polyethylene [176], and rubber [177] have all been used. Detailed reviews of PMMA composites have recently been published [157,178]. The salient points of these studies are summarized in Table 5.

In general, the factors affecting the processing and properties of reinforced PMMA are the type, dimensions, volume fraction, and distribution of the second phase, interaction between the different phases, energy dissipation mechanisms, mixing technique, and workability.

Chemical Modifications.   Although most improvements of bone cement have focused on mechanically modifying PMMA, some studies have evaluated chemical modifications of PMMA [179,180]. One cement is based on an *n*-butyl methacrylate monomer instead of methylmethacrylate [180]. In another, polybutylmethacrylate (PBMA) is used but the PMMA powder is replaced rather than the monomer, leading to a composite cement of PBMA beads in a methylmethacrylate matrix [179]. The results of these studies indicate that PBMA has a peak temperature lower than that of PMMA, a modulus 25–50% less than that of PMMA, and a higher ductility and apparent fracture toughness. At low strain rates, PBMA tears in a ductile manner whereas PMMA fails by brittle fracture. This difference in fracture mechanisms may be attributed to the fact that PBMA has a glass transition temperature of 27°C and is in a rubbery state at body temperature. The rationale for a lower-modulus cement is that there will be better compatibility at the cement–bone interface. It is unclear though whether the mechanics of the cement–metal interface will be compromised.

Bone Cements with Biologically Active Second Phases.   Another method of improving the properties of bone cement by a composites approach is the use of bone particle impregnated cement [181]. Partial bonding between the cement and bone particles results in increased axial and shear moduli with increasing bone particle concentration, but not to the extent that composites theory predicts [181]. Although crack propagation rates are reduced, tensile and impact strengths are also reduced, due to either a weak bone particle–cement bond or the inherent weakness of the bone particles themselves [181]. *In.vivo* studies show impregnated cement has a greater bone–cement interfacial shear strength than nonimpregnated cement, but impregnation with demineralized bone matrix results in a higher interfacial strength than impregnation with inorganic phases [182].

The most recent thrust in bone cement research is the development of bioactive and

Table 5 Mechanical Properties of Reinforced PMMA Bone Cements

Ref.	Type	Reinforcing material dimensions	Fraction	Important results[a]
Knoell et al. [165]	Graphite	$l = 6$ mm	1, 2, 3, & 10 w/o	Increase in modulus, UCS, flexural strength
Pilliar et al. [166]	Carbon	$l = 6$ mm $d = 7\ \mu$m	2 v/o	60% increase in UTS 100% increase in modulus
Pilliar et al. [214]	Carbon	$l = 6$ mm $d = 10–15\ \mu$m	1 & 2 v/o	Increase in static and dynamic moduli
Robinson et al. [215]	Carbon	$l = 1.5$ mm $d = 10\ \mu$m	2 v/o	5% increase in UCS, 30% increase in K_{Ic}
Wright and Robinson [167]	Carbon	$l = 1.5$ mm	2 v/o	10% decrease in da/dN
Saha and Pal [216]	Carbon		2 w/o	10% increase in UCS 20% increase in shear strength 30% increase in UTS, bending strength 40% increase in modulus
Saha and Pal [168]	Carbon Aramid	$l = 6$ mm $l = 8$ mm	1 w/o 2–4 w/o	20–30% increase in UTS
Pourdeyhimi et al. [169]	Carbon Aramid	$l = 3.2$ mm	1–7 w/o	100% increase in K_{Ic} 360% increase in J_{Ic}
Wright and Trent [170]	Aramid	$l = 13$ mm	1–7 w/o	30% increase in UTS 75% increase in K_{Ic}
Taitsman and Saha [171]	316L SS Vitallium	$d = 1$ mm $d = 1$ mm		45% increase in UTS
Fisbane and Pond [172]	316L SS	$l = 0.5–6$ mm $d = 65–90\ \mu$m	6.5 v/o	25% increase in UCS
Schnur and Lee [173]	Ti	$d = 1$ mm	16 v/o	380% increase in modulus 65% increase in UCS 160% increase in YS
Topoleski et al. [174,178]	Ti	$l = 1.5, 5$ mm $d = 18, 22$ mm	5 v/0	50% increase in K_{Ic} 5–10% increase in σ_{fat}
Pourdeyhimi et al. [176]	PE	$l = 3.2$ mm $d = 38$ mm	1–7 w/o	E, flexural strength, K_{Ic} only increase up to 1 w/o
Murkami et al. [177]	Rubber			10% increase in ϵ_F 75% increase in K_{Ic}

Source: Adapted from Ref. 63

[a]da/dn = fatigue crack propagation rate; K_{Ic} = mode I fracture toughness; J_{Ic} = critical value of (mode I) J-integral; UCS = ultimate compressive strength; UTS = ultimate tensile strength; YS = yield strength; ϵ_F = failure strain; σ_{fat} = fatigue strength

biodegradable cements. The rationale for such systems is that the cements are workable; can be molded to conform to the interstices of bone; can provide immediate structural support, augment normal bone healing and remodeling; and, over time, be replaced by host bone, or, with more stable bioactive fillers, form a direct bond with bone without resorbing. Candidate cements are PMMA linked with apatite fillers [183], bioactive glass powders with ammonium phosphate [184] or bis-GMA 2,2-*bis*[4(2-hydroxy-3 methacryl-oyloxy-propyloxy)-phenyl]propane [185], and powdered tricalcium phosphate (TCP) in a gelatin matrix [186].

2. Bioactive Ceramics

The concept of bioactivity was introduced with respect to bioactive glasses via the following hypothesis: *The biocompatibility of an implant material is optimal if the material elicits the formation of normal tissues at its surface, and in addition, if it establishes a contiguous interface capable of supporting the loads that normally occur at the site of implantation* [42]. Three classes of ceramics fulfill these requirements: bioactive glasses and glass ceramics, calcium phosphate ceramics, and bioactive glasses and ceramics with inert second phases. Detailed reviews have been published [37,38,63,187].

Bioactive Glasses and Glass Ceramics.   Bioactive glasses were first developed by Hench et al. [42], who synthesized glasses containing mixtures of silica, phosphate, calcia, and soda. Bioactive glasses and glass ceramics are proposed as both bulk implant materials and coatings on metal or ceramic implants [42,109,112].

Chemical reactions are limited to the surface (about 300–500 μm) of the glasses and bulk properties are not affected by surface reactivity. The implant surface releases Na^+ ions and subsequently also Ca^{2+} and P^{5+} ions. The degree of activity (and physiologic response) is dependent on the chemical composition of the glass and may vary by over an order of magnitude [112]. For example, the substitution of CaF for CaO decreases the solubility of the glass, whereas the addition of B_2O_3 increases the solubility of the glass [112].

Ceravital is another glass, with different alkali oxide concentrations from Bioglass. The physiological responses of Bioglass and Ceravital are similar though [188]. It is hypothesized that the general biologic response to both glasses is the nucleation of hydroxyapatite crystals at the implant surface within an ordered collagen matrix, followed by the formation of mineralized bone [112].

A glass–ceramic containing crystalline oxyapatite and fluorapatite [$Ca_{10}(PO_4)_6$-(O,F_2)] and β-wollastonite (SiO_2–CaO) in an MgO–CaO–SiO_2 glassy matrix (denoted glass–ceramic A-W) is a third bioactive glass [189]. If the physiological environment is correctly simulated in terms of ion concentration, pH, and temperature, this layer consists of carbonate containing hydroxyapatite of small crystallites with a defective structure, and the composition and structural characteristics are similar to those of bone [190]. A-W glass–ceramic bonds to living bone, through a thin calcium and phosphorus-rich layer that is formed at the surface of the glass–ceramic [189].

Calcium Phosphate Ceramics.   Calcium phosphate ceramics are ceramic materials with varying calcium-to-phosphate ratios. Among them, the apatites are the most studied. The most common apatitic ceramic used in medicine is hydroxyapatite (HA), a material with a hexagonal crystal lattice; an ideal chemical formula—$Ca_{10}(PO_4)_6(OH)_2$; ideal weight percents of: 39.9% Ca, 18.5% P and 3.38% OH; and an ideal calcium/phosphate ratio of 1.67. The crystal structure and crystallization behavior of HA are dependent on the substitutional nature of the ionic species and the ordering.

The impetus for using synthetic HA as a biomaterial stems from the perceived advantage of using a material similar to the mineral phase in bone and teeth for replacing these materials. Better tissue bonding is therefore expected. Additional advantages of bioactive ceramics include low thermal and electrical conductivity, elastic properties similar to those of bone, control of *in vivo* degradation rates through control of material properties, and the possibility of the ceramic functioning as a barrier when it is coated onto a metal substrate [191].

Two points about the crystal chemistry of natural and synthetic apatites need to be recognized. First, the hydroxyapatite in bone is nonstoichiometric; has a Ca/P ratio less than 1.67; and contains carbonate ions, sodium, magnesium, fluorine, and chlorine [192]. Second, most synthetic hydroxyapatites contain substitutions for the phosphate and/or hydroxyl groups and vary from the ideal stoichiometry and Ca/P ratios. Oxyhydroxyapatite [$Ca_{10}(PO_4)_6O$], α-tricalcium phosphate (α-TCP), β-tricalcium phosphate (β-TCP), or β-Whitlockite [$Ca_3(PO_4)_2$], tetracalcium phosphate ($Ca_4P_2O_9$), and octocalcium phosphate [$Ca_8(HPO_4)_2(PO_4)_4 5H_2O$) have all been detected, postprocessing, in varying amounts via x-ray diffraction, FTIR, and chemical analyses [193,194]. These compounds are not apatites per se, since the crystal structure differs from that of actual apatite.

Differences in the structure, chemistry, and composition of apatites arise from differences in material processing techniques, time, temperature, and atmosphere. Understanding the processing–composition–structure–processing synergy for calcium phosphate ceramics helps us understand the *in vivo* function of these materials. It is therefore important to understand the thermal behavior and solubility of apatites.

The dissolution behavior of hydroxyapatite in an aqueous media is also dependent on the chemical composition of the crystal. The ion exchanges occurring at the apatite surface are dependent on the rate of formation and dissolution of the various phases, the powder weight to liquid volume ratio, pH, specific surface area, crystal defects, impurities and vacancies, and substitutional ions.

Related to these general properties are specific properties: (1) powder particle size, (2) particle shape, (3) pore size, (4) pore shape, (5) pore size distribution, (6) specific surface area, (7) phases present, (8) crystal structure, (9) crystal size, (10) grain size, (11) hardness, (12) coating thickness, (13) surface roughness, and (14) density.

Analysis can be accomplished with solution chemical methods, such as atomic absorption spectroscopy; physical methods, such as thin-film x-ray diffraction, electron microprobe analysis (EMP), energy dispersive x-ray analysis (EDXA), Fourier transform infrared spectroscopy (FTIR); and surface methods, such as Auger electron spectroscopy (AES), electron spectroscopy for chemical analysis (ESCA); and secondary ions mass spectroscopy (SIMS). AES, ESCA, and SIMS are true surface analysis techniques, having sampling depths of several atomic layers, while the other techniques sample depths on the order of microns (Fig. 7).

Calcium phosphate coatings are deposited onto porous metals to accelerate and enhance fixation of the prosthesis to bone and to shield the tissues from metallic corrosion products [17]. The results of these studies vary with respect to implant–tissue bond strength, ceramic solubility, and *in vivo* function. Some studies [17] report increased bone–porous implant shear strengths at early time periods (4 weeks) over non-ceramic-coated controls, while others [195] report no significant differences in the early stabilization of porous-surfaced implants. The discrepancies in data suggest material and processing induced differences in both the ceramic and metal [191]. Despite the differences in

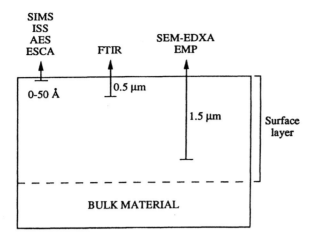

Figure 7 Schematic of sampling depths for different surface analysis techniques. (From Kohn and Ducheyne, Ref. 63.)

short-term results, all studies indicate that long-term stabilization and fixation strength do not depend on the ceramic coating.

Results of *ex vivo* push-out tests indicate that the ceramic–metal bond fails before the ceramic–tissue bond [196]. Thus, there is reason for concern about the weak ceramic-metal bond and integrity of that interface over a lengthy service life of functional loading. No fatigue testing of either the ceramic alone or of the ceramic–metal interface has been conducted. Material behavior under dynamic loading is a critical parameter and is a much needed research area [191]. Although a number of tests are available for studying ceramic–metal bond strength, such as pullout, lap-shear, three- and four-point bending, double cantilever beam, double torsion, indentation, and scratch tests [191], there are inherent difficulties in performing each of these tests, particularly for thin, brittle coatings. A more fundamental fracture mechanics approach has been taken through the use of an interfacial "fracture toughness" test [22], with a resultant reduction in data variability.

Properties important to understanding the implant–tissue bond and reactions at the implant surface and in tissues have been outlined: (1) characterization of surface activity, including surface analysis, biochemistry and ion transport; (2) physical chemistry, pertaining to strength and degradation, stability of the tissue–ceramic interface, and tissue resorption; and (3) biomechanics, as related to strength, stiffness, design, wear, and tissue remodeling [38]. These properties are time dependent and must therefore be characterized as functions of loading and environmental history. The importance of this characterization is underscored by the variability in results, discussed above, and potential limitations of bioactive materials, such as fatigue, fracture, coating delamination, and unwanted material degradation.

3. Composites

Many times, one material cannot meet all of the design and property requirements for a specific application. For such cases, composite materials are developed. Biomaterial composites may improve the properties and service life of femoral stems, fracture plates, bioactive ceramics, and bone cement. Composite materials are formed by combining two or more materials, resulting in a material that possesses a combination of properties that neither material can meet individually. The individual constituents of a composite are physically and mechanically separate, so the combined materials and properties can be controlled.

The motivation for using composite materials in total joint replacements is based on several concepts. Composite materials can be very strong, since materials in fiber form exhibit strengths near the theoretical values. As a result, advanced composites can be as strong as metals and, in some cases, more flexible [197]. The properties of composites can be more easily tailored than with metals. A specific example is that the modulus of composites can be tailored to some extent to be close to that of bone. The rationale for designing "isoelastic" prostheses is based on observations of proximal bone resorption in the presence of stiff metal femoral stems [4,34]. The rationale is also based on the hypothesis that a prosthesis that matches the elastic properties of the proximal femur will result in a more physiological stress distribution than can be attained with higher-modulus metallic implants. As a result, it is believed that less adverse tissue remodelling and aseptic loosening will arise [1,6]. Interestingly, there is no clearly documented data that demonstrates that a total joint replacement with a reduced modulus and stiffness will represent an improvement over a higher-modulus implant [198].

Summary of Materials. Candidate biomedical composites are either polymer-based (fiber-reinforced plastics) or ceramic-based (carbon fiber reinforced carbon). The matrix that has found the largest initial following is polysulfone [198–200]. Less common matrices include polycarbonate [199], carbon [201,202], silicon carbide [202], polyetheretherketone (PEEK) [198], epoxy [203], and triazin [204]. Fibers are either carbon/graphite [198,200–202] or polyamide (Kevlar) [198,199].

Polysulfone is a thermoplastic polymer with a glass transition well above body temperature and a modulus similar to that of trabecular bone. The chemical and mechanical properties of polysulfone (Table 6) are a function of the chemical structure. For example, the benzene rings permit dissipation of energy, without loss of structural integrity [198]. Polysulfone will, however, be swollen by polar organic solvents and, therefore, cannot be used in conjunction with PMMA [198].

Carbon-based materials are also strong candidates for use as biomedical composites, because of their biocompatibility. Carbon fiber reinforced carbon (CFRC) composites offer several advantages over the more conventional carbon fiber reinforced plastics — they do not release soluble products, they are less susceptible to stress corrosion, they do not degrade with time, and they are more suitable to surface modifications [202].

Both carbon and Kevlar fibers exhibit good tensile strength in the longitudinal direction, but have low transverse strength (Table 6). The compressive and tensile strengths of carbon are nearly equal, but the compressive strength of Kevlar is only 20% of the tensile strength. The important difference between the fibers is the brittle nature of carbon (< 1% elongation), compared to Kevlar's ductile failure mechanisms.

Properties of Selected Composite Materials. The properties of a composite are dependent on the fibers, the matrices, and interaction between the two. Generalizations about the properties of composite systems, even for the same fiber embedded in different matrices, or different fibers embedded in the same matrix, cannot be made. Each individual composite system, as well as each constituent within a given system, must be evaluated. In this regard a dual problem exists. First, is the difficulty in characterizing the

Table 6   Properties of Biomedical Composite Constituents

	Matrix material		
Property	Polysulfone	PEEK	UHMWPE
ρ(g/cc)	1.3	1.3	0.9
UTS (MPa)	70	92	20
UCS (MPa)	96	118	15
E (GPa)	2.5	3.6	0.6
%EL	50–100	50	200–525
σ_{flex} (MPa)	106	170	13
σ_{fat} (MPa)	7	70	16

	Fiber		
Property	Carbon: PAN-based type 1	Carbon: PAN-based type 2	Kevlar
Diam. (μm)	7–10	8–9	12
E_1 (GPa)	390	250	125
E_2 (GPa)	12	20	–
UTS (MPa)	2200	2700	2800–3600

Source: Modified from Ref. 198

in-plane and out-of-plane stiffness and strengths of composites. Second, the *in vivo* loading conditions that these composite structures will be exposed to are unknown.

Fibers can only carry tensile loads and therefore, alone, they are of little structural value. However, when incorporated into a matrix, fibers are also able to carry compressive and shear loads. The properties (stiffness and tensile, compressive, flexural, and fatigue strength) of composites vary with fiber volume fraction, dimensions, orientation and, flaw distribution.

Since an implant is subjected to axial, bending, and torsional loads, unidirectional reinforcement is clearly insufficient. Therefore, most current composite implants are laminates, with the individual layers either unidirectional or randomly oriented. In laminated composites, strength and stiffness are highest if reinforcement is unidirectional. Laminated composites, with each layer having a different fiber orientation, can result in resistance to both in-plane and out-of-plane stresses. Woven, continuous fiber reinforced composites have less directional dependence than ordered composites but offer the advantage of having a greater balance in properties with respect to direction. The properties of woven composites depend on weave direction, spacing, and density.

Modulus.   Bounds on the elastic modulus of composites are defined by two limiting cases. For unidirectional long-fiber composites, the modulus in the direction of fiber orientation approaches the modulus of the fibers as the volume fraction of fibers increases. Similarly, as fiber fraction decreases, the modulus approaches that of the matrix. In the transverse direction, unidirectional fibers do not have any stiffening effect and the composite modulus is similar to that of the matrix.

In general, the modulus of chopped-fiber composites is significantly less than that of long-fiber composites. Calculating the modulus of laminated composites is more rigorous

[197]. More detailed mathematical models, such as Hashin–Shtrikman bounds, composite sphere assembly models, composite cylinder assembly models, periodic array models, theories of rigid inclusions in rigid and nonrigid matrices, and approximation methods have been developed [29,30,205,206]. In this regard, we have recently applied homogenization theory to calculate effective stiffness of composites and of tissue–implant interfacial zones [29,30,207]. These concepts are discussed later in this section.

Strength. Composite materials derive their beneficial mechanical properties through two primary mechanisms: The generally brittle fibers demonstrate their tensile strength, while their brittleness is shielded by being incorporated in a more ductile matrix. The strength, stiffness, and energy absorption mechanisms of the weaker matrix are increased by the inclusion of the fibers.

In any given layer of a laminate, for low fiber volume fractions, the tensile strength of the layer is dictated by the strength of the matrix. As volume fraction increases, the tensile strength is governed by the strength of the fibers. In unidirectional composites strength is maximized if loading is in the direction of the fibers. The fibers carry the majority of the load and no damage occurs until fiber fracture. Upon fracture, energy is released from the fiber into the matrix. Energy release is proportional to fiber diameter; thus composites with smaller diameter fibers, which release less energy, are more damage resistant [199].

For a given set of fiber characteristics, the more ductile the matrix, the stronger the composite, since ductile materials exhibit greater crack propagation resistance following fiber fracture. A strong fiber–matrix interface transfers load directly to the matrix, resulting in stress concentrations in the matrix and a greater propensity for failure. A weak interfacial bond results in debonding around the fiber end as a secondary means of energy absorption following fiber fracture. Thus, a weakly bonded interface would appear preferable. However, too weak an interfacial bond reduces the overall strength of the composite. Therefore, to optimize tensile strength, an intermediate interfacial bond strength is recommended, as it creates a means to maintain damage at only a local level [208].

Tensile strength transverse to the direction of fiber orientation is governed by the properties of the matrix and interface [209]. The fibers act as rigid inclusions in a sandwich of alternating compliant and stiff layers [199]. The strain levels are much higher in the more compliant matrix and at the interface with the more rigid fibers. At the fiber–matrix interface are sites of stress concentration and crack initiation. In general, more ductile matrix materials are more resistant to transverse cracking since they can plastically deform ahead of the crack tip.

Compressive strength is a more important property than tensile strength, because of the inability of some fibers to withstand compressive forces, and the propensity for fiber buckling. Under compressive loading, fibers must rely on the matrix and interface for lateral support. Therefore, the fibers, matrix, and interface synergistically determine compressive strength [199]. If the buckling strength of the fiber is greater than the shear strength, as is the case with carbon and Kevlar fibers, compressive strength is dependent on the shear moduli of the fiber and matrix [198]. Therefore a brittle matrix with a high shear modulus best resists lateral deformation of the fibers and provides the best composite compressive strength.

Based on the discussion above, it is clear that determining the failure strength of laminated composites is complicated, since the fiber direction may vary in each layer. Additionally, each layer has a different failure mode and failure criteria. Catastrophic compressive failures have been the observed failure modes in laminated carbon fiber reinforced polysulfone total hip replacements [198]. There are two general failure modes in laminated composites: in-plane and out-of-plane failure. Matrix fracture, fiber fracture, fiber buckling and fiber–matrix shear are all associated with in-plane failure, whereas out-of-plane failures are related to delamination [197].

Interfacial Bond Strength. The fiber–matrix interfacial bond is the most important microstructural parameter with respect to the mechanical performance of fiber reinforced composites. The integrity of this interface dictates the ability of the composite to transmit tensile and shear forces across the interface and to dissipate energy during deformation processes. Without sufficient bonding, only compressive stresses are transferred across the fiber–matrix interface. The fracture properties of the interface can also influence the overall composite fracture resistance and structural stability.

The fiber–matrix bond enables reinforcement to be beneficial by providing structural support and a load transfer mechanism. This bond may be either mechanical or chemical in nature. Most bonds are mechanical in nature, achieved through interlocking via the microroughness and porosity of the fiber surface. In general, carbon fibers are much rougher than Kevlar fibers. Thus, the greater surface area available for micromechanical interlocking provides greater frictional resistance to interfacial deformation. Another mechanism for enhancing bond strength is to wet the fiber surface with the matrix material. Kevlar fibers are typically treated in this fashion, because of their weak bonding with thermoplastics. Molecular weight, functionality, and steric factors of the matrix determine the degree of fiber–matrix adhesion strength of the interfacial bond [198].

Single-fiber pull-out tests show that carbon fiber interfaces possess greater ultimate and fatigue strengths than Kevlar fiber interfaces for both polysulfone and polycarbonate matrices [199,210]. For a given fiber type, the interfacial bond strengths are similar for both matrix types. During static loading, adhesive failure of the fiber–matrix interface occurs, whereas during fatigue loading, debonding occurs by a combination of adhesive failure and matrix cohesive failure.

Static and dynamic strengths are reduced by 40% and 60%, respectively, when tested in an aqueous environment [210,211]. However, no significant differences between testing in saline and in inflammatory exudate are found, implying that either water or salt ions mediate degradation. Moisture-induced material degradation represents an important consideration in composite implant design. Moisture-induced reductions in strength and stiffness are a result of interfacial bond degradation, which is believed to occur as a result of water molecules competing for adhesive bonding sites and matrix swelling [210,211].

Biological Response. In assessing the biological response to composite materials, the biological reactions of each constituent must be analyzed individually and in both bulk and particulate form. The effects of any wetting agents must also be assessed. Since polysulfone cannot be used with bone cement, most composite total hips are press-fit designs. As a result, the potential exists for the generation of wear debris resulting from abrasion between the composite and bone. Little is known about the biological reaction to particulate polysulfone, but in light of the adverse reactions and consequences of polyethylene and PMMA debris, studies are warranted.

4. Coupled Global/Local Finite Element Modeling of Implant–Tissue Interfaces

Osseointegration into orthopedic and dental implants is heterogeneous and often limited to the outer regions of the implant surface [8,34,49]. These biological facts make it

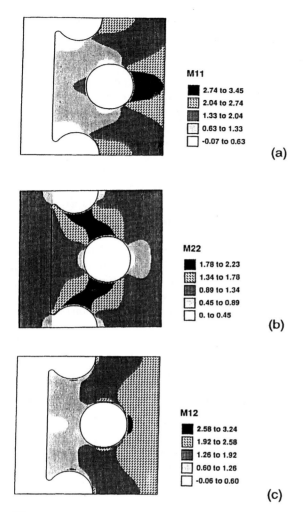

(a)

(b)

(c)

Figure 8 Plots of local structure matrices M_{ij}, which indicate local strain distributions: (a) M_{11} distribution of strain across interface; (b) M_{22} distribution of strain along interface; (c) M_{12} distribution of strain in shear.

important to quantify stresses and strains within the interfacial zone accounting for the specific local architecture and structure of the implant surface and adjacent tissue. We hypothesize that the architecture and structure of the implant surface–tissue composite is the major factor determining local stresses and strains, and influences tissue ingrowth and ultimately implant function.

Previous global or whole-implant finite element models have treated the interfacial zone as either a bonded or contact surface with no details of local structures [3,32]. Localized models, or submodels, analyze the structure of the interfacial zone and quantify local stresses, but these models do not connect the local and global analyses [139]. Our objective, therefore, has been to model the interfacial zone with a level of specificity

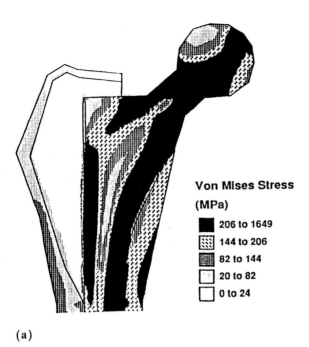

Von Mises Stress
(MPa)

■ 206 to 1649

▨ 144 to 206

▦ 82 to 144

▢ 20 to 82

☐ 0 to 24

(a)

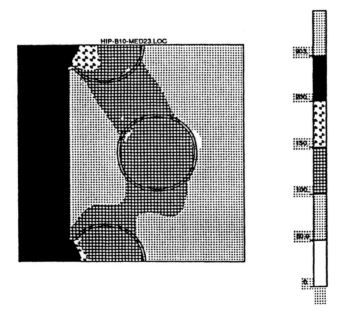

(b)

Figure 9 Von Mises stress distributions for (a) global whole-implant model of proximally porous-coated total hip replacement; (b) local unit cell model extracted from medial side of global model.

capable of accounting for local histological variations. Such detailed microscopic modeling is a necessary advancement, but it is not sufficient. The results of localized models must also be coupled with whole-implant models in a systematic fashion. We have therefore developed more physiologically realistic models of orthopaedic and dental implants to predict stresses and strains in the interfacial zone and combine global analyses of whole implants with local analyses of selected regions of the interfacial zone [29,30,209]. This modeling is performed using homogenization theory [29,30,209,212]. The advantage of this modeling technique is that it offers the ability to construct a whole-implant model without losing the details of local heterogeneous architecture.

The elastic properties of the composite interfacial zone are directionally dependent, with the zone being almost an order of magnitude stiffer in the longitudinal direction. Strain fields around individual microspheres are inhomogeneous (Fig. 8). For strain normal to the direction of loading, strain decreases from the exterior to the interior regions of the coating (Fig. 8a). Strain is concentrated at the point where bone contacts the outer edge of the microsphere. The highest strains in the interfacial zone are more than triple the strains predicted by the global analysis. For normal loads directed along the interface, strain is concentrated in the tissue between the microspheres, and the peak strains are more than 2 times higher than what is predicted by the global model (Fig. 8b). For shear loads, strains are also concentrated at the point where the tissue contacts the outer edge of the microsphere and the peak strains are 3 times greater than what is predicted by a global model (Fig. 8c).

Using the results of these local unit cell models, global stresses in a whole implant and local stresses in selected regions of the interfacial zone are calculated. Global analyses do not vary much with increasing stiffness of bone or with the incorporation of fibrous tissue, and are therefore insufficient to predict variations in interfacial stresses. Local stresses, however, are quite heterogeneous and strongly dependent on tissue properties. Comparing local stresses to global values at the same location indicates that the maximum stresses in the metal are higher than the global values at the same location (Fig. 9).

Based on the material and stress inhomogeneity of the interfacial zone, traditional global finite element models, which typically assume average material properties for the interfacial zone, cannot accurately quantify local micromechanical behavior in this region, and modeling at multiple levels of structural hierarchy is needed.

IV. SUMMARY

In this chapter some current problems with implants for hard tissue replacement have been outlined. Following a fundamental materials engineering approach of relating material processing to material composition, structure, and properties, some of the mechanisms underlying these problems have been addressed and potential solutions cited. In materials engineering, a discussion of properties generally means physical, chemical, and mechanical properties. In biomaterials, we must also include analyses of the effect of the physiological environment on the materials, as well as the effect of the material on its surrounding biological milieu. The material properties discussed in this chapter are by no means exhaustive, but some basic materials engineering mechanisms related to biomaterials applications have been outlined, and a lengthy reference list is provided.

REFERENCES

1. Crowninshield, R.D., Brand, R.A., Johnston, R.C., and Milroy, J.C., *J. Bone Joint Surg.*, *62A*, 68–78 (1980).
2. Delport, P., Ducheyne, P., and Martens, M., in *Biomaterials and Biomechanics* (Ducheyne, P., Vander Perre, G., and Aubert, A.E., eds.), Amsterdam: Elsevier, 1983, pp. 43–48.
3. Ducheyne, P., Aernoudt, E., De Meester, P., Martens, M., Mulier, J.C., and Van Leeuwen, D., *J. Biomech.*, *11*, 297–307 (1978).
4. Engh, C.A., and Bobyn, J.D., *Clin. Orthop.*, *231*, 7–28 (1988).
5. Ferguson, A. B., Jr., Laing, P. G., and Hodge, E. S., *J. Bone Joint Surg.*, *42A*, 77–90 (1960).
6. Huiskes, R., in *Functional Behavior of Orthopaedic Biomaterials*, Vol. II, *Applications* (Ducheyne, P., and Hastings, G.W., eds.), Boca Raton, FL : CRC Press, 1984, pp. 121–162.
7. Klawitter, J.J., and Hulbert, S.F., *J. Biomed. Mater. Res. Symp.*, *2*, 161–229 (1971).
8. Goldstein, S.A., Matthews, L.S., Kuhn, J.L., and Hollister, S.J., *J. Biomech.*, *24*(S1), 135–150 (1991).
9. Kohn, D.H., and Ducheyne, P., *J. Mater. Sci.*, *26*, 328–334 (1991).
10. Kohn, D.H., and Ducheyne, P., *J. Biomed. Mater. Res.*, *24*, 1483–1501 (1990).
11. Connally, G.M., Rimnac, C.M., Wright, T.M., Hertzberg, R.W., and Manson, J.A., *J. Orthop. Res.*, *2*, 119–125 (1984).
12. Cook, S.D., Georgette, F.S., Skinner, H.B., and Haddad, R.J., Jr., *J. Biomed. Mater. Res.*, *18*, 497–512 (1984).
13. Freitag, T.A., and Cannon, S.L., *J. Biomed. Mater. Res.*, *10*, 805–828 (1976).
14. Pilliar, R.M., and Weatherly, G.C., in *CRC Critical Reviews in Biocompatibility* (Williams, D.F., ed.), Boca Raton, FL: CRC Press, 1986, Vol. 1, pp. 371–403.
15. Galante, J., Restoker, W., Lueck, R., and Ray, R.D., *J. Bone Joint Surg.*, *53A*, 101–114 (1971).
16. Albrektsson, T., Branemark, P.I., Hansson, H.A., Kasemo, B., Larsson, K., Lundstrom, I., McQueen, D.H., and Skalak, R., *Ann. Biomed. Engr.*, *11*, 1–27 (1983).
17. Ducheyne, P., Hench, L.L., Kagan, A., II, Martens, M., Bursens, A., and Mulier, J.C., *J. Biomed. Mater. Res.*, *14*, 225–237 (1980).
18. Healy, K.E., and Ducheyne, P., *J. Biomed. Mater. Res.*, *26*, 319–338 (1992).
19. Thomas, K.A., Cook, S.D., Renz, E.A., Anderson, R.C., Haddad, R.J., Jr., Haubold, A.D., and Yapp, R., *J. Biomed. Mater. Res.*, *19*, 145–159 (1985).
20. Kohn, D.H., Ducheyne, P., and Awerbuch, J., in *Titanium Science and Technology* (Lacombe, P., Tricot, R., and Beranger, G., eds.), Paris: Les Editions de Physique, 1989, pp. 789–794.
21. Kohn, D.H., Ducheyne, P., and Awerbuch, J., *J. Biomed. Mater. Res.*, *26*, 19–38 (1992).
22. Filiaggi, M.J., Coombs, N.A., and Pilliar, R.M., *J. Biomed. Mater. Res.*, *25*, 1211–1229 (1991).
23. Klawitter, J.J., Bagwell, J.G., Weinstein, A.M., Sauer, B.W., and Pruitt, J.R., *J. Biomed. Mater. Res.*, *10*, 311–323 (1976).
24. Raab, S., Ahmed, A.M., and Provan, J.W., *J. Biomed. Mater. Res.*, *16*, 679–704 (1982).
25. Bobyn, J.D., Pilliar, R.M., Cameron, H.U., and Weatherly, G.C., *Clin. Orthop.*, *150*, 263–270 (1980).
26. Anderson, R.C., Cook, S.D., Weinstein, A.M., and Haddad, R.J., Jr., *Clin. Orthop.*, *182*, 242–257 (1984).
27. Martens, M., Ducheyne, P., De Meester, P., and Mulier, J.C., *Acta Orthop. Traumat. Surg.*, *97*, 111–116 (1980).
28. Pilliar, R.M., Lee, J.M., and Maniatopoulos, C., *Clin. Orthop.*, *208*, 108–113 (1986).
29. Kohn, D.H., Ko, C.C., and Hollister, S.J., in *1992 Advances in Bioengineering*, BED-Vol. 22 (M.W. Bidez, ed.), New York: American Society of Mechanical Engineers, 1992, pp. 297–300.

30. Kohn, D.H., Ko, C.C., and Hollister, S.J., *Advances in Bioengineering 1993*, BED-Vol. 26 (J.M. Tarbell, ed.), New York: American Society of Mechanical Engineers, 1993, pp. 231–224.

31. Ducheyne, P., Martens, M., De Meester, P., and Mulier, J., in *ASTM STP 796 Titanium Alloys in Surgical Implants* (Luckey, H.A., and Kublsi, F., Jr. eds.), Baltimore, MD: ASTM, 1983, pp. 265–279.

32. Rohlmann, A., Cheal, E.J., Hayes, W.C., and Bergmann, G., *J. Biomech.*, *21*, 605–611 (1988).

33. Ducheyne, P., De Meester, P., Aemoudt, E., Martens, M., and Mulier, J.C., *J. Biomed. Mater. Res.*, *11*, 811–838 (1977).

34. Bobyn, J.D., Pilliar, R.M., Binnington, A.G., and Szivek, J.A., *J. Orthop. Res.*, *5*, 393–408 (1987).

35. Black, J., *Biological Performance of Materials—Fundamentals of Biocompatibility*, New York: Dekker, 1992.

36. Stauffer, R.N., *J. Bone Joint Surg.*, *64A*, 983–990 (1982).

37. Ducheyne, P., and Lemons, J.E. (eds.), *Bioceramics: Material Characteristics versus In vivo Behavior*, New York: NY Acad. Sci., 1987.

38. Ducheyne, P., *J. Biomed. Mater. Res.: Appl. Biomat.*, *21*(A2), 219–236 (1987).

39. Merget, M., and Aldinger, F., in *Titanium, Science and Technology* (Lutjering, G., Zwicker, U., and Bunk W., eds.), Oberursel, Germany: Deutsche Gesellschaft für Metallkunde, 1985, pp. 1393–1398.

40. Homsy, C.A., Cain, T.E., Kessler, F.B., Anderson, M.S., and King, J.W., *Clin. Orthop.*, *89*, 220–235 (1972).

41. Spector, M., Davis, R.J., Lunceford, E.M., and Harmon, S.L., *Clin. Orthop.*, *176*, 34–41 (1983).

42. Hench, L.L., Splinter, R.J., Allen, W.C., and Greenlee, T.K., Jr., *J. Biomed. Mater. Res. Symp.*, *2*, 117–141 (1972).

43. Rijke, A.M., and Rieger, M.R., *J. Biomed. Mater. Res.*, *11*, 373–394 (1977).

44. Smith, L., *Arch. Surg.*, *87*, 653–661 (1963).

45. Ducheyne, P., Martens, M., Aemoudt, E., Mulier, J., and De Meester, P., *Acta Orthop. Belg.*, *40*, 799–805 (1974).

46. Hirschhorn, J.S., and Reynolds, J.T., in *Research in Dental and Medical Materials* (Korostoff, E., ed.), New York: Plenum Press, 1969, pp. 137–150.

47. Welsh, R.P., Pilliar, R.M., and Macnab, I., *J. Bone Joint Surg.*, *53A*, 963–977 (1971).

48. Hahn, H., and Palich, W., *J. Biomed. Mater. Res.*, *4*, 571–577 (1970).

49. Morscher, E., in *The Cementless Fixation of Hip Endoprostheses* (Morscher, E., ed.), Berlin: Springer-Verlag, 1984, pp. 1–8.

50. Chandler, H., Reineck, F.T., Wixson, R.L., and McCarthy, J.C., *J. Bone Joint Surg.*, *63A*, 1426–1434 (1981).

51. Kavanagh, B.F., Ilstrup, D.M., and Fitzgerald, R.H., *J. Bone Joint Surg.*, *67A*, 517–526 (1985).

52. Friedman, R.J., Black, J., Galante, J.O., Jacobs, J.J., and Skinner, H.B., *J. Bone Joint Surg.*, *75A*, 1086–1109 (1993).

53. Kohn, D.H., Ducheyne, P., Cuckler, J.M., Chu, A., and Radin, S., *Medical Progress Through Technology*, *20*, 169–177 (1994).

54. Chao, E.Y.S., and Coventry, M.B., *J. Bone Joint Surg.*, *63A*, 1078–1094 (1981).

55. Cameron, H.U., and McNeice, G.M., *Clin. Orthop.*, *150*, 154–158 (1980).

56. Topoleski, L.D.T., Ducheyne, P., and Cuckler, J.M., *J. Biomed. Mater. Res.*, *24*, 135–154 (1990).

57. Hood, R.W., Wright, T.M., and Burstein, A.H., *J. Biomed. Mater. Res.*, *17*, 829–842 (1983).

58. Charnley, J., *Low Friction Arthroplasty of the Hip: Theory and Practice*, Berlin: Springer-Verlag, 1979.

59. Collier, J.P. Surprenant, V.A., Jensen, R.E., and Mayor, M.B., *Clin. Orthop.*, *271*, 305–312 (1991).
60. Willert, H.G., and Semlitsch, M., *J. Biomed. Mater. Res.*, *11*, 157–164 (1977).
61. McKellop, H. A., Sarmiento, A., Schwinn, C. P., and Ebramzadeh, E., *J. Bone Joint Surg.*, *72A*, 512–517 (1990).
62. Maloney, W.J., Jasty, M., Harris, W.H., Galante, J.O., and Callaghan, J.J., *J. Bone Joint Surg.*, *72A*, 1025–1034 (1990).
63. Kohn, D.H., and Ducheyne, P., in *Medical and Dental Materials* (D.F. Williams, ed.), *Materials Science and Technology—A Comprehensive Treatment* (R.W. Cahn, P. Haasen, and E.J. Kramer, ser. eds.), Germany: VCH Verlagsgesellschaft, 1992, pp. 29–109.
64. Maloney, W.J., Jasty, M., Rosenberg, A., and Harris, W.H., *J. Bone Joint Surg.*, *72B*, 966–970 (1990).
65. Jasty, M.J., Floyd, W.E., III, Schiller, A.L., Goldring, S.R., and Harris, W.H., *J. Bone Joint Surg.*, *68A*, 912–919 (1986).
66. Jacobs, J.J., Urban, R.M., Schajowicz, F., Gavrilovic, J., and Galante, J.O., in *Biocompatibility of Particulate Implant Materials* (St. John, K., ed.), Philadelphia: ASTM, 1992.
67. Willert, H.G., Bertram, H., and Buchhorn, G.H., *Clin. Orthop.* *258*, 108–121 (1990).
68. Anthony, P.P., Gie, G.A., Howie, D.W., and Ling, R.S., *J. Bone Joint Surg.*, *72B*, 971–979 (1990).
69. Schmalzried, T.P., and Harris, W.H., *J. Bone Joint Surg.*, *74A*, 1130–1139 (1992).
70. Goldring, S.R., Schiller, A.L., Roelke, M., Rourke, C.M., O'Neil, D.A., and Harris, W.H., *J. Bone Joint Surg.*, *65A*, 575–584 (1983).
71. Goodman, S.B., Chin, R.C., Chiou, S.S., Schurman, D.J., Woolson, S.T., and Masada, M.P., *Clin. Orthop.*, *244*, 182–187 (1989).
72. Howie, D.W., Vernon-Roberts, B., Oakeshott, R., and Manthey, B., *J. Bone Joint Surg.*, *70A*, 257–263 (1988).
73. Shanbhag, A.S., Jacobs, J.J., Glant, T.T., Gilbert, J.L., Black, J., and Galante, J.O., *Trans. Soc. Biomat.*, *15*, 29 (1993).
74. Ducheyne, P., De Meester, P., Aernoudt, E., Martens, M., and Mulier, J.C., *J. Biomed. Mater. Res. Symp.*, *6*, 199–219 (1975).
75. Pilliar, R.M., *Clin. Orthop.*, *176*, 42–51 (1983).
76. Yue, S., Pilliar, R.M., and Weatherly, G.C., *J. Biomed. Mater. Res.*, *18*, 1043–1058 (1984).
77. Ranawat, C.S., Johanson, N.A., Rimnac, C.M., Wright, T.M., and Schwartz, R.E., *Clin. Orthop.*, *209*, 244–248 (1986).
78. Morrey, B.F., and Chao, E.Y.S., *Clin. Orthop.*, *228*, 182–189 (1988).
79. Cook, S.D., and Thomas, K.A., *J. Bone Joint Surg.*, *73B*, 20–24 (1991).
80. Rosenqvist, R., Bylander, B., Knutson, K., Rydholm, U., Rooser, B., Egund, N., and Lidgren, L., *J. Bone Joint Surg.*, *68A*, 538–542 (1986).
81. Wevers, H.W., and Cooke, T.D.V., Bead loosening in porous coated orthopaedic implants: A case study, *Clin. Mater.*, *2*, 67–74 (1987).
82. Black, J., *Biomaterials*, *5*, 11–18 (1984).
83. Jacobs, J.J., Skipor, A.K., Black, J., Urban, R.M., and Galante, J.O., *J. Bone Joint Surg.*, *73A*, 1475–1486 (1991).
84. Sunderman, F.W., Jr., Hopfer, S.M., Swift, T., Rezuke, W.N., Ziebka, L., Highman, P., Edwards, B., Folcik, M., and Gossling, H.R., *J. Orthop. Res.*, *7*, 307–315 (1989).
85. Bianco, P.D., and Ducheyne, P., *Trans. Orthop. Res. Soc.*, *39*, 295 (1993).
86. Williams, D.F. (ed.), *Biocompatibility of Clinical Implant Materials*, Boca Raton, FL: CRC Press, Vol. 1, 1980.
87. Lalor, P.A., Revell, P.A., Gray, A.B., Wright, S., Railton, G.T., and Freeman, M.A.R., *J. Bone Joint Surg.*, *73B*, 25–28 (1991).
88. Gil-Albarova, J., Lacleriga, A., Barrios, C., and Canadell, J., *J. Bone Joint Surg.*, *74B*, 825–830 (1992).

89. Penman, H.G., and Ring, P.A., *J. Bone Joint Surg.*, *66B*, 632–634 (1984).
90. Ward, J.J., Thornbury, D.D., Lemons, J.E., and Dunham, W.K., *Clin. Orthop.*, *252*, 299–306 (1990).
91. Brien, W.W., Salvati, E.A., Healey, J.H., Bansal, M., Ghelman, B., and Betts, F., *J. Bone Joint Surg.*, *72A*, 1097–1099 (1990).
92. Lang, B.R., Morris, H.F., and Razzoog, M.E. (eds.), *International Workshop—Biocompatibility, Toxicity and Hypersensitivity to Alloy Systems Used in Dentistry*, Ann Arbor, MI, 1985.
93. St. John, K. (ed.), *The Biocompatibility of Particulate Implant Materials*, Philadelphia: ASTM, 1992.
94. Kovacs, P., and Davidson, J. A., *Trans. Soc. Biomat.*, *16*, 198 (1990).
95. McKellop, B., Clarke, I., Markolf, K., and Amstutz, H., *J. Biomed. Mater. Res.*, *15*, 619–653 (1981).
96. McKellop, B.A., and Rostlund, T.V., *J. Biomed. Mater. Res.*, *24*, 1413–1425.
97. Hsu, H.P., and Walker, P.S., *Clin. Orthop.*, *246*, 260–265 (1989).
98. Rose, R.M., Ries, M.D., Paul, I.L., Crugnola, A.M., and Ellis, E., *J. Biomed. Mater. Res.*, *18*, 207–224 (1984).
99. McKellop, H.A., Clarke, I.C., Markolf, K.L., and Amstutz, H.C., *J. Biomed. Mater. Res.*, *12*, 895–927 (1978).
100. Rose, R.M., Nusbaum, H.J., Schneider, H., Ries, M., Paul, I., Crugnola, A., Simon, S.R., and Radin, E.L., *J. Bone Joint Surg.*, *62A*, 537–549 (1980).
101. Charnley, J., and Halley, D., *Clin. Orthop.*, *112*, 170 (1975).
102. Hastings, G.W., *Wear*, *55*, 1 (1979).
103. Nagy, E. V., and Li, S., *Trans. Soc. Biomat.*, *16*, 109 (1990).
104. Eyerser, P., Kurth, M., McKellop, H.A., and Mittlmeier, T., *J. Biomed. Mater. Res.*, *21*, 275–291 (1987).
105. Bartel, D.L., Bicknell, V.L., and Wright, T.M., *J. Bone Joint Surg.*, *68A*, 1041–1051 (1986).
106. Farling, G., and Bardos, D., *Proc. 3rd Conf. on Materials for Use in Medicine and Biology*, Keele University, 1978.
107. Stretcher, R.M., *Trans. Soc. Biomat.*, *17*, 181 (1991).
108. Li, S., and Howard, E.G., *Trans. Soc. Biomat.*, *16*, 190 (1990).
109. Griss, P., Silber, R., Merkle, B., Haehner, K., Heimke, G., and Krempien, B., *J. Biomed. Mater. Res. Symp.*, *7*, 519–528 (1976).
110. Salzer, M., Zweymuller, K., Cocke, H., Zeibig, A., Stark, N., Plenk, H., Jr., and Punzet, G., *J. Biomed. Mater. Res.*, *10*, 847–856 (1976).
111. Boutin, P., Christel, P., Dorlot, J.M., Meunier, A., de Roquancourt, A., Blanquaert, D., Herman, S., Sedel, L., and Witvoet, J., *J. Biomed. Mater. Res.*, *22*, 1203–1232 (1988).
112. Hench, L.L., and Ethridge, E.C., *Biomaterials: An Interfacial Approach*, New York: Academic Press 1982.
113. Frakes, J.T., Brown, S.D., and Kenner, G.H., *Am. Ceram. Soc. Bull.*, *53*, 183–187 (1974).
114. Walter, A., and Lang, W., in *Biomedical Materials*, Mater. Res. Soc. Symp. Proc. Vol. 55 (Williams, J.M., Nichols, M.F., and Zingg, W., eds.), Pittsburgh, PA: Materials Research Society, 1986, pp. 181–190.
115. Plitz, W., and Hoss, H.U., in *Biomaterials 1980* (Winter, G.D., Gibbons, D.F., and Plenk, H., eds.), New York: Wiley, 1980, pp. 187–196.
116. Christel, P., Meunier, A., Heller, M., Tome, J.P., and Peille, C.N., *J. Biomed. Mater. Res.*, *23*, 45–61 (1989).
117. Kumar, P., Oka, M., Ikeuchi, K., Shimizu, K., Yamamuro, T., Okumura, H., and Kotoura, Y., *J. Biomed. Mater. Res.*, *25*, 813–828 (1991).
118. Restoker, W., and Galante, J.O., *Biomaterials*, *2*, 221–224 (1981).
119. Peterson, C.D., Hillberry, B.M., and Heck, D.A., *J. Biomed. Mater. Res.*, *22*, 887–903 (1988).

120. Hirvonen, J.K., Carosella, C.A., Kant, R.A., Singer, I., Vardiman, R., and Rath, B.B., *Thin Solid Films, 63*, 5-10 (1979).

121. Streicher, R.M., Weber, H., Schon, R., and Semlitsch, M., *Biomaterials, 12*, 125-129 (1991).

122. Ducheyne, P., and Healy, K.E., in *Surface Characterization of Biomaterials* (Ratner, B., ed.), Amsterdam: Elsevier, 1988, pp. 175-192.

123. Ratner, B., Johnston, A.B., and Lenk, T.J., *J. Biomed. Mater. Res.: Appl. Biomat., 21*(A1), 59-90 (1987).

124. Kasemo, B., *J. Pros. Dent., 49*, 832-837 (1983).

125. Healy, K.E., and Ducheyne, P., *J. Colloid Interface Sci.*, in press.

126. Kilner, T., Pilliar, R.M., Weatherly, G.C., and Allibert, C., *J. Biomed. Mater. Res., 16*, 63-79 (1982).

127. Sullivan, C.P., Donachie, M.J., Jr., and Moral, F.R., *Cobalt Based Superalloys*, Brussels: Centre de Information de Cobalt 1970.

128. Dobbs, H.S., and Robertson, J.L.M., *J. Mater. Sci., 18*, 391 (1983).

129. Spires, W.P., Kelman, D.C., and Pafford, J.A., in *ASTM STP 953: Quantitative Characterization and Performance of Porous Implants for Hard Tissue Applications* (Lemons, J.E., ed.), Philadelphia, PA: ASTM, 1987, pp. 47-59.

130. Devine, T.M., and Wulff, J., *J. Biomed. Mater. Res., 9*, 151-167 (1975).

131. Ducheyne, P., Kohn, D., and Smith, T.S., *Biomaterials, 8*, 223-227 (1987).

132. Stubbington, C.A., and Bowen, A.W., *J. Mater. Sci., 9*, 941-947 (1974).

133. Stubbington, C.A., *AGARD Conf. Proc.*, No. 185, 1976, pp. 3.1-3.19.

134. Peters, M., Gysler, A., and Lutjering, G., in *Titanium '80: Science and Technology* (Kimura, H., and Izumi, O., eds.), Warrendale, PA: The Metallurgical Society of AIME, 1980, pp. 1777-1786.

135. Margolin, H., Williams, J.C., Chesnutt, J.C., and Lutjering, G., in *Titanium '80: Science and Technology* (Kimura, H., and Izumi, O., eds.), Warrendale, PA: The Metallurgical Society of AIME, 1980, pp. 169-216.

136. Lutjering, G., and Gysler, A., in *Titanium, Science and Technology* (Lutjering, G., Zwicker, U., and Bunk W., eds.), Oberursel, Germany: Deutsche Gesellschaft für Metallkunde, 1985, pp. 2065-2083.

137. Lutjering, G., Gysler, A., and Wagner, L., in *Titanium Science and Technology* (Lacombe, P., Tricot, R., and Beranger, G., eds.), Paris: Les Editions de Physique, 1989, pp. 71-80.

138. Georgette, F.S., and Davidson, J.A., *J. Biomed. Mater. Res., 20*, 1229-1248 (1986).

139. Wolfarth, D., Filiaggi, M., and Ducheyne, P., *J. Appl. Biomat., 1*, 3-12 (1990).

140. Kohn, D.H., and Ducheyne, P., *J. Mater. Sci., 26*, 534-544 (1991).

141. Soltesz, S.M., Smickley, R.J., and Dardi, L.E., in *Titanium, Science and Technology* (Lutjering, G., Zwicker, U., and Bunk, W., eds.), Oberursel, Germany: Deutsche Gesellsehaft für Metallkunde, 1985, pp. 187-194.

142. Kerr, W.R., Smith, P.R., Rosenblum, M.E., Gurney, F.J., Mahajan, Y.R., and Bidwell, L.R., in: *Titanium '80: Science and Technology* (Kimura, H., and Izumi, O., eds.), Warrendale, PA: The Metallurgical Society of AIME, 1980, pp. 2477-2486.

143. Levin, L., Vogt, R.G., Eylon, D., and Froes, F.H., in *Titanium, Science and Technology* (Lutjering, G., Zwicker, U., and Bunk ,W., eds.), Oberursel, Germany: Deutsche Gesellschaft für Metallkunde, 1985, pp. 2107-2114.

144. Eylon, D., and Pierce, C.M., *Met. Trans. A, 7A*, 111-121 (1976).

145. Kohn, D.H., in *Handbook of Advanced Materials Testing* (Cheremisinoff, N.P., and Cheremisinoff, P.N., eds.), New York: Marcel Dekker, 1995, pp. 593-627.

146. Kohn, D.H., Ducheyne, P., and Awerbuch, J., *J. Mater. Sci., 27*, 3133-3142 (1992).

147. Kohn, D.H., Ducheyne, P., and Awerbuch, J., *J. Mater. Sci., 27*, 1633-1641 (1992).

148. Hoar, T.P., and Mears, D.C., *Proc. R. Soc., London, A294*, 486 (1992).

149. Lacombe, P., in *Titanium and Titanium Alloys* (Williams, J.C., and Belov, A.F., eds.), New York: Plenum Press, 1982, pp. 847-880.

150. Koegel, A., and Black, J., *J. Biomed. Mater. Res., 18,* 513–522 (1984).
151. Brown, S.A., Merritt, K., Farnsworth, L.J., and Crowe, T.D., in *ASTM STP 953: Quantitative Characterization and Performance of Porous Implants for Hard Tissue Applications* (Lemons, J.E., ed.), Philadelphia, PA: ASTM, 1987, pp. 163–181.
152. Brown, S.A., Farnsworth, L.J., Merritt, K., and Crowe, T.D., *J. Biomed. Mater. Res., 22,* 321–338 (1988).
153. Merritt, K., Crowe, T.D., and Brown, S.A., *J. Biomed. Mater. Res., 23,* 845–862 (1989).
154. Wapner, K.L., Morris, D.M., and Black, J., *J. Biomed. Mater. Res., 20,* 219–233 (1986).
155. Ducheyne. P., Willems, G., Martens, M., and Helsen, J., *J. Biomed. Mater. Res., 18,* 293–308 (1984).
156. Ducheyne, P., and Healy, K.E., *J. Biomed. Mater. Res., 22,* 1137–1163 (1988).
157. Saha, S., and Pal, S., *J. Biomed. Mater. Res., 18,* 435–462 (1984).
158. Krause, W., and Mathis, R.S., *J. Biomed. Mater. Res.: Appl. Biomat.,* 22(A1),: 37–53 (1988).
159. de Wijn, J. R., Slooff, T.J.J.H., and Driessens, F.C.M., *Acta. Orthop. Scand., 46,* 38–51 (1975).
160. Wixson, R.L., Lautenschlager, E.P., and Novak, M., *Trans. 31st Orthop. Res. Soc.,* 1985.
161. Burke, D.W., Gates, E.I., and Harris, W.H., *J. Bone Joint Surg., 66A,* 1265–1273 (1984).
162. Davies, J.P., Burke, D.W., O'Connor, D.O., and Harris, W.H., *J. Orthop. Res., 5,* 366–371 (1987).
163. Topoleski, L.D.T., Ducheyne, P., and Cuckler, J.M., *Trans. Soc. Biomat., 17,* 48 (1991).
164. Rimnac, C. M., Wright, T.M., and McGill, D.L., *J. Bone Joint. Surg., 68A,* 281–287 (1986).
165. Knoell, A., Maxwell, H., and Bechtol, C., *Ann. Biomed. Eng., 3,* 225–229 (1975).
166. Pilliar, R.M., Blackwell, R., Macnab, I., and Cameron, H.U., *J. Biomed. Mater. Res., 10,* 893–906 (1976).
167. Wright, T.M., and Robinson, R.P., *J. Mater. Sci., 17,* 2463–2468 (1982).
168. Saha, S., and Pal, S., *J. Biomech., 17,* 467–478 (1984).
169. Pourdeyhimi, B., Robinson, H.H., IV, Schwartz, P., and Wagner, H.D., *Ann. Biomed. Eng., 14,* 277–294 (1986).
170. Wright, T.M., and Trent, P.S., *J. Mater. Sci., 14,* 503–505 (1979).
171. Taitsman, J.P., and Saha, S., *J. Bone Joint Surg., 59A,* 419–425 (1977).
172. Fishbane, B.M., and Pond, R.B., *Clin. Orthop., 128,* 194–199 (1977).
173. Schnur, D. S., and Lee, D., *J. Biomed. Mater. Res., 17,* 973–991 (1983).
174. Topoleski, L.D.T., Ducheyne, P., and Cuckler, J.M., *J. Biomed. Mater. Res., 26,* 1599–1617 (1992).
175. Beaumont, P.W.R., *J. Mater. Sci., 12,* 1845–1852 (1977).
176. Pourdeyhimi, B., and Wagner, H.D., *J. Biomed. Mater. Res., 23,* 63–80 (1989).
177. Murakami, A., Behiri, J. C., and Bonfield, W., *Trans. 3rd World Biomat. Cong.,* 1988, p. 334.
178. Topoleski, L.D.T., Ph.D. Dissertation, University of Pennsylvania, 1990.
179. Litsky, A.S., Rose, R.M., and Rubin, C.T., in *Biomedical Materials,* Mater. Res. Soc. Symp. Proc., Vol. 55 (Williams, J.M., Nichols, M.F., and Zingg, W., eds.), Pittsburgh, PA: Materials Research Society, 1986, pp. 171–179.
180. Weightman, B., Freeman, M.A.R., Revell, P.A., Braden, M., Albrektsson, B.E.J., and Carlson, L.V., *J. Bone Joint Surg., 69B,* 558–564 (1987).
181. Park, H.C., Liu, Y.K., and Lakes, R.S., *J. Biomech. Eng., 108,* 141–148 (1986).
182. Henrich, D.E., Cram, A.E., Park, J.B., Liu, Y.K., and Reddi, H., *J. Biomed. Mater. Res., 27,* 277–280 (1993).
183. Dandurand, J., Delpech, V., LeBugle, A., Lamure, A., and Lacabanne, C., *J. Biomed. Mater. Res., 24,* 1377–1384 (1990).
184. Nishimura, N., Yamamuro, T., Taguchi, Y., Ikenaga, M., Nakamura, T., Kokubo, T., and Yoshihara, S., *J. Appl. Biomat., 2,* 219–229 (1991).
185. Kawanabe, K., Tamura, J., Yamamuro, T., Nakamura, T., Kokubo, T., and Yoshihara, S., *J. Appl. Biomat., 4,* 135–141 (1993).

186. Gerhart, T.N., Miller, R.L., Kleshinski, S.J., and Hayes, W.C., *J. Biomed. Mater. Res., 22*, 1071–1082 (1988).
187. Van Raemdonck, W., Ducheyne, P., and De Meester, P., in *Metal and Ceramic Biomaterials*, Vol. 2, *Strength and Surface* (Ducheyne, P., and Hastings, G.W., eds.), Boca Raton, FL: CRC Press, 1984, pp. 143–166.
188. Gross, U.M., and Strunz, V., *J. Biomed. Mater. Res., 14*, 607–618 (1980).
189. Nakamura, T., Yamamuro, T., Higashi, S., Kokubo, T., and Ito, S., *J. Biomed. Mater. Res., 19*, 685–698 (1985).
190. Kokubo, T., Ito, S., Huang, Z.T., Hayashi, T., Sakka, S., Kitsugi, T., and Yamamuro, T., *J. Biomed. Mater. Res., 24*, 331–343 (1990).
191. Koeneman, J., Lemons, Ducheyne, P., Lacefield, W., Magee, F., Calahan, T., and Kay, J., *J. Appl. Biomat., 1*, 79–90 (1990).
192. Posner, A.S., *Clin. Orthop., 200*, 87–99 (1985).
193. Ducheyne, P., Van Raemdonck, W., Heughebaert, J.C., and Heughebaert, M., *Biomaterials, 7*, 97–103 (1986).
194. Ducheyne, P., Radin, S., Heughebaert, M., and Heughebaert, J.C., *Biomaterials, 11*, 244–254 (1990).
195. Berry, J.L., Geiger, J.M., Moran, J.M., Skraba, J.S., and Greenwald, A.S., *J. Biomed. Mater. Res., 20*, 65–77 (1986).
196. Teske, D.A., Mayor, M.B., Collier, J.P., and Surprenant, V.A., *Trans. 35th Orthop. Res. Soc.*, 1989, p. 333.
197. Chang, F.K., Perez, J.P., and Davidson, J.A., *J. Biomed. Mater. Res., 24*, 873–899 (1990).
198. Skinner, H.B., *Clin. Orthop., 235*, 224–236 (1988).
199. Latour, R.A., Jr., Black, J., and Miller, B., *J. Comp. Mater., 26*, 256–273 (1991).
200. Magee, F.P., Weinstein, A.M., Longo, J.A., Koeneman, J.B., and Yapp, R.A., *Clin. Orthop., 235*, 237–252 (1988).
201. Adams, D., Williams, D.F., and Hill, J., *J. Biomed. Mater. Res., 12*, 35–42 (1978).
202. Christel, P.S., *CRC Crit. Rev. Biocompat., 2*, 189–218 (1986).
203. Iyer, L.S., Jayasekaran, T., Blunck, C.F.J., and Selvam, R.P., *Biomed. Sci. Instrum., 19*, 57 (1983).
204. Esper, F.J., Harms, J., Mittlemeier, H., and Gohl, W., in *Biomedical Materials*, Mater. Res. Soc. Symp. Proc., Vol. 55 (Williams, J.M., Nichols, M.F., and Zingg, W. eds.), Pittsburgh, PA: Materials Research Society, 1986, pp. 203–210.
205. Hollister, S.J., and Kikuchi, N., *Comput. Mech., 10*, 73–95 (1992).
206. Ahmed, S., and Jones, F.R., *J. Mater. Sci., 25*, 4933–4942 (1990).
207. Kohn, D.H., Ko, C.C., and Hollister, S.J., in *1992 Advances in Bioengineering*, BED-Vol. 22 (M. W. Bidez, ed.), New York: American Society of Mechanical Engineers, 1992, pp. 607–610.
208. Berlin, A.A., Volfson, S.A., Enikolopian, N.S., and Negmatov, S.S., *Principles of Polymer Composites*, New York: Springer-Verlag, 1986.
209. Broutman, L.J., *J. Adhesion, 2*, 147 (1970).
210. Latour, R.A., Jr., and Black, J., *J. Biomed. Mater. Res., 26*, 593–606 (1992).
211. Latour, R.A., Jr., and Black, J., *J. Biomed. Mater. Res., 27*, 1281–1291 (1993).
212. Hollister, S.J., Fyhrie, D.P., Jepsen, K.J., and Goldstein, S.A., *J. Biomech., 24*, 825–839 (1991).
213. Cook, S.D., Thongpreda, N., Anderson, R.C., and Haddad, R.J., Jr., *J. Biomed. Mater. Res., 22*, 287–302 (1988).
214. Pilliar, R.M., Bratina, W.J., and Blackwell, R., in ASTM STP 636, *Fatigue of Filamentary Composite Materials* (Reifsnider, K.L., Lauraitis, K.N., eds.), Philadelphia: ASTM, 1977, pp. 206–227.
215. Robinson, R.P., Wright, T.M., and Burstein, A.H., *J. Biomed. Mater. Res., 15*, 203–208 (1981).
216. Saha, S., and Pal S., *J. Biomed. Mater. Res., 20*, 817–826 (1986).

5

Failure Analysis of Metallic Orthopedic Devices

Lyle D. Zardiackas and Lance D. Dillon
The University of Mississippi Medical Center
Jackson, Mississippi

I. INTRODUCTION

Failure, as defined by *Webster's* [1], is paraphrased as the omission or inability to perform a function. This definition provides an interesting dilemma to the scientist or engineer when retrieved implanted devices that have reportedly failed are examined. Since the function of implanted metallic orthopedic devices may or may not be to serve as definitive substitutes for bone, assessment of success or failure is often dependent on the intended application rather than only on whether or not the device has fractured or deteriorated to the point at which it is no longer useful. It is, therefore, imperative to carefully consider the function of the device when assessing success or failure. Additionally, unlike many other devices such as automobile crankshafts, train axles, aircraft wings, etc., prediction of the physiological loads that will be placed on the implant by an individual patient and the biological changes that may occur is not possible. If these factors do not make analysis difficult enough, success or failure of the implant to fulfill its intended function over the life cycle for which it was designed is often tied to the psychology and compliance of the patient. When assessing the adequacy of a device, especially a fracture fixation device, it is important, therefore, to correlate the "failure" of the device with patient record information, which is useful in determining the patient's physiology and psychology during healing.

The intended function of the implant and the degree to which it fulfills its purpose will certainly affect the outcome of the patient's recovery. In establishing intended function it is necessary to point out that metallic orthopedic devices may be separated into two categories: (1) Fracture fixation devices are used to anatomically align and, in some cases, to compress the bone at the fracture site to promote healing. Since fracture fixation devices are not designed as definitive replacements for the bone, it is generally anticipated that they will serve their intended purpose for periods of up to approximately 6 months in a load-sharing capacity as bone heals. Sometimes devices are removed after bone healing occurs. (2) Metallic prostheses are devices designed for long-term replacement of hard tissue (bone). Generally, these devices are used as replacements for joints and are intended to remain in the patient for extended periods (years) without the need for replacement.

II. IMPLANTS FOR FRACTURE FIXATION AND JOINT REPLACEMENT

Implants for fracture fixation are designed to provide for stabilization in cases in which bone fracture has occurred, bone is missing due to osteotomy or trauma, or fusion at joints is desired. These devices are placed by orthopedic surgeons to anatomically align the bone as it heals, and/or they are placed to both align and compress the opposing sides of the fractured bone in cases where this is possible and advisable. Since the sites at which fixation are needed is highly variable and since it is not possible to design and manufacture fracture fixation devices for each individual application or patient, great versatility and adaptability of these implants are required. Various sizes and types of plates, nails, screws, wires, etc., which may be further customized during surgery to meet specific anatomical conditions, have been developed; but this array of devices cannot be infinite.

Prostheses are designed to be replacements for bone. Metallic prostheses are most often designed to be replacements for joints and are often thought of as permanent. They should not, however, be considered permanent replacements since they are subject to the same physiological environment that caused failure of the original biological joint. While the intent is that they will be as permanent as possible, it is recognized that implant degradation begins once it is placed or, at least, as soon as it is loaded. As is the case with fracture fixation devices, there are numerous manufacturers of prosthetic implants. Various sizes, types, and material combinations are used in the manufacture of prostheses such as hip, knee, shoulder, and finger joints. Unlike the situation with fracture fixation devices, there has been success in providing custom prostheses. This success has been possible for a variety of reasons but primarily it is related to economics and the fact that joints are used for a single specific application. As an example, a hip prosthesis is not used to replace a knee; but a fracture fixation plate may be used for various applications and on more than one type of bone.

Regardless of the stringent requirements placed upon the manufactured implants, environmental variations placed upon them by biology, coupled with the demands placed upon them by biomechanics and patient motion, will sometimes lead to fracture of an implant. Fracture of the implant does not necessarily mean that the implant has failed to provide its primary function. Complications arising from any one or more of the following factors may contribute to or cause fracture prior to healing of the bone:

1. Loosening of the implant due to bone resorption
2. Delayed union or nonunion due to biological considerations
3. Secondary trauma at or near the original fracture site
4. Overloading of the implant by the patient
5. Inadequate reduction or alignment
6. Improper implant handling during placement
7. Implant degradation due to biological considerations
8. Implant wear

Great care has been taken here to elucidate these concepts because of the use or misuse of the term *implant failure*. This terminology is used by those knowledgeable in the field to describe the failure of an implant to achieve its intended function due to inadequacy of materials, design, or manufacturing defects that render the device unusable. Material defect levels must be compared with values defined by the appropriate specifications for the specific material of which the implant is made. The existence of manufacturing defects must be determined based upon the appropriate manufacturing documents for the specific device, as well as upon American Society for Testing and Materials (ASTM) [2] and the International Standards Organization (ISO) specifications, where appropriate. Design defects are much more difficult to determine and must be examined based upon consideration of research data documenting the fundamental development, *in vitro* evaluation, and probably more importantly, the use of the device under controlled conditions in patients. Input from experts in biomaterials, biomechanics, and certainly from orthopaedic surgeons is required to evaluate the suitability of a device for its intended application. It must always be recognized that fracture of a device does not necessarily mean failure or even inadequate design, faulty material, or surgical error. In the instances of failed fracture fixation devices that have been examined in our laboratories, the patient, more often than not, failed to heal in a reasonable time period or placed mechanical stresses on the implant beyond its design capabilities. The reasons for delayed union and nonunion of bone are varied and numerous; they are generally not in the control of the surgeon, implant, or device manufacturer; and patient noncompliance is often not easily discernible. In the case of failed prostheses, bone resorption, cement fracture, and fracture and/or wear of polymeric materials that constitute one side of a bearing surface are often responsible for, or at least contribute to, failure of the implant.

III. MATERIALS

A number of metallic materials are currently accepted for use in implants for orthopedics. These materials have been found to be appropriate based upon their physical, mechanical, electrochemical, and biological properties. The metals and alloys have been scrutinized; and evaluation and specification of their composition, and physical, mechanical, and electrochemical properties are delineated by the ASTM and ISO. Since these specifications are revised periodically and the material should be evaluated according to the document pertaining to that material and implant, it is important that the appropriate document be referenced. Determination of such characteristics as the composition, grain structure, level and type of nonmetallic inclusions, existence and type of foreign phases, mechanical properties, and corrosion susceptibility is a key part of the overall evaluation of the failure of an implant. If any of the parameters are found to deviate from the appropriate specifications, there is just cause to find the device faulty.

Most of the stainless steel currently used for fracture fixation devices is implant quality, grade 2/316L austenitic stainless steel. The specifications for this material are specifically covered by ASTM F138 and F139. The structure of austenitic stainless steel, which is face-centered cubic, defines the mechanism of atomic motion and thus crack propagation. Most of this material is supplied to device manufacturers in the work- or strain-hardened condition to achieve higher strength. The grain structure of the work-hardened material, therefore, shows a highly twinned, single-phase microstructure (Fig. 1a). While sensitization and grain boundary precipitation of carbides is a rare occurrence in this material, due to the low level of carbon ($<0.03\%$ for grade 2), examination of the microstructure for grain boundary precipitates is a necessity. Should carbide precipitates

(a)

(b)

Figure 1   (a) Microstructure of cold-worked 316L stainless steel (100×). (b) Globular oxide (Type D) and sulfide stringer (Type A) inclusions in 316L stainless steel (100×).

in the grain boundaries exist, they would be the first indication of increased corrosion susceptibility of the material. The material should be relatively free of inclusions; and it is important that inclusions be rated in both transverse and longitudinal directions since inclusions such as sulfide, alumina, and silicate types are elongated during cold working (Fig. 1b). Inclusions at too high a level may result in premature crack initiation, since they may act as stress concentrators. Several other stainless steel alloys are available and are currently in use. These alloys include 22-13-5 and Ortron 90, both of which have a higher concentration of Cr and lower concentration of Ni than is found in 316L stainless steel.

Titanium and titanium alloys constitute the second major material used in the manufacture of fracture fixation devices. α-Titanium exists at equilibrium at room temperature in the hexagonal close-packed structure (hcp). The structure is transformed to body-centered cubic (bcc), known as the β-structure, at 883°C. Commercially pure (CP) titanium is supplied in four grades, and the properties and composition are governed by ASTM F67. As the grade number increases from 1 to 4, the oxygen concentration increases and, therefore, the strength increases. The strength of this material may also be appreciably increased by work-hardening. The grain structure of CP titanium in the annealed condition and the grain structure in the transverse direction of cold-worked material show equiaxed grains with a structure free of appreciable inclusions (Fig. 2a). The titanium alloys generally used in orthopedic implants are Ti-6Al-4V and Ti-6Al-7Nb. These titanium alloys are two-phase α-β alloys whose properties are governed by ASTM F136 and ASTM F1295, respectively. Typical grain structures are shown in Figs. 2b and 2c. The alloys are significantly stronger than is CP titanium, but there continue to be questions concerning the biocompatibility of the vanadium-containing alloys.

Metals with Co and Cr as the primary alloying elements constitute the final major metallic system used in orthopedics. The cast alloy is governed by ASTM F75; and the wrought alloy, depending on composition, is governed by ASTM F90 or ASTM F799. These alloys also form single-phase microstructures. The grains in the as-cast condition are very large, and only a few grains may be visible in a transverse section of a casting (Fig. 3a). The grain structure of annealed-wrought ASTM F90 alloy is similar to that of the F75 cast alloy with rather large grains (Fig. 3b). The structure of ASTM F799 work-hardened wrought alloys is generally equiaxed with much smaller grains than either the cast alloy or the other wrought alloy (Fig. 3c).

IV. STRUCTURE AND BIOLOGY OF BONE

One of the most important aspects to consider when examining the failure of any type of orthopedic implant is how the host differs from nonliving systems. Although it is true that all systems change with environment and time (expand, contract, corrode, change phase, etc.), none changes with such dynamics as does a living, growing system such as bone. In addition to the functioning of the bone itself, the presence and interaction of soft tissues (muscles, ligaments, tendons, blood vessels, etc.) guide and often limit the implanted device in size, composition, properties, and form. It is the biology of the individual in which the device is implanted that controls design and limits the restoration of function. Failure to consider these factors can—and will, in many cases—lead to failure of function of the host, which is a far more profound consideration than failure of the device.

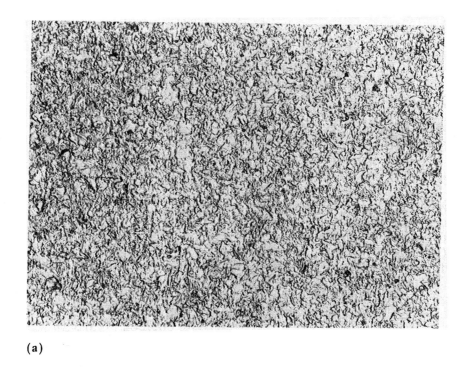

(a)

(b)

Figure 2   (a) Grain structure of cold-worked Grade 4 CP titanium (200×). (b) Grain structure of cold-worked Ti–6Al–4V alloy (200×). (c) Grain structure of cold-worked Ti–6Al–7Nb alloy (200×).

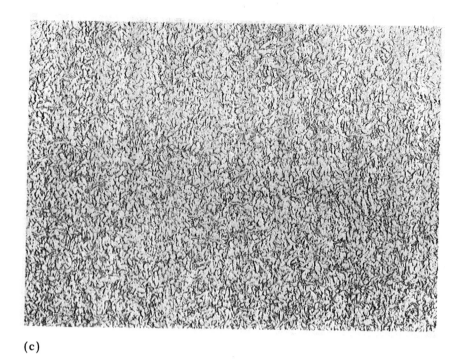

(c)

A. Ultrastructure of Bone

Bone can be defined as a connective tissue in a highly complex form that is composed of intertwined cells in an intercellular composite material of collagen fibrils, ground substance, and a mineral phase [3]. Osteoclasts, osteoblasts, and osteocytes are three major components of bone at the cellular level. A thorough discussion of bone on the cellular level can be found in many texts [3–5]. The bone matrix consists of between 35% [6] and 50% [7] collagen by volume. Bone mineral is described as very small crystals of hydroxyapatite. The mineral phase accounts for about 65% of the volume of bone matrix [3]. Once this tissue reaches maturity, hard, compact bone called *cortical bone* and porous, lamellar bone called *cancellous bone* exist.

The inside of the long bones has a cavity lined with a vascular areolar membrane called the *endosteum*. The cavities are filled with bone marrow. Haversian systems, which can be seen in a cross-sectional view of bone, consist of a central hole—or Haversian canal, lamellae, lacunae, canaliculi, and Volkmann's canals. The 0.05 mm diameter Haversian canals primarily house the one or two blood vessels, nerve filaments, and lymphatic vessels. Crosschannels, the Volkmann's canals, connect adjacent Haversian canals. The periosteum, a fibrous membrane enclosing the bone, provides a way for vessels to reach the hard tissue.

B. Mechanical Properties of Bone

Bone is elastic, hard, and tough in compression and tension. Cortical bone, which is the outer layer of bone, is dense and compact, and is often compared to reinforced concrete. The inner, or cancellous, bone consists of trabeculae and lamellae, which are tiny, slender

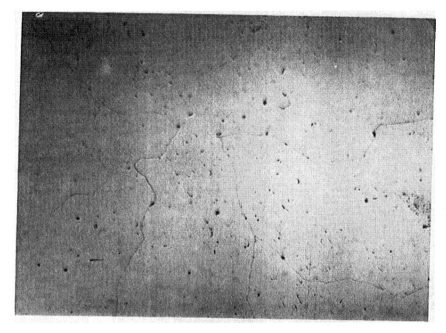

(a)

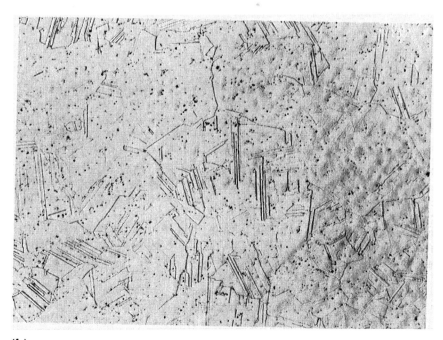

(b)

Figure 3 (a) Grain structure of cast Co–Cr ASTM F75 alloy (50×). (b) Grain structure of wrought Co–Cr ASTM F90 alloy (100×). (c) Grain structure of wrought Co–Cr ASTM F799 alloy (200×).

(c)

spicules. Both cortical and cancellous bone are porous; however, the difference in structure between the two depends upon the amount of solid matter and the size and spacing of the pores. The outside of most long bones is always cortical bone. The interior, however, may consist of cortical bone (shaft or diaphysis) or cancellous bone (metaphysis and epiphysis). The proportions of each type of bone varies from bone to bone and throughout the different parts of a single bone, depending on its particular use or function.

The elastic properties of bone can be defined by Hooke's law (elastic behavior). Physical stresses formed biologically are an absolute necessity for positive change in hard tissue, as well as soft tissue mechanical properties. Sufficient stress is required to stimulate adequate bone healing. The cellular response associated with bone growth is not fully understood. Other factors that significantly affect bone growth are time and strain. Therefore, *strain rate* becomes an important parameter when determining the mechanical stimulus [7]. Sometimes, the bone receives an insufficient amount of stress or strain, which hinders the bone remodeling activity. In some cases a fracture fixation device or prosthesis may adversely alter the mechanical distribution of load to the fracture site, joint, or other area in need of adequate bone remodeling. This phenomenon is commonly known as *stress or strain shielding*. Strain shielding may reduce the bone mineral content by an amount ranging from 7% to 78%, depending on factors such as age, activity level, and disease. The fact that there is persistent strain shielding of bone with time means that there is also persistent stress shielding. Persistent stress shielding, which increases with time, implies that the resorptive bone remodeling may not necessarily be in a state of equilibrium but may be progressive as healing occurs [8].

Important material properties inherent to all bone include *viscoelastic* and *anisotropic* behavior. Viscoelastic behavior describes the response dependence of the material over a specific period of time during loading and unloading of that material. In cortical bone, this response to change in loading is not very large. Bone is also anisotropic, which means that the strength of the bone varies with change in orientation of the bone [9]. In trabecular bone, mechanical properties are controlled by the apparent density. The strength of trabecular bone is related to the square of the apparent density and modulus to the cube of the apparent density.

Other parameters affecting remodeling are mineralization and demineralization (chemical work), which are controlled by nutrition, activity, hormones, and rest. Biological response to mechanical loading occurs not only axially, due to walking and exercise, but also transversely or circumferentially. The transverse biological response usually occurs in or around joints where forces on the bone are all but uniaxial. This response can sometimes appear in the form of cortical bone hypertrophy near the ends of a mechanically loaded intramedullary device or joint prosthesis. The nonsymmetrical loading seen in the shoulder, hip, and knee joints will sometimes generate localized bone remodeling near the tips of the prosthesis in the diaphyseal areas where the forces are concentrated. Consequently, other areas of the bone around the joint prosthesis may undergo stress shielding, which hinders bone remodeling. Cortical bone thickening in diaphyseal areas has been shown to be a result of new lamellar bone formation (periosteal bone). The degree of mineralization in the newly formed bone is lower than that of cortical bone.

C. Bone Growth

Many biological and physiological mechanisms are activated by bone fracture. The actual nature of the stimulus for new bone formation following trauma or arthroplasty is unknown. However, it is known that, when a bone is broken or sectioned, blood from ruptured medullary, periosteal, and adjacent soft tissue vessels extravasates so that a hematoma, or clot, is formed around the fractured or sectioned location. Periosteal and intraosseous osteoblasts are activated, and bone stem cells form new osteoblasts. Within a short period of time, a callus is formed between the two ends. The callus formation that occurs between two or more bones during the healing process includes cartilage and fibrocartilage. In the case of a fracture or osteotomy, the osteoblastic activity is accelerated by mechanical internal fixation. The principle that bone stress aids in the healing mechanism of bone fracture is utilized during treatment. When fractures are bridged with implants—i.e., compression plates, bone screws, K-wires, intramedullary rods, etc.—the patient may realize immediate use of the fractured or osteotomized bone. This use of the bone prior to healing creates biomechanical stresses on opposing ends of the bones, which may accelerate the remodeling process. *Rigid stability* and an intact vascular supply to fractured bone are two essential criteria for primary bone union. In some cases, bone heals so well that the fracture location is almost impossible to find once fully healed.

It is important to note that compression between fragments alone does not promote the remodeling of bone. Compression only stabilizes a fracture or sectioned piece to keep it rigid enough to assist in primary bone healing. Motion and micromotion or cyclical loading and unloading appear to stimulate or enhance bone healing. For primary bone healing to occur, however, macromotion must not occur. If macromotion takes place, a nonunion will be precipitated, or loosening of a prosthesis may occur.

Many experiments using rigid and flexible internal fixation have been performed to observe the patterns of bone healing. The remodeling of bone due to static compression and tension of cortical bone has been observed extensively [10]. It has been shown that, in some cases, remodeling of bone that occurs next to internal fixation devices may not be a result of a foreign-body effect nor static axial compression, but rather a combination of biological factors and dynamic loading.

In the instance of arthroplasty where various prostheses are introduced to replace major joints, previously discussed principles of bone remodeling are necessary for adequate healing. While it is true that fracture fixation devices are bent during surgery to fit the contour of the bone, for joints, the "fit" of the device to the contour of the bone becomes an increasingly important factor. Bone–implant interface in joint systems is important since the fit of the device, as well as the type of surface that the device has, will determine bone adherence. Since joint prostheses are not designed for short-term use, bone healing and bone quality around the device are essential criteria for the promotion of longevity as well as the prevention of loosening.

V. FAILURE ANALYSIS OF FRACTURE FIXATION DEVICES

It is necessary to ensure that retrieved implants are properly sterilized prior to performing failure analysis. Before viewing the fracture surfaces using light and scanning electron microscopy (SEM), it is often necessary to perform an additional thorough cleaning of the fracture surfaces to permit complete examination and prevent charging in the scanning electron microscope. Cleaning is generally accomplished by sonication of the pieces containing the fracture surfaces in a mild detergent solution in an ultrasonic cleaner to remove blood and biological debris that may adhere to the irregular fracture surface.

While light microscopy can be used to aid in fracture analysis, especially in cases in which the parts are very large or only a general identification of the fracture mode is required, this technique is limited by magnification and depth of field. Scanning electron microscopy is usually used to examine the fracture surface in order to increase the depth of field at higher magnifications. Viewing in the SEM usually allows the source of crack initiation and precise mode of crack propagation to be identified. Sample size is a limiting factor in using the SEM; however, chamber size has increased in recent years and samples as large as 50 mm and even in excess of 75 mm may now be viewed while allowing enough movement to scan the entire sample. It is often necessary to examine only one of the fracture surfaces since opposing fracture surfaces are mirror images of one another. If the surface is covered with debris that is not readily removable, or if the morphological characteristics that delineate the mode of fracture have in some way been obliterated, examination of the opposing fracture surface is required.

A. Failure Analysis of Dynamic Compression Plate

Full documentation for a specific implant is necessary to provide a complete and thorough failure analysis. It is, therefore, necessary to examine the application of the device as used for the specific patient. Determination of how the device has been used is done most easily through examination of x rays and the patient record. Figure 4a shows the position of the fracture in the bone, the condition of the bone around the fracture site, and the relative position of the fracture of a plate in relation to the fracture of the bone. Figure 4b shows the plate after removal from the patient. The patient record and the markings on the plate were used to identify the manufacturer. This information was used to make a preliminary assessment that the material was implant-quality grade 2/316L

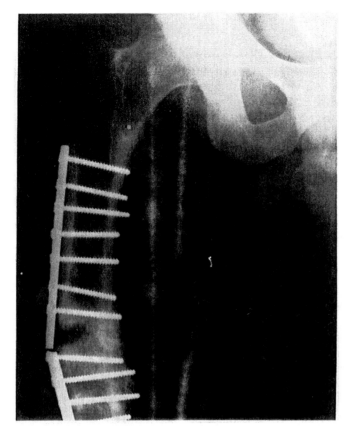

(a)

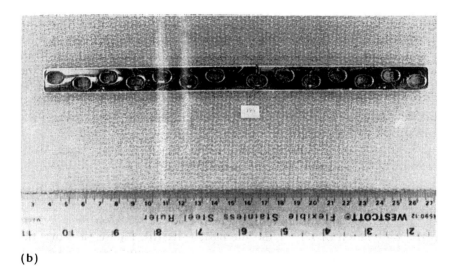

(b)

Figure 4 (a) X-ray of dynamic compression plate *in situ*. (b) Photograph of dynamic compression plate after retrieval.

134

stainless steel. After sonication for 30 min in a solution of a mild laboratory detergent to remove the bulk of the biological debris, the plate was rinsed in water and ethanol, and air-dried. The plate was then sectioned below the fracture surface to provide a piece small enough to fit into the SEM. Care was taken not to disturb any of the screw holes or the fracture surface. An additional piece was sectioned for quantitative X-ray fluorescence analysis to determine the composition of major alloying elements, and for metallography. Quantitative X-ray fluorescence analysis (Fig. 5) determined that the major alloying elements (Fe, Cr, Ni, Mo, Mn, Si), were within specification according to ASTM F138. Examination of inclusion content on a transverse section, as described by ASTM E45, showed the level of inclusions to be acceptable (Fig. 6a). Evaluation of the grain size according to ASTM E112 showed the grain size to be 5.5, which is within specification according to ASTM F138. The structure was also free of carbide precipitates in the grain boundaries (Fig. 6b), thus indicating an acceptable microstructure. Since examination of the surface, the screw holes, and the microstructure showed no signs of excess corrosion

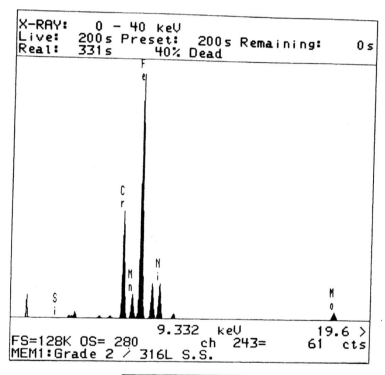

Element	Weight %
Fe	62.6440
Mn	1.8115
Ni	14.8306
Mo	2.7440
Cr	17.7222
Si	.2379

Figure 5 Quantitative X-ray fluorescence analysis of dynamic compression plate.

(a)

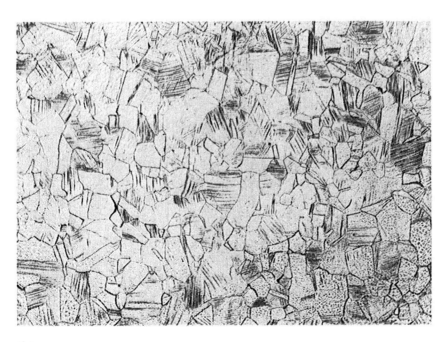

(b)

Figure 6 (a) Light micrograph showing transverse inclusions in dynamic compression plate of 316L stainless steel (100×). (b) Light micrograph showing grain structure and ASTM grain size of 5.5 (100×). (c) Light micrograph showing etch pits and discontinuous grain boundary ditching in 316L stainless steel after screening test according to ASTM A262.

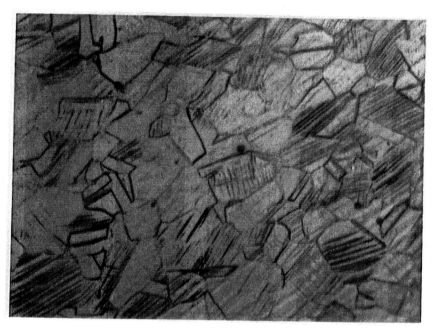

(c)

or a suspect microstructure, evaluation of intergranular corrosion was deemed unnecessary; however, should corrosion be suspect, the test for intergranular corrosion (ASTM A262) should be performed. An example of an acceptable microstructure for 316L stainless steel after the screening test for intergranular corrosion as described in ASTM A262 is seen in Fig. 6c.

Evaluation of the Vickers microhardness (H_v) on the polished surface of the transverse sample used for inclusion evaluation gave a value of $H_v = 350$. Since 316L stainless steel work hardens readily during testing, hardness tests cannot be used to precisely judge mechanical properties. Microhardness can, however, be used as a guide to determine acceptability of mechanical properties. The value obtained for this sample is within the range expected for implant-quality, grade 2/316L stainless steel in the work-hardened condition.

It is necessary to examine the inclusion content of stainless steel in the longitudinal direction of material fabrication. The reason for evaluation of longitudinal inclusion content, as well as evaluation for foreign phases in the longitudinal direction, is that during processing or drawing of the metal, inclusions and foreign phases such as δ-ferrite in austenitic stainless steel are elongated. These inclusions and foreign phases become more visible and attain their elongated appearance when viewed in the longitudinal direction. Figure 7a shows the inclusion content prior to etching and Fig. 7b shows the same sample after etching with a solution of $CuCl_2$ in HCl and ethanol. The levels of both oxide-type (spherical) and elongated sulfide-type stringers seen in the micrographs are within the limits as specified by ASTM F138. The size of the inclusions has been exacerbated by the etching, which is the reason that inclusions are to be rated without etching. The specific type of inclusions can be distinguished by examination in the SEM and by

(a)

(b)

Figure 7 (a) Light micrograph showing globular oxide and sulfide-type stringer inclusions in longitudinal section of dynamic compression plate (100×). (b) Light micrograph showing no δ-ferrite visible in etched longitudinal sample (100×). (c) SEM micrograph showing morphology of sulfide-type stringer and alumina-type inclusions.

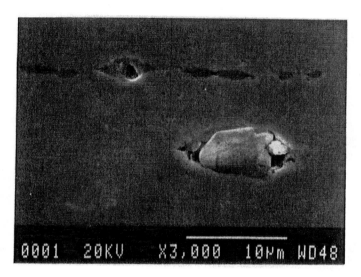

(c)

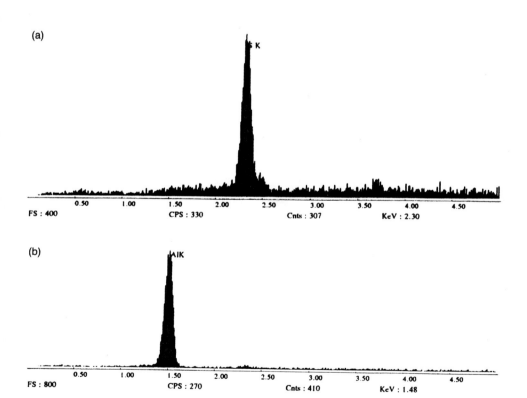

Figure 8 (a) Energy-dispersive spectra of sulfide-type inclusion. (b) Energy-dispersive spectra of alumina-type inclusion

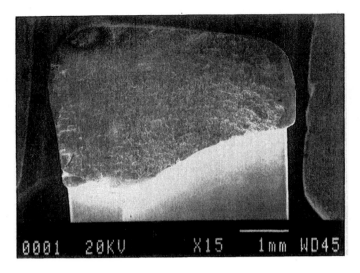

(a)

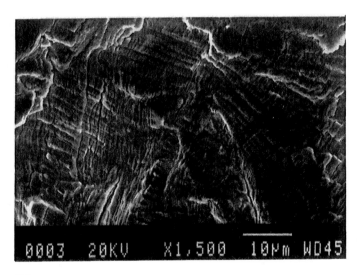

(b)

Figure 9 (a) SEM micrograph of fracture surface of dynamic compression plate on one side of screw hole — crack initiation at lower right. (b) SEM micrograph showing fine striations and secondary fatigue cracks — Stage II fatigue over fracture surface in (a). (c) SEM micrograph showing fretting corrosion and wear in screw hole.

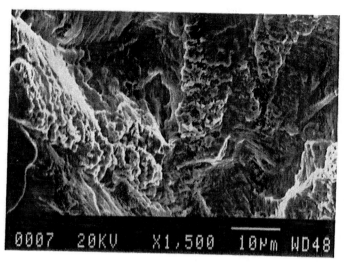

(c)

compositional analysis using either an energy-dispersive or a wavelength-dispersive analyzer coupled to the SEM. Figure 7c is an SEM micrograph of two inclusions having different morphologies. Using energy-dispersive spectroscopy, the upper inclusion was identified as a sulfide-type inclusion (Fig. 8a) and the lower inclusion was identified as an alumina-type inclusion (Fig. 8b). Figure 7b shows that there is no δ-ferrite visible in the sample.

As previously stated, it is often not necessary to examine opposing fracture surfaces since they are mirror images of each other. In the case where fracture occurs through a screw hole, it is, however, necessary to examine both fracture surfaces to evaluate the mechanism of fracture on both sides of the screw hole. Figure 9a shows the fracture surface on one side of the screw hole of the plate. The orientation of crack arrest marks indicates that the crack initiated in the area of intersection of the screw hole and the upper plate surface (lower right, Fig. 9a). Figure 9b shows well-defined fatigue striations and multiple secondary cracking indicative of Stage II fatigue crack propagation. This morphology was noted over most of the fracture surface except in those areas where the metal was smeared due to repeated rubbing of opposing fracture surfaces. Figure 9c shows an example of fretting corrosion and wear in the screw hole due to motion between the plate and screws. Fretting and corrosion is often observed in areas where rubbing has occurred. Examination of the fracture surface on the other side of the screw hole showed an almost identical morphology, with the crack initiating at the upper left in Fig. 10a and propagating radially toward the lower right. Striations and secondary fatigue cracks indicative of cyclical loading and Stage II fatigue crack propagation were observed over greater than 90% of the fracture surface (Fig. 10b). Final fracture of the plate on this side of the screw hole occurred due to ductile tensile overload in the area marked with an arrow in Fig. 10a. This area exhibited equiaxed dimples (Fig. 10c) indicative of Stage III fatigue fracture (ductile tensile overload failure), and was in all probability the area of final fracture.

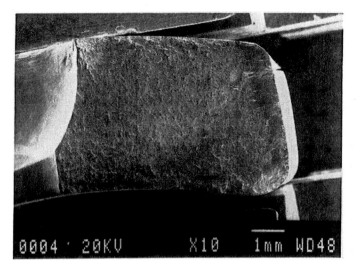

(a)

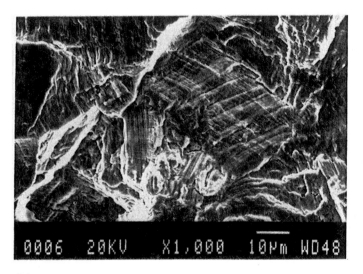

(b)

Figure 10   (a) SEM micrograph of fracture surface of dynamic compression plate on opposite side of screw hole from Fig. 9a—crack initiation at upper left. (b) SEM micrograph showing striations over fracture surface in (a). (c) SEM micrograph showing area of final Stage III fatigue (tensile overload) at lower right in (a).

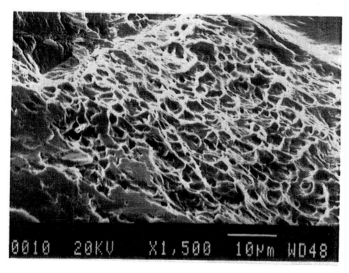

(c)

Evaluation of the X-rays and patient record indicated nonunion of the bone. Further examination of the patient record indicated that this was the second fracture fixation device implanted and that the first implant had also fractured due to a nonunion. This information, along with the medical history of the patient and the length of time to fracture of the plate, provided the explanation for fracture of the device, which was found to be free of metallurgical and manufacturing defects. Based upon all tests, X-rays, and patient records it was concluded that failure of this device was due to loading at levels above the fatigue limit over a prolonged period by the patient. Failure was not related to deficiencies in the plate.

B. Failure Analysis of Stainless Steel Screws

Determination of grain structure and grain size, inclusion content of both transverse and longitudinal samples, evaluation and identification of foreign phases, compositional analysis, and hardness testing are required for all evaluations of fractured devices of 316L stainless steel. It is, however, not necessary to repeat the discussion of each of these tests for each failure analysis described herein. Therefore, the description of each test and analysis is not included in further discussion except in those areas where they shed further light on the failure analysis.

Screws used in fracture fixation fail due to the application of both single-cycle stresses, which are most often applied during insertion and removal, and by fatigue. Figure 11a is an X-ray showing two screws at the distal end of a femoral intramedullary nail. Upon removal, both screws were found to be broken in the area below the screw head where they intersected the screw hole. This case illustrates the importance of good-quality x rays. Undetectability of fracture of the screws in X-rays of this patient may have been due to the crack location; however, broken implants may not be detected *in situ* due to the poor quality of the X-rays. Figure 11b shows the fracture surface with the site of

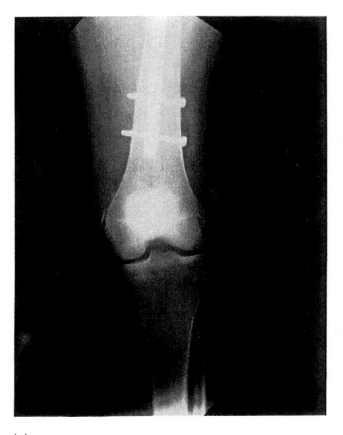

(a)

Figure 11   (a) X-ray showing screws in femoral intramedullary nail. (b) SEM micrograph of fractured screw—crack initiation at left. (c) SEM micrograph showing pitting corrosion and wear near crack initiation site. (d) SEM micrograph showing fatigue striations on screw fracture surface. (e) SEM micrograph showing area of final tensile overload at far right in (a).

crack initiation at the left marked with an arrow. The clamshell marks associated with crack propagation are readily visible in this micrograph. Examination of the fracture surface in the area of crack initiation showed wear and surface pitting caused by removal of the passive layer and subsequent corrosion (Fig. 11c). While there is often significant wear of the fracture surface, especially in cases where the device remains in the patient for a prolonged time period after fracture, careful examination most often reveals the mechanism of crack growth. In this case, nearly all areas showed fatigue striations and secondary cracking indicative of fracture due to cyclical loading (Fig. 11d). The spacing of the striations in all areas of the surface where they were still visible indicates that crack propagation proceeded due to high-cycle fatigue ($> 10^5$ cycles). The area of final fracture at the far right in Fig. 11a showed the presence of dimples indicative of Stage III or

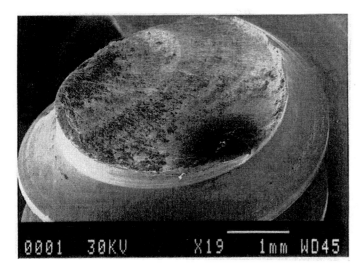

(b)

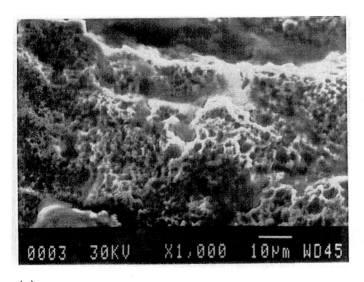

(c)

ductile tensile overload fracture (Fig. 11e). Fracture analysis of the second screw was similar to that of the first scew and is, therefore, not included here.

Examination of the patient record and X-rays indicated several factors that could have contributed to or induced fracture of the screws. The first of these contributing factors was that the patient was significantly overweight. The second was that this was a case where union of the bone still had not taken place after 6 months (nonunion). Since no defects in the materials were found and no manufacturing defects in the screws could

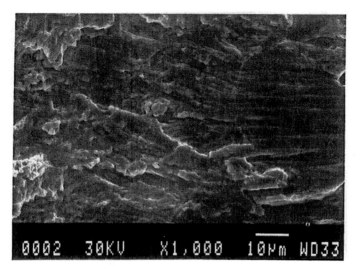

(d)

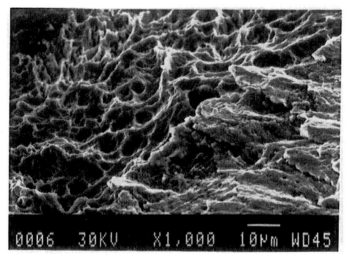

(e)

Figure 11   Continued

be detected, the indication was that factors relating to the patient and the lack of sufficient healing led to fracture of the screws.

There are cases where device failure does not occur due to patient loading and is also in no way due to faulty materials, manufacturing, or design. Figure 12a shows the fracture surface of a 316L stainless steel screw viewed toward the screw head. As with all retrieval analysis, prior to SEM evaluation, the fracture surface of the screw was sonicated in a mild detergent solution to remove the bulk of the biological debris, rinsed in water and ethanol, and air-dried. Figure 12b is a higher-magnification SEM micrograph of the area of the fracture surface marked with an arrow toward the top of Fig. 12a. The orientation of the oblated shear dimples indicates torsional fracture caused during removal of the screw. The area marked with an arrow toward the bottom right of Fig. 12a shows fracture due to tensile overload (Fig. 12c). The orientation of the surface morphology seen clearly in the thread root adjacent to the fracture surface (*S* pattern) indicates that the screw had been permanently deformed during insertion, as well as during removal (Fig. 12a). Overtorquing of the screw during insertion will enhance fatigue fracture as well as contribute to fracture during removal. As a consequence of the effects of the handling of the device prior to and during implantation, careful attention should be paid, not only to the fracture surface morphology, but also to areas of the surface. Special attention should be paid to the surface areas adjacent to the fracture surface in the area of crack initiation.

C.   Failure Analysis of an Intramedullary Nail

The failure analysis of intramedullary (IM) nails is often hampered by severely worn fracture surface since the nail is often secured with screws at both the proximal and distal ends to keep the bone in compression. Figure 13a shows an X-ray of a fractured slotted femoral intramedullary nail. Examination of the surface for corrosion and manufacturing defects, compositional analysis, and microstructure revealed no deviations from ASTM F139. Figure 13b shows the nail fracture surface on the side of the screw hole that does not contain the slot. While there is significant wear of the fracture surface, the orientation of the crack arrest marks indicates that a crack began at the intersection of the outside surface of the intramedullary nail and the screw hole at the far left. Analysis of the area at the intersection of the outside surface and the screw hole at the left in Fig. 13b is shown at increased magnification in Fig. 13c. Examination of the surface of the IM nail in this area revealed the presence of multiple intersecting slip bands indicative of a high state of stress. Figure 13d shows fatigue, striations, secondary fatigue cracks, and wear in the area outlined by the white box in Fig. 13a. The region on the IM nail surface at the screw hole showed a high degree of strain, fretting, and pitting corrosion caused by relative motion of the locking bolt and the nail (Fig. 13e). Inspection of the locking screws confirmed that significant wear had occurred between the locking screws and the screw hole surface. Motion of this type can cause removal of the passive oxide layer, leading to fretting and/or pitting corrosion.

In addition to showing wear, the area of the fracture surface between the screw holes and both sides of the slot (Fig. 14a) exhibited striations and secondary cracks typical in Stage II fatigue crack propagation (Fig. 14b). Figure 14c shows the remnants of striations, wear, and corrosion pits precipitated by wear. Within the screw hole, a significant number of intersecting slip bands and additional cracking were observed (Fig. 14d). Evaluation of the patient record and X-rays revealed that the patient had healed uneventfully, with no fracture of the nail detected. The X-ray shown in Fig. 13a was taken 15 months after initial injury and no refracture of the bone had occurred. The IM nail was removed uneventfully, and it was surmised that a crack had initiated sometime during the healing process but that propagation had continued due to load sharing after healing.

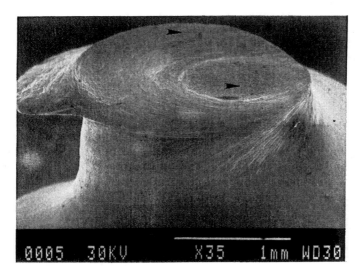

(a)

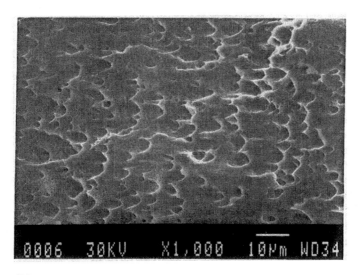

(b)

Figure 12 (a) SEM micrograph of 316L stainless steel screw. (b) SEM micrograph of area at top of (a) showing orientation of sheer dimples. (c) SEM micrograph of area of final tensile overload toward bottom right of (a).

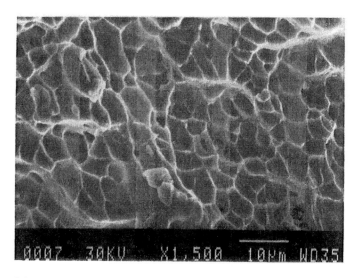

(c)

D.   Failure Analysis of a Titanium Screw

In addition to stainless steel, the use of titanium and titanium alloys for fracture fixation devices continues to increase. Plates, screws, wire, intramedullary nails, etc., are available from a number of manufacturers in both CP titanium and titanium alloys. Since there are four grades of CP titanium, it is necessary to determine which grade is present. This may be done by evaluation of the oxygen concentration since this increases as the grade number increases, or it may be done by evaluation of the hardness. As an example, the Vickers microhardness reading for the fractured screw described in the following paragraphs was in the range of 249. This microhardness value, along with the compositional analysis, indicates that the material is work-hardened Grade 4 CP titanium.

Figure 15a is a low-magnification SEM micrograph of the entire fracture surface of the CP titanium screw. The site of initiation of a fatigue crack, marked with an arrow in Fig. 15a, is defined by the orientation of the arrest marks. Examination of the root of the screw thread at the initiation site of a crack showed slip bands on the surface (Fig. 15b). Very fine fatigue striations, typical in high-cycle Stage II fatigue fracture, were noted over much of the central area of the fracture surface (Fig. 15c). Other areas of the fracture surface nearer the periphery exhibited tearing or shear structures and fluting as well as the presence of some fatigue striations (Fig. 15d). This type of morphology is not atypical for metals having a hexagonal crystal structure and may be indicative of a triaxial state of stress, or transition from high cycle/low load to low cycle/high load fatigue. The mixed morphology of this fracture surface indicates that a complex and variable load spectrum was in operation.

Quantitative X-ray fluorescence spectroscopy for analysis of major alloying elements showed the presence of titanium and a minor amount of iron (Fig. 16). Since no other major alloying elements were present, these results indicate that the material of which the screw was made is CP titanium.

The more macroscopic morphology seen on the fracture surface of failed titanium

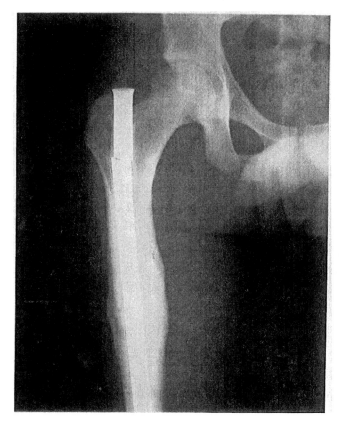

(a)

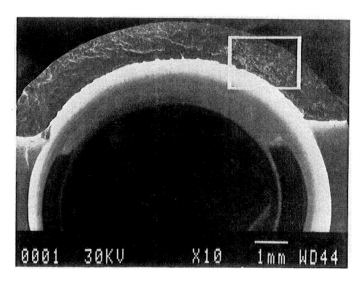

(b)

Figure 13 (a) X-ray of fractured slotted femoral IM nail. (b) SEM micrograph of fracture surface of IM nail. (c) SEM micrograph showing slip bands in screw hole. (d) SEM micrograph showing fatigue striations, secondary cracks, and wear in boxed area of panel (a). (e) SEM micrograph showing fretting and pitting corrosion in screw hole.

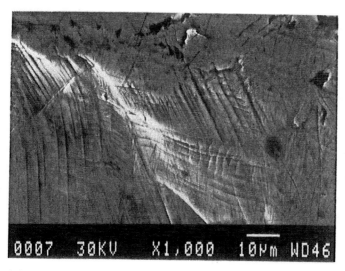

(c)

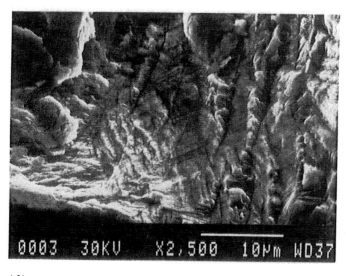

(d)

plates and IM nails is similar to that discussed in the sections on those types of devices composed of stainless steel. As an example, assuming a similar load spectrum and similar site of the bone fracture, crack initiation of a CP titanium or titanium alloy plate will begin in the area of reduced cross section on the side of the plate away from the bone (tension side), and the fracture surface morphology will be nearly identical to that seen in Figs. 9a and 10a. The morphology of fatigue crack propagation will be similar to that seen for the CP titanium screw in Figs. 15c and 15d.

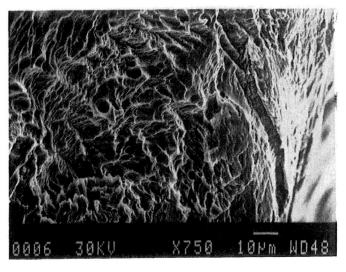

0006   30KV   X750   10μm   WD48

(e)

Figure 13   Continued.

VI.   FAILURE ANALYSIS OF PROSTHESES

Failure analysis of prostheses has very little difference from that of fracture fixation devices. The primary differences are that the prosthesis is often composed of cast rather than wrought material, and that the prosthesis has been in the patient for a much greater period of time. Therefore, it is often difficult, if not impossible, to obtain patient records and X-rays documenting the device history. Additionally, as previously stated, there are a number of factors other than fracture of the metal components that may have contributed to the failure of the prosthesis.

A.   Failure Analysis of a Co–Cr Hip Stem

Fracture of the hip prosthesis discussed in the following paragraphs had occurred transversely through the stem approximately two thirds of the distance from the distal end. Prior to microstructural evaluation, a piece was cut from the stem, polished with 1-micron diamond, and qualitatively analyzed using energy-dispersive X-ray analysis in the scanning electron microscope to verify elemental composition. The energy-dispersive X-ray spectrum (Fig. 17) indicates that the primary element is cobalt (Co), with chromium (Cr) being next highest in concentration, then molybdenum (Mo), and a minor amount of silicon (Si). All of these alloying elements, in their relative proportion, are in agreement with those to be expected for implant-quality casting alloy conforming to ASTM F75. This same polished sample was evaluated for Vickers hardness (H_v) and a mean value of $H_v = 347.1$ was recorded. This value is in the range expected for cast Co-Cr-Mo alloy (ASTM F75).

The inclusion content and grain structure were examined on the sample used for hardness testing. Evaluation of inclusions showed typical carbide distribution (Fig. 18a) and pores typical of castings. After evaluation of inclusion content, the sample was etched using Fe_2Cl_3 in HCl and HNO_3 to reveal the grain structure (Fig. 18b). This grain structure is typical of cast Co–Cr–Mo alloys with large grains and dendritic grain growth.

The sample containing the fracture surface was ultrasonically cleaned in mild detergent solution, rinsed in water and ethanol, and air-dried. Figure 19a shows the fracture surface tilted so that the entire surface may be viewed from the lateral toward the medial. Of particular interest is the multifaceted appearance of most of the fracture surface. This type of morphology is indicative of a fatigue crack that has propagated primarily due to Stage I fatigue. Stage I fatigue occurs at relatively low values of stress. This observation was further corroborated by observations of the microscopic fracture morphology of the majority of the fracture surface. Figure 19b shows the "staircase" or "sawtooth" type markings that are often seen and are indicative of Stage I fatigue fracture in cast Co–Cr–Mo hip prostheses. Careful note should be taken of the presence of multiple secondary fatigue cracks and the orientation of slip on either side of these cracks, with the absence of continuous alignment of these markings across the microcracks. Material separation has taken place along preferred glide planes, which is typical for fatigue fracture in this alloy. Also, the small voids normally present in this type of casting should be noted. Figure 19c is a SEM micrograph of the fracture surface at a different orientation. The fracture surface appears to have a different morphology; however, the sawtooth pattern is discernable, and multiple secondary fatigue cracks are again visible. Fatigue striations may also be visible on areas of the fracture surface at high magnification (Fig. 19d). This type of morphology is indicative of crack propagation due to repeated cyclical loading above the endurance limit during Stage II fatigue crack propagation. Stage II fatigue crack propagation generally occurs at higher stress rates in a given system than Stage I and propagation may shift between the two stages. During Stage II fatigue, striations are often contained on plateaus at different levels and are joined by ledges containing striations or by tear ridges.

The area of major fatigue crack initiation on the lateral surface of the prosthesis is seen in Fig. 20a. This area shows the presence of multiple cracks on the stem surface, which appear to have been precipitated by fatigue loading. The area of the crack initiation at the intersection of the lateral surface of the stem and the fracture surface, as identified by the orientation of the radial clamshell marks, is indicated with an arrow in Fig. 20a. Careful examination of the fracture surface, clearly seen in Figs. 20b and 20c, showed numerous discontinuous secondary fatigue cracks. This is typical of fatigue fracture in hip prostheses since stresses are not applied uniaxially during movement by the patient. The area in close proximity of the crack near the stem surface appears to be reasonably planar when the sample is oriented as seen in Fig. 20d. Striations, indicative of Stage II fatigue crack propagation, are clearly defined on both sides of the secondary crack. Because the striations do not appear to be aligned across the crack in this orientation of the sample, the conclusion could be drawn that the crack was preexisting and was, therefore, a manufacturing defect. Examination at several orientations revealed that the area above the secondary crack is not in the same plane as the area below the crack. Another view of the fracture surface, but with significant tilting, can be seen in Fig. 20e. The fracture surface orientation seen in Fig. 20e clearly shows that the area above the crack is at a significant angle to the area below, which accounts for the apparent lack of fatigue striation alignment across the crack due to a difference in slip in different

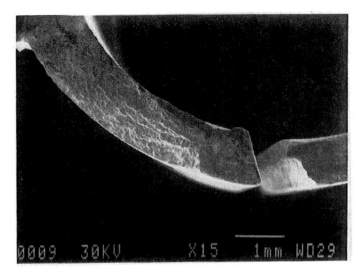

(a)

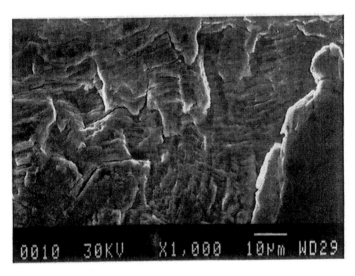

(b)

Figure 14 (a) SEM micrograph of fracture surface of IM nail near slot. (b) SEM micrograph showing fatigue striations and secondary cracks. (c) SEM micrograph showing corrosion pits on striations and wear on fracture surface. (d) SEM micrograph showing slip bands and additional fatigue crack in screw hole.

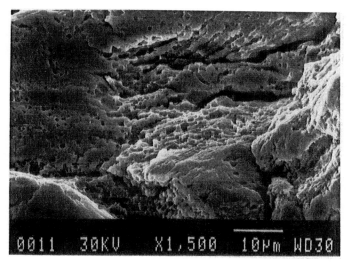

(c)

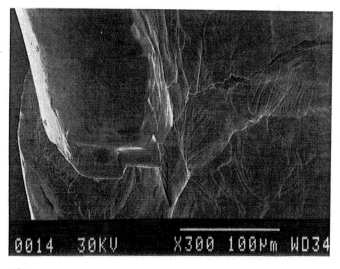

(d)

crystallographic directions. The two planes are therefore joined together by a ledge or wall containing fatigue striations.

Neither the X-rays nor the patient record was available, but discussion with the patient indicated that the prosthesis had been in place for in excess of 15 years. In addition, significant fracture and deterioration of the cement was noted as well as bone resorption. This information, along with the failure analysis previously described, and

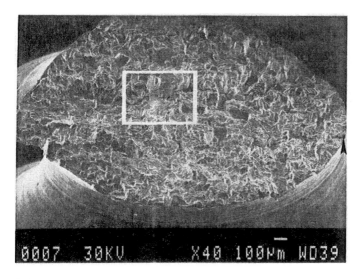

(a)

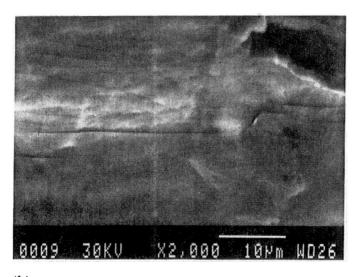

(b)

Figure 15   (a) SEM micrograph showing oblique view of fracture surface and threads of titanium screw. (b) SEM micrograph showing slip bands at crack initiation site. (c) SEM micrograph of central area of fracture surface showing fatigue striations. (d) SEM micrograph of area near periphery of fracture surface showing flutes and tear structures.

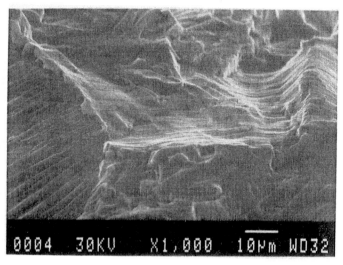

(c)

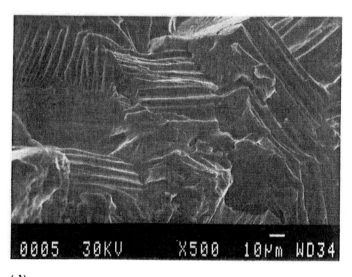

(d)

the age and weight of the patient indicated that fatigue of the hip stem was related to factors other than the prosthesis itself.

B. Failure Analysis of Ti–6Al–4V Tibial Tray

The fractured tibial tray that is the subject of this fracture analysis is seen in Fig. 21a. Compositional analysis of major alloying elements using X-ray fluorescence analysis (Fig. 21b) showed that the material was Ti–6Al–4V. Vickers microhardness testing in

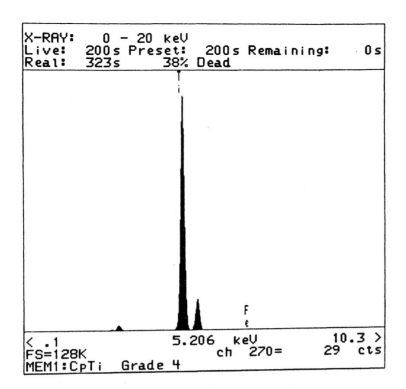

Element	Weight %
Ti	99.7978
Fe	.1943

Figure 16 Quantitative X-ray fluorescence spectra of CP titanium screw.

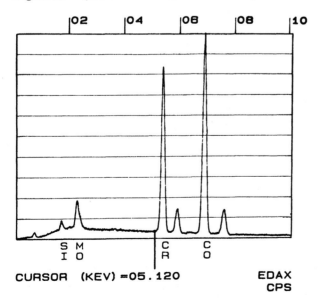

Figure 17 Quantitative energy-dispersive X-ray spectra of Co–Cr–Mo hip.

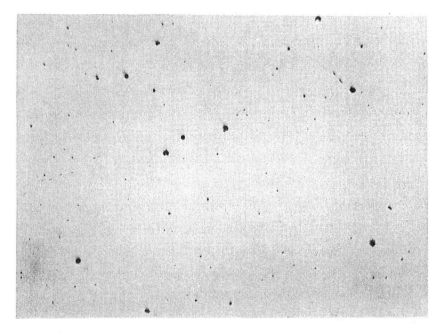

(a)

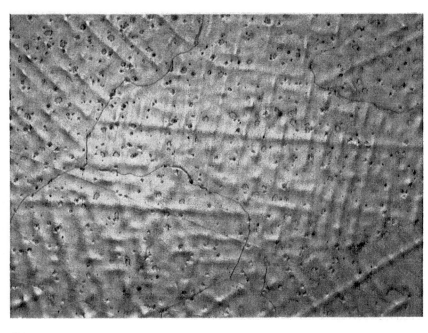

(b)

Figure 18   (a) Light micrograph showing carbide distribution in ASTM F75 Co–Cr–Mo hip stem (100×). (b) Light micrograph showing large-grain microstructure and dendritic grain growth in ASTM F75 Co–Cr–Mo hip stem (50×).

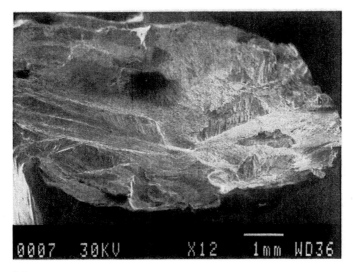

(a)

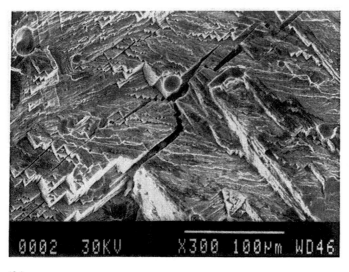

(b)

Figure 19   (a) SEM micrograph of fracture surface of Co–Cr–Mo hip stem. (b) SEM micrograph showing saw tooth pattern on fracture surface indicative of Stage I fatigue crack growth. (c) SEM micrograph of fracture surface tilted; note secondary fatigue cracks. (d) SEM micrograph of fracture surface showing striations typical in Stage II fatigue crack growth.

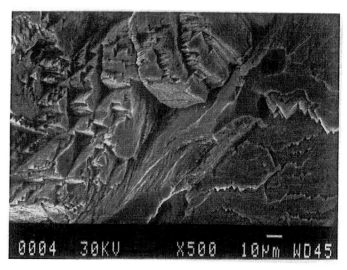

(c)

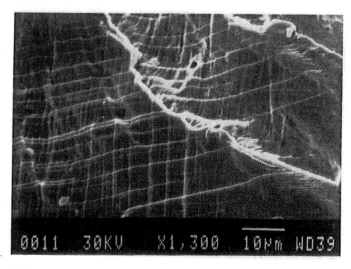

(d)

three areas of a transverse sample gave a mean H_v value of 313. This value is within the range expected for Ti–6Al–4V. Examination of the microstructure of the transverse piece used for microhardness testing (Fig. 21c) showed a large-grained microstructure and additional microcracks in the section. This large-grain microstructure indicates a cast rather than wrought tibial tray.

SEM examination of an area of the fracture surface toward one of the ends of the smaller piece seen at the left in Fig. 21a is shown in Fig. 22a. The morphology in this

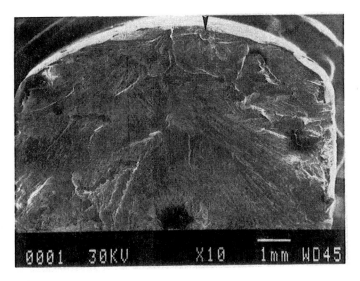

(a)

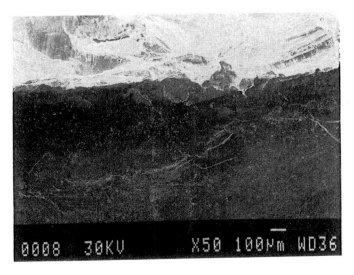

(b)

Figure 20   (a) SEM micrograph showing cracks on lateral surface of stem. (b) SEM micrograph showing fracture surface morphology in area of crack initiation. (c) Higher-magnification SEM micrograph of area of crack initiation showing multiple secondary cracks. (d) Higher-magnification SEM micrograph showing striations on both sides of a secondary crack. (e) SEM micrograph of crack and striations in (d) at different orientation.

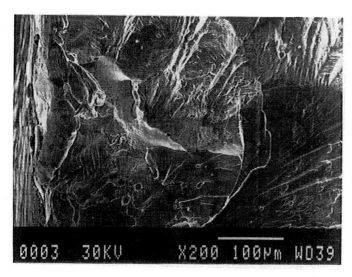

(c)

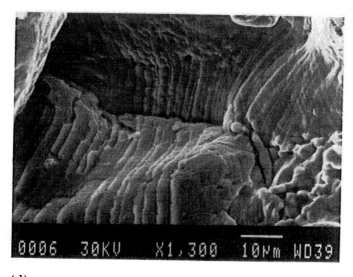

(d)

micrograph is typical of fatigue fracture through a piece of this alloy having a large-grained microstructure. The area toward the far lower left is seen at higher magnification in Fig. 22b. This area showed fluting and cleavage common in fracture of Ti–6Al–4V alloys. The area of the fracture surface marked with an arrow in Fig. 22c showed more fluting and tongues typical in fatigue fracture of hcp metals. The area of the fracture surface toward the top center of Fig. 22a showed the presence of striations typical in Stage II fatigue crack propagation.

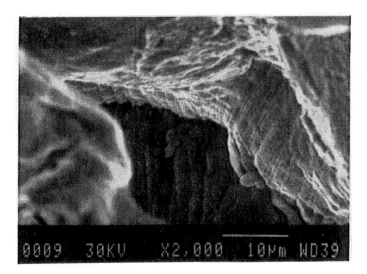

(e)

Figure 20 Continued.

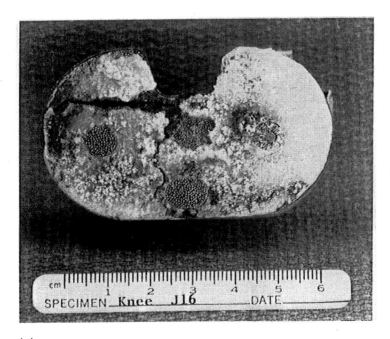

(a)

Figure 21 (a) Photograph of fractured tibial tray. (b) Quantitative X-ray fluorescence spectra of Ti–6Al–4V fractured tibial tray. (c) Light micrograph showing large-grained microstructure of Ti–6Al–4V tibial tray – note microcrack (35 ×).

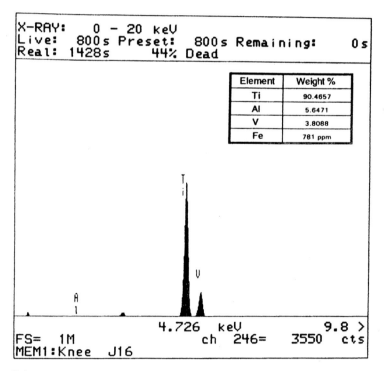

(b)

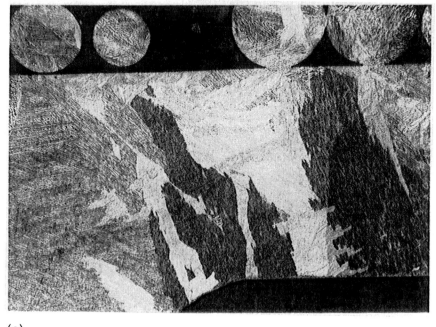

(c)

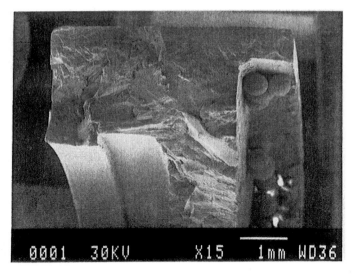

(a)

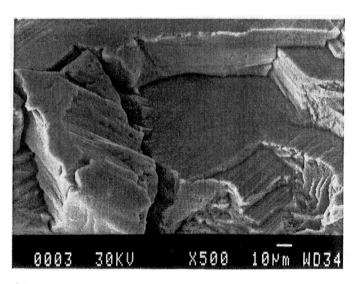

(b)

Figure 22   (a) SEM micrograph of fracture surface of end of small piece at left in Fig. 21a. (b) SEM micrograph of area of fracture surface at lower left in (a) − note fluting and cleavage. (c) SEM micrograph of area of fracture surface marked with arrow in (a) − note fluting and tongues indicating complex fatigue stresses. (d) Higher-magnification SEM micrograph of area toward top center in (a) − note striations.

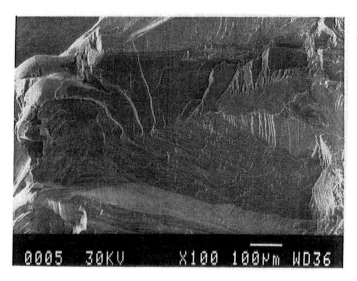

(c)

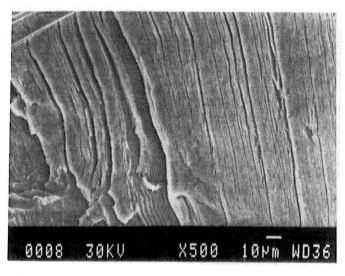

(d)

The area of the fracture below that seen in Fig. 22a, where the metal cross section is not as great, is seen in Fig. 23a. This area showed fatigue striations, and multiple secondary fatigue cracks (Fig. 23b). The area at the other end of this fractured piece is seen in Figs. 24a and 24b. Figure 24b shows the area in the approximate center of the end (marked with arrow). This area showed the presence of a sawtooth structure indicative of crack propagation due to Stage I fatigue.

Examination of the patient record and X-rays showed significant bone resorption below the tibial tray. This resorption would account for excessively high stresses being

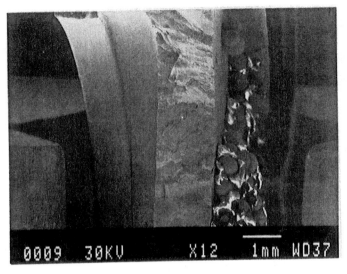

(a)

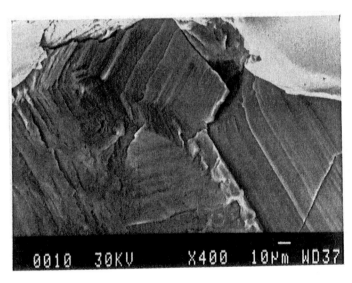

(b)

Figure 23 (a) SEM micrograph of area of fracture surface below that in Fig. 22a. (b) Higher-magnification SEM micrograph of area marked with arrow in (a) — note striations and secondary fatigue cracks.

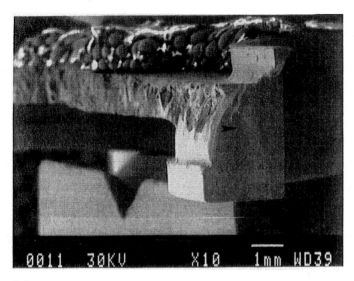

(a)

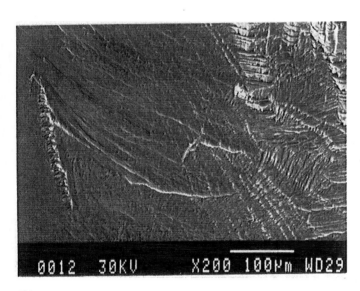

(b)

Figure 24 (a) SEM micrograph of fracture surface at end opposite from that shown in Fig. 22a. (b) Higher-magnification SEM micrograph of fracture surface in (a) showing Stage I fatigue.

placed on the tibial tray. In addition to the bone resorption, the very large grain structure would have contributed to the fracture; however, even if the material had been a wrought alloy, the missing bone below the tibial tray, which left the component unsupported, would have led to fracture.

VII. CONCLUSIONS

Analysis of any failed device requires careful attention to detail. Precise information concerning the history of the specific device is often needed in order to render an accurate opinion. Because implants have a direct and very personal impact on people, failure analysis information is especially important. Through failure analysis, recommendations of materials, design, and manufacturing modifications can be prescribed. Great care is required to ensure that analysis is documented and that the results are tracked to statistically determine the advisability of any changes.

Failure analysis should not be thought of as a method to prove or disprove the adequacy of a device. Rather, the scientist should embark on the analysis with the express intent of determining:

1. If the device is faulty
2. What contributing factors could have led to failure if no materials, manufacturing, and/or design faults are noted

As stated in the introduction to this chapter, failure does not necessarily indicate that the implant is faulty. We as humans do not control the biology of the patient and certainly cannot change patient physiology to fit a device. This fact often predisposes an implant to failure, given the wide variability of circumstances that it may experience.

REFERENCES

1. *Webster's Ninth New Collegiate Dictionary*, Merriam-Webster, Springfield, MA, 1986, p. 445.
2. *Annual Book of ASTM Standards*, American Society for Testing and Materials, Philadelphia, PA, 1993.
3. Mears, D. C., Materials and orthopaedic surgery, in *Tissues of the Musculo-skeletal System*, Williams & Wilkins, Baltimore, MD, 1979, pp. 142–150.
4. Anthony, C. P., and N. J. Kolthoff, *Textbook of Anatomy and Physiology*, C. V. Mosby, St. Louis, 1971.
5. Hole, J. W., *Essentials of Human Anatomy and Physiology*, 2nd ed., W. C. Brown, Dubuque, IA, 1986.
6. Barnes, M. J., Biochemistry of collagens from mineralized tissues, in *Hard Tissue Growth Repair and Remineralization*, Excerpta Medica, Amsterdam, 1973, p. 247.
7. Wainwright, S. A., W. D. Biggs, J. D. Currey, and J. M. Gosline, *Mechanical Design in Organisms*, Princeton University Press, Princeton, New Jersey, 1976, p. 169.
8. Engh, C. A., D. O'Connor, M. Jasty, T. F. McGovern, J. D. Bobyn, and W. H. Harris, Quantification of implant micromotion, strain shielding, and bone resorption with porous-coated anatomic medullary locking femoral prostheses, *Clin. Orth. Rel. Res., 285*, 13 (1992).
9. Schmid-Schönbein, G. W., S. L-Y. Woo, and B. W. Zweifach, *Frontiers in Biomechanics*, Springer-Verlag, New York, 1986, pp. 197–201.
10. Perren, S. M., P. Matter, R. Ruedi, and M. Allgöwer, Biomechanics of fracture healing after internal fixation, in *Surgery Annual* (L. M. Nyhus, ed.), Appleton-Century-Crofts, New York, 1975, p. 361.

6

Design, Analysis, and Material Considerations of a Composite Material Artificial Hip Implant

James B. Koeneman,* Mary K. Overland,† and Joseph A. Longo III

Harrington Arthritis Research Center
Phoenix, Arizona

I. INTRODUCTION

Bone resorption has been widely observed around artificial joint implants in human clinical studies [1] and in animal models [2,3]. These bone changes have been implicated as a major contributing factor to the increased loosening rate of joint implants 10 years postsurgery [4]. Although the etiology of this aseptic loosening is incompletely understood [5], reduced bone stress due to implant insertion, death of bone cells caused by reaction to wear debris, and motion of the implant caused by inadequate fixation have all been identified as major factors contributing to bone loss around implants and subsequent implant loosening. The reduction in bone stress around implants has been attributed to the high elastic modulus of metals as compared to bone, consequently, the use of composite materials that have lower elastic moduli has been investigated as a method of preventing "periprosthetic stress shielding." Carbon, glass, quartz, and polymeric fibers have been considered for the reinforcing phase and carbon (carbon–carbon composites), epoxy, polyetheretherketone (PEEK), polybutadiene, and polysulfone have been used as matrices [6-18]. Initially the interest in composites was generated by the ability of these materials to have adequate strength at low modulus, but other characteristics such as the ability to vary stiffness within the material and the anisotropic nature of their mechanical properties may be the ultimate reasons for composite use in the future. One of the first applications of structural composites as implant materials was in the femoral stems of artificial hip joints. To use structural polymeric composites in this application the

*Current affiliation: Orthologic, Phoenix, Arizona
†Current affiliation: Telectronics Pacing Systems, Englewood, Colorado

strength of the composite in the body environment, the strength of any particular design configuration, and the resistance of the surface to degradation must be examined. The purpose of this chapter is to describe the design of a composite material hip stem, describe studies that evaluate the effectiveness of design characteristics, and determine the environmental resistance of candidate materials.

II. DESIGN

Most composite hip designs have been machined from flat or curved laminates constructed by alternating layers of continuous fibers [12,16]. Part of the design process is to specify the sequence of ply fiber orientation that will meet the strength and stiffness objectives. Although laminate construction has proven effective when used for beams where the loading is mainly bending in one plane, *in vivo* loads are biplanar and torsional. This complex loading increases the intra- and interlaminar shear stresses and thus challenges a traditional weak link of composite materials. Additionally, difficulties arise with laminate construction when attempting to vary the material stiffness through the construct. The innovative design that was chosen for the Harrington Arthritis Research Center (HARC) hip is shown in Fig. 1 (canine) and Fig. 2 (human). It consists of a cylindrical core of unidirectional carbon fibers embedded in a polymer matrix. The core is enclosed in a braid of carbon fibers using the same polymer matrix and, finally, this structure is encased with pure polymer. Canine implants were manufactured using a polysulfone matrix, whereas the human design has utilized both polysulfone and, more recently, PEEK matrices. The unidirectional core and braid follow the axis of the implant. This type of design provides for maximum strength for the unsupported neck, bending and torsion loads carried by fibers, and reduced reliance on composite interface bonding. In the human design, tapering of the unidirectional core directly below the point of insertion into the femur forces proximal load transfer to the surrounding bone due to

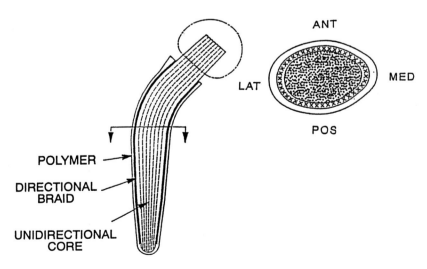

Figure 1   HARC canine composite femoral stem.

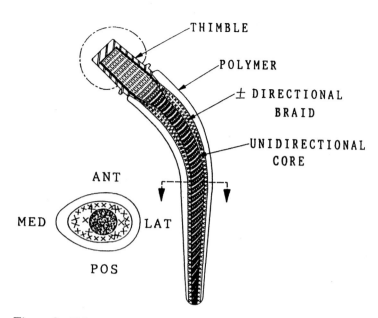

Figure 2   HARC human composite implant design.

the reduction in bending stiffness along the length of the stem. Table 1 lists the advantages and disadvantages of each type of design.

The shape of the Harrington hip implant was selected so that the composite stem would be supported by the internal tube of condensed cancellous bone within the proximal femur. This stem shape was determined by removing the femoral head and the low-density cancellous bone inside the tube with a curette. Next, a mold of the cavity was made using a room-temperature curing silicone rubber. Computer-generated solid models of both the canine and human proximal femoral cavities were constructed from measurements of the mold and contact X rays of femora, and also from physical sections of bones. In addition, a proximal flare was incorporated in the implant's design geometry to generate circumferential (hoop) stresses in the cancellous bone in an attempt to prevent the proximal–medial bone resorption that has been observed around other hip implants. The complex geometry and proximal flare eliminated the need for a collar. The level of the neck cut was very high. This was chosen to provide implant stability, especially to torsion loads.

Table 1   Comparison of Composite Designs

Type of design	Advantages	Disadvantages
Laminate	Established design and manufacturing methods Extensive aerospace use	Primarily for in-plane loading Exposed fiber ends Reduced neck strength
Tubular	High neck strength Continuous fibers Variable elastic modulus	Manufacturing methods not well established

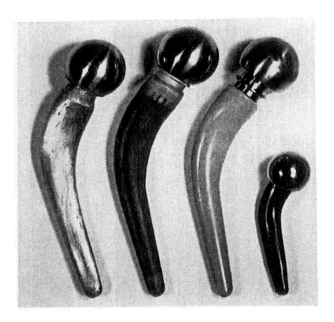

Figure 3   HARC human femoral stems; Co–Cr, carbon fiber/polysulfone, carbon fiber/PEEK; and canine femoral stem (left to right).

III.   FABRICATION

The canine implants were fabricated by compression molding, under vacuum, unidirectional carbon fiber–polysulfone plates that had the lateral–medial curvature of the stem incorporated. Unidirectional cores were then machined from the compression-molded plates. A sheath of dry fibers was braided around a mandrel that duplicated the shape of the unidirectional core. The machined unidirectional cores were inserted into the dry sheaths and the system was dipped in a solution of methylethylketone solvent and polysulfone. The solvent was allowed to evaporate and the dipping process repeated several times until the braid was fully impregnated with polysulfone. The system was then compression molded. The resultant implant had a thin coating of pure polysulfone. The braided cores of the polysulfone human implants were constructed in a similar manner. However, in the final fabrication step the pure polymer coating was injection molded around the cores. Cores of carbon fiber–PEEK for the human design were fabricated by molding comingled fibers of carbon fiber and PEEK. The outside coating was injected molded around the core. Figure 3 is a photo showing the canine hip and the polysulfone, PEEK, and cobalt–chrome human hips.

IV.   EFFECTS OF DESIGN FEATURES

There is a disruption of the path of load transfer in the femur when the femoral head is cut off and an implant inserted. Typically the bone immediately below the cut has a significantly reduced strain and this results in a reduction in bone mass. Away from the neck cut, the strain in the femur is reduced because the implant stiffens the implant–bone

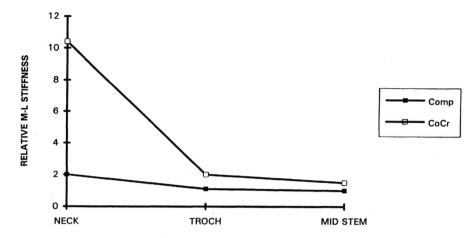

Figure 4 Canine femur relative stiffness; implanted section stiffness divided by unimplanted section stiffness.

system and there often are reductions in bone mass because of this. The maintenance of bone strain around an implant can be enhanced through consideration of two concepts: load sharing and load transfer [19]. In the Harrington design the portion of the load shared by the composite implant relative to the surrounding bone was minimized by keeping both the moment of inertia (I) and modulus of elasticity (E) of the implant relatively small. The bending stiffness (EI) of the implant–bone construct was calculated at three levels along the femur (at the neck cut, halfway down the greater trochanter, and at midstem). The calculated ratio of implanted to unimplanted stiffness in the medial–lateral direction (about the anterior–posterior axis) of the canine femur is shown in Fig. 4 and that of the human in Fig. 5. Although considerably less than that of the metallic

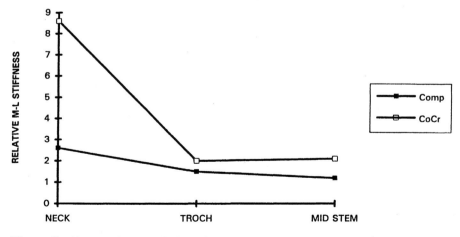

Figure 5 Human femur relative stiffness; implanted section stiffness divided by unimplanted section stiffness.

Co–Cr stem, it can be seen that even with the use of a composite stem, the stiffness in the region of the neck is doubled by the insertion of an implant.

Changing the mechanism of load transfer can be used to increase the bone strain in this proximal region. A unique and critical aspect of the Harrington design compensates for the reduction in axial strains by increasing circumferential strains by use of a proximal flare and taper. Care must be taken, however, since increased hoop strains can split a femur. In the human design a change in stiffness along the length of the implant adds to the proximal load transfer and reduces stress shielding. The effect of load-sharing and load-transfer differences was demonstrated by axial strain gauge measurements in cadaver dog femora subjected to simulated canine midstance loading. Composite and metal implants of the tubular Harrington design and standard straight-stem designs were compared [20]. Figure 6 shows the measured average percentage change in the axial bone strain on the medial aspect of the femora. Although the higher neck cut associated with the Harrington implant skews the results, the composite implants of both designs have higher proximal bone strains. Also, when compared to the straight-stemmed composite hip implants, the lower bending stiffness and proximal flare of the Harrington design produce higher bone strains than the straight stem at comparable distances below the neck cut.

The effectiveness of the proximal load transfer was demonstrated by hoop strain gauge measurements of dog cadaver femora [21]. Immediately after sacrifice of three dogs that were 78 months postimplantation of HARC stems, strain gauges were attached to both proximal femora (one implanted and one control) and the strain distribution due to a head load was measured. The strain distribution of zero-time implanted femora were also measured. Figure 7 shows that the hoop strains in just-implanted femora were over three times the normal femur; however, after 6 years of implantation the proximal bone had increased in thickness so the strains were reduced to approximately the level of the unimplanted bone. A thickened femoral cortex in this region was visually evident on all implanted femora, as shown in Fig. 8. Cortical wall thickness changes between the implanted and unimplanted sides were measured on transverse sections cut from the two

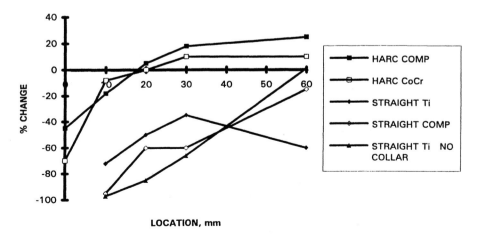

Figure 6   Percent change in cortical bone strains on medial aspect of canine femur; ratio of implanted to unimplanted strains.

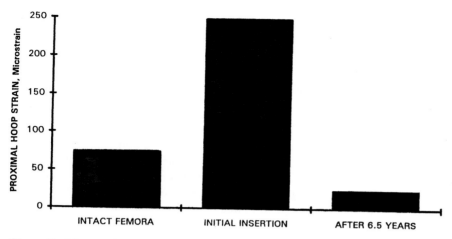

Figure 7   Measured canine femur proximal–medial hoop strains.

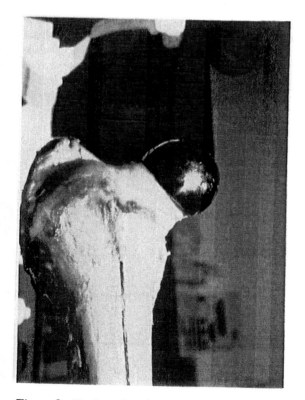

Figure 8   Explanted canine femur 78 months postsurgery showing proximal bone enhancement.

femora at identical levels. An increase in the average proximal thickness of 30% was observed for the implanted femur over the normal, as seen in Fig. 9. In the proximal medial region, cortical wall thickness increased by as much as 100%.

To analyze the effect of implant stiffness, implant geometry, location of neck cut, and interface bonding, three-dimensional finite element models of the proximal femur of the canine and human were constructed. Computer tomography (CT) scans and images from sectioned bones were used to define the geometry. The nonbonded interface condition that existed with most Harrington composite implants was modeled using nonlinear gap elements. Three loading conditions were applied: paw-off, mid-stance, and paw-strike. The muscle loads of the abductors, gluteals, and obturators were included, and all loads including the joint reaction force satisfied equilibrium with force plate measurements. ANSYS, a general-purpose finite element program, was used for the stress calculations. The results showed that the elastic modulus of the implant had a small effect on bone strain in the canine model. This indicates that the significant proximal load-sharing effect of implant modulus (Fig. 4) is counteracted by the load-transfer mechanism. Another factor investigated using the finite element method (FEM) of analysis was the effect of implant geometry and location of neck cut. It was anticipated that a high neck cut would provide stiffer proximal support and produce higher proximal bone strains and thus have better bone retention, but this was not the case. For any one geometry and interface condition, there was little difference in the bone stresses between the high (subcapital) and normal neck cuts. However, implant shape and interface conditions had significant effect on the proximal periprosthetic cancellous and cortical bone stresses, and thus significantly affected long-term bone changes. The proximal flare on the implant changed the cortical bone strain to a more circumferential direction. The anatomic HARC design had the highest proximal bone stresses of any evaluated. This is demonstrated by Fig. 10, which shows the direction and magnitude of the cortical bone principal stresses for the HARC design and a straight stem. Distal stem load transfer was assessed by summing the vertical loads on the cancellous bone supporting the distal tip. Figure 11

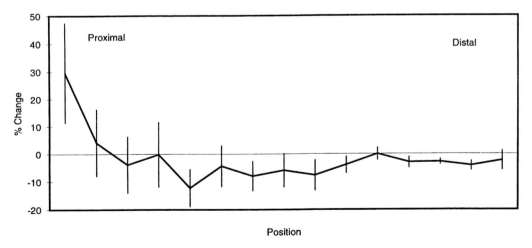

Figure 9   Average cortical thickness as percent of contralateral control; canine femur with composite implant at 78 months postsurgery.

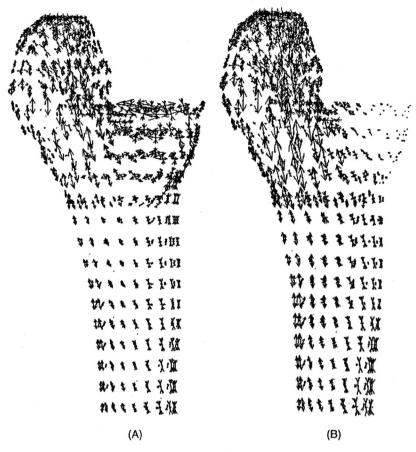

(A)   (B)

Figure 10   Principal stress magnitudes and directions in an implanted canine femur: (A) Co–Cr anatomic stem, (B) Co–Cr straight stem, both nonbonded.

shows the summation of vertical loads as a percentage of the vertical component of the applied head load. The specific implant designs modeled were: (*a*) HARC anatomic composite, (*b*) HARC Co–Cr, (*c*) HARC Comp without proximal wedge, (*d*) straight-stem Co–Cr with medial wedge, (*e*) straight Co–Cr stem. This demonstrates the importance of proximal geometry on load transfer.

An experimental assessment of the effect on bone response of distal load transfer as a function of proximal geometry was performed by comparing the area of bone in the medullary canal around the distal stem of the HARC prosthesis and a straight-stem prosthesis [22]. The straight-stem design had over three times the increase in distal tip bone compared to the HARC implant. It has been proposed that nonbonded stems in general will gradually subside and find distal support that will cause proximal "stress bypass" and thus have proximal cortical bone loss in the longer term [23]. Our results demonstrate that proximal geometry can substitute for proximal interface bonding and provide high proximal bone stresses and maintenance of proximal bone.

Most of the HARC dog implants had a smooth surface. Much research has been

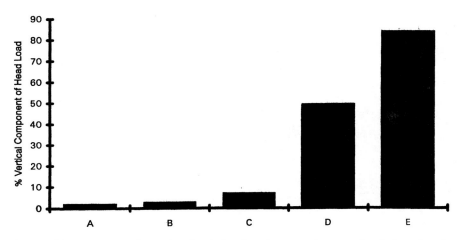

Figure 11   Load transfer under distal tip of canine stem (see text for designations).

done on attaining direct biological attachment to prostheses with porous coatings and/or bioactive coatings such as hydroxyapatite (HA). However, this direct bonding of bone to implant affects the local stress distribution around the implant. This in turn can affect periprosthetic bone changes. The finite element calculations described above were used to compare the effects of bonded and nonbonded implants. All bonded cases, no matter which stem design, had significant reduction in the proximal cortical bone stresses, although distal load transfer was reduced with proximal bonding. Figures 12a and 12b show the principal stress distributions for the bonded and nonbonded interface conditions, which show proximal bone strain reduction with bonding. An animal study was used to evaluate the effect of interface bonding [24]. Cobalt–chrome HARC implants with four different interface conditions (smooth, porous beads, HA on smooth, HA on beads) were implanted. Bone resorption at 13 months was significantly greater for the HA-beaded implant. One HA-beaded implant went to 28 months. It had such significant proximal anterior and posterior bone resorption that beads of the coating were exposed through the cortex (Fig. 13). Analysis of bone changes around the few HARC composite implants that had proximal HA coating also showed a slight increase in cortical porosity on the endosteal surface [25].

V. MATERIALS

A. Materials Selection

Four criteria are considered in the selection of candidate materials for use in implantable composite devices: (1) the materials must possess the mechanical and physical properties specified by the prosthetic design; (2) the materials must retain these properties after sterilization; (3) the materials must exhibit long-term biostability, i.e., resistance to mechanical and chemical degradation by the physiological environment; and (4) the materials must exhibit acceptable long-term biocompatibility after implantation.

Two morphologically distinct thermoplastic polymers have been evaluated for use in the HARC composite hip implant: polysulfone (PSF) and PEEK. Historically, PSF is the older of the two polymers, having been considered as early as 1976 for biomedical

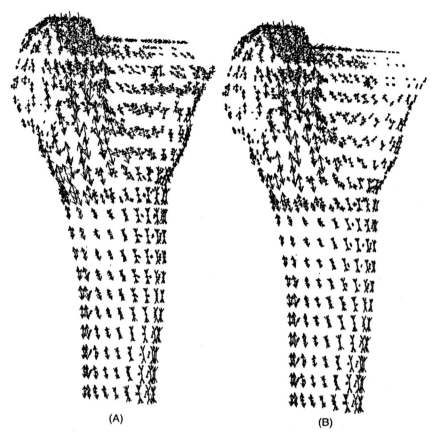

(A)   (B)

Figure 12 Principal stress directions in implanted canine femur: (A) nonbonded stem and (B) proximally bonded stem.

applications, and it has been more extensively evaluated [26]. PSF is an amorphous thermoplastic exhibiting ease of processing, good mechanical properties (Table 2), and good biocompatibility [27]. The structural repeat unit of PSF consists of phenylene units linked by three different chemical groups: isopropylidene, ether, and sulfone (Fig. 14). The high bond strength imparted by the resonance of this structure gives good chemical stability and resistance to hydrolysis. Additionally, the aromatic nature of the ring structure lends polysulfone some resistance to crosslinking and chain scission, which can result when exposed to ionizing radiation.

PEEK is a semicrystalline thermoplastic possessing good mechanical properties (Table 2) and good biocompatibility [28,29]. The repeating structural unit of PEEK consists of phenylene units linked by two different chemical groups: two ethers and one ketone linkage (Fig. 14). Replacing the bulky sulfone group found in polysulfone with a more compact ketone group linkage allows crystallization to occur in PEEK and a range of polymer crystallinity can be achieved. The semicrystalline structure of PEEK gives the polymer good chemical stability and better resistance to tensile strength degradation after gamma-irradiation [30].

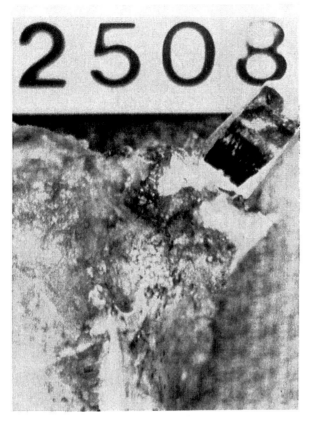

Figure 13   Explanted canine femur, proximal porous bead with HA coating (28 months post-surgery).

PAN-based, AS-4 carbon fibers were used as the reinforcing phase for the HARC composite hip implants. Both PSF/CF and PEEK/CF composite materials form strong carbon fiber–polymer matrix interfacial bonds and exhibit good interlaminar fracture toughness.

B.   Effects of Sterilization on Candidate Materials

Sterilization is required of all medical devices implanted within the body. As such polymer matrix–carbon fiber composite hip implants must be able to undergo sterilization without subsequent degradation of their mechanical, physical, or chemical properties. Three methods are commonly used to sterilize medical devices: steam sterilization, exposure to an ethylene oxide atmosphere, and gamma-irradiation using a Co-60 source. The effects of various sterilization regimens on the diametral tensile strength of unidirectional polysulfone–carbon fiber composite specimens have been tested [31]. In the study, the failure strength of steam-sterilized PSF/CF specimens was found to increase with repeated autoclave exposures of 270°F and 30 psi. Also, slight increases in failure strength were observed in the PSF/CF specimens exposed to repeated cycles of ethylene oxide at 150°F and 15 psi. However, the failure strength of PSF/CF specimens sterilized by repeated

Table 2   Room Temperature Properties of Polysulfone (PSF) and PEEK

Property	PSF	PEEK
Tensile yield strength (MPa)	70.3	92
Tensile modulus (GPa)	2.48	3.6
Compressive yield strength (MPa)	96	119
Tensile elongation to break (%)	50–100	50
Poisson's ratio	0.37	0.42
Density (g/cc)	1.25	1.32

cycles of 2.5 Mrad gamma-irradiation (Co-60 source) was found to decrease with each exposure.

A second study evaluated the long-term effects of gamma-irradiation on the tensile strength of PSF/CF and PEEK/CF, which were subsequently environmentally conditioned in either saline or lipid solutions [30]. After a single dosage of 3.5 Mrads of Co-60 gamma-radiation, neither the tensile strength of the unconditioned PSF/CF nor that of the unconditioned PEEK/CF specimens was significantly degraded. However, after 6 months conditioning in both saline and lipid solutions, the tensile strength of the PSF/CF specimens decreased significantly. In contrast, the tensile strength of the gamma-irradiated, environmentally conditioned PEEK/CF specimens was not significantly affected.

The results indicate that sterilization by gamma-irradiation followed by long-term exposure to physiologic fluids may compromise the mechanical properties of PSF/CF composite implants, and therefore, alternative sterilization methods should be used.

C.   Effects of Environmental Exposure on Candidate Materials

Once implanted the PSF/CF or PEEK/CF composite hips are subjected to a complex physiological environment that has the potential to degrade the polymer matrix. Various parts of the implant are exposed either to bone, to the articular cartilage covering the

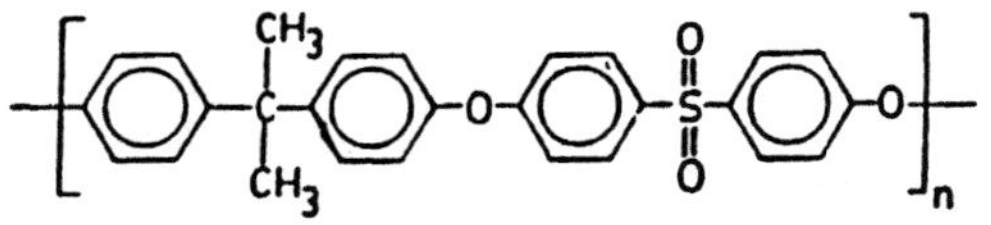

(a) Polysulfone Structural Repeat Unit

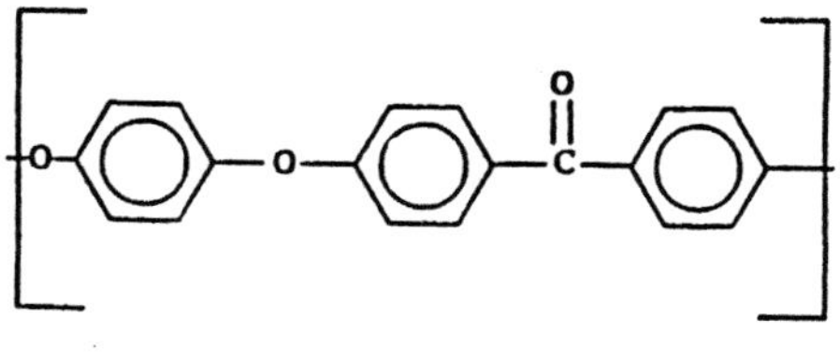

(b) PEEK Structural Repeat Unit

Figure 14   Structural repeat units of (a) polysulfone and (b) polyetheretherketone (PEEK).

Table 3   Transverse Tensile Strength of PSF/CF and PEEK/CF
Composites Conditioned in Palm Oil (MPa)

	PSF/CF	PEEK/CF
Lipid (6 months)	37.6 ± 9.5	85.1 ± 3.5
Control	49.1 ± 7.4	82.6 ± 8.0
Single-factor ANOVA (F critical: 5.3)	3.9	0.410

load-bearing surfaces of the joints, to the synovial fluids that lubricate the joints, or to the bone marrow contained within the femoral cavities. In particular, the effect of the lipid component of bone marrow on the mechanical properties of PSF and PEEK is a concern.

1.   In Vitro Environmental Effects

The effects of long-term, *in vitro* conditioning in a simulated physiological bone marrow lipid (palm oil) on the transverse tensile strength of PSF/CF and PEEK/CF composite specimens have been reported [30]. The experimentally determined transverse tensile strengths are listed in Table 3. The tensile strength of the two composite systems has not been significantly degraded by environmental conditioning in lipids.

Gel permeation chromatography (GPC) and nuclear magnetic resonance (NMR) analyses were performed on unreinforced PSF resins exposed to the same simulated physiological bone marrow lipids to evaluate the chemical resistance to PSF to environmental degradation. As seen in Table 4, GPC revealed no significant changes in the molecular weight of PSF after 6-month conditioning in lipids. Comparison of the ^{13}C-NMR spectra show them to be nearly identical. These results indicate that the chemistry of the polysulfone has not been significantly altered by 6 months conditioning in a simulated bone marrow lipid.

2.   In Vivo Environmental Effects

The HARC PSF/CF steam sterilized composite hip was first implanted in canines in 1984. Unilateral femoral arthroplasties were performed on three skeletally mature greyhounds. After 6½ years clinical performance, the contralateral and implant-containing femurs were harvested and cross-sectioned into widths of 2 to 3 mm. Consecutive femoral sections were prepared either for histologic or morphologic materials evaluation. Histological specimens of the bone–composite interface were prepared with the composite section in place by embedding, polishing, and staining with mineralized bone stain. Histo-

Table 4   Gel Permeation Chromatography Analyses of the Molecular
Weight of Lipid-Conditioned Polysulfone Resins

	M_n	M_w	M_z
Palm oil (6 months)	15,200	48,200	86,100
Implant (6.5 years)	14,500	48,900	87,000
Control	15,600	47,700	86,600

Note. Calibration: polystyrene

logic evaluation showed 90% of the implant outer surfaces to be in direct contact with a circumferentially striated, organized fibrous membrane having an average thickness of 250 μm. In areas of direct bone apposition, a nearly continuous circumferential shell of lamellar trabecular bone was surrounded by densified cancellous bone, which demonstrated active remodeling as determined by UV fluorescence.

Composite specimens for morphologic materials evaluation were prepared by removing the implant section from the surrounding bone. (This surrounding bone was then used to calculate the changes in the cortical bone thickness and density as described earlier.) The morphological condition of the outer PSF coating of the HARC hip after 6½ years implantation in the physiologic environment was evaluated using both light microscopy and scanning electron microscopy. Overall, the implants demonstrated excellent long-term clinical performance. No gross structural flaws were observed. The interfaces of the braid and unidirectional core maintained good integrity and showed no evidence of separation. Although the majority of the composite hips outer surfaces appeared smooth when viewed both by light and scanning electron microscopy, some cracking in isolated areas of the outer PSF surfaces was observed.

The molecular structure of the outer PSF coating was analyzed using GPC in order to determine if observed cracking was associated with environmentally induced changes in the polymer's molecular structure. As seen in Table 4, no significant alteration of molecular weight was observed. Additionally, the molecular weight distribution remained unimodal, with no evidence for the presence of the smaller polymer species typically associated with structural degradation.

The effects of the physiologic environment on the chemical structure of the carbon atoms that make up the backbone and side chains of the outer polysulfone coating were analyzed using ^{13}C-NMR. Six and one-half years following implantation, no significant spectral differences were seen by NMR analysis. The results indicate that the PSF coating of the HARC composite hip has excellent resistance to chemical degradation by the physiologic environment during long-term implantation.

VI. DISCUSSION

The stiffness of an implant is determined by both its material elastic moduli and its geometry. The HARC implant has both comparatively low material and geometric stiffness. However, stiffness determines the upper limit of how much of the applied load can possibly be removed from the bone. It is not, however, the only factor in determining the change in cortical bone changes. Proximal load-transfer mechanisms can induce bone strains that compensate for loss of load being carried. Also, rigid bonding of an implant to bone has the potential to significantly reduce bone strains. The HARC composite implant utilizes a lower-modulus material that has maximum strength in the unsupported region, does not require high interface strength, and has geometry and material stiffness variations that create proximal load transfer. The effectiveness of these design features has been demonstrated by *in vitro* and *in vivo* tests.

The PEEK and PFS polymer-based composite implants demonstrated adequate biostability and biocompatibility properties in these studies. The HARC PSF/CF composite hip was manufactured with the materials and processing technology available in 1984. The cracking observed in the 6½-year implants is believed to result from residual stresses that were induced during the implant manufacture. Since that time, technological advances in polymer molding techniques and the development and availability of new high-performance semicrystalline polymers have allowed for the reduction of the residual stresses found in the original HARC composite hip.

This development program has demonstrated the effectiveness of the stem design concepts of (1) proximal wedging load transfer, (2) lower-modulus implants, and (3) nonbonded implant surfaces. The viability of the HARC implant system is thus demonstrated.

ACKNOWLEDGMENTS

A number of people have made significant contributions to this research project over the past 10 years. Among these are: Tom Hansen, Allan Weinstein, Janson Emmanual, Ron Yapp, Frank Magee, Roger Johnson, Bob Poser, Tom Murray, Ed Koeneman, Debbie Lumbardo, Roy Gealer, Tony Hedley, John Szivek, and Tony Villaneuva.

REFERENCES

1. Huiskes, R., Biomechanics of artificial-joint fixation, in *Basic Orthopaedic Biomechanics* (V. C. Mow and W. C. Hayes, eds.), Raven Press, New York, 1991.
2. Sumner, D. R., Turner, T. M., Urban, R. M., and Galante, J. O., Remodeling and ingrowth of bone at two years in a canine cementless total hip-arthroplasty model, *J. Bone Joint Surg.*, *74-A*(2), 239–250 (February 1992).
3. Bobyn, J. D., Mortimer, E. S., Glassman, A. H., Engh, C. A., Miller, J. E., and Brooks, C. E., Producing and avoiding stress shielding, *Clin Orthop. Rel. Res.*, May 1991, pp. 79–96.
4. Page, A., Jasty, M., Bragdon, C., Ito, D., and Harris, W. H., Alterations in femoral and acetabular bone strains immediately following cementless total hip arthroplasty: An *in vitro* canine study, *J. Orthop. Res. 9*, 738–748 (January 1990).
5. Fornasier, V., Wright, J., and Seligman J., The histomorphologic and morphometric study of asymptomatic hip arthroplasty, *Clin. Orthop. Rel. Res.*, No. 271, October 1991, pp. 272–282.
6. Magee, F. P., Weinstein, A. M., Longo III, J. A., Koeneman, J. B., and Yapp, R. A., A canine composite femoral stem, *Clin. Orthop. Rel. Res.*, No. 235, October 1988, pp. 237–252.
7. Christel, P., Meunier, A., Leclercq, S., Bouquet, Ph., and Buttazzoni, B., Development of a carbon–carbon hip prosthesis, *J. Biomed. Mater. Res.: Appl. Biomater. 21*(A2), 191–218 (1987).
8. Devanathian, D., and Levine, D., *Composites in orthopaedics*, Technical Paper, Society of Manufacturing Engineers, Autocom '86, Dearborn, MI, EM86-362, 1986, pp. 3–7.
9. Musikant, S., Quartz and graphite filament reinforced polymer composites for orthopaedic surgical application, *J. Biomed. Mater. Res. Symp., 1*, 225–235 (1971).
10. Hastings, G. W., Carbon fibre composites for orthopaedic implants, *Composites*, 1978, pp. 193–197.
11. McKenna, G. B., Statton, W. O., Dunn, H. K., Johnson, K. D., Bradley, G. W., and Daniels, A. U., *The development of composite materials for orthopaedic implant devices*, presented at Meeting of Society of Aerospace Materials and Process Engineers, 1976, pp. 232–241.
12. Chang, F. K., Perez, J. L., and Davidson, J. A., Stiffness and strength tailoring of a hip prosthesis made of advanced composite materials, *J. Biomed. Mater. Res., 24*, 873–899 (1990).
13. Davidson, J. A., The challenge and opportunity for composites in structural orthopaedic applications, *J. Comp. Technol. Res., 9*(4), 151–161 (1987).
14. Kwarteng, K. B., and Stark, C., Carbon fiber-reinforced PEEK (APC-2/AS-4) composites for orthopaedic implants, *SAMPE Q.*, October 1990, pp. 10–14.

15. Skinner, H. B., Composite technology for total hip arthroplasty, *Clin. Orthop. Rel. Res.*, No. 235, October 1988, pp. 224–236.

16. Tarr, R. R., and McLaren, A., *The design of canine THR for the biological evaluation of human THR*, presented at Second World Congress on Biomaterials, 10th Annual Meeting of the Society for Biomaterials, Washington, DC, April 27–May 1, 1984.

17. Roffman, M., Mendes, D. G., Charit, Y., and Hunt, M. S., *Total hip arthroplasty in dogs using carbon fibers reinforced polysulfone implants*, presented at Second World Congress on Biomaterials, 10th Annual Meeting of the Society for Biomaterials, Washington, DC, April 27–May 1, 1984.

18. Hulbert, S. F., and Wack, M. A., *A composite hip prosthesis*, presented at 15th Annual Meeting of the Society for Biomaterials, Lake Buena Vista, FL, April 28–May 2, 1989.

19. Koeneman, J. B., Fundamental aspects of load transfer and load sharing, in *Quantitative Characterization and Performance of Porous Implants for Hard Tissue Applications* (J. E. Lemons, ed.), American Society for Testing and Materials, Philadelphia, ASTM STP 953, 241–248, 1987.

20. Poser, R. D., O'Connor, D. O., Koeneman, J. B., Jasty, M., Longo, J. A., and Harris, W. H., *Material and geometric effect on femoral strain restoration and micromotion: An* in-vitro *comparison of canine femoral components*, presented at 4th World Biomaterials Congress, Berlin, April 24–28, 1992.

21. Koeneman, J. B., Lumbardo, D. F., Hansen, T. M., Poser, R. D., and Longo III, J. A., *Comparison of initial stress stimuli with six year cortical bone changes around a unique hip implant*, presented at Bioengineering Conference, American Society of Mechanical Engineers, Breckenridge, Colorado, June 25–29, 1993, 24, 546–548.

22. Lumbardo, D. F., Koeneman, J. B., Hansen, T. M., Longo III, J. A., and Poser, R. D., *The effect of interface bonding and geometry on long term periprosthetic bone changes*, presented at 40th Annual Meeting of the Orthopaedic Research Society, New Orleans, LA, February 21–24, 1994.

23. Van Rietbergen, B., Huiskes, R., Weinans, H., Sumner, D. R., Turner, T. M., and Galante, J. O., The mechanism of bone remodeling and resorption around press-fitted THA stems, *J. Biomech.*, 26(4/5), 369–382 (1993).

24. Poser, R. D., Magee, F. P., Longo III, J. A., Koeneman, J. B., Emmanual, J., and Hedley, A. K., *Comparison of four femoral stem surface coatings in a canine model*, presented at 4th World Biomaterials Congress, Berlin, April 24–28, 1992.

25. Longo III, J. A., Magee, F. P., Mather, S. E., Emmanual, J. E., Koeneman, J. B., and Weinstein, A. M., *An interface comparison between a press-fit and HA-coated composite hip prosthesis*, presented at Interfaces '90, 1990.

26. McKenna, G. B., *The development of fiber reinforced polymer composites for orthopedic applications*, Ph.D., Dissertation, University of Utah, 1976.

27. Spector, M., *Basic biocompatibility of polysulfone*, Union Carbide Internal Report.

28. Jockisch, K., et al., *J. Biomed. Mater. Res., 26*, 133–146, 1992.

29. Williams, D. F., et al., *J. Mater. Sci. Lett., 6*, 188, 1987.

30. Overland, M. K., *The Environmental Resistance of Three Orthopedic Composite Materials Conditioned in an In Vitro Environment*, Ph.D. Dissertation, Arizona State University, 1993.

31. Koeneman, J. B., Orthomatrix Internal Report, November 1985.

II
ORTHOPEDIC BIOMATERIALS

7

Crystallographic and Spectroscopic Characterization and Morphology of Biogenic and Synthetic Apatites

B. Ben-Nissan, C. Chai, and L. Evans
University of Technology
Sydney, Australia

I. INTRODUCTION

Apatite is the name given to a group of crystals of the general formula $M_{10}(RO_4)_6X_2$, where R is most commonly phosphorus, M could be one of several metals, although it is usually calcium, and X is commonly hydroxide or a halogen such as fluorine or chlorine. The mineral was first called apatite in 1788 by Werner, having been earlier confused with other minerals such as aquamarine, olivine, and fluorite. Similarity in composition to calcined bone was established by the analysis of Proust and Klaproth in 1788 (Deer, Howie, and Zussman 1985).

Since DeJong's (1926) publication of the first x-ray diffraction (XRD) study of bone, it has been recognized that the inorganic phase of bone closely resembles the mineral structures known as apatites. Even though there is a general agreement that the biogenic materials are a basic calcium phosphate with apatitic structure, disagreements have continued for many years due to the following problems: the presence of impurities and isomorphous substitutional changes, the pre- and coexistence of other calcium phosphates, and the nonstoichiometry of biogenic apatites.

Bone is the best known example of a biogenic apatite and, like most biologically formed materials, is a complex structure. It is a specific connective tissue consisting of closely packed bundles of collagen fibers containing very small crystallites of a material resembling calcium hydroxyapatite. The microarchitecture of these components influences the mechanical properties of bone. Within the skeletal system, bone also incorporates soft vascular interstices and macroscopic pores (Herring 1968).

The chemical composition of bone consists of 25% by weight of organics and the remainder is inorganic matter (Boskey and Posner 1984; LeGeros 1993). Most of the organic matter is collagen Type I (about 90%) (Gay and Miller 1978; Termine et al. 1981), the remainder being acidic glycoproteins (Leaver, Triffit, and Holbrook 1975),

Table 1   Typical Composition of the Mineral Phases of Human Femoral Bone[a]

CaO	P$_2$O$_5$	Na$_2$O	CO$_2$	H$_2$O	MgO	K$_2$O	F	Cl
51.31	36.65	1.04	5.86	3.78	0.77	0.32	0.23	0.01

Source: From Dallemagnes and Richelle 1973
[a]Weight percentage after removal of organic fraction by glycerine per 6% KOH

phosphoproteins (Shuttleworth and Veis 1972), serum proteins (Ashton, Hohling, and Triffit 1976), lipids, and small proteoglycans (Boskey 1984). The composition of collagen is relatively constant, but minor variations in the amino acid components may be observed as a function of species and tissue. The nature of the sequence of the amino acid residues in bone collagens is given by Hanning and Nordwig (1965) and Fietzek and Kuhn (1976).

Bone mineral can contain several types of hydrated calcium phosphates, with the most common form being calcium hydroxyapatite Ca$_{10}$(PO$_4$)$_6$(OH)$_2$ (HA). The typical composition of the mineral phases of human femoral bone is given in Table 1 (Dallemagnes and Richelle 1973).

From a chemical perspective, it is now quite well established that kinetic factors may be considerably more important in determining the nature of calcium phosphate phases present during a precipitation reaction than considerations based solely upon equilibrium data (Brown and Fulmer 1991). The initial formation of an amorphous calcium phosphate (ACP) at high pH may be followed by its transformation to HA via the formation of octacalcium phosphate (OCP), which may serve as a template for HA growth. As the acidity of the solution is increased, other precursor phases such as dicalcium phosphate dihydrate (DCPD) may participate in accordance with Oswald's rule, which predicts that the least stable phase having the highest solubility is formed preferentially during a sequential precipitation.

It has also been shown by Nancollas (1982a) and LeGeros (1981) that different calcium phosphate phases may be stabilized or destabilized by the presence of various cations and anions, which may not be significantly incorporated into the calcium phosphate crystal lattice, but may markedly influence nucleation and subsequent growth processes.

Another complicating factor in the mechanism of calcium phosphate crystallization is that mixed solids may form by the growth of one phase upon another in the metastable supersaturated solutions. The formation of these solid phases in supersaturated physiological fluids such as serum and saliva is mediated not only by biological restraints, but also by the nucleation and growth mechanisms. It is also important to consider both the role and the effect of the organic matrix in the nucleation and growth of the apatite crystallites in biological environments.

II.   CALCIUM PHOSPHATE PHASES

Although hydroxyapatite (HA) is usually assumed to be a model structural component for biological apatites, there is wide acceptance that other phases (Table 2) may also participate in the crystallization reaction. It is generally recognized that the crystallization of many sparingly soluble salts involves the formation of metastable precursor phases that subsequently dissolve as the precipitation reaction proceeds.

Table 2 Calcium Phosphate Phases

	Mineral	Empirical formulas	Ca/P
Dicalcium phosphate dihydrate	Brushite	$CaHPO_4 \cdot 2H_2O$	1.00
Dicalcium phosphate	Monetite	$CaHPO_4$	1.00
Octacalcium phosphate		$Ca_8H_2(PO_4)_6 \cdot 5H_2O$	1.33
β-Tricalcium phosphate	Whitlockite	$\beta\text{-}Ca_3(PO_4)_2$	1.50
Hydroxyapatite		$Ca_{10}(PO_4)_6(OH)_2$	1.67
Tetracalcium phosphate monoxyde		$Ca_4(PO_4)_2O$	2.0
Defect apatites		$Ca_{10-x}(HPO_4)_x(PO_4)_{6-x}(OH)_{2-x}$ $0 < x < 2$	$(10\text{-}x)\text{:}6$

Source: Modified from Nancollas 1989

Unstable amorphous calcium phosphate (ACP) is formed when calcium phosphate is precipitated from highly supersaturated solutions (Brecevic and Furedi-Milhofer 1972). This is usually characterized by the absence of definite peaks in the x-ray diffraction pattern (Fig. 1), a lower resolution in the infrared (IR) absorption spectra, and some degree of short-range order in the radial distribution pattern. The composition of ACP appears to depend upon the precipitation conditions and it is usually formed in calcium phosphate solutions of pH greater than 7.

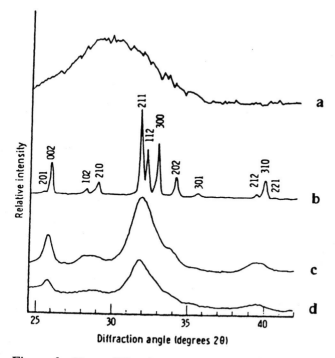

Figure 1 X-ray diffraction patterns: (a), amorphous calcium phosphate (ACP); (b), well-crystallized hydroxyapatite (HA); (c), small-crystallite-size synthetic HAp; and (d), powdered human femur diaphysis. (From Posner, Betts, and Blumenthal 1979.)

When HA is precipitated from solutions of low saturation (Moreno and Varughese 1981), very fine crystals of hydroxyapatite, smaller than those formed at high supersaturation, precipitate directly with no amorphous precursor (Boskey and Posner 1976).

Crystalline HA can be prepared either by allowing ACP to transform in aqueous slurries or by direct precipitation under conditions of low supersaturation from metastable solutions (Boskey and Posner 1976). ACP is also known to transform to HA in water and upon exposure to high humidity in air.

Dicalcium phosphate dihydrate (DCPD) regularly forms in slightly acidic calcium phosphate solutions near or below room temperature (Nancollas 1984; Brown and Fulmer 1991). These monoclinic crystals have been found in immature bone and in dental and renal calculi. DCPD consists of parallel interconnected continuous chains of $CaHPO_4$ groups in a sheetlike arrangement with water molecules between the sheets (Young and Brown 1982).

Octacalcium phosphate (OCP) has also been found in dental calculi, bone, and immature teeth (Tung and Brown 1985). It can also be prepared by hydrolysis of DCPD in solutions of pH 5–6 (Brown et al. 1962) and can also be heterogeneously precipitated directly upon tricalcium phosphate (TCP) (Heughebaert et al. 1988). OCP crystals consist of distinct alternating layers, one having a structure similar to that of HA, and the other consisting of more widely spaced phosphate and calcium ions with interspersed water molecules (Young and Brown 1982). The similarity between HA and OCP structures supports the suggestions of OCP acting as a precursor phase to the precipitation of HA in the formation of many biogenic calcium phosphates (Tung and Brown 1983).

Detailed studies on apatite formation have been made at low temperatures in order to understand the mechanisms of bone mineralization. At medium or high supersaturation, growth of the apatite structure involves the formation of one or more precursors with a formation rate that is higher than that of apatite. The most commonly reported precursor is amorphous tricalcium phosphate (ATCP), characterized by a calcium/phosphate (Ca/P) ratio of 1.50. Ca/P ratios lower than the stoichiometric HA have been attributed to the adsorption of HPO_4^{2-} ions onto ATCP particles.

Work on water-alcohol solutions has shown the existence of another amorphous calcium phosphate phase characterized by a Ca/P ratio of 1.33, corresponding to the composition of OCP. Amorphous octacalcium phosphate (AOCP) and ATCP can often be found simultaneously; it has been postulated that the first-formed precipitate is generally a mixture of two amorphous compounds showing a Ca/P ratio ranging from 1.33 to 1.50 (Rey et al. 1991). AOCP appears essentially in neutral and slightly basic solutions, whereas ATCP forms in basic media.

These metastable amorphous phases can be transformed into poorly crystalline apatite at rates that depend on the temperature and composition of the solution. Several mechanisms have been proposed for the transformation of amorphous phases into apatite. The formation of transient phases such as crystalline OCP has been postulated on the basis of solubility measurements (Brown et al. 1962; Young and Brown 1982).

III. SUBSTITUTED APATITES

Most of the published work suggests that bone phosphate exists almost entirely as hydroxyapatite (HA). However, the relative deficiency of calcium and the presence of substantial CO_3^{2-} and HPO_4^{2-} in bone phosphate indicates modification of the ideal HA structure. The hexagonal crystal structure, constructed from columns of divalent metal ions and oxygen atoms forming parallel channels in the lattice, makes it particularly prone to ion substitution (Kibby and Hall 1972). This is a major cause of the complexity of the precipitating apatite system.

In biological mineralization, substitutions may involve ions of the same charge, such as F^- or Cl^- for OH^- (Moreno and Varughese 1981), Sr^{2+} and other divalent metal ions for Ca^{2+}, or might involve ions of other charges, such as carbonate or sulfate for phosphate, and trace constituents such as iron, copper, zinc, and so on. In all cases, crystal surfaces play an important role and maturation processes may be strongly altered by surface adsorption of ions or molecules. A number of reviews on the possible roles of the minor constituents and some trace elements are given in Table 3. Ions like Mg^{2+}, CO_3^{2-}, $P_2O_7^{4-}$ and several bone proteins (osteocalcine, proteoglycan) have been shown to inhibit apatite maturation and growth (Blumenthal, Betts, and Posner 1975).

HA has been extensively studied and a number of reviews have described its physical chemistry (Kanazowa and Monma 1973; Nancollas 1982a; Driessens 1983; LeGeros and LeGeros 1984; Arends et al. 1987). There have also been extensive investigations of the precipitation of HA or its precursor phases from aqueous solutions. Studies have been carried out at low (Boskey and Posner 1976), moderate (Feenstra and deBruyn 1979), and high supersaturations (Brecevic and Furedi-Milhofer 1972), and at constant composition (Koutsoukos et al. 1980). Kinetics of calcium-deficient hydroxyapatite formation were studied by Brown and Fulmer (1991).

Table 3 Various Substitutions Occurring in Apatites

Impurities	Substituent for	Reference
Na^+	Ca^{2+}	LeGeros 1967
K^+	Ca^{2+}	Driessens 1982
Mg^{2+}	Ca^{2+}	LeGeros 1981
Li^+		LeGeros et al. 1990
Carbonate, CO_3^{2-}	PO_4^{3-}	McConnell 1973
Fluoride, F^-	OH^-	LeGeros 1981
Chloride, Cl^-	OH^-	LeGeros 1974
Pyrophosphate $P_2O_7^{4-}$	PO_4^{3-}	LeGeros 1981
Citrate, $C_6H_5O_7^{3-}$	PO_4^{3-}	Driessens 1982
Acid phosphate, HPO_4^{2-}	PO_4^{3-}	Trautz 1967
Sr^{2+}	Ca^{2+}	LeGeros et al. 1990
Pb^{2+}	Ca^{2+}	Neumans and Neuman 1958
Ba^{2+}	Ca^{2+}	Brudevold and Soremark 1967
Fe^{3+}	Ca^{2+}	LeGeros et al. 1980
Cd^{2+}	Ca^{2+}	LeGeros et al. 1980
Mn^{2+}	Ca^{2+}	Mayer et al. 1993
Zn^{2+}	Ca^{2+}	Guggenheim and Caster 1973
Co^{2+}		Blumenthal et al. 1975
Ni^{2+}		LeGeros 1981
Al^{3+}	Ca^{2+}	Blumenthal and Posner 1984
AlO_4^{3-}	PO_4^{3-}	LeGeros 1981
$Cr3^+$	PO_4^{3-}	LeGeros et al. 1980

Table 4 Basic Lattice Constant Differences in Various Apatites

Apatite series	Formulas	a	c	c/a
Carbonated apatite	$Ca_{10}(PO_4)_6(CO_3)H_2O$	9.34	6.88	0.736
Fluorapatite	$Ca_5(PO_4)_3F$	9.36	6.88	0.7346
Chlorapatite	$Ca_5(PO_4)_3Cl$	9.64	6.77	0.702
Hydroxyapatite	$Ca_5(PO_4)_3(OH)$	9.41	6.88	0.731

According to LeGeros (1967, 1981), the inorganic or mineral phase of bone should be regarded as carbonate-substituted apatite, which has Ca/P ratio below or above 1.67 depending upon the species, age, and type of bone.

Carbonate- and fluorine-substituted apatites are the most commonly encountered in natural and biogenic apatites and are called dahllite and fluorapatite, respectively, while francolite is the name used for an apatite containing appreciable amounts of carbonate and greater than about 1% of fluorine. The most common substitution in HA occurs in the (OH) position, yielding fluorapatite and chlorapatite. The chemical stability of these compounds varies due to the presence of these substitutions, with fluorapatite being more chemically stable than HA, which is in turn more stable than chlorapatite. Young and Elliot (1966) have attributed this to the fact that there is no polar moment associated with Ca^{2+} and F^- in fluorapatite, which is not the case for hydroxyapatite and chlorapatite. The lattice parameters and the c/a ratios are given in Table 4.

As stated earlier, mammalian hard tissue is an impure form of the calcium phosphate, hydroxyapatite. Hydroxyapatite exists over a compositional range that may be characterized in terms of its Ca/P ratio. Stoichiometric hydroxyapatite, $Ca_{10}(PO_4)_6OH_2$ has a Ca/P ratio of 1.67, while calcium-deficient hydroxyapatite, $Ca_{(10-x)}(HPO_4)_x(PO_4)_{(6-x)}(OH)_{2-x}$ may have a Ca/P ratio as low as 1.5. Biological apatites are known to be calcium deficient. Bone apatites contain carbonate, while teeth contain substantial amounts of fluoride as well (Table 5).

IV. BONE MINERALIZATION

The factors initiating the deposition of mineral in the calcification of bone are not well understood. There is evidence that the earliest extracellular mineral deposited in the chick embryo is a noncrystalline calcium phosphate (Landis, Paine, and Glimcher 1981; Lee, Landis, and Glimcher 1986). Some investigators report that the first phase that appears in the mineralization of extracellular matrix vesicles in the growth plates of long bones is an amorphous calcium phosphate (Wuthier and Eanes 1975), while others report HA as the first phase (Ali, Wisby, and Gray 1978; Hertzfeld et al. 1980; Murphree, Hsu, and Anderson 1982) have suggested that, in early bone formation in the chick embryo, the mineral $CaHPO_4 \cdot 2H_2O$ is a precursor to bone apatite (Lee, Landis, and Glimcher 1986). Mineralization occurs extracellularly and involves the initial formation of apatite crystals in specific sites along collagen fibers, followed by the replacement of much of the water in the tissue with mineral.

Many theories have been proposed to explain the initiation of mineralization, including local elevations of phosphate via hydrolysis of organic phosphates by alkaline phosphatase, enzymatic removal of inhibitors of mineral deposition, and direct nucleation of

Table 5 Composition of Human Bone Dentine
and Enamel

Constituents[a]	Bone	Dentine	Enamel
Ca^{2+}	24.5	27.0	36.0
PO_4^{3-} as P	10.5	13.0	17.7
Na^+	0.7	0.3	0.5
K^+	0.03	0.05	0.08
Mg^{2+}	0.55	1.1	0.44
CO_3^{2-}	5.8	4.5	2.3
F^-	0.02	0.05	0.01
Cl^-	0.10	0.01	0.30
$P_2O_7^{4-}$	0.05	0.08	0.022
Ash[b]	65	70	97.0
Organic	25	20	1.0
H_2O[c]	8.7	10	1.55

Source: LeGeros 1981
[a]Percentage of total dry weight
[b]Total inorganic
[c]Adsorbed water

hydroxyapatite or other calcium phosphate minerals onto bone collagen fibers. However, it should be noted that most of the published work states that the mineral deposited in ossification is formed by epitaxial growth on existing crystals.

Many detailed studies on calcium phosphates and collagen have been previously undertaken. Glimcher and Krane (1967) studied the mineral contents of bone and the effects of phosphoproteins on the bonding of phosphates onto organic matrices. Nancollas (1982b) performed growth experiments of calcium phosphate on ceramic surfaces under different conditions and analyzed the chemistry of crystallization in terms of ionic strength, degree of supersaturation, and acidity. Klein, Driessens, and de Groot (1984) looked at the biodegradability and macropore tissue ingrowth of different calcium-phosphate-based ceramics. Clarke et al. (1993) reported on the nucleation and kinetics of growth of phosphate on Type I collagen and HA at different concentrations, acidities, and temperatures, with special emphasis on the crystallographic characteristics of the crystals obtained.

Dalas and Koutsoukos (1989), in their investigations based on HA-containing metal oxides, found that only those containing ZrO_2 stabilized with 8% Y_2O_3 were able to induce calcium phosphate formation upon immersing into calcium phosphate supersaturated solutions. Ebrahimpour, Perez, and Nancollas (1991) have demonstrated the possibility of calcium oxalate monohydrate (COM) growth on HA and showed that the human serum albumin promoted the growth, while citrate and magnesium acted as inhibitors.

Crystallization of HA on phosphorous-containing copolymers was carried out by Dalas, Kallitsis, and Koutsoukos (1991). A biomaterial composite was produced by precipitation of calcium phosphate onto collagen by Clarke et al. (1991). These authors have found that the addition of 1 millimole (mM) of O-phosphoserine causes the morphology of the brushite crystals to change from large to small needles. Osteoblastic differentiation was promoted on the surface of the material and new bone growth was observed.

V.   THE MORPHOLOGY OF BONE AND BIOGENIC APATITES

Morphologically, there are three types of bone cells: the osteoblast, osteocyte, and osteoclast. The osteoblast, described in detail by Pritchard (1976a) and Robinson, Doty, and Cooper (1973), is a mononucleated cell, typically 20 to 30 micrometers (μm) in length in humans, with a variable shape. These cells are usually located adjacent to the surface of the bone matrix. Their function is the production and secretion of components of this bone matrix, forming a precollagen material within the ribosomes of the endoplasmic reticulum, which are accumulated in the Golgi vesicles, being organized into collagen chains on secretion from the cell.

The osteoblasts themselves eventually become osteocytes, which are basically osteoblasts that have become buried by the bone they have synthesized (Pritchard 1976b). The osteoclast is a large, multinucleated cell, typically with 20 nuclei and with extensive Golgi membranes (Hancox 1976). The function of the osteoclast is that of bone resorption, probably through the extracellular degradation of collagen by enzymes that are synthesized and released from the osteoclasts (Robinson et al. 1973).

Pritchard (1976a) has identified three basic categories of structure in relation to human bone, these being termed bundle bone, woven bone, and fine-fibered bone. In bundle bone, coarse fiber bundles are arranged in a regular form. The fiber bundles are similarly coarse in woven bone, but are more loosely packed, running an irregular pathway through the matrix and being associated with high organic binder content. In fine-fibered bone, the collagen fibrils are arranged in much finer bundles with a minimum amount of binder. The fine-fibered bone predominates in the adult mammalian skeleton, but bundle and woven bone are found in the growing skeleton, at tendon and ligament attachment sites, and in fracture callus.

Mammalian bone morphologically is arranged in the skeleton as either cortical or cancellous bone. Compact or cortical bone consists of fine-fibered bone that has, as its basic structure, the osteon. These are cylinders of bone that have small blood vessels running along their axes. In the long bone, these axes are usually parallel to the long axis of the bone itself. The osteon and blood vessel arrangement is referred to as a *haversian system*, and the canal containing the blood vessel is known as a haversian canal. The bone within the osteon is usually lamellated, with concentric layers of bone easily visible. There is also a circumferential lamellated pattern and a further arrangement of bone within the spaces between the haversian system, known as interstitial bone (Van Mullem and Maltha 1983).

Cancellous bone has the same microstructure as compact bone, but differs in morphology, existing as trabeculae that are comprised of osteon fragments and interstitial bone. These are meshlike (trabeculae) arrangements with the bone itself being interspersed with intertrabecular marrow spaces. The structure of concentric cylinders of osteons has been compared by Ascenzi and Bonucci (1976) to cross-ply laminates, indicating that the fibrous structure of each lamella is oriented at a different angle to the long axis of the osteons. Scanning electron microscopy (SEM) investigations have shown that the concentric cylinders of hydroxyapatite are separated from each other by organic phase filled spaces with some mineral cross-linking (Piekarski 1973, 1984).

Currey (1962) considered bone as a two-phase composite material. Using the theoretical scheme of Cox (1952), he quantified the dependence of the longitudinal Young's modulus of bone by the basic conception of cylindrically shaped apatite crystals embedded in a collagen matrix and aligned with the long axis of collagen fibrils.

Lang (1969) and Reilly and Burnstein (1975) considered bone to be a transversally isotropic material. Katz (1980) proposed a two-level hierarchal fiber-reinforced composite model in which a single osteon is treated as a coherent entity and is modeled as a laminated circle surrounding the haversian canal. The osteons are packed in a pseudohexagonal arrangement. Sasaki, Ikawa, and Fukuda (1991) incorporated structural information on the differing orientation of the crystals in alternating bone lamellae. Weiner, Arad, and Traub (1991), using a more refined micromechanical model of bone based on rat bone lamellae, proposed the structure of bone in terms of three hierarchal levels: the collagen crystal composite, the plywoodlike lamellae, and the cylindrical structures (Weiner, Arad, and Traub 1991; Weiner and Traub 1991).

The exact location of apatite crystals in the organic matrix has been a source of controversy for many years (Bocciarelli 1970). It has been suggested that the long axes of the crystals are parallel to the collagen fibrils and are arranged at 640 Å intervals around, but not in the fibrils (Robinson 1952; Robinson, Doty, and Cooper 1973), while others have suggested the crystals nucleate within holes in the tropocollagen (Glimcher and Krane 1967).

In mature bone, the apatite crystals are observed as irregularly shaped thin plates or rodlike structures of carbonate apatite that are rarely stoichiometric or structurally perfect, and are typically 450 Å to 500 Å in length, up to 250 Å in width and with thicknesses of 20 Å to 30 Å (Weiner, Arad, and Traub 1991). These crystallites are arranged in parallel layers within the fibril, with the distance between layers 40 Å to 50 Å (Hohling, Ashton, and Koster 1974). It has been proposed that the *c* crystallographic axes of the crystals are aligned with the collagen fibrils (Schmidt 1936; Moradian-Oldak et al. 1991).

Regardless of which model is correct, the apatite of bone should be accepted as a living mineral since it undergoes continual growth, dissolution, and remodeling involving mineralization and resorption. The structure and mechanical properties of bone are derived from the organized mineralization of hydroxyapatite within a matrix of collagen fibrils, proteoglycans, and many other proteins. The combination of the organized structure of the collagen and the hardness of the apatite gives bone its desirable mechanical properties.

The mineralization occurs within holes between adjacent collagen molecules and the platelike crystals are crystallographically oriented in parallel arrays across the fibrils. The long-range order observed may be responsible for much of the unusual fracture properties of bone (Jackson, Cartwright, and Lewis 1978).

As early as 1926, bone, tooth enamel, and dentine were observed to have x-ray diffraction patterns similar to those of mineral apatites, while urinary or dental calculi and abnormal calcifications in soft tissues have been identified as apatite or apatitelike materials (LeGeros 1991). The nonstoichiometry of biogenic apatites, especially that of enamel apatite, has been partially attributed to the presence of HPO_4^{2-}. HPO_4^{2-} is believed to be either adsorbed on the apatite surface (Neumans and Neuman 1958), partially substituting for the PO_4^{3-} in the apatite lattice (Trautz 1967), a constituent of interlayered OCP (Brown et al. 1962), a constituent of DCPD, or a precursor of apatite.

Mature human tooth enamel differs from cortical bone in that it contains of some 96% inorganic material, 1% organic material, and 3% water by weight (Berkovitz, Holland, and Moxham 1978). The inorganic phase is mainly carbonated HA, while the organic phase is made up of a protein unique to tooth enamel. As such, tooth enamel is the hardest tissue in the human body, able to withstand the loads encountered during mastication while at the same time protecting the underlying dentine (Kerebel, Daculsi, and Kerebel 1979). The hardness of the enamel layer increases toward the surface. The thickness of the enamel layer varies from about 2–2.5 mm thick at the crown of the tooth, to a knife edge at the neck of the tooth (Yaeger 1980).

Like bone, many studies have been carried out to try to establish the morphology of tooth enamel crystallites. Jensen and Moller (1948) used XRD and determined the size of enamel crystallites to lie in the range of 250 Å to 600 Å. The morphology was determined to be roughly spherical and the size was found to increase toward the surface. Conversely, Grove, Judd, and Ansell (1972) used dark field electron microscopy to show that the long, rodlike crystals, observed by many, consist of smaller rectangular crystallites having dimensions of approximately 321 Å long and 366 Å wide.

VI. SYNTHETIC HYDROXYAPATITE

Hydroxyapatite (HA) has been synthesized by a solid-state reaction between Ca^{2+} and PO_4^{3-} bearing compounds and/or under solution conditions in the form of powders that are eventually sintered to a dense polycrystalline body by firing. Single crystals of HA have been grown under hydrothermal conditions or from the melt (Makishima and Aoki 1984), while details of the crystal growth from gels has been reviewed by Henisch (1970).

The growth of HA and other calcium phosphate crystals using the gel system has been reported by LeGeros and Tung (1983) and Kamiya et al. (1989). They prepared HA in the agar gel system, in which Ca^{2+} ions were incorporated in the gel and PO_4^{3-} solution was layered over the gel.

HA can be obtained through various routes (Table 6). The reason for the many alternatives arises from the conceptually simple but rich and complicated thermal chemistry of HA (Jarcho 1981).

The method by which the calcium phosphate is produced and the stoichiometry can also affect the transformation of hydroxyapatite to high-temperature phases such as tricalcium phosphate. For example, at 700–1125°C, a calcium-deficient HA produces β-$Ca_3(PO_4)_2$ (β-TCP), but, at temperatures greater than 1450°C, stoichiometric HA promotes α-$Ca_3(PO_4)_2$ (α-TCP). Calcium phosphate materials of different composition or materials of identical composition with different isomorphs (e.g., α-TCP versus β-TCP) may differ in their crystallographic structure, depending on their methods of production and sintering conditions. Modification in their internal bonding strength due to the crystallographic changes influences their stability and solubility or dissolution properties (Driessens, van Dijk, and Borggrevan 1978; Driessens 1988). The order of relative solubility of some calcium phosphate compounds is as follows:

$$ACP > DCP > TTCP > \alpha\text{-TCP} > \beta\text{-TCP} > HA$$

where TTCP is tetracalcium phosphate ($Ca_4P_2O_9$).

It has been reported by Klein, Driessens, and de Groot (1984) and LeGeros (1988) that *in vitro* dissolution of β-TCP is 3 to 12 times faster than stoichiometric HA. The production of HA influences the chemical, physical, and crystallographic characteristics of calcium phosphates and hence the biological behavior (Driessens, van Dijk, and Borggrevan 1978; Ducheyne et al. 1980; LeGeros 1993). For example, the crystal morphology can vary from a platelike, to needlelike, to a spherical morphology, depending on the production route and conditions chosen.

The most popular method of HA production is the wet method, used since 1955 (Hayek and Stadlmann 1955). All documented wet processes suggest adding phosphate-

Table 6   Different Processes Available for the Production of Hydroxyapatite

Process	Reactants	Reference
Hydrolysis	$Ca_9(PO_4)_6H(OH)$	Schleede, Schmidt, and Kindt 1932
	$Ca_4(PO_4)_2O$	Schleede, Schmidt, and Kindt 1932
	$Ca_8H_2(PO_4)_25H_2O$	Nancollas 1982a
Hydrothermal synthesis	$CaHPO_4$, H_3PO_4 and $CaHPO_4$, $2H_2O$	Kanazawa and Monma 1973
	$Ca(CH_3COO)_2H_2O$ and $(C_2H_5O)_3PO$	Hattori, Iwadate, and Kato 1988
	$Ca(NO_3)_2$ and $(NH_4)_2HPO_4$	Somiya, Ioku, and Yoshimura 1988
	$Ca_2P_2O_7$ and CaO	Hattori and Iwadate 1990
Hydrothermal exchange	$CaCO_3$ and $(NH_4)_2HPO_4$ with H_2O	Roy and Linnehan 1974
Solid process	Bovine bone	Webster et al. 1987
Sol-gel	$Ca(OC_2H_5)_2$ and $P(OC_2H_5)_3$	Masuda, Matubaram, and Sakka 1990
	$Ca(CH_3CH_2COO)_2$ and $P(OEt)_3$	Chai et al. 1993
Spray pyrolysis	$Ca(NO_3)_2$ and $(NH_4)_2HPO_4$	Hayek and Stadlmann 1955
	$Ca(NO_3)_2$ and H_3PO_4 in $MeOH_2O$-HNO_3	Tiselius, Hjerten, and Levin 1956
Wet chemistry	$CaCl_26H_2O$ and $(NH_4)_2HPO_4$	Kanazawa and Monma 1973
	$CaCl_2$ and Na_2HPO_4	Jarcho et al. 1976
	$Ca(OH)_2$ and H_3PO_4	Tagai and Aoki 1978
	CaO, $Ca(OH)_2$ $CaCO_3$, CaF_2, $CaCl_2$ and $Ca(NO_3)_2$ powder with H_3PO_4 solution	Aoki 1978
	$Ca(NO_3)_2$ and Na_2HPO_4	Jarcho 1981
	$Ca_3(PO_4)_2$ and H_2O	De Groot 1984
	$Ca(OC_2H_5)_2$-EtOH and H_3PO_4-EtOH	Ozaki 1986
	CaO(or $Ca(OH)_2$) and $CaHPO_42H_2O$	Nakaso and Nakahara 1986
	$CaHPO_4 \cdot 2H_2O$ and $CaCO_3$	Hakamazuka 1987
	$Ca(CH_3COO)_2$ and $(C_2H_5O)_3PO$	Hattori et al. 1987
	$CaHPO_4$ and $Ca_4(PO_4)_2O$	Brown and Chow 1987
	$CaCl_2$ and H_3PO_4	Inoue and Ono 1987
	$Ca(NO_3)_2$ and $(NH_4)_2PO_4$	Suzuki and Matsuda 1988
	$Ca(NO_3)_24H_2O$ and $(NH_4)_2HPO_4$	Kamiya et al. 1989
Natural coralline (hydrothermal)	Coral exoskeleton (*Porites geniopora*)	Holmes et al. 1984

Source: Modified from Gross 1990

containing solution dropwise to the stirred calcium-ion-containing solution (Akao, Aoki, and Kato 1981). The reason for this is that precipitated anions (PO_4^{3-}) are generated slowly in solutions containing the metal ion (Ca^{2+}) to be precipitated. This is controlled by hydrolysis of suitable compounds under the condition for formation of insoluble $Ca_{10}(PO_4)_6(OH)_2$. The exception is with triethyl phosphate and calcium acetate. The reactants are mixed together and droplets are formed in liquid nitrogen, dried by sublimation under reduced pressure, and then spray dried.

The simplest production route of all the wet processes involves the use of orthophosphoric acid and calcium hydroxide. Earlier formulations used the reactants in concentrated 4M $Ca(OH)_2$ and an 8 weight percent (wt%) solution of H_3PO_4 (Tagai and Aoki 1978, 1980). This has been modified by Aoki in 1988 and the modified technique is more reproducible because it allows the reactants to be mixed thoroughly. A solution of 0.3M H_3PO_4 in 1000 milliliters (ml) of distilled water is usually added as drops over 1 to 2 hours (h) to 0.5M $Ca(OH)_2$ in 1000 ml of distilled water at 40°C to produce a gelatinous precipitate (Aoki 1988). The addition rate of the phosphate solution to the calcium-containing solution determines the crystal size of the apatites. A slower rate will produce a larger particle size. The reaction mixture is stirred for a few hours and aged at room temperature for a period of a day up to a week. The precipitate is dried between 80°C and 120°C, and then calcined at 800°C.

Higher purity HA with these methods may only be obtained in small quantities and only after using time-consuming and tedious methods. Recently, a new method has been reported to accelerate the production rate by using microwave irradiation to produce HA powders (Lerner, Sarig, and Azoury 1991).

Based on composition and origin, commercially available calcium phosphate materials may be classified as tricalcium phosphate, β-$Ca_3(PO_4)_2$ (β-TCP); calcium hydroxyapatite $Ca_{10}(PO_4)_6(OH)_2$ (HA); biphasic calcium phosphate consisting of mixed β-TCP and HA phases; unsintered calcium phosphate powders; coralline HA; and bone-derived materials (LeGeros 1993).

VII. THERMAL DECOMPOSITION OF APATITES

The thermal behavior of apatites have been extensively investigated. Decomposition temperatures for pure HA have been reported to be as low as 1100°C (Hayek and Newesely 1963) and as high as 1400°C (Driessens et al. 1980). The decomposition temperature has been reported to be dependent on several factors, including the method and conditions of formation (Newesley and Osborn 1980), amount and type of impurities present (Krajewski et al. 1984), atmosphere of sintering (Yokogawa et al. 1992, Wang and Chaki 1993), additives (Ruys et al. 1992), and other factors such as sample size, particle size, and heating rate of the sample.

When nonstoichiometric apatites are heated above 200°C, several reactions may occur (Table 7) involving thermally unstable species such as HPO_4^{2-} and CO_3^{2-}. The first reaction occurring between 250°C and 600°C is dissociation of HPO_4^{2-} to $P_2O_7^{4-}$ and H_2O. The $P_2O_7^{4-}$ ions remain in the apatite lattice in a very distorted form. At 700°C, $P_2O_7^{4-}$ ions react with the OH^- ions of the apatite to generate PO_4^{3-} groups. Pyrophosphate ions will then form a separate phase of β-TCP.

In carbonate-containing apatites, several reactions with HPO_4^{2-} and $P_2O_7^{4-}$ may occur, leading to the formation of CO_3^{2-} and PO_4^{3-} groups. In addition, carbonate ions substituted for phosphate in the apatite structure begin to decompose at 600°C. The decomposition of carbonate ions substituted for hydroxide ions requires higher temperatures and longer times to reach completion. At 1000°C, according to the Ca/P ratio and composition, several phases may be observed (Table 8).

Apatites containing CO_3^{2-} and Na^+ ions may form a mixture of stoichiometric HA, sodium, and calcium oxides at 1000°C. It has been reported by Rey, Trombe and Montel

Table 7 Thermal Decomposition Reactions of Stoichiometric Apatites

Temperature	Reactions		Reference
25–200°	Loss of adsorbed H_2O		Arends et al. 1987
250–550°	$2HPO_4^{2-} \rightarrow P_2O_7^{4-} + H_2O$		Arends et al. 1987
550–700°	$P_2O_7^{4-} + 2OH^- \rightarrow 2PO_4^{3-} + H_2O$		Arends et al. 1987
700–850°	$2OH^- \rightarrow O^{2-} + H_2O\uparrow$	No	Arends et al. 1987
	$Ca_{10}(PO_4)_6(OH)_{2-2x}O_x$	H_2O	
	$Ca_{10}(PO_4)_6(OH)_2 \rightarrow Ca_{10}(PO_4)_6(OH)_{1-x}O_{x/2} + H_2O$		Trombe and Montel 1978a, 1978b
	$Ca_{10}(PO_4)_6(OH)_{0.50}O_{0.75}$	H_2O Cool	Trombe and Montel 1978a, 1978b
1100–1200°	$Ca_{10}(PO_4)_6O \rightarrow 2\beta\text{-}Ca_3(PO_4)_2 + Ca_4P_2O_9$		Shimbayashi and Nakagaki 1978
	$Ca_{10}(PO_4)_6(OH)_2 \rightarrow 3\beta\text{-}Ca_3(PO_4)_2 + CaO + H_2O$		
1125°	$\beta\text{-}Ca_3(PO_4)_2 \rightarrow \alpha\text{-}Ca_3(PO_4)_2$		Hayek and Newesely 1963
1300°	$Ca_{10}(PO_4)_6(OH)_2 \rightarrow 2\alpha\text{-}Ca_3(PO_4)_2 + Ca_4P_2O_9 + H_2O$		Hayek and Newesely 1963
1400°	$2Ca_3(PO_4)_2 + Ca_{10}(PO_4)_6(OH)_2 \rightarrow 4\,Ca_4P_2O_9 + P_2O_5$ $+ H_2O$		Newesely and Osborn 1980
1570°	Liquid Phases		
1700°	CaO		

(1973) that, on heating to 1000°C, some of the sodium ions may enter into the lattice-producing nonstoichiometric apatites containing vacancies on OH^- sites. Above 850°C, in a water-free atmosphere, it is impossible to obtain stoichiometric hydroxyapatite due to the decomposition of the hydroxide ions, which leads to the formation of an oxyhydroxyapatite, $Ca_{10}(PO_4)_6(OH)_{2-2x}O_x[\quad]_x$, where [ ] is a vacancy on the hydroxyl site. These OH^- vacancies are thought to be responsible for electrical conduction through ionic transport. This oxyhydroxyapatite (OHA) seems to exist only at high temperatures, takes up water very rapidly after cooling, and a nonstoichiometric compound is formed in air containing small amounts of OH^- ions, $Ca_{10}(PO_4)_6(OH)_{0.5}O_{0.75}$.

Trombe and Montel (1978a, 1978b) have successfully stabilized oxyhydroxyapatite and observed a large number of vacancies. The substitution of two OH^- by one O^{2-} ion and one vacancy induces no structural modifications but a slight decrease of the unit cell *a* dimension and slight increase of *c*. HA and OHA, due to their crystallographic

Table 8 Phases Observed at 1000°C According to their Ca/P Ratio

Ca/P	Phases
1.33–1.50	α-TCP, β-TCP, β-calcium pyrophosphate
1.50	Pure β-TCP
1.50–1.67	β-TCP and stoichiometric HA
1.67	Stoichiometric HA
>1.67	CaO and stoichiometric HA

arrangement, cannot be easily differentiated by using XRD; however, the presence of OHA in HA has been detected by infrared spectroscopy. Kijima and Tsutsumi (1979) reported that the peak at 3572 cm^{-1}, corresponding to the OH$^-$ stretching mode, begins to decrease between 900°C and 1050°C due to the loss of hydroxyl groups and therefore the creation of vacancies (Fig. 2). At temperatures higher than 1300°C, hydroxyapatite decomposes to α-TCP and TTCP (Van Raemdonck et al. 1984).

On heating at temperatures above 1570°C, a liquid phase begins to form and above 1700°C the only solid phase to exist is calcium oxide. These decomposition reactions explain why calcium oxide and other high-temperature calcium phosphate phases are frequently found in plasma-sprayed coatings. This is a major drawback as the hydrolysis of CaO into Ca(OH)$_2$ in air at low temperatures is associated with a volume increase that creates strains in the ceramic layer and may lead to its fracture (Rey et al. 1991) and, in the long term, dissolution in physiological environments.

The decomposition of pure HA to TCP and TTCP that occurs during sintering has been widely reported. Tricalcium phosphate exists in two crystalline forms, α-Ca$_3$(PO$_4$)$_2$ and low-temperature β-Ca$_3$(PO$_4$)$_2$ (Mackay 1953). Above 1125°C, the most likely phase to exist is α-Ca$_3$(PO$_4$)$_2$ (Mathew et al. 1977). The TCP formation is complex and is temperature, time, and atmosphere dependent. TCP is bioresorbable and undesirable for mechanically stable load-bearing applications (Jarcho 1981; Hench 1986).

Impurities, reinforcing phases, or additives have been found to decrease the tempera-

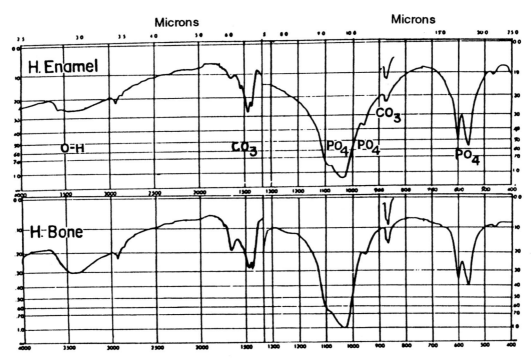

Figure 2   Infrared absorption spectra of biogenic apatites showing CO$_3$ ν doublet at 869 and 879 cm^{-1}. (From LeGeros et al. 1970.)

ture at which the decomposition begins (Uematsu et al. 1989; Ribeiro and Barbosa 1991; Ruys et al. 1992; Ji and Marquis 1992; Chai and Ben-Nissan 1993). It has been reported by Ioku, Somiya, and Yoshimura (1989, 1990) that zirconia additions decrease the decomposition temperature significantly. The addition of silica has also been shown to induce the reaction at approximately 900°C (Monma and Kanazawa 1975).

Yamashita et al. (1988) attempted to control the decomposition reaction through the use of water vapor at 1400°C, and reported complete suppression of decomposition to TCP. Recent studies by Ruys et al. (1992) showed that an overpressure of inert gas in a graphite furnace resulted in a higher dehydration temperature for HA-based composites than the samples sintered in air at ambient pressure.

During the last decade, plasma-sprayed hydroxyapatite coatings have become increasingly popular in the field of prosthetic replacements. Hydroxyapatite is susceptible to both dissolution and ion substitution when immersed in various solutions (Lee 1988; Radin and Ducheyne 1990; Berndt et al. 1990; Albrektsson 1993).

Radin and Ducheyne (1990, 1992) have reported that all commercially obtained plasma-sprayed HA coatings underwent plasma-induced changes in crystal structure, phase composition, specific surface area, and morphology. These plasma-induced transformations have been found to depend on the starting powder properties. Examples of these transformations include β-TCP to α-TCP, dehydroxylation of HA to OHA, and partial decomposition of α-TCP to TTCP.

The carbonate content of plasma-sprayed HA coatings has been found by Fourier transform infrared (FTIR) spectroscopy to increase after immersion into physiological simulated solutions. Increased intensity of the carbonate vibrational band observed after one week might be due to some type of dissolution-precipitation reaction. Such dissolution mechanisms have been proposed for bulk HA materials by LeGeros and Tung (1983), LeGeros et al. (1987), and Heughebaert et al. (1988). It is possible that, as the calcium phosphate material dissolves, the calcium could have combined with the phosphate and carbonate ions in solution to form a carbonated calcium phosphate. Another possibility for the increase in the carbonate vibrational band in the FTIR spectra is CO_3^{2-} substitution into the apatite lattice. The affinity for such substitutions and substitutional effects is well documented (LeGeros and Tung 1983) and it has been generally assumed to decrease the solubility of the HA coating.

VIII. SPECTROSCOPY AND CRYSTALLOGRAPHY

A large number of studies compare crystallographic analysis of human bone, dentine, and enamel structures using x-ray diffraction, infrared and laser Raman spectroscopies, electron spin and nuclear magnetic resonance, radial distribution function analysis, small-angle x-ray scattering, and electron diffraction with varying degrees of success.

The IR absorption spectra of whole bone consists of absorption bands from both the mineral phase and the organic matrix. Most of the published work on the IR spectra focuses on the deproteinated bone and related synthetic calcium phosphates. The final properties of apatites (both biogenic and synthetic) largely depend on preparation methods and conditions. Therefore, for the purpose of comparison, we have studied bovine tibia, human tooth enamel, and synthetic HA powders.

Ground bovine tibia (BT) samples were deproteinated using a 2.6 wt% sodium hypochlorite (NaOCl) solution (Weiner and Price 1986). The samples were washed with distilled water and ethanol and then dried prior to analysis.

Human tooth enamel samples were prepared using caries-free adult human teeth. A tetrabromoethane flotation method (density 2.7 g·cm^{-3}) was employed to separate the enamel from the dentine (Nelson and Williamson 1982).

The first type of synthetic HA powder (PA) was prepared using the method of Tagai and Aoki (1978). This involved preparing a 200-ml suspension of Ca(OH)$_2$ and slowly adding 200 ml of 0.28M H$_3$PO$_4$. The solution was maintained at a temperature of 50 ± 1°C and agitated with a magnetic stirrer for the duration of the addition process and for a subsequent 24 h after acid addition had ceased. The resulting precipitate was allowed to settle out for a period of days and some of the water was permitted to evaporate. After this, the powder was dried in an air oven at 110°C.

High-temperature stoichiometric (HTS) hydroxyapatite was prepared using Nelson and Williamson's (1982) method. Monocalcium phosphate monohydrate and analytical reagent calcium carbonate were ground separately and thoroughly mixed in a stoichiometric molar ratio of 3:7. The mixture was sintered for 18 hours at 1100–1200°C under a wet nitrogen atmosphere. The material was allowed to cool under the gas stream and 5-g portions of the ground product were extracted twice with neutral 0.3 M triammonium citrate (50 ml) at 70°C for 1 hour. The product was then washed with double-distilled water and dried overnight at 110°C.

All powder samples were examined using a Siemens D5000 x-ray diffractometer, with CuKα radiation, running at 40 kilovolts (kV) and 50 milliamperes (mA). Samples were scanned from 20° to 50°, with a step size of 0.02° and a step time of 2.5 seconds.

For FTIR analysis, approximately 1 milligram (mg) of apatite powder was mixed intimately with about 100 mg of KBr powder. The mixture was then pressed into pellets and analyzed using a Perkin Elmer 1720/X spectrometer.

The two biogenic apatite samples produced vastly different diffraction patterns (Fig. 3). The bovine tibia scan displayed no distinct peaks, rather a single broad peak was

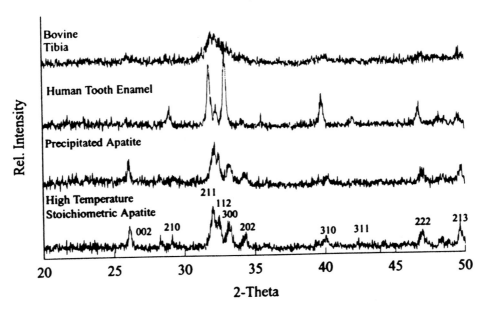

Figure 3   X-ray diffraction patterns of biogenic and synthetic apatites.

displayed from about 30° to 35°, which actually encompasses the three major HA peaks. This behavior is indicative of an amorphous or poorly crystalline material and/or a material with a very small crystallite size. Blumenthal, Betts, and Posner (1975) have attributed the poor resolution from x-ray diffraction to a combination of small crystallite size plus internal disorder brought about by CO_3^{2-} substitution. In addition, younger bone appears less crystalline than more mature bone, which indicates that younger bone contains a larger amorphous fraction or possesses smaller crystallites that may be more distorted than those in more mature bones (Currey 1979; Neumans 1980; Piekarski 1984).

Conversely, the human tooth enamel sample produces very sharp peaks, even more so than the two synthetic apatites. This indicates that the apatite present in human tooth enamel is highly crystalline, and demonstrates the differences that occur in biogenic apatites. In addition, the peaks corresponding to the planes parallel to the c-axis in the apatite unit cell are very intense, indicating that the apatite in human tooth enamel is not only highly crystalline, but also well oriented in the z-direction.

The two synthetic HAs produce diffraction patterns that are almost identical. These patterns also correspond closely to the Joint Committee on Powder Diffraction Standards (JCPDS) 9-432 card for HA. None of the patterns show any extraneous peaks that would indicate the presence of a second phase.

The infrared absorption spectra of biological apatites display characteristic bands due to OH^-, PO_4^{3-}, and CO_3^{2-} (Fig. 4). Stoichiometric synthetic HA shows bands due to OH^- and PO_4^{3-} groups only. This material is characterized by a sharp band at 3572 cm^{-1} that is due to an OH stretching vibration. Note that the increased absorption at 634 cm^{-1} (hydroxyl librational band) for stoichiometric synthetic hydroxyapatite, when compared with the biological apatites, has been attributed to hydroxyl ion deficiencies in the structure of carbonated apatites (Nelson and Williamson 1982). The strong peak at 3572 cm^{-1} confirms the presence of OH ions in the apatite crystal lattice. This band is due to the characteristic O-H stretching mode of the hydroxyl ion vibration in the crystal. The OH librational 630-cm^{-1} mode is missing in the bone pattern, but present in the synthetic HA pattern, although OH is present in both materials. The strong- and medium-absorption peaks at 1040, 1093, 733, 692 cm^{-1} and so on confirm the presence of the tetrahedral orthophosphate ion PO_4^{3-} in the apatite crystal lattice.

Adsorbed water appears as a broad band between 3700 and 3500 cm^{-1}, and as a sharper band at 1620 cm^{-1}. While these bands are always present in biological apatites, they may be greatly reduced in synthetic hydroxyapatite, depending on the method of preparation (Arends et al. 1987). However, adsorbed water is present in all the apatites examined in this study in similar degrees. Human tooth enamel shows marginally less amounts of adsorbed water than the other apatites.

The most intense bands associated with PO_4^{3-} vibrations in calcium phosphate materials are the antisymmetric stretching mode at 1100–1000 cm^{-1} (ν_3 band) and the antisymmetric bending mode at 600–550 cm^{-1} (ν_4 band) (Termine 1973) (Fig. 5). In amorphous calcium phosphate (ACP) the latter band appears as a single broad peak, while in biological apatites two bands of unequal intensity usually appear (Fig. 6). In contrast, synthetic stoichiometric apatites will show three bands for each of the ν_3 and ν_4 modes, with precipitated synthetic hydroxyapatite behaving more like a biological apatite displaying two unequal bands.

Carbonate ion is the main impurity in biological apatites, and much evidence exists to show that CO_3^{2-} substitutes for PO_4^{3-} in the crystal lattice structure (LeGeros et al. 1970; LeGeros 1981). Biogenic apatites show characteristic absorption bands due to

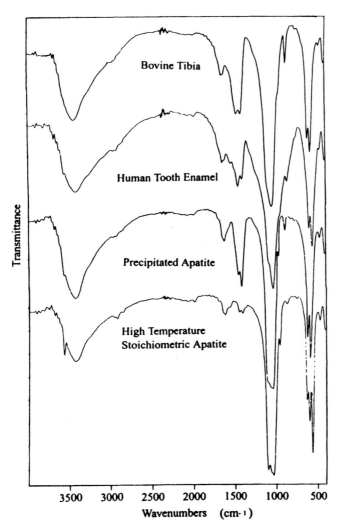

Figure 4 Fourier transform infrared (FTIR) absorption spectra of biogenic and synthetic apatites.

CO_3^{2-} at 1450, 1410, and 870 cm^{-1}. Bands produced by the presence of carbonate ions are clearly evident in the spectra of precipitated synthetic HA.

The CO_3^{2-} ν_2 vibration is normally nondegenerate. The appearance of the anomalous ν_2 doublet at 869 and 879 cm^{-1} in the spectra of biogenic apatites has been explained by Emmerson and Fischer (1962) as indicating the CO_3^{2-} to be present in two different environments. Elliot (1964) defined these environments as being outside the lattices and within the lattice substituting for OH$^-$. Several other alternative explanations based on PO_4^{3-} substitution and due to coupling between neighboring CO_3^{2-} groups have also been proposed (Decius 1955).

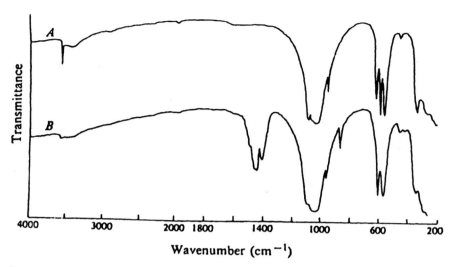

Figure 5   Infrared spectra showing antisymmetric stretching (ν_3) and bending (ν_4) modes: (*A*), high-temperature stoichiometric hydroxyapatite (HA); and (*B*), high-temperature carbonated apatite with 6.7 wt% carbonate. (From Nelson and Williamson 1982.)

Apart from CO_3^{2-} for PO_4^{3-} substitution, other anions such as Cl^- and F^- can readily substitute for OH^- in the lattice structure of biological apatites. Fluoride-substituted apatites are quite common in living organisms, such as the carbonate-containing fluorapatites in brachiopod shells (LeGeros et al. 1985), fish enameloid (Suga 1984), and chiton teeth (Evans, Macey, and Webb 1992). F^- and Cl^- substituted apatites typically show a distinct shoulder in their infrared absorption spectra at about 575 cm^{-1}.

Thus, the precipitated apatite is chemically similar to the apatite in bovine tibia, while being significantly more crystalline. Human tooth enamel is the most crystalline apatite of those examined, displaying a distinct *c*-axis orientation, although being chemically similar to the bovine tibia. Conversely, the stoichiometric synthetic apatite is closer to a true HA than the other three apatites investigated.

The space group of HA has been determined by x-ray diffraction methods (Kay Moi, Tiyng, and Posner 1964) to be $P6_3/m$ and results of infrared and Raman studies of HA at room temperature seems to confirm this (Nelson and Williamson 1982). However, theoretical considerations suggest the space group should be $P6_3$. It has been proposed that the hydroxyl ions in HA are displaced by some 0.3 Å along the hexagonal screw axis, destroying the mirror plane and consequently altering the space group from $P6_3/m$ to $P6_3$.

It has been reported by Posner, Perloff, and Diorio (1958) and Park and Lakes (1992) that there are two types of crystallographically independent calcium atoms in the synthetic HA unit cell. Of the ten calcium ions in a unit cell, six which are called Ca(II) are associated with two hydroxyl ions on the corners, resulting in strong interactions among them. Each Ca(II) atom is surrounded by 6 oxygen atoms belonging to PO_4 groups and an OH group, whereas each of the other 4 calcium ions, called Ca(I), is nearly octahedrally surrounded by 6 oxygen atoms from PO_4 groups (Mayer et al. 1993).

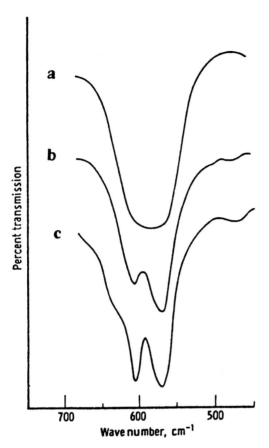

Figure 6   Infrared spectra showing the antisymmetric bending mode ν_4: (a), 100% amorphous calcium phosphate (ACP); (b), ACP-hydroxyapatite (ACP-HA) mixture; and (c), 100% HA. (From Posner et al. 1979.)

Dental enamel is a carbonated hydroxyapatite (Young 1975) containing approximately 2–5 weight percent carbonate, which is crystallographically disordered. It has been proposed that this disorder is the result of carbonate substitution in the apatite crystal structure (Blumenthal and Posner 1973). LeGeros (1965) proposed that, in synthetic and biological apatites, carbonate ions replace phosphate ions in the apatite structure, causing a contraction of the *a*-axis unit cell dimensions and a slight expansion of the *c*-axis unit cell dimension.

The appearance of two $\nu_1(CO_3)$ bands, four $\nu_4(CO_3)$ bands, and three $\nu_3(CO_3)$ bands in the Raman spectrum of synthetic carbonated apatites suggests that carbonate ions have two distinct site symmetries, and hence occupy two crystallographically distinct sites in the apatite structure. Of the various models presented for carbonate substitution in apatite (McConnell 1965; McConnell 1973; Trautz 1955), the model presented by McConnell (1973) appears to explain the spectroscopic data best. This suggests that three phosphate ions are replaced by four carbonate ions, essentially leaving the oxygen lattice intact. The carbonate ions then take two sites, one parallel to the *c*-axis and one perpendicular to the *c*-axis. If random substitution of carbonate ions by replacement of phosphate ions in the apatite structure occurs, then long-range translational symmetry of the apatite structure is destroyed.

It is possible that the poor resolution of the IR pattern of bone mineral is due in large part to small crystal size and internal disorder caused by the CO_3 normally found in bone apatite. In an IR study of calcium-deficient HA, no absorption bands due to octacalcium phosphate were observed. Instead, bands at 1210 cm $^{-1}$ from hydrogen-bonded HPO_4 at 1133 cm $^{-1}$ from a component of the HPO_4 vibration and at 870 cm $^{-1}$ from a P-O(H) vibration were observed, confirming the presence of hydrogen ions.

Since the early years of the XRD study of bone, there has emerged a body of literature on possible mineral phases in bone other than HA (Table 9). The limitations of XRD techniques that have prevented definitive characterization of the structure of bone are its inability to resolve closely spaced lines in fine-grained materials, coupled with the limited periodicity of thin crystals. Thermodynamically stable HA and its analogs, such as fluorapatite and chlorapatite, are reviewed by Elliott, Mackie, and Young (1973) and Young (1975).

When synthetic HA is formed at 25°C, the crystals are small with a large specific surface of about 150–200 m^2·g^{-1}, while higher preparation temperatures yield larger crystals with smaller specific surface (at 100°C, the value is about 50 m^2·g^{-1}) (Blumenthal and Posner 1973). As the pH at which HA is prepared is increased from about 6 to 10, the average crystal size decreases.

The use of electron diffraction has aided in characterization of the larger individual crystals and aggregates of smaller crystals (Lee, Landis, and Glimcher 1986; Ji and

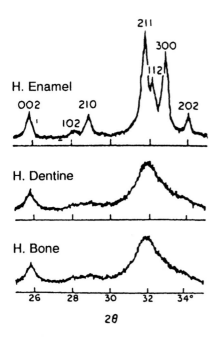

Figure 7 Comparative x-ray diffraction patterns of human enamel, dentine, and bone showing major peaks. (From LeGeros 1981.)

Table 9 Comparison of Lattice Parameters of Various Apatites

Name	Empirical formulas	JCPDS number	Structure	a (Å)	b (Å)	c (Å)	Density ($g \cdot cm^{-3}$)
Dicalcium phosphate dihydrate	$CaHPO_4 \cdot 2H_2O$	11-293	Monoclinic	5.837	15.192	6.265	2.30
Dicalcium phosphate dihydrate (syn.)	$CaHPO_4 \cdot 2H_2O$	9-77	Monoclinic	6.363	15.19	5.815	2.31
Dicalcium phosphate	$CaHPO_4$	9-80	Triclinic	6.906	8.577	6.634	2.92
Octacalcium phosphate	$C_8H_2(PO_4)_6 \cdot 5H_2O$	26-1056	Triclinic	9.529	18.994	6.855	2.673
β-Tricalcium phosphate	$\beta\text{-}Ca_3(PO_4)_2$	9-169	Rhomobohedral (hex)	10.429	–	37.38	3.07
Hydroxyapatite (syn.)	$Ca_{10}(PO_4)_6(OH)_2$	9-432	Hexagonal	9.418	–	6.884	3.15
Tetracalcium phosphate monoxide	$Ca_4(PO_4)_2O$	25-1137	Monoclinic	7.018	11.980	9.469	3.056
α-Tricalcium phosphate	$\alpha\text{-}Ca_3(PO_4)_2$	29-359	Monoclinic	12.887	27.280	15.219	2.863
α-Tricalcium phosphate	$\alpha\text{-}Ca_3(PO_4)_2$	9-348	Orthorhombic	15.22	20.71	9.109	2.870
Calcium fluoride phosphate	$Ca_5F(PO_4)_3$	15-876	Hexagonal	9.3684	–	6.8841	3.20
Calcium chloride fluoride phosphate hydroxide	$Ca_5(PO_4)_3(OH,Cl,F)$	25-166	Hexagonal	9.490	–	6.851	3.12
Calcium chloride phosphate	$Ca_5(PO_4)_3Cl$	24-214	Monoclinic	19.210	6.785	9.605	3.19
Calcium chloride phosphate (syn.)	$Ca_5(PO_4)_3Cl$	33-271	Hexagonal	9.641	–	6.771	3.17

Marquis 1991). Using computer deconvoluted x-ray diffraction, Germine and Parsons (1988) tried to resolve component overlapped (002) profiles from mixtures of synthetic and biogenic apatites. The (002) HA peak is most favorable for description of c-axis parameters (Fig. 7) due to its isolation and relative intensity (Bonar et al. 1983). Studies have been performed relating the half-breadth of this reflection to density and composition of bone (Menczel, Posner, and Harper 1965; Quinaux and Richelle 1967).

Measurements of human enamel apatite by x-ray diffraction show that its *a*-axis is about 0.02 Å longer than that observed in mineral HA, while its *c*-axis is not significantly different (Carlstroem 1955; Trautz 1955; LeGeros 1967). The observed expansion of the *a*-axis dimension of human enamel apatite has been attributed to partial substitutions of CO_3^{2-} for OH^- (Elliott 1964, 1969), Cl^- for OH^- (Trautz 1955; LeGeros 1967), HPO_4^{2-} for OH^- (McConnell 1965), and combined water or partial substitution of H_3O^+ for Ca^{2+} (McConnell 1973), or partial substitution of HPO_4^{2-} for PO_4^{3-} or H_3O^+ for OH^-, and Cl^- for OH^- (LeGeros 1974).

IX. SUMMARY

The crystallography and characterization of biogenic and synthetic apatites are very complex and clearly, after so many years, the data and interpretations are still of a preliminary nature. This review has attempted to cover nearly four decades of research on one of the most intriguing and fascinating fields of research. The total analysis of the results observed and obtained suggests that, with newer scientific tools and with refinement and further study, we will succeed to address problems relating to the structure and analysis of the biogenic materials and hopefully produce synthetic apatites or composites that will try to emulate the structure and characteristics of natural bone.

REFERENCES

Akao, M., Aoki, H., and Kato, K. (1981). Mechanical Properties of Sintered Hydroxyapatite for Prosthetic Applications, *J. Mater. Sci.*, 16:809–812.

Albrektsson, T. (1993). In Current Issues Forum: What Is Your Opinion Concerning the Long-Term Consequences of HAp Coating within Bone? *Int. J. of Oral and Maxillo. Imp.*, 8(6): 707–711.

Ali, S.Y., Wisby, A., and Gray, J.C. (1978). Electron Probe Analysis of Cryosections of Epiphyseal Cartilage, *Met. Bone Dis. Rel. Res.*, 1:97.

Aoki, H. (1978). $CaO-P_2O_5$ Apatite, Japanese Patent JP 78110999.

Aoki, H. (1988). Hydroxyapatite of Great Promise for Biomaterials, *Proc. Strategy of Innovation in Materials Processing*, 99–104.

Arends, J., Christoffersen, J., Christoffersen, M.R., Eckert, H., Fowler, B.O., Heughebaert, J.C., Nancollas, G.H, Yesinowski, J.P., and Zawacki, S.J. (1987). A Calcium Hydroxyapatite Precipitated from an Aqueous Solution, *J. Cryst. Gr.*, 84:515–532.

Ascenzi, A., and Bonucci, E. (1976). Mechanical Similarities Between Alternate Osteons and Crossply Laminates, *J. Biomechanics*, 9:65–68.

Ashton, B.A., Hohling, H.J., and Triffitt, J.T. (1976). Plasma Proteins Present in Human Cortical Bone: Enrichment of the α-2HS-Glycoprotein, *Calcif Tiss. Res.*, 22:27–33.

Berkovitz, B.K., Holland, G.R., and Moxham, B.J. (1978). In *A Colour Atlas and Textbook of Oral Anatomy*, Wolfe Medical Pub., London, pp. 79–88.

Berndt, C.C., Haddad, G.N., Farmer, A.J.D., and Gross, K.A. (1990). Review: Thermal Spraying for Bioceramic Applications, *Materials Forum*, 14:161–173.

Blumenthal, N.C., Betts, F., and Posner, A.S. (1975). Effect of Carbonate and Biological Macromolecules on Formation and Properties of Hydroxyapatite, *Calc. Tiss. Res.*, 18:81–90.

Blumenthal, N.C., and Posner, A.S. (1973). Hydroxyapatite: Mechanism of Formation and Properties, *Calc. Tiss. Res.*, 13:235.

Bluementhal, N.C., and Posner, A.S. (1984). In vitro model of aluminium induced osteomalacia: Inhibition of hydroxyapatite formation and growth, *Calc. Tiss. Int.*, 36:439–441.

Bocciarelli, D.S. (1970). Morphology of Crystallites in Bone, *Calc. Tiss. Res.*, 5:261–269.

Bonar, L.C., Roufosse, A.H., Sabine, W.K., Grynpas, M.D., and Glimcher, M.J. (1983). X-Ray Diffraction Studies of the Crystallinity of Bone Mineral in Newly Synthesized and Density Fractioned Bone, *Calc. Tiss. Int.*, 35:202–209.

Boskey, A.L. (1984). Overview of Cellular Elements and Macromolecules Implicated in the Initiation of Mineralisation. In *The Chemistry and Biology of Mineralised Tissues*, W.T. Butler, Ed., Pub. SN, Birmingham, AL, pp. 335–343.

Boskey, A.L., and Posner, A.S. (1976). Formation of Hydroxyapatite at Low Supersaturation, *J. Phys. Chem.*, 80:40–44.

Boskey, A.L., and Posner, A.S. (1984). Structure and Formation of Bone Mineral. In *Natural and Living Biomaterials*, G.W. Hastings and P. Ducheyne, Eds., CRC Press, Boca Raton, FL, pp. 27–42.

Brecevic, L.J., and Furedi-Milhofer, H. (1972). Precipitation of Calcium Phosphates from Electrolyte Solutions, *Calcif Tiss. Res.*, 10:82–90.

Brown, P.W., and Fulmer, M. (1991). Kinetics of Hydroxyapatite Formation at Low Temperature, *J. Am. Ceram. Soc.*, 74:934–940.

Brown, W.E., and Chow, L.C. (1987). A New Calcium Phosphate, Water Setting Cement. In *Cements Research Progress—1987*, P.W. Brown. Ed., American Ceramic Society, Westerville, OH.

Brown, W.E., Smith, J.P., Lehr, J.R., and Frazier, A.W. (1962). Crystallographic and Chemical Reactions Between Octacalcium Phosphate and Hydroxyapatite, *Nature*, 196:1051–1055.

Brudevold, F., and Soremark, R. (1967). In *Structural and Chemical Organisation of Teeth*, Miles, Ed., Academic Press, New York, p. 251.

Carlstroem, D. (1955). X-Ray Crystallographic Studies on Apatite and Calcified Structures, *Acta Radiol. Suppl.*, 121.

Chai, C., and Ben-Nissan, B. (1993). Interfacial Reactions Between Hydroxyapatite and Titanium, *J. Aust. Ceram. Soc.*, 29, 81.

Chai, C., Ben-Nissan, B., Pyke, S., and Evans, L. (1994). Sol Gel Derived Hydroxyapatite Coatings for Biomedical Applications, *In Surface Modification Technologies VII*, T.S. Suddshan, K. Ishizaki, M. Takata and K. Kamata, Eds., Cambridge University Press, Cambridge, UK, pp. 509–524.

Clarke, K.I., Graves, S.E., Wong, A.T.-C., Triffitt, J.T., Francis, M.J.O., and Czernuszka, J.T. (1993). Investigation into the Formation and Mechanical Properties of a Bioactive Material Based on Collagen and Calcium Phosphate, *J. Mat. Sc., Mat. in Medicine*, 4:107–110.

Clarke, K.I., Wong, A.T.-C., Czernuszka, J.T., Dowling, B., and Triffitt, J.T. (1991). Crystallographic Aspects of the Growth of Calcium Phosphate on Type I Collagen and Hydroxyapatite. In *Bioceramics*, Vol. 4, W. Bonfield, G.W., Hastings, and K.E. Tanner, Eds., Butterworth-Heinemann., London, pp. 107–113.

Cox, H.L. (1952). The Elasticity and Strength of Paper and Other Fibrous Materials, *Brit. J. Appl. Phys.*, 3:72–79.

Currey, J.D. (1962). The Relationship Between the Stiffness and the Mineral Content Bone, *J. Biomechanics*, 2:477–480.

Currey, J.D. (1979). Changes in the Impact Energy Absorption of Bone with Age, *J. Biomechanics*, 12:459.

Dalas, E., Kallitsis, J.K., and Koutsoukos, G.P. (1991). Crystallisation of Hydroxyapatite on Polymers, *Langmuir*, 7:1822–1826.

Dalas, E., and Koutsoukas, P.G. (1989). The Growth of Calcium Phosphate on Ceramic Surfaces, *J. Mater. Sci.: Letters*, 24:999–1004.

Dallemagnes, M.J., and Richelle, L.J. (1973). Inorganic Chemistry of Bone. In *Biological Mineralisation*, I. Zipkin, Ed., John Wiley and Sons, New York, p. 23.

Decius, J.C. (1955). Coupling the Out-of-Plane Bending Mode in Nitrates and Carbonates of the Aragonite Structure, *J. Chem. Phys.*, 23:1290-1294.

Deer, W.A., Howie, R.A., and Zussman, J. (1985). *An Introduction to the Rock Forming Minerals*, Longman, Hong Kong, pp. 504-509.

De Groot, K. (1984). Degradable Ceramics. In *Biocompatibility of Clinical Implant Materials*, Vol. 1, D.F. Williams, Ed., CRC Press, Boca Raton, FL, p. 199.

DeJong, W.F. (1926). La Substance Material dans lesos, *Rec. Tav. Chim.*, 45:415-448.

Driessens, F.C.M. (1982). Mineral Aspects of Dentistry. In *Monographs in Oral Science*, Vol. 10, S. Karger, Basel, Switzerland.

Driessens, F.C.M. (1983). Formation and Stability of Calcium Phosphates in Relation to the Phase Compositions of the Mineral in Calcified Tissues. In *Bioceramics of Calcium Phosphate*, K. de Groot, Ed., CRC Press, Boca Raton, FL, p. 1-32.

Driessens, F.C.M. (1988). Physiology of Hard Tissues in Comparison with Solubility of Synthetic Calcium Phosphates. In *Bioceramics: Materials Characteristics versus In Vivo Behaviour*, P. Ducheyne and J. Lemons, Eds., Ann. N.Y. Acad. Sci., 523:131.

Dreissens, H.W., deGroot, K., Driessens, A.A., Wolke, J.G.C., Peelan, J.G.J., van Dijk, H.J.A., Gehring, A.P., and Klopper, P.J. (1980). Hydroxyapatite Implants: Preparation, Properties and Use in Alveolar Ridge Preservation, *Science of Ceramics*, 10:63-69.

Driessens, F.C.M., van Dijk, J.W.E., and Borggreven, J.M.P.M. (1978). Biological Calcium Phosphates and Their Role in the Physiology of Bone and Dental Tissues I. Composition and Solubility of Calcium Phosphates, *Calc. Tiss. Res.*, 26:127-137.

Ducheyne, P., Hench, L.L., Kagan, A., II, Martens, A., Bursens, A., and Mulier, J.C. (1980). Effect of Hydroxyapatite Impregnation on Skeletal Bonding of Porous Coated Implants, *J. Biomed. Mater. Res.*, 14:225-242.

Ebrahimpour, A., Perez, L., and Nancollas, G. H. (1991). Induced Crystal Growth of Calcium Oxalate Monohydrate at Hydroxyapatite Surfaces. The Influence of Human Serum Albumin, Citrate and Magnesium, *Langmuir*, 7:577-583.

Elliot, J.C. (1964). The Crystallographic Structure of Dental Enamel and Related Apatites, Ph. D. thesis, University of London.

Elliot, J.C. (1969). Recent Progress in the Chemistry, Crystal Chemistry and Structure of Apatites, *Calc. Tiss. Res.*, 3:293.

Elliot, J.C., Mackie, P.E., and Young, R.A. (1973). Monoclinic Hydroxyapatite, *Science*, 180:1055-1057.

Emmerson, W.H., and Fischer, E.E. (1962). The Infrared Spectra of Carbonate in Calcified Tissues, *Arch. Oral Biol.*, 7:671-683.

Evans, L.A., Macey, D.J., and Webb, J. (1992). Calcium Mineralization in the Radular Teeth of the Chiton *Acanthopleura hirtosa*, *Calcif. Tiss. Int.*, 51:78-82.

Feenstra, T.P., and deBruyn, P.L. (1979). Formation of Calcium Phosphates in Moderately Supersaturated Solutions, *J. Phys. Chem.*, 83:475-479.

Fietzek, P.P., and Kuhn, K. (1976). The Primary Structure of Collagen. In *International Review of Connective Tissue Research*, D.A. Hall and D.S. Jackson, Eds., Academic Press, New York, 7, p. 1.

Gay, S., and Miller, E.J. (1978). *Collagen in the Physiology and Pathology of Connective Tissue*, Gustav-Fisher Verlag, Stuttgart.

Germine, M., and Parsons, J.R. (1988). Deconvoluted X-Ray Analysis of Bone and Mixtures of Bone and Particulate Hydroxyapatite, *J. Biomed. Mater. Res.: Appl. Biomater.*, 22:55-67.

Glimcher, M.T., and Krane, S.M. (1967). In *Treatise on Collagen*, Vol. 1, G.N. Ramachandran, Ed., Academic Press, New York, p. 17.

Gross, K.A. (1990). Surface Modification of Prosthesis, M.Sc. thesis, Monash University, Melbourne, Australia.

Grove, C.A., Judd, G., and Ansell, G.S. (1972). Determination of Hydroxyapatite Crystallite Size in Human Dental Enamel by Dark Field Electron Microscopy, *J. Dent. Res.*, 51(1):22-29.

Guggenheim, K., and Caster, D. (1973). In *Biological Mineralisation*, I. Zipkin, Ed., J. Wiley and Sons, New York, pp. 443–462.

Hakamazuka, K. (1987). Manufacture of Calcium Phosphate-Containing Hydroxyapatite, Japanese Patent JP 62191410.

Hancox, N.M. (1976). The Osteoclast. In *The Biochemistry and Physiology of Bone*, Vol. 1, G. Bourne, Ed., Academic Press, London, pp. 45.

Hanning, K., and Nordwig, A. (1965). General Sequence Studies on Collagen. In *Structure and Function of Connective and Skeletal Tissue, Proc. NATO Conf. St. Andrews, June, 1964*, Butterworths, London, p. 7.

Hattori, T., and Iwadate, Y. (1990). Hydrothermal Preparation of Calcium Hydroxyapatite Powders, *J. Am. Ceram. Soc.*, 73(6):1803–1805.

Hattori, T., Iwadate, Y., Inai, H., Sato, K., and Imai, Y. (1987). Preparation of Hydroxyapatite Powder Using a Freeze Drying Method, *Yogyo-Kyokai-Shi*, 95(8):71–73.

Hattori, T., and Iwadate, Y. (1990). Hydrothermal Preparation of Calcium Hydroxyapatite Powders, *J. Am. Ceram. Soc.*, 73(6):1803–1805.

Hattori, T., Iwadate, Y., and Kato, T. (1988). Hydrothermal Synthesis of Hydroxyapatite from Calcium Acetate and Triethyl Phosphate, *Adv. Ceram. Mater.*, 3(4):426–428.

Hayek, E., and Newesely, H. (1963). Pentacalcium Monohydroxyorthophosphate, *Inorg. Synth.*, 7:63–65.

Hayek, E., and Stadlmann, W. (1955). Preparation of Pure Hydroxyapatite for Adsorption Uses, *Angew. Chem.*, 67:327

Hench, L.L. (1986). Ceramic Implants for Humans, *Adv. Ceram. Mater.*, 1:306–324.

Hennisch, H.K. (1970). *Crystal Growth in Gels*, Pennsylvania State University Press, University Park.

Herring, G.M. (1968). The Chemical Nature of Tendon, Cartilage, Dentin and Bone Matrix, *Clin. Orthop.*, 60:261–299.

Hertzfeld, J., Ronfosse, A., Haberkorn, R.A., Griffin, R.G., and Glimcher, M.J. (1980). Magic Angle Sample Spinnings in Inhomogeneously Broadened Biological Systems, *Phil. Trans. R. Soc. Lond.*, B289:459.

Heughebaert, M., LeGeros, R.Z., Gineste, M., Guilhem, and Bonel, G. (1988). Physico-Chemical Characterisation of Deposits Associated with HA Ceramics Implanted in Non-Osseous Sites, *J. Biomed. Mater. Res.: Appl. Biomat.*, 22(A3):257–268.

Hohling, H.J., Ashton, B.A., and Koster, H.D. (1974). Quantitative Electron Microscope Investigations of Mineral Nucleation in Collagen, *Cell. Tiss. Res.*, 148:11–26.

Holmes, R., Mooney, V., Bucholz, R., and Tencer, A. (1984). Coralline Hydroxyapatite Bone Graft Substitute. Preliminary Report, *Clin. Orthopaed.*, 199:252–262.

Inoue, S., and Ono, A. (1987). Preparation of Hydroxyapatite by Spray Pyrolysis Technique, *Yogyo Kyokaishi*, 95(8):759–763.

Ioku, K., Somiya, S., and Yoshimura, M. (1989). Dense/Porous Layered Apatite Ceramics Prepared by HIP Post Sintering, *J. Mater. Sci.: Letters*, 8:1203–1204.

Ioku, K., Yoshimura, M., and Somiya, S. (1990). Microstructure and Mechanical Properties of Hydroxyapatite Ceramics with Zirconia Dispersion Prepared by Post-Sintering, *Biomaterial*, 11:57–61.

Jackson, S.A., Cartwright, A.G., and Lewis, D. (1978). The Morphology of Bone Mineral Crystals, *Calc. Tiss. Res.*, 25:217–222.

Jarcho, M. (1981). Calcium Phosphate Ceramics as Hard Tissue Prosthetics, *Clin. Orthop. Rel. Res.*, 157:259–278.

Jarcho, M., Bolen, C.H., Thomas, M.B., Bobick, J.F., Kay, J.F., and Doremus, R.H. (1976). Hydroxyapatite Synthesis and Characterisation in Dense Polycrystalline Form, *J. Mater. Sci.*, 11:2027–2035.

Jensen, A.T., and Moller, A. (1948). Determination of the Size and Shape of the Apatite Particles in Different Dental Enamels and in Dentin by the X-Ray Powder Method, *J. Dent. Res.*, 27(4):524–531.

Ji, H., and Marquis, P.M. (1991). Modification of Hydroxyapatite During Transmission Electron Microscopy, *J. Mater. Sci. Letters*, 10:132–134.

Ji, H., and Marquis, P.M. (1992). Sintering Behaviour of Hydroxyapatite Reinforced with 20wt% Al₂O₃, *J. Mater. Sci.*, 28:1941–1945.

Kamiya, K., Yoko, T., Tanaka, K., and Fujiyama, Y. (1989). Growth of Fibrous Hydroxyapatite in the Gel System, *J. Mater. Sci.*, 24:827–832.

Kanazawa, T., and Monma, H. (1973). Recent Progress in the Chemistry of Calcium Phosphate, Especially Apatites – Their Composition, Structure and Properties, Part 1, *Kagaku-no-Ryoiki*, 27:22–32.

Katz, J.L. (1980). Anisotropy of Young's Modulus of Bone, *Nature*, 283:106–107.

Kay Moi, I., Tiyng, R.A., and Posner, A.S. (1964). The Crystal Structure of HAp, *Nature*, 204:1050–1152.

Kerebel, B., Daculsi, G., and Kerebel, L.M. (1979). Ultrastructural Studies of Enamel Crystallites, *J. Dent. Res.*, 58(B):844–850.

Kibby, C.L., and Hall, W.K. (1972). In *The Chemistry of Biosurfaces*, Vol. 2, M.L. Hair, Ed., Dekker, New York, p. 663.

Kijima, T., and Tsutsumi, M. (1979). Preparation and Thermal Properties of Dense Polycrystalline Oxyhydroxyapatite, *J. Amer. Ceram. Soc.*, 62:455–460.

Klein, C.P.A.T., Driessens, A.A., and de Groot, K. (1984). Relationship Between the Degradation Behaviour of Calcium Phosphate Ceramics and their Physical Chemical Characteristics and Ultrastructural Geometry, *Biomaterials*, 5:157–160.

Koutsoukos, P., Amjad, Z., Tomson, M.B., and Nancollas, G.H. (1980). Crystallisation of Calcium Phosphates: A Constant Composition Study, *J. Am. Chem. Soc.*, 102:1553–1557.

Krajewski, A., Ravaglioli, A., Riva di Sanseverino, L., Marchetti, F., and Monticelli, G. (1984). The Behaviour of Apatite Based Ceramics in Relation to the Critical 1150–1250°C Temperature Range, *Biomaterials*, 5:105–108.

Landis, W.S., Paine, M.C., and Glimcher, M.J. (1981). Considerations for the Electron Optical Identification of Matrix Vesicles and Mineral Phase Particles Possibly Associated with them in Calcifying Tissues, *Trans. Orthop. Res. Soc.*, 6:59.

Lang, S.B. (1969). Elastic Coefficients of Animal Bone, *Science*, 165:287–288.

Leaver, A.G., Triffitt, J.T., and Holbrook, I.B. (1975). Newer Knowledge of Noncollageous Protein in Dentin and Cortical Bone Matrix, *Clin. Orthop.*, 110:269–292.

Lee, D.R. (1988). Dissolution Characterization of Commercially Available Hydroxyapatite Particulate, M.Sc. thesis, University of Alabama, Birmingham.

Lee, D.R., Landis, W.J., and Glimcher, W.J. (1986). The Solid, Calcium Phosphate Phases in Embryonic Chicken Bone Characterized by High Voltage Electron Diffraction, *J. Bone. Min. Res.*, 1:425–432.

LeGeros, R.Z. (1965). Effect of Carbonate on the Lattice Parameters of Apatite, *Nature*, 206:403.

LeGeros, R.Z. (1967). Crystallographic Studies on the Carbonate Substitution in the Apatite Structure, Ph.D. thesis, New York University, New York.

LeGeros, R.Z. (1974). The Unit Cell Dimensions of Human Enamel Apatite: Effect of Chlorine Incorporation, *Arch. Oral. Biol.*, 20:63–71.

LeGeros, R.Z. (1981). Apatites in Biological Systems. In *Inorganic Biological Crystal Growth*, Part 2, B.R. Pamplin, Ed., Pergamon Press, New York, pp. 1–45.

LeGeros, R.Z. (1988). Calcium Phosphate Materials in Restorative Dentistry: A Review, *Adv. Dent. Res.*, 2:164–183.

LeGeros, R.Z. (1991). Calcium Phosphates in Oral Biology and Medicine, In *Monographs in Oral Sciences*, Vol. 15, H. Myers, S. Karger, Basel, Switzerland.

LeGeros, R.Z. (1993). Biodegradation and Bioresorption of Calcium Phosphate Ceramics, *Clin. Mater.*, 14:65–88.

LeGeros, R.Z., Kijkowska, R., Tung, M., and LeGeros, J.P. (1990). Effect of Strontium on Some Properties of Apatites. In *Tooth Enamel V*, R.W. Feanhead, Ed., Florence Publishers, Tokyo, Japan, pp. 393–401.

LeGeros, R.Z., and LeGeros, J.P. (1984). Phosphate Minerals in Human Tissues. In *Phosphate Minerals*, J.O. Nriagen and P.M. Moore, Eds., Springer-Verlag, Berlin, pp. 351–385.

LeGeros, R.Z., LeGeros, J.P., Trautz, O.R., and Klein, E. (1970). Spectral Properties of Carbonate in Carbonate-Containing Apatites, *Dev. Appl. Spectrosc.*, 7:3–12.

LeGeros, R.Z., Orly, I., Gregoire, M., Agergas, T., Kazimroff, J., and Tarpley, T. (1987). Physico-Chemical Properties of Calcium Phosphate Biomaterials Used as Bone Substitutes, *Trans. 13th Annual Meeting of the Society for Biomaterials*, 84.

LeGeros, R.Z., Pan, C.-M., Suga, S., and Watabe, N. (1985). Crystallo-Chemical Properties of Apatite in Atremate Brachiopod Shells, *Calcif. Tiss. Int.*, 37:98–100.

LeGeros, R.Z., Taheri, M.H., Quirolgico, G.M., and LeGeros, J.P. (1980). Formation and Stability of Apatites: Effects of Some Cationic Substituents, *Proc. 2nd Int. Congr. on Phosphorus Compounds*, 89–103.

LeGeros, R.Z, and Tung, M.S. (1983). Chemical Stability of Carbonate and Fluoride Containing Apatites, *Caries Res.*, 17:419–429.

Lerner, E., Sarig, S., and Azoury, R. (1991). Enhance Maturation of Hydroxyapatite from Aqueous Solutions Using Microwave Irradiation, *J. Mater. Sci.: Mater. in Med.*, 2:138–141.

McConnell, D.J. (1965). Crystal Chemistry of Hydroxyapatite. Its Reaction to Bone Mineral, *Archs. Oral. Biol.*, 10:421.

McConnell, D. (1973). Apatite: Its Crystal Chemistry, Mineralogy, Utilisation and Geologic and Biologic Occurrences. In *Applied Mineralogy*, Vol. 5, Springer-Verlag, Berlin.

Mackay, A.L. (1953). A Preliminary Examination of the Structure of α-$Ca_3(PO_4)_2$, *Acta Crystallogr.*, 6:743–744.

Makashima, A., and Aoki, H. (1984). In *Bioceramics*, T. Yamaguchi and H. Yanagida, Eds., Gihodo, Japan, p. 267.

Masuda, Y., Matubaram, K., and Sakka, S. (1990). Synthesis of Hydroxyapatite from Metal Alkoxides through Sol-Gel Technique, *J. Ceram. Soc. Japan, Int. Ed.*, 98:1266–1277.

Mathew, M., Schroeder, L.W., Dickens, B., and Brown, W.E. (1977). The Structure of α-$Ca_3(PO_4)_2$, *Acta Crystallogr.*, B33:1325–1333.

Mayer, I., Diab, H., Reinen, D., and Albrecht, C. (1993). Manganese in Apatites, Chemical Ligand Field and Electron Paramagnetic Resonance Spectroscopy Studies, *J. Mater. Sci.*, 28:2428–2432.

Menczel, J., Posner, A.S., and Harper, R.A. (1965). Age Changes in the Crystallinity of Rat Bone Apatite, *Israel J. Med. Sci.*, 1:251–252.

Monma, H., and Kanazawa, T. (1975). The Mechanism of Thermal Reactions in Apatites-Silica Water Systems, *Bull. Chem. Soc. Japan*, 46:1816–1819.

Moradian-Oldak, J., Weiner, S., Addadi, L., Landis, W.J., and Traub, W. (1991). Electron Imaging and Diffraction Study of Individual Crystal of Bone, Mineralised Tendon and Synthetic Carbonate Apatite, *Conn. Tiss. Res.*, 25:219–228.

Moreno, E.C., and Varughese, K. (1981). Crystal Growth of Calcium Apatites from Dilute Solution, *J. Cryst. Growth*, 53:20–30.

Murphree, S., Hsu, H.H.T., and Anderson, H. C. (1982). *In Vitro* Formation of Crystalline Apatite by Matrix Vesicles Isolated from Rachitic Rat Epiphyseal Cartilage, *Calcif Tiss. Int.*, 34:562.

Nakaso, Y., and Nakahara, H. (1986). Manufacture of Hydroxyapatite, Japanese Patent JP 61151010.

Nancollas, G.H. (1982a). In *Biological Mineralisation*, G.H. Nancollas, Ed., Dahlem Konferenzen, Springer-Verlag, Berlin, pp. 79–99.

Nancollas, G.H. (1982b). Phase Transformations During Precipitation of Calcium Salts. In *Biological Mineralisation and Demineralisation*, G.H. Nancollas, Ed., Springer-Verlag, Berlin, pp. 79–100.

Nancollas, G.H. (1984). The Nucleation and Growth of Phosphate Minerals. In *Phosphate Minerals*, J.O. Nriagu and P.P. Moore, Eds., Springer-Verlag, Berlin, pp. 137–154.

Nancollas, G.H. (1989). In vitro Studies of Calcium Phosphate Crystallization. In *Biomineralization: Chemical and Biochemical Perspectives*, S. Mann, J. Webb and R. J. P. Williams, Eds., VCH Verlagsgesellschaft, Weimheim, pp. 157–187.

Nelson, D.G.A., and Williamson, B.E. (1982). Low-Temperature Laser Raman Spectroscopy of Synthetic Carbonated Apatites and Dental Enamel, *Aust. J. Chem.*, 35:717–727.

Neumans, W.F. (1980). Bone Materials and Calcification Mechanisms. In *Fundamental and Clinical Bone Physiology*, M.R. Urist, Ed., J.R. Lippincott, Philadelphia, pp. 83–107.

Neumans, W.F., and Neuman, M.W. (1958). *The Chemical Dynamics of Bone Mineral*, University of Chicago Press.

Newesely, H., and Osborn, J.F. (1980). Structural and Textural Implications of Calcium Phosphates in Ceramics. In *Advances in Biomaterials*, Vol. 2: *Mechanical Properties of Biomaterials*, G.W. Hastings and D.F. Williams, Eds., John Wiley and Sons, New York, pp. 457–464.

Ozaki, K. (1986). Preparation of Hydroxyapatite as a Prosthetic Material, Japanese Patent JP 61295215.

Park, J.B., and Lakes, R.S. (1992). *Biomaterials: An Introduction*, 2nd Ed., Plenum Press, New York.

Piekarski, K. (1973). Analysis of Bone as a Composite Material, *Int. J. Eng. Sci.*, 11:557.

Piekarski, K. (1984). Fractography of Bone. In *Natural and Living Biomaterials*, G.W. Hastings and P. Ducheyne, Eds., CRC Press, Boca Raton, FL, pp. 99–117.

Posner, A.S., Betts, F., and Blumenthal, N.C. (1979). Bone Mineral Composition and Structure. In *Skeletal Research*, Academic Press, New York, pp. 167–192.

Posner, A.S., Perloff, A., and Diorio, A.D. (1958). Refinement of the Hydroxyapatite Structure, *Acta Crystallogr.*, 11:308–309.

Pritchard, J.J. (1976a). General Anatomy and Histology of Bone. In *The Biochemistry and Physiology of Bone*, Vol. 1, G. Bourne, Ed., Academic Press, London, p. 1.

Pritchard, J.J. (1976b). The Osteoblast. In *The Biochemistry and Physiology of Bone*, Vol. 1, G. Bourne, Ed., Academic Press, London, p. 21.

Quinaux, W., and Richelle, L.J. (1967). X-Ray Diffraction and Infrared Analysis of Bone Specific Gravity Fractions in the Growing Rat, *Israel J. Med.*, 3:677–691.

Radin, S., and Ducheyne, P. (1990). The Effect of Plasma Sprayed Induced Changes in the Characteristics on the *In Vitro* Stability of Calcium Phosphate Ceramics, *Trans. 16th Ann. Meeting of the Soc. for Biomaterials*, 13:128.

Radin, S., and Ducheyne, P. (1992). Plasma Spraying Induced Changes of Calcium Phosphate Ceramic Characteristics and the Effect on *In Vitro* Stability, *J. Mater. Sci.: Mater. in Med.*, 3:33–42.

Reilly, D., and Burnstein, A.H. (1975). The Elastic and Ultimate Properties of Compact Bone Tissue, *J. Biomechanics*, 8:393–405.

Rey, C., Freche, M., Heughebaert, M., Heughebaert, J.C., Lacout, J.L., Lebugle, A., Szilagyi, J., and Vignoles, M. (1991). Apatite Chemistry in Biomaterial Preparation, Shaping and Biological Behaviour. In *Bioceramics*, Vol. 4, W. Bonfield, G.W. Hastings, and K.E. Tanner, Eds., Butterworth-Heinemann, London, pp. 57–64.

Rey, C., Trombe, J.C., and Montel, G. (1973). Retention of Molecular Oxygen by the Lattice of Certain Alkaline Earth Apatites, *C.R. Acad. Sci.*, Ser. C., 276:1385–1388.

Ribeiro, C.C., and Barbosa, M.M. (1991). Influence of Metal Ions on the Dissolution Behaviour of Hydroxyapatite. In *Bioceramics*, Vol. 4, W. Bonfield, G.W. Hastings, and K.E. Tanner, Eds., Butterworth-Heinemann, London, pp. 146–153.

Robinson, M. (1952). An Electron Microscope Study of the Crystalline Inorganic Component of Bone and Its Relationship to the Organic Matrix, *J. Bone Jnt. Surg.*, 34A:389.

Robinson, R.A., Doty, S.B., and Cooper, R.R. (1973). Electron Microscopy of Mammalian Bone. In *Biological Mineralisation*, I. Zipkin, Ed., John Wiley and Sons, New York, pp. 273.

Roy, D.L., and Linnehan, S.K. (1974). Hydroxylapatite Formed from Coral Skeletal Carbonate by Hydrothermal Exchange, *Nature*, 247:220–222.

Ruys, A.J., Wei, M., Brandwood, A.A., Milthorpe, B.K., and Sorrell, C.C. (1992). The Effect of Excessive Sintering on the Properties of Hydroxyapatite. In *Ceramics Adding the Value. Proc.*

Int. Ceram. Conf. Austceram '92, M.J. Bannister, Ed., CSIRO Pub., Melbourne, Australia, pp. 586–590.

Sasaki, N., Ikawa, T., and Fukuda, A. (1991). Orientation of Mineral in Bovine Bone and the Anisotropic Mechanical Properties of Plexiform Bone, *J. Biomechanics*, 24:57–61.

Schleede, A., Schmidt, W., and Kindt, H. (1932). Zur Kennlni's der Calcium Phosphate und Apatite, *Elektrochem.*, 38:633.

Schmidt, W.S. (1936). Uber die Kristallorientierung im Zahnschmelz, *Naturwissensch*, 24:361.

Shimbayashi, S., and Nakagaki, M. (1978). Dehydration and Change in the Structure of HA by Heating, Nippon Kagaku Kaishi, 3:326–331.

Shuttleworth, A., and Veis, A. (1972). The Isolation of Anionic Phosphoproteins from Bovine Cortical Bone via the Periodate Solubilisation of Bone Collagen, *Biochin. Biophys. Acta*, 257: 414–420.

Somiya, S., Ioku, K., and Yoshimura, M. (1988). Hydrothermal Synthesis and Characterisation of Fine Apatite Crystals. In *Ceramic Developments*, C.C. Sorrell and B. Ben-Nissan, Eds., *Materials Science Forum*, 34–36:371–378.

Suga, S. (1984). The Role of Fluoride and Iron in Mineralization of Fish Enameloid. In *Tooth Enamel IV*, R.W. Fearnhead and S. Suga, Eds., Elsevier, Amsterdam, pp. 472–477.

Suzuki, O., and Matsuda, Y. (1988). Continuous Manufacture of Hydroxyapatite, Japanese Patent JP 63170205.

Tagai, H., and Aoki, H. (1978). Preparation of Synthetic Hydroxyapatite and Sintering of Apatitic Ceramics, *Bioceramics Symposium*, 16, University of Keele, United Kingdom.

Tagai, H., and Aoki, H. (1980). Preparation of Synthetic Hydroxyapatite and Sintering of Apatite Ceramics. In *Mechanical Properties of Biomaterials*, G.W. Hastings and D.F. Williams, Eds., John Wiley and Sons, New York, pp. 477–488.

Termine, J.D. (1973). In *Biological Mineralization*, I. Zipkin, Ed., John Wiley and Sons, New York, pp. 397–411.

Termine, J.D., Kleinman, H.K., Whitson, S.W., Conn, M.K., McGarvey, M.L., and Martin, G.R. (1981). Osteonectin, A Bone-Specific Protein Linking Mineral to Collagen, *Cell*, 26:99–105.

Tiselius, A., Hjerten, S., and Levin, O. (1956). Protein Chromatography on Calcium Phosphate Columns, *Arch. Biochem. Bio Phys.*, 65:132–155.

Trautz, O.R. (1955). X-Ray Diffraction Studies of Biological and Synthetic Apatites, *Ann. N.Y. Acad. Sci.*, 109:696.

Trautz, O.R. (1967). The Crystalline Organisation of Dental Enamel. In *Structural and Chemical Organisation of Teeth*, Vol. 2, A.E.W. Miles, Ed., Academic Press, New York, Ch. 16.

Trombe, J.C., and Montel, G. (1978a). Some Features of the Incorporation of Oxygen in Different Oxidation States in the Apatite Lattice, I. On the Existence of Calcium and Strontium Oxyapatites, *Inorg. and Nucl. Chem.*, 40:15–21.

Trombe, J.C., and Montel, G. (1978b). Some Features of the Incorporation of Oxygen in Different Oxidation States in the Apatite Lattice, II. On the Synthesis and Properties of Calcium and Strontium Perioxiapatites, *J. Inorg. and Nucl. Chem.*, 40:23–26.

Tung, M.S., and Brown, W.E. (1983). An Intermediate State in Hydrolysis of Amorphous Calcium Phosphate, *Calcif. Tiss. Int.*, 35:783–790.

Tung, M.S., and Brown, W.E. (1985). The Role of Octacalcium Phosphate in Subcutaneous Heterotopic Calcification, *Calcif Tiss. Int.*, 37:329–331.

Uematsu, K., Takagi, M., Honda, T., Uchida, N., and Saito, K. (1989). Transparent Hydroxyapatite Prepared by Hot Isostatic Pressing of Filter Cake, *J. Amer. Ceram. Soc.*, 72:1476–1478.

Van Mullem, P.J., and Maltha, J.C. (1983). Histology of Bone: A Synopsis. In *Bioceramics of Calcium Phosphate*, K. de Groot, K., Ed., CRC Press, Boca Raton, FL, pp. 53–78.

Van Raemdonck, W., Ducheyne, P., and De Meester, P. (1984), Calcium Phosphate Ceramics. In *Metal and Ceramic Biomaterials*, Vol. 2, P. Ducheyne and G.W. Hastings, Eds., CRC Press, Boca Raton, FL, pp. 143–166.

Wang, P.E., and Chaki, T.K. (1993). Sintering Behaviour and Mechanical Properties of Hydroxyapatite and Dicalcium Phosphate, *J. Mater. Sci.: Mat. in Medicine*, 4:150–158.

Webster, A.V., Cooper, J.J., Hampson, C.J., and Cubbon, P.R.C. (1987). The Properties of Milled Bone, *Brit. Ceram. Soc. Trans. J.*, 86:91–98.

Weiner, S., Arad, T., and Traub, W. (1991). Crystal Organisation in Rat Bone Lamellae, *FBBS Lett.*, 285:49–54.

Weiner, S., and Price, P.A. (1986). Disaggregation of Bone into Crystals, *Calc. Tiss. Int.*, 39:365–375.

Weiner, S., and Traub, W. (1991). In *Organisation of Crystal Bone. Mechanisms and Phylogeny of Mineralisation in Biological Systems*, S. Suga and H. Nakahara, Eds., Springer-Verlag, Berlin, pp. 247–253.

Wuthier, R.E., and Eanes, E.D. (1975). Effect of Phospholipids on the Transformation of Amorphous Calcium Phosphate to Hydroxyapatite *In Vitro*, *Calc. Tiss. Res.*, 23:135.

Yaeger, J.A. (1980). In *Orban's Oral Histology and Embryology*, S.N. Bhaskar, Ed., C.V. Mosby, St. Louis, pp. 46–106.

Yamashita, K., Kobayashi, T., Kitamura, M., Umegaki, T., and Kanazawa, T. (1988). Effect of Water Vapour on the Solid-State Reaction Between Hydroxyapatite and Zirconia of CaO-PSZ, *J. Ceram. Soc. Japan*, 96:616–619.

Yokogawa, Y., Toriyama, M., Kawamoto, Y., Suzuki, T., and Kawamura, S. (1992). Apatite Coating on Yttria Doped Partially Stabilized Zirconia Plate in the Presence of Water Vapour, *J. Ceram. Soc. Japan, Int. Ed.*, 100:599–601.

Young, R.A. (1975). Biological Apatites vs. Hydroxyapatite at the Atomic Level. *Clin. Orthop.*, 113:249–256.

Young, R.A. and Brown, W.E. (1982). In *Structures in Biological Minerals in Biological Mineralisation and Demineralisation*, G.H. Nancollas, Ed., Springer-Verlag, Berlin, pp. 104.

Young, R.A., and Elliot, J.C. (1966). Atomic Scale Bases for Several Properties of Apatites, *Arch. Oral Biol.*, 11:699–707.

8
Biomaterials in the
Fixation of Bone Fractures

Allan F. Tencer
The University of Washington
Seattle, Washington

I. INTRODUCTION

In this chapter the properties of materials used for the stabilization of bone fractures are discussed. These include metals, principally stainless steels and titanium alloys, that are used for load-bearing fracture hardware; adhesives such as cyanoacrylates and fibrin for repositioning of small, non-load-bearing fragments; biodegradable polymers for fixation where removal of the implant is difficult or undesirable; and allografts or ceramics that can be used to fill bone defects.

II. METALS

A. Methods of Fabrication of Implants

The characteristics of metals used for fracture implants have been well defined. Stainless steel (316L) and titanium (6Al-4V ELI), which are commonly used for screws and hardware, are governed by national standards for maximum content of alloys and impurities [1] and mechanical properties [2]. These standards are necessary to define the compositional requirements of the material and the maximum allowable percentage of impurities.

The actual mechanical properties of the metal are a function partly of its composition and partly of its grain structure, shown in Fig. 1. In general a finer-grained metal is both stronger and more ductile, which are useful attributes in fracture implants that frequently must be shaped to the geometry of the bone in the operating room. Grain structure is affected by the method of fabrication of the implant. Casting consists of heating the metal to a molten state and pouring it into a mold. Few fracture implants, if any, are currently fabricated in this manner because the act of pouring the molten metal into a mold results in internal impurities, pores, and other defects that reduce the fatigue life of the finished part. In addition, the grains in the cast part are large, resulting in low strength

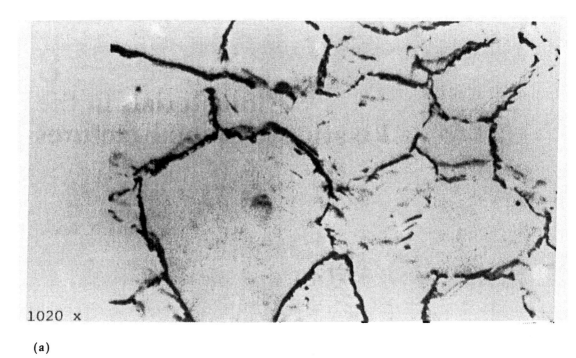

(a)

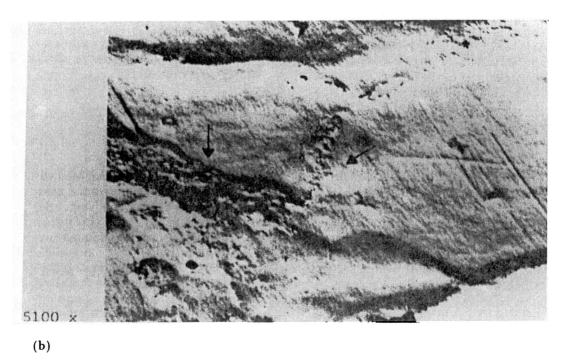

(b)

Figure 1 An example of carbide precipitations within the grain boundaries of the surface of a fixation plate: (a), ×1020; (b), ×5100. (From Ref. 4 with permission.)

and brittleness. An improvement to regular casting is hot isostatic pressing, forming the part under high pressure in an inert gas filled chamber, which reduces the sizes of defects in the casting. The part may then be machine finished in various ways.

Mechanical forming techniques are currently in wide use for forming fracture implants. Rolling (between rollers) and drawing (through a hole in a hardened plate) are methods used to form bar and wire. The material is plastically deformed in the process and the grains become elongated in the direction of deformation. Machining, which includes drilling, lathe turning, milling, and grinding, is used on parts that require holes, grooves, or other geometric features. Machining may work-harden the surface of the material but does not change its grain structure. Forging consists of gradually shaping a metal by compressive impact between die pairs, in conjunction with controlled heating or cooling. After forming, metal parts undergo heat treatment to alter structure and properties. In particular, annealing (heating to about half the melting point followed by controlled cooling) reverses the effects of work hardening and restores ductility and toughness to the metal. Finishing the surface by polishing removes scratches that could act as local stress risers. Acid treatment is used to passivate the surface of stainless steels by creating an oxide layer on the surface, which protects against corrosion. Nitriding, or allowing the surface to react with ammonia or potassium cyanate, is used to harden the surface of titanium implants. The following sections discuss specifics of stainless steels and titanium alloys, the most common metals used in fracture implants.

B. Stainless Steel

Stainless steel, an alloy primarily of iron, chromium, and nickel (Table 1), is protected from corrosion primarily by the addition of chromium. The chromium forms a passivating chromium oxide layer on the surface, which aids in preventing oxidation of the iron (corrosion) [3]. The carbon component increases strength but the implant may be subject to corrosion if carbon, which is diffused throughout the alloy, is allowed to precipitate at the grain boundaries, a result of improper heat treatment, Fig. 1. It can react with chromium to form carbides [4].

When immersed in an electrolytic solution, the alloy will corrode anodically while the carbides at the grain boundaries act as cathodes, a form of galvanic corrosion. (Galvanic corrosion requires the presence of two dissimilar materials immersed in an electrolyte, with one giving up ions and the other receiving them.) Also, the carbides degrade the mechanical properties of the material. The addition of small quantities of titanium or niobium reduces the formation of intergranular carbides by competing for carbon. Stainless steel is protected from corrosion by a protective surface chromium oxide layer, which is enhanced by the addition of small quantities of molybdenum. This can decrease the rate of slow passive dissolution by up to 1000-fold [5]. Molybdenum also hardens the alloy and makes it more difficult to work [3]. Surface treatment also reduces corrosion. Implants are surface finished by grinding and polishing to a specified roughness, which reduces the exposed surface area, and then cleaned with an alkaline cleaner. The oxide layer is then produced by immersion in 20–40% nitric acid by volume for a minimum of 30 min [6].

Several stainless steels are currently used for fracture implants. The commonly designated AISI (American Iron and Steel Institute) 316L (carbon content < 0.03%), has the composition shown in Table 1. Its strength can be greatly altered by the method of manufacture, and it can be extremely ductile (up to 55% strain to failure), as indicated in

Table 1 Compositions and Mechanical Properties of Some Stainless Steels Used in Fracture Fixation Implants

A. Compositions

Alloy				
ASTM	F 55°, F 138°	F 745		
ISO	5832-1			
Other	AISI 316L		22–13–5	Ortron 90[b]
Elements (w/o)				
C	<0.03	<0.06	<0.03	0.05
Cu	<0.5		<0.5	
Cr	17–20	17–19	22.5–23.5	21.5
Fe		balance (>58%)		
Mn	<2	<2	<2	4
Mo	2.25–3.5	2–3	2–3	2.6
N				0.39
Nb			0.1–0.3	0.3
Ni	13–16	11–14	11.5–13.5	9
P	<0.025	<0.045	<0.025	0.017
S	<0.01	<0.03	<0.01	0.005
Si	<0.75	<1	<0.75	0.25
V	<0.75		0.1–0.3	

B. Mechanical Properties[c]

Alloy				
ASTM	F 55, F 138	F 745		
ISO	5832-1			
Other	AISI 316L		22-13-5	Ortron 90
Mechanical properties				
Tensile modulus (γ, GPa)	193	—[d]	—[d]	—[d]
0.2% yield strength ($\sigma_{0.2\%}$, min, MPa)	170a 250hf 310cw 1,200cf[c]	205c	785hf 1,175cw	479a 928cw
Ultimate strength (σ_u, min, MPa)	480a 550hf 655cw 1,300cf[e]	480c	930hf 1,300cw	834a 1,035cw
Strain to failure (ϵ_u, min, %)	40a 55hf 28cw 12cf[e]	30c	37hf 15cw	72a 64cw
Hardness	85RBa 30RCcw			

Source: Ref. 3
[a]Grade 2
[b]See Table 7
[c]Annealed; c, as cast; cw, 30% cold worked; cf, cold forged; hf, hot forged; RB, Rockwell B; RC, Rockwell C
[d]Not reported, close to F 55
[e]F 138

Table 2. The alloy designated F 745 is a high-strength casting material, while alloy 22-13-5 possesses a much greater yield strength than 316L with the same treatment method, Table 1. Stainless steels are popular for use as fracture implants because the base materials are relatively inexpensive, they can be formed using common techniques, and their strength and ductility properties can be adjusted over a wide range [3].

C. Titanium

Titanium derives its excellent resistance to corrosion from the formation of an oxide layer that binds tightly to its surface. Impurities such as oxygen, hydrogen, and nitrogen tend to make it brittle, which is why only minimal amounts are acceptable in titanium alloys used in surgical implants, Table 2. Aluminum stabilizes the alpha form of the material, while vanadium has the same effect on the beta form. (*Alpha form* and *beta form* are commonly used to describe different phases of an alloy that have different properties.)

Table 2 Compositions and Mechanical Properties of Titanium and Alloys Used in Fracture Fixation Implants

	A. Composites		
Alloy			
ASTM	F 67°	F 136	
ISO		5832-3	
Other	Pure Ti	Ti–6Al–4V	Ti–5Al–2.5Fe
Elements (w/0)			
Al	—	5.5–6.5	4.5–5.5
C	<0.1	<0.08	<0.08
Fe	<0.5	<0.25	2–3
H	<0.01	<0.015	<0.0125
N	<0.05	<0.05	<0.05
O	<0.4	<0.2	<0.2
Ti	>99	←————Balance————→	
V	—	3.4–4.5	—
	B. Mechanical Properties[b]		
Alloy			
ASTM	F 67[a]	F 136	
ISO		5832-3	
Other	Pure Ti	Ti–6Al–4V	Ti–5Al–2.5Fe
Mechanical properties			
Tensile modulus γ (GPa)	100	105	—[c]
0.2% Yield strength	485ac	795a	818a
($\sigma_{0.2\%}$, min)			900f,a
Ultimate strength	550af	860af	963a
σ_u, min (MPa)			985f,a
Strain to failure	15af	10af	36a
ϵ_u, min (%)			33f,a

Source: Ref. 3
[a]Grade 4
[b]a, annealed; af, as fabricated; f, forged
[c]Similar to F 138

The higher strength beta form normally exists only at higher temperatures. Combinations of both components form a two-phase alloy with good strength properties and one that can be heat treated [2]. In general the elastic moduli of titanium and its alloys are about half those of stainless steel alloys, Table 2. It is important to note that the ductility of titanium alloy is considerably lower than that of most forms of stainless steels [3]. The alloy Ti-5Al-2.5Fe is more ductile than Ti-6Al-4V (Table 2) and the absence of vanadium may be of biologic benefit [3].

D. Corrosion of Metals

Corrosion describes a chemical reaction in which material is removed from an object. Passivation occurs when an oxide layer is formed on the surface that reduces corrosion. A number of corrosion processes can occur in fracture implants. In general corrosion requires the components of a galvanic cell; two different conducting solids, with an electrically conductive path between them, immersed in an electrolyte solution containing free ions, Fig. 2. Galvanic corrosion, shown in Fig. 3, may occur at the surface of an implant having an impurity. Stress corrosion involves both chemical and mechanical effects. Figure 3 demonstrates how a scratch or crack acts as both a stress concentrator and as a small corrosion cell. The implant is passivated by the oxygen layer formed on its surface. At the tip of an opening crack oxygen availability may be limited, preventing formation of the oxide layer. In the area near the crack there exist effectively two dissimilar materials. The galvanic corrosion effect accentuates the progression of the crack through the material. Crevice corrosion occurs in a similar manner but between components that may have some relative motion between them, such as a screw head within a plate, Fig. 3. Pitting corrosion occurs when abrasion creates a pit and allows the entrance of foreign materials through the oxide layer. The pit area is anodic with respect to the rest of the material, Fig. 3. The ability of a material to repassivate or regenerate its protective oxide film after scratching or abrasion is important in reducing its susceptibility to corro-

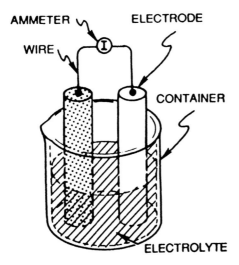

Figure 2 A basic galvanic cell, consisting of two different metals, an electrically conductive path between them, and an electrolyte containing free ions.

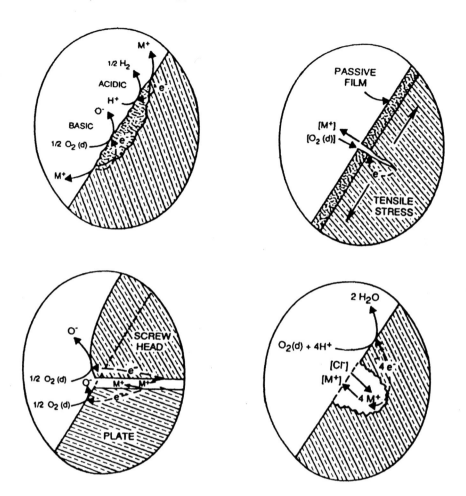

Figure 3 *Top left*: Example of a galvanic cell formed by an impurity in the surface of an implant (M^+ = metal ions, different reactions depending on the pH of the electrolyte). *Top right*: A surface scratch on a metal implant acts as both a stress riser, and as the crack opens, a galvanic corrosion cell, causing stress corrosion. (From Ref. 3 with permission.) *Bottom left*: Crevice corrosion results from relative movement between two surfaces, such as a screw head in a plate hole, which removes the passivating layer from the surface. *Bottom right*: Pitting corrosion is a local form of crevice corrosion. (From Ref. 3 with permission.) At the anode metal ions (Me^+) are released, while at the cathode the metal ions form oxides with available ions from the solute. (Adapted from Ref. 2.)

sion. As shown in Fig. 4, titanium and its alloys can repassivate considerably more quickly than can stainless steels [5].

E. Ion Release

Another consideration in use the of metallic implants is the potential for release of metal ions into surrounding tissues, and their long-term effects. Table 3 demonstrates that there

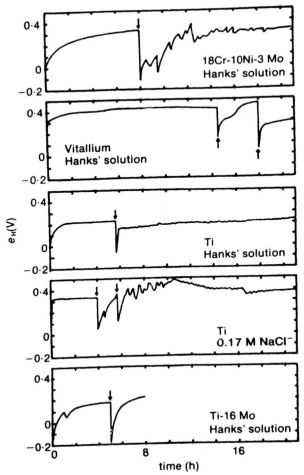

Figure 4 Electrical potential of various implant alloys in Hank's solution or sodium chloride before and after scratching the surface (indicated by the arrow). (From Ref. 5 with permission.)

can be significant increases in the concentrations of metal ions in tissues surrounding implants compared with controls. In particular, the concentration of titanium in animal studies was found to increase from a mean of 11.4 parts per million (ppm) to 236.8 ppm, a 20-fold gain [5]. *In vivo* effects of ion release from implants is controversial. French et al. [7] studied the reactions of tissues in patients undergoing hardware removal and concluded that tissue reaction decreases with time, and that since tissue reaction is not a major clinical factor, internal fixation devices need not be removed routinely. In a study by Brunet et al. [8], the ultrastructure of tissues covering an implant was found to consist of a single layer of lining cells over fibroblasts with an outer layer of fibrofatty tissue having few inflammatory cells. These results would suggest that ion release *in vivo* is not a major concern. However, McNamara and Williams [9] embedded disks of various materials in the paraspinal muscles of rats and showed that cobalt produced an intense

Table 3 Concentrations (in ppm) of Elements Found in Tissues Next to Metallic Implants of Various Types, in Rabbits, Compared with Controls

Element	Alloy[a]	No. of specimens	Mean concentration[b]	Standard deviation
Fe	Control	97	37.9	34.6
	AISI 316	61	76.8	45.7
	A 286	16	46.1	19.0
	Inconel X	14	39.3	18.0
	Hastelloy C	18	17.2	6.6
Ni	Control	132	8.0	9.3
	AISI 316	66	40.5	41.2
	A 286	16	54.9	20.2
	Inconel X	14	41.5	19.4
	Hastelloy C	18	15.7	8.2
Cr	Control	75	3.7	4.9
	AISI 316	63	76.0	55.7
	A 286	16	26.9	24.9
	Inconel X	14	7.6	1.6
	Hastelloy C	18	7.3	3.8
	Co–Cr–Mo	37	67.0	43.6
	Co–Cr–Ni–W	9	74.9	99.8
Mo	Control	124	1.8	3.2
	AISI 316	65	8.4	9.2
	A 286	19	2.6	3.2
	Hastelloy C	18	3.2	1.8
	Co–Cr–Mo	46	11.5	8.9
Co	Control	280	2.9	6.4
	Hastelloy C	18	4.7	7.6
	Co–Cr–Mo	54	76.7	45.9
	Co–Cr–Ni–W	9	63.8	77.8
Ti	Control	225	11.4	17.4
	A 286	17	27.1	32.4
	Titanium	25	236.8	168.8

Source: From Ref. 3
[a]AISI 316, stainless steel, surgical grade; A 286, stainless steel containing Tl; Inconel X, Ni 80%, Cr 14%, Fe 6%; Hastelloy C, Mo 17%, Fe 5%, Cr 14%, W 5%, Ni balance; Co–Cr–Mo, cast cobalt-chromium alloy; Co–Cr–Ni–W, wrought cobalt-chromium alloy
[b]The figures give the concentration of metallic dissolution products in parts per million dry ash of the various elements found in the tissues surrounding implants of selected alloys in rabbits.

toxic reaction while nickel induced polymorph activity in perivascular areas along with some cell necrosis, demonstrating the potential toxicity of these materials.

As discussed by Black [3], the literature reports the presence of implant-site tumors associated with fracture fixation devices. However, many of the implants reported on were pre-1980 vintage or even older. Patients may be sensitive to chromium or nickel found in stainless steel implants. Black reported on a study in which, of 32 patients presenting for internal fixation, 16 were found to be sensitive to implant metals. After

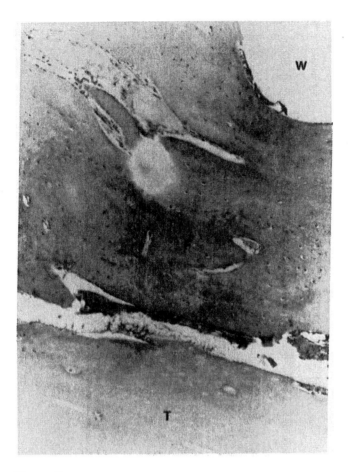

Figure 5 Histological appearance of an osteotomy of the tibiofibular junction in the rabbit that was bonded using isobutyl-2-cyanoacrylate. The fracture gap is occupied by glue with no healing across it. The periosteal callus heals normally. (From Ref. 17 with permission.)

removal, 3 more had become sensitive [3]. At this time there are both risks and benefits to implant removal. The most obvious risks are the high cost and potential morbidity associated with a second operative procedure for removal. The procedure may be complex because bone remodeling around the implant makes removal difficult. On the other hand, the long-term effects of retention of the implant are unclear. One solution may be the further use of titanium materials, which appear to be more biologically benign.

F. Comparison of Stainless Steel and Titanium

Both materials have benefits and deficiencies when used for bone fracture fixation devices. Stainless steel has greater elastic modulus and ductility than titanium alloy, and an equivalent endurance limit (mean stress at which fatigue failure does not occur). Ductility is an important property for implants such as wires or plates, which must be contoured during an operative procedure. The machinability and lower cost of the base metals result in stainless steel implants potentially costing less. Significant advantages of titanium alloy are its corrosion resistance and the fact that it does not release potentially toxic ions such as chromium and nickel, which are present in stainless steels, into surrounding tissues.

III. ADHESIVES

A. General Properties

Adhesives are not commonly used in orthopedic fracture treatment at present; however they represent a potentially useful alternative method of fixation, particularly for small fragments that are difficult to hold in position by mechanical or other means. The two adhesives that have received the majority of attention in orthopedic fracture surgery are cyanoacrylate and fibrin. Clinical results using these materials have been variable, which may be partly due to the lack of attention paid to surface preparation, a critical aspect in the use of any adhesive system, and the problem that some adhesives cannot tolerate a

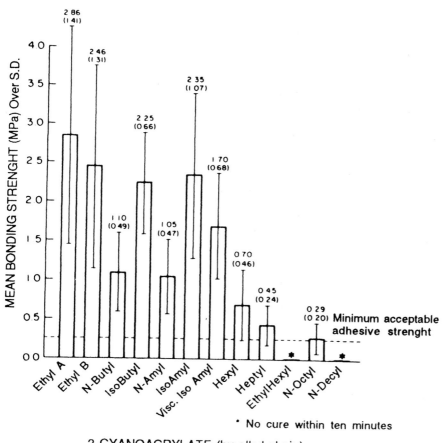

Figure 6 Bond strengths achieved in cortical bone tested in tension using various cyanoacrylates. (From Ref. 10 with permission.)

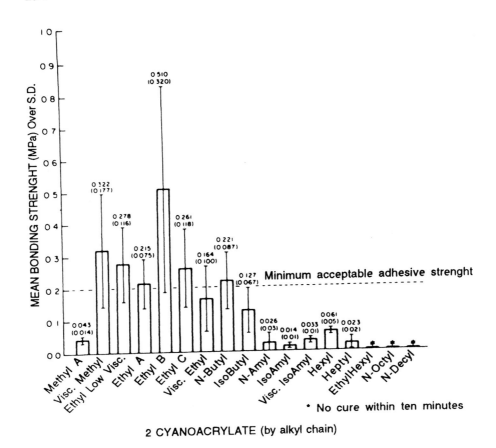

Figure 7 Bond strengths achieved in cancellous bone tested in tension using various cyanoacrylates. (From Ref. 10 with permission.)

gap between the mating surfaces. Any bonding agent to be used surgically should possess the following;

1. Sufficient bond strength
2. Biocompatability
3. The ability to adhere to moist surfaces
4. Ability to heal across the bond line
5. Sterilizability [10]

Methylmethacrylate, though commonly termed "bone cement" does not meet enough of these criteria to be defined as a true adhesive.

B. Cyanoacrylates

N-Butyl cyanoacrylates have been widely used in general surgery, opthalmology, gynecology, and dentistry [11–13]. However, their application to bone fractures has been controversial. Cyanoacrylates have fallen out of favor because of concerns of tissue toxicity

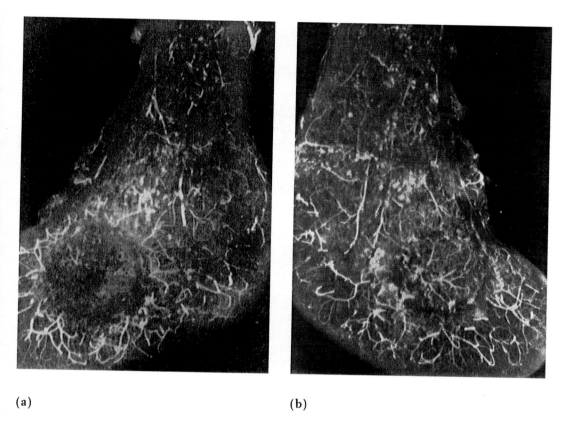

(a)   (b)

Figure 8   In experimental cancellous bone grafting of the femoral condyle of the dog, the graft with fibrin adhesive (a) demonstrates more vascularity than the contralateral without adhesive (b) 3 days postoperatively. (From Ref. 28 with permission.)

leading to high rates of nonunion and infection, and problems with redisplacement of bonded fracture fragments [14–16]. Hampel et al. [17] reported that in oblique cortical fractures at the tibiofibular junction in rabbits, periosteal healing took place around the glue line but no healing occurred across the bonded fracture, Fig. 5. Bond strengths achieved, even in carefully prepared *in vitro* bone specimens, have been highly variable [18], which may be due to sensitivity to surface preparation techniques and the requirement for intimate contact between bonded surfaces without gaps. These observations may help to explain some of the problems encountered clinically.

In an extensive study by Weber and Chapman [10] the bonding strengths of various cyanoacrylates applied to bovine cortical and cancellous bone specimens were determined. Figure 6 shows the results of bonding strength tests in cortical bone specimens. The longer alkyl chain cyanoacrylates did not cure within the 10-min time period considered by the authors as the maximum acceptable in surgical use and therefore had very low bonding strengths. They also noted large standard deviations in their results, although most of the adhesives surpassed bonding strengths that they defined to be clinically the minimum acceptable. Surface treatments using chloroform and acetone increased bond

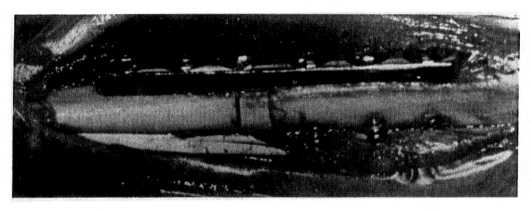

(a)

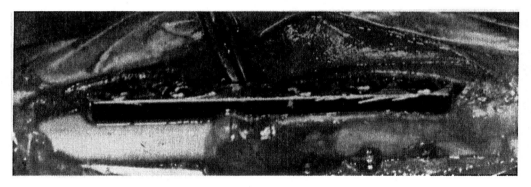

(b)

Figure 9   Response of an osteotomized segment of bone in the rabbit: (a), control bone; (b), bone with fibrin adhesive. (From Ref. 29 with permission.)

strengths, although not sufficiently to establish statistical significance, while the use of Tween 50 reduced strengths. The bond strengths of cancellous specimens, shown in Fig. 7, were much lower than those of cortical bone, with only 4 of the cyanoacrylates achieving minimum acceptable strengths. Again, the longer-chain adhesives demonstrated poorer performance and the scatter in the data was large. Considering the sensitivity of bond strength to both surface preparation and intimate contact of the bone surfaces, these adhesives were not considered practical for fracture surgery use in their present forms.

Recently Harper [19] described the use of a viscous adhesive, isoamyl-2-cyano-acrylate, which allows bonding across surface gaps. In an experimental model, an oseo-tomized section of the femoral condyle in the rabbit was bonded using this adhesive applied only to the perimeter regions, to allow healing across the central part of the defect. In 23 of the 24 animals, reductions were maintained and healing proceeded with no abnormal histologic appearances. The author attributed the success of this experiment to the ability of the viscous adhesive to act as a gap filler and possibly produce mechanical interlock as well as true adhesion. Also, the concept of applying the bonding agent in

Table 4   Tensile Bonding Strength of Fibrin Adhesive Compared with Equivalent Samples Bonded Using Isobutyl Cyanoacrylate or Polymethylmethacrylate, and the Tensile Strength of Intact Bone

Adhesive	Bonding strength (MPa)	
	Mean	(SD)
Bovine fibrinogen in solution[a] Thrombin (in Ringer's sol.)[b] Factor XIII[c]	0.016	(0.005)[d]
Bovine fibrinogen (dry) Thrombin (in Ringer's sol.) Factor XIII	0.017	(0.005)
Bovine fibrinogen in solution Thrombin (in calcium sol.) Factor XIII	0.016	(0.007)
Human cryoprecipitate Thrombin (in calcium sol.) No Factor XIII	0.005	(0.002)
Human cryoprecipitate Thrombin (in calcium sol.) Factor XIII	0.006	(0.003)
Isobutyl cyanoacrylate	0.127	(0.067)[e]
Polymethylmethacrylate	1.01	(0.51)[d,e]
Intact bone	5.77	(2.19)

Source: From Ref. 10
[a]Fibrinogen made up 90 mg/ml
[b]Thrombin made up 600 NIH U/ml in either CaCl or Ringer's lactate
[c]Factor XIII made up 65 U/ml
[d]$t = 6.14; p < 0.001$
[e]$t = 5.52; p < 0.001$

limited regions is important since it has been shown that bone will appose but not grow through the adhesive, as Fig. 5 shows. Since applying the adhesive to a greater area will improve the immediate strength of fixation but will inhibit long-term bone healing, the decision of how much adhesive to apply in fragment fixation is important. The long-term fate of the adhesive has not been addressed.

C.   Fibrin

A second adhesive that has been extensively investigated for use in fracture fixation is fibrin, which plays an important role in the natural coagulation of blood and in wound healing. Fibrin has found use in the sealing of defects in visceral organs [20] and in cardiac surgery [21]. Fibrin glue simulates the last step in the process of coagulation [22]. As discussed by Lerner and Binur [23], fibrinogen and factor XIII are activated by thrombin in the presence of calcium ions. The fibrinogen converts to fibrin, which polymerizes to form a stable clot. Factor XIII stimulates fibroblast proliferation, which is

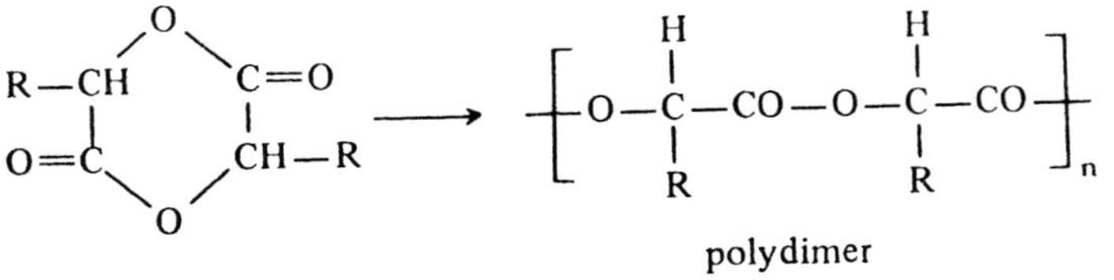

R = H : glycolide
R = CH₃ : lactide

Figure 10   Basic molecular structure of glycolide and lactide and the polydimer. (From Ref. 32 with permission.)

assisted also by fibronectin. Cold insoluble globulin encourages the adhesion of fibroblasts to the clot. Bosch [24] demonstrated that optimal clotting occurred with a 5:1 ratio of fibrinocryoprecipitate with 600 NIH units of thrombin in a 250-mmol calcium chloride solution.

Fibrin adhesive has been described for the repair of osteochondral defects [25], and in bone grafting [26,27]. Faster revascularization of a cancellous bone graft was found if a thin layer of fibrin was used to adhere the graft within the defect, Fig. 8. However, a thicker layer of fibrin, similar to a clot, must be fragmented before revascularization can proceed [28]. Results of an experimental study of osteotomy healing have also demon-

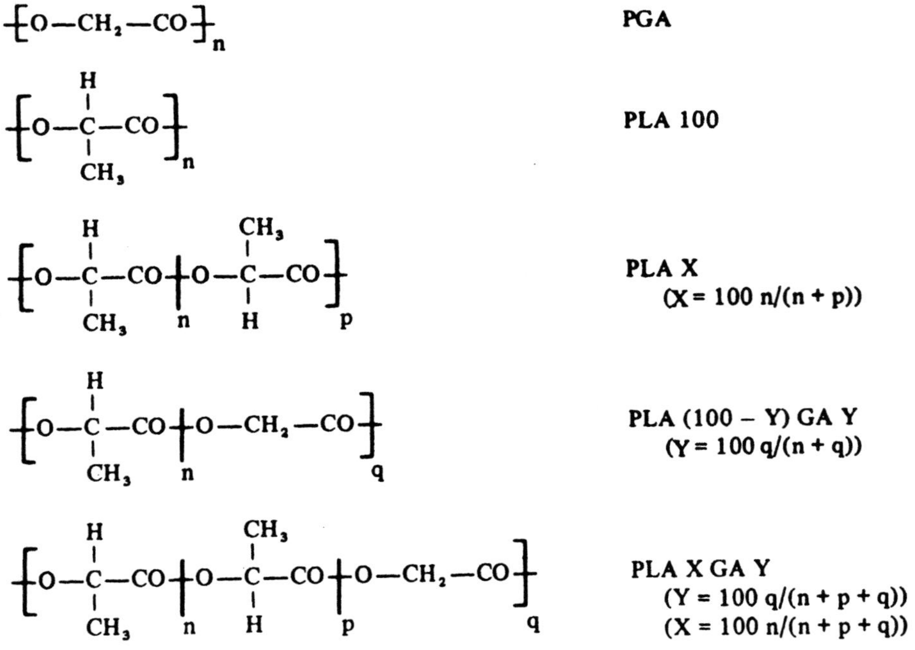

Figure 11   Structure of the polymers poly(lactic acid) and poly(glycolic acid), and their copolymers, PLA (100-Y)GA Y, and PLA X GA Y. (From Ref. 32 with permission.)

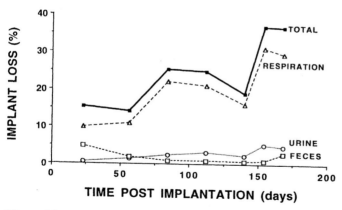

Figure 12 Proportion of PLA implants eliminated by various routes during *in vivo* degradation in the rat. (Adapted from data of Ref. 35.)

strated better callus bridging, faster reconstruction of the osteotomy site, and greater bending strength with the use of fibrin adhesive [29], Fig. 9.

Weber and Chapman [10], in their extensive testing of osteoadhesives, also reported on the tensile strengths of bone bonds using fibrin adhesives after clamping the bonded pieces for 10 min. The results, shown in Table 4, indicate that the bond strength formed by fibrin was significantly lower than that produced by cyanoacrylate. They concluded that fibrin adhesives should find use only for fracture fragments with considerable inherent stability or for those that would be non-load bearing.

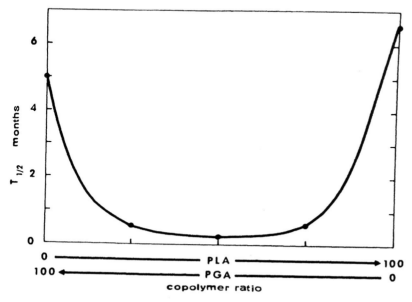

Figure 13 Half-life, in months, of implants formed from various ratios of PLA and PGA. (From Ref. 41 with permission.)

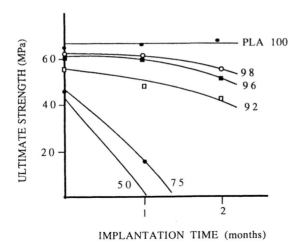

Figure 14   Ultimate tensile stress (MPa) of samples of various stereocopolymers after *in vivo* implantation for varying periods of time. (From Ref. 32 with permission.)

IV.   BIODEGRADABLE POLYMERS

A.   General Comments

Degradable polymers represent an area of increasing interest in orthopedic fracture fixation. Their attractiveness lies in the potential that implants made from these materials will hydrolyze *in situ* and therefore make hardware removal unnecessary. This would present a significant advantage in many clinical situations since no secondary procedure with its associated trauma, potential morbidity, and additional cost would be necessary.

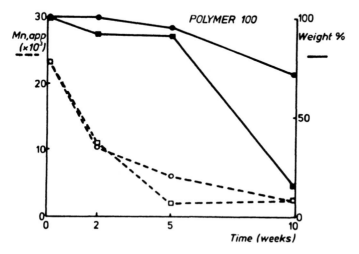

Figure 15   *In vivo* (○) and *in vitro* (□) degradation profiles of polyhydroxyacid copolymers of different molecular weights. Solid line: % weight change; dashed line: molecular weight. (From Ref. 43 with permission.)

While a large number of degradable polymers have been identified [30], the polyesters, poly(lactic acid) (PLA), poly(glycolic acid) (PGA), and their copolymers have received the most study. These materials were initially proposed for use as degradable sutures [31] and are commonly used today under tradenames such as Vicryl and Dexon. In order to find use in fracture fixation, a fixation implant made of a biodegradable material should:

1. Possess adequate mechanical strength for the application
2. Retain sufficient strength over an appropriate time period to maintain stability of the fracture components during healing and prevent loss of reduction
3. Degrade into products that do not encourage an adverse biological reaction, and that can be easily eliminated from the body

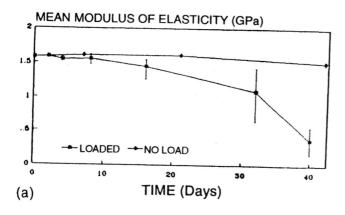

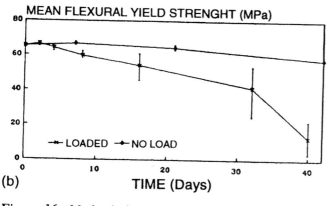

Figure 16 Mechanical properties of samples of the degradable polymer, poly(orthoester), immersed and loaded in 3-point bending at 10% of flexural yield load for 630 cycles at 1 Hz: (a), modulus of elasticity; (b), flexural yield strength, both plotted as a function of time. (From Ref. 44 with permission.)

Table 5 Comparison of the Mechanical Properties of Metals and Resorbable Polymers Used in Orthopedic Surgery

Material	Young's modulus (GPa)	Tensile strength (GPa)
Bone	7–40	0.09–0.12
Steel 316L	200	0.80
Titanium (0% porosity)	100	0.70
Ti–Al–V (0% porosity)	124	0.90
Polylactides	3–5	0.06
Polylactides (oriented)	6–14	0.3–2.5
Polylactides (resorbable)		
Glass fiber	8–30	0.20

Source: Ref. 36

B. Structure and Degradation Processes

Poly(α-hydroxy-acids) form a class of polyesters with repeating units [O—CO—CH—R], derived from glycolic acid (where, R = H) and lactic acid (where, R = CH$_3$), as shown in Fig. 10. Lactic acid has two enantiomeric forms, L and D, which have opposite configurational structures. The structures of PGA, PLA, and its copolymers are shown in Fig. 11 [32]. Degradation of polyhydroxyacids occurs in aqueous media via

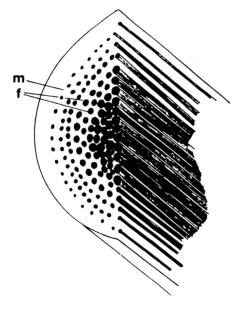

Figure 17 A schematic diagram of the construction of a self-reinforced PGA rod formed from axially aligned PGA sutures (f) fused into an amorphous PGA matrix (m). (From Ref. 50 with permission.)

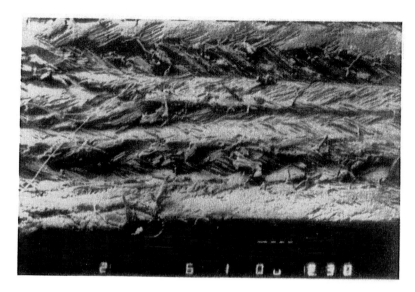

(a)

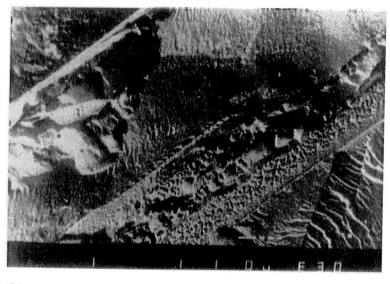

(b)

Figure 18   Scanning electron micrographs of sections of (a), a self-reinforced PGA rod; and (b), an injection-molded PGA rod. (From Ref. 50 with permission.)

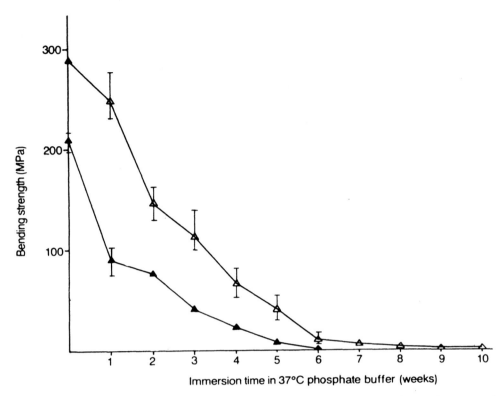

Figure 19 A comparison of the initial bending strengths and the change in bending strength with time for (upper curve) 3.2 mm diam self-reinforced and (lower curve) injection-molded PGA rods. (From Ref. 50 with permission.)

bulk hydrolysis of the ester bonds in the polymer chain. Chu [33] proposed that PGA sutures consist of alternate regions of crystalline and amorphous structures with polymer tie chains passing between regions. He observed that degradation did not proceed at the same rate throughout the whole material, and considered that the process began in the amorphous regions, which were more permiable to water, and specifically in the backbone ester linkages of the polymer tie chains. This process dominated the initial degradation procedure.

In vivo degradation proceeds in a similar fashion however enzymatic action may also be involved [34]. The degradation process converts PLA to lactic acid and glycine, which are incorporated into the tricarboxylic acid cycle. Brady et al. [35] showed that implants in rats were ultimately eliminated primarily in respiration, and secondarily in the feces and urine, Fig. 12. The biocompatability of polyhydroxyacids and the intensity of the tissue response to their degradation depends on their purity, shape, size, and rate of degradation [36]. In general, inflammatory reactions have been reported as mild in experimental investigations [32,37,38]. In contrast, using PGA or PLA-Co-PGA rods for fracture or osteotomy fixation, Bostman et al. [39] reported a 7.9% rate of clinically manifest foreign-body reactions that produced a fluctuant swelling at the implant site after 12 weeks (41/516 patients). Daniels et al. [40] explained the toxicity of rapidly degrading PGA as due to the production of significant quantities of acid, when maintained in a confined space. In their experiments, the pH in a water bath surrounding rapidly degrading PGA specimens decreased to less than 3, while the pH of fluid around more slowly degrading PLA samples stayed between 7 and 5 at 12 weeks.

C. Mechanical Properties

Both the degradation rate and mechanical properties of polyhydroxyacids are affected by a number of parameters. Degradation is dependent on the polymer–copolymer ratio of PLA to PGA. As shown in Fig. 13, a 50/50 PLA/PGA copolymer produces implants with the lowest half-life, while implants of pure PLA exhibit the greatest half-life [41].

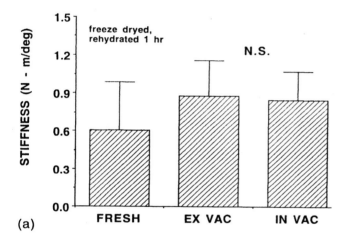

(a)

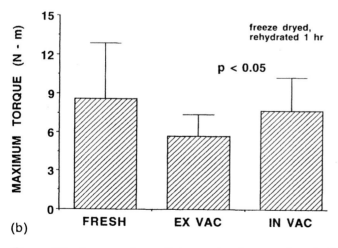

(b)

Figure 20 A comparison of the torsional properties of allograft bone, fresh or freeze dried followed by rehydration either *ex vacuo* or *in vacuo* for 1 h: (a), stiffness; (b), maximum torque. (From Ref. 65.)

Similarly, the ultimate tensile stress of 100% PLA samples is greater than that of any stereocopolymer (PLA/PGA) of less than 100% PLA content, Fig. 14 [32]. The pH of the solution in which the implant is immersed affects degradation properties, with the slowest loss of mass and mechanical properties occurring at a solution pH of 7.5 [42]. As discussed above, slower degradation rates may be beneficial in terms of reducing the potential for tissue reaction to the implant.

Lower molecular weight samples also degrade more rapidly, Fig. 15. It is also noteworthy that the rate of degradation for the same samples was found to be similar at most time points tested both *in vivo* and *in vitro* [43]. However, as Fig. 16 shows, the *in vitro* decrease in mechanical properties of dynamically loaded degradable polymers is much more rapid than is found for specimens immersed in solution but not exposed to mechanical loads [44]. This is an important consideration in designing implants for load-bearing

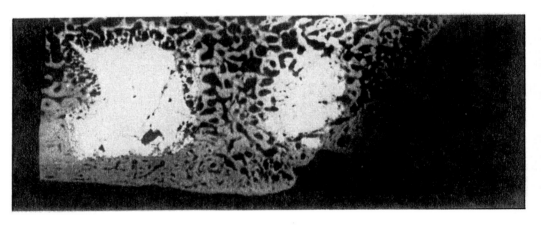

(a)

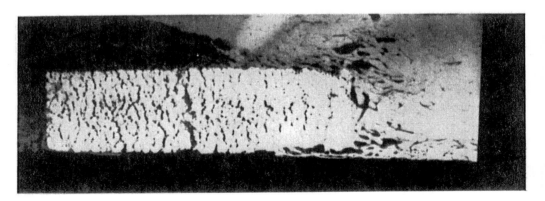

(b)

Figure 21   A microradiograph of a porous tricalcium phosphate implant 1 year after implantation into the middiaphyseal cortex of the dog femur showing (a) fragmentation and (b) bone ingrowth. (From Ref. 80 with permission.)

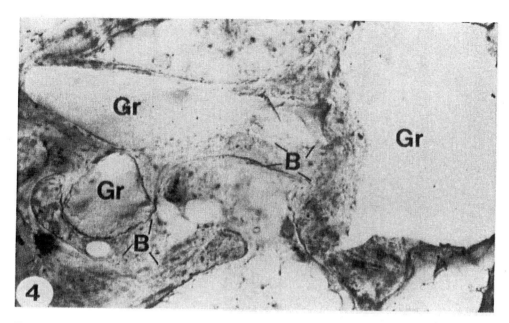

Figure 22 Histologic appearance of hydroxyapatite granules (Gr) placed within cancellous bone (B). Bone connects the granules and there is an absence of inflammatory cells (human specimen, ×5). (From Ref. 82 with permission.)

situations in orthopedic surgery and has not been fully explored. Sterilization can also alter the properties of degradable polymers due to depolymerization and the breaking of crosslinks [45,46]. Rozema et al. [46] studied 7 different protocols for steam sterilization and found that all reduce the mechanical strength of PLA to some extent; however, the minimum effect was produced using a sterilization cycle with lower temperature and smaller exposure time.

D. Development of Practical Implants

Given the concern that biodegradable materials have initially poorer material properties than metals commonly used for load-bearing orthopedic fracture applications, Table 5, and that these properties are affected by factors such as sterilization, loading, pH, and time of implantation, practical biodegradable implants have been designed using the methods of composite materials to improve strengths. Using this approach, stiffer fibers of various materials are incorporated in a more flexible polymer matrix. The fibers improve strength properties while the matrix provides the implant with flexibility and fracture toughness. An early attempt to build composite fixation plates utilized carbon fibers preimpregnated with PLA, which were then cut and placed in a mold at specific orientations between 45° and 0° (parallel to the long axis of the plate), and molded under pressure and elevated temperatures [47]. Plates made in this way had significantly improved mechanical properties, compared with plates of solid polymer without reinforcement, and were further enhanced by molding instead of machining the screw holes, since machining the holes exposes the internal matrix. However, concern for the fate of

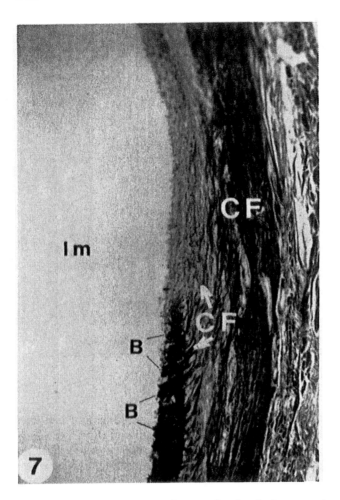

Figure 23 Detailed light micrograph of a hydroxyapatite–tissue interface, showing bone (B) deposited directly against the implant (Im), and collagen fibers (CF) within the bone tissue. (From Ref. 82 with permission.)

the nonresorbable carbon fibers has led others to explore different methods for increasing the strength of implants fabricated from these materials.

Several groups have developed biodegradable implants with increased strength, compared to the basic polymer. One approach is to produce a material with extremely high molecular weight, up to 1×10^6, by careful control of polymerization using low catalyst concentrations and formation temperatures [48,49]. Polymers with tensile strengths of up to 83 MPa have been fabricated using these techniques. The self-reinforcement approach utilizes a composite material in which the reinforcing fibers are of the same base material as the matrix but have a greater molecular weight. As shown schematically in Fig. 17 and by scanning electron micrography in Fig. 18, this technique consists of laying PGA sutures in a mold, after which the exterior surface is melted and internally the sutures are fused together. The molecular chains of the sutures are highly oriented axially.

This construction has been demonstrated to significantly increase bending strengths, shown in Fig. 19, in comparison to injection-molded rods of the same materials [50]. The modulus of elasticity of this material is 10–15 GPa, compared to pure PGA, at 6.5 GPa [50]; titanium, at 100 GPa; and stainless steel used in conventional implants, at 200 GPa. The fact that the modulus, and hence for the same size and shape of implant, the bending stiffness of implants of stainless steel is 20 times that of self-reinforced PGA indicates that these devices should be considered for low-load applications; otherwise, larger-diameter implants would be required.

E.   Other Benefits

Apart from eliminating metal toxicity, and the requirement for hardware removal, degradable polymer implants may have another potential advantage in fracture fixation. Polyhydroxyacids have been extensively used for the controlled delivery of drugs. Recent experiments have described the use of controlled release of agents for bone formation delivered from a biodegradable intramedullary (IM) rod placed in the femur in rabbits [51–53]. Ultimately, these devices may, apart from providing fixation stability, be used to deliver antibiotic agents or stimuli to bone healing.

V.   BONE GRAFT SUBSTITUTES

A.   Introduction

While ceramics and allograft bone are not used as materials in fracture implants, they have found use as defect fillers and buttressing devices in fracture fixation situations. Therefore, they can constitute a significant mechanical component of the fracture construct. Their properties are reviewed here briefly. Autogenous bone remains the graft material of choice because of its inherent biocompatability and demonstrated osteogenic capacity, yet complications can occur with the harvest of bone from the iliac crest. These can include additional blood loss [54,55], sepsis and pelvic instability [54,56], fatigue fracture [54,57], iliac hernia [56,58,59], ureteral injury [60], and heterotopic bone formation [54]. Younger and Chapman noted an overall major complication rate of 8.6% with an additional minor rate of 20.6% with iliac crest bone grafting [61].

B.   Allograft Bone

Damien and Parsons [62] presented a comprehensive review of bone graft substitutes. Allogeneic bone is one alternative bone graft substitute for autograft bone. Freeze drying of harvested grafts is commonly used for preservation and storage; however, this procedure alters mechanical properties, increasing stiffness by 175% and decreasing torsional strength to 80% of that of fresh fibular bone [63–65]. Drying that occurs during freezing, in effect, makes bone more brittle. Rehydration either *in vacuo* for 1 h or *ex vacuo* for 24 h returned the torsional strength of fibular grafts to that of fresh bone, Fig. 20; however the stiffness remained 135% greater compared with fresh bone [65]. *In vacuo* rehydration can be accomplished by injecting saline into the storage container in which the graft is packaged before surgery. Cancellous allograft mechanical properties in compression are similarly affected by freeze drying [66]. Apart from the differences in mechanical properties, bone formation occurs at a slower rate in allogeneic bone grafts compared with autografts [67–69], and there is a potential for the transmission of viral infections from the donor to the recipient [70].

C. Reaction of Bone to Ceramics

Historically, plaster of Paris was the first ceramic proposed and extensively studied as a bone substitute [71–73]. As early as 1892, Dreesman reported its use in nine bone defect sites with healing occurring in six [71]. This material is the β-hemihydrate form of calcium sulfate [$(CaSO_4)_2 \cdot H_2O$]. The addition of water results in setting of the material with the generation of heat [62]. However, plaster is brittle and has poor strength and abrasion resistance [74], as well as being resorbed rapidly [75], and therefore may be better suited as a method for the short-term delivery of antibiotics [72,76] or bone morphogenic protein [77] than as a structural defect filling material.

Ceramics can be classified by material or structure. Typical materials used as bone defect fillers are tricalcium phosphates, hydroxyapatites, and composites containing a polymer component. Structurally, these materials come in block or particulate forms with varying degrees of porosity. Porosity is probably their most important property, since increasing porosity increases the potential for bone ingrowth and the rate of dissolution, while at the same time it decreases mechanical strength. In general, ceramics can be classified as being very brittle with little tensile strength, and as being susceptible to rapid crack propagation and fatigue. Ceramics have been found to be highly biocompatable [78] but function mainly as a scaffold for new bone growth across a void (termed *osteoconductive*) as opposed to actually stimulating bone formation (*osteoinductive*).

Tricalcium phosphate (TCP) is one of the two most widely used ceramic materials in bone fracture fixation. Its chemical composition is $Ca_3(PO_4)_2$, with a calcium-to-phosphorous ratio of 1:5. The more stable form is β-TCP. which has been reported to be highly biocompatible [79]. Klein et al. [80] reported that of implants of hydroxyapatite (HA) and TCP in dense, microporous, and macroporous form, only the porous TCP degraded, with disintegration occurring by breaking of the material into smaller particles that were transported to neighboring tissues as well as being digested by phagocytes. The pores of TCP implants were filled with new bone, in direct apposition to the implants, and had the morphologic appearance of osteons with haversian canals. By 12 months postimplantation, only fragments of the TCP implants remained, Fig. 21.

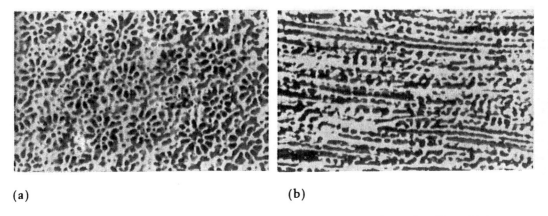

(a)   (b)

Figure 24   Oriented porosity of the coral, genus *Porities*, showing (a) haversian-like voids in cross section and (b) oriented channels with cross-fenestrations in longitudinal section. (From Ref. 85 with permission.)

Synthetically formed hydroxyapatite is similar to the naturally occurring mineral component of bone although in bone the crystals are usually smaller, being 100 μm or less in dimension [78]. Hydroxyapatite has a nominal composition of the form: Ca_{10} $(PO_4)_6(OH)_2$ with a calcium-to-phosphorous ratio of 1:67. It is an attractive material for use with bone because of its chemical similarity to bone mineral. Several reports have demonstrated direct apposition and bonding of bone to hydroxyapatite implants [81–83], as shown in Figs. 22 and 23. The biological reactions to implantation of HA have been described as initial roughening of the surface of the implant by macrophages, followed by migration of osteoblasts to the surface where osteoid is laid down and progressively mineralized [83]. The responses of osteoblasts to various orthopedic materials, including Ti–6Al–4V alloy, 316L stainless steel, and hydroxyapatite have been compared. Cell growth was found to be significantly lower on HA surfaces than any other the surfaces of the other materials in the first 4-day period, indicating some initial hesitation by osteoblasts to respond to implanted HA.

Porosity is a key property of both HA and TCP implants. One method of fabrication of porous HA is sintering of granules, which form pores between them as they fuse. The granule size and sintering temperature control the size of the pore produced [78]. The internal pore structure produced by this method is random, however, and is not similar in geometry to the oriented porosity of bone. A process of hydrothermal exchange has been described in which calcium carbonate is converted to pure hydroxyapatite [84]. This technique has been applied to the exoskeletons of several corals, which were selected based on the similarity of their pore size and structure to that of bone. The implant material produced demonstrates oriented porosity with longitudinal channels and cross-fenestrations, Fig. 24. As shown by Holmes [85], in addition to the direct apposition of bone to the intersticies of the implant, the cross-fenestrations permit vascular formation, Fig. 25. Morphometric studies have demonstrated that the microstructure of the coral, genus *Goniopora*, is very similar to that of cancellous bone derived from the iliac crest, as shown in Table 6 [86].

Three properties affected by pore size are bone ingrowth, mechanical strength, and possibly biodegradation. Bone ingrowth was found to be more rapid in porous coralline implants having a void fraction averaging 70% (pore size 260–600 μm), compared with 60% (pore size 190–230 μm) [87], Fig. 26. In implants with random instead of oriented porosity, the relation of pore size to the quantity of bone ingrowth has been found to be similar [88]. The degradation of HA implants is thought to be dependent on pore size [89]; however, up to 48 months postimplantation *in vivo*, significant degradation of HA implants has not been demonstrated [90].

D. Mechanical Properties of Ceramics

Defining the mechanical properties of ceramic bone substitutes is complex because the ingrowth of bone effectively decreases porosity and increases the strength of the implant, while degradation, if it occurs, has the opposite effect. Thus, like a healing fracture, the properties of a bone substitute, placed *in vivo*, change with time. The lowest strength can be anticipated to occur at the time of implantation before ingrowth occurs. De Putter et al. [91] described a relationship between the ultimate compressive stress (CS) and the total volume occupied by pores in the implant (VP) as follows:

$$CS = 700\,[\exp(-5\,VP)] \qquad \text{(with compressive stress (CS) in megapascals)}$$

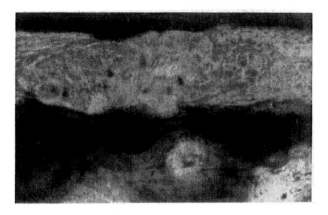

(a)

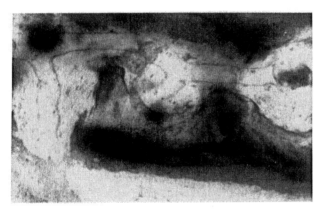

(b)

Figure 25 Bone formation within a porous hydroxyapatite implant with oriented porosity. (a) At 4 months both woven and lamellar bone are present in the implant. (b) A vascular channel can be seen bridging a cross-fenestration. (c) At 6 months, haversian osteons occupy the implant pores with (d) interchannel communication. (From Ref. 85 with permission.)

This relationship demonstrates a strong dependence of strength on pore volume. Table 7 provides mechanical property data for hydroxyapatite implants of varying porosity. The compressive and tensile strengths of ceramics encompass those of bone; however, their moduli range from about 3 to 8 times that of bone [92]. For implants with oriented porosity, the orientation of the longitudinal channels significantly affects properties, as shown in Fig. 27, with a more than 50% decrease in strength for only a 20° difference between pore channel axis and load axis [93].

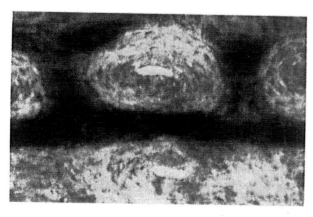

(c)

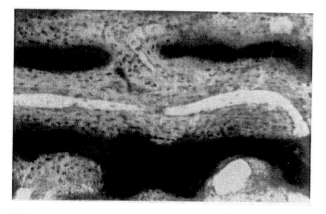

(d)

As discussed above, the strength and stiffness of a ceramic implant can be expected to increase as bone invades it. The incorporation of porous HA into the metaphyseal bone of the dog tibia, shown in Fig. 28, can be well appreciated. Detailed scanning electron microscopy clearly distinguishes how new bone directly apposes the internal surfaces of the implant, Fig. 29 [94]. As shown in Table 8, 6 months postimplantation, the ultimate strength of a cancellous autograft is about twice that of normal cancellous bone, while an incorporated hydroxyapatite implant (ingrown with bone) increases by about 6 times from its preimplantation compressive strength, from 60% of that of cancellous bone to more than 300% [95].

Although the compressive strength of solid ceramics has been shown to be in the range of that of bone, the use of materials of greater porosity to enhance ingrowth also

Table 6 Morphometric Comparison (Mean and Standard Error) of the Microstructure of the Hydroxyapatite Bone Substitute Derived from Coral, Genus *Goniopora* (IP500), and Human Iliac Crest Cancellous Bone

	IP500	Iliac bone	Iliac bone
Volume fraction (%)	35.1 ± 1.5	20.5 ± 0.4	20.3 ± 0.4
Surface area (mm^2/mm^3)	5.3 ± 0.2	3.0 ± 0.1	3.4 ± 0.1
Ratio of surface area to volume fraction	15.3 ± 0.6	14.6 ± 0.6	17.3 ± 0.2
Mean trabecular width (μm)	131.9 ± 4.4	136.6 ± 4.5	120.3 ± 1.6
Mean pore width (μm)	245.0 ± 9.0	529.6 ± 22.9	468.2 ± 27.2

Source: Ref. 86

Table 7 Mechanical Properties of Hydroxyapatite Materials Compared with Cancellous and Cortical Bone

Material	Compressive strength (MPa)	Tensile strength (MPa)	Modulus (GPa)
Bone			
Cortical	137.8	68.9	13.8
Cancellous	41.4	3.5	—
Calcium phosphates			
Porous	6.9–68.9	2.48	
Dense	206.7–895.7	68.9–192.9	34.5–103.4

Source: Ref. 62

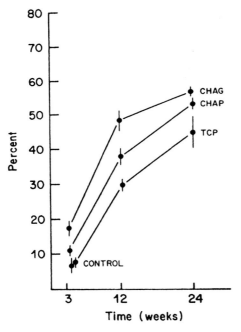

Figure 26 Bone ingrowth (percent of total volume) into porous coralline implants with different pore size ranges as a function of time postimplantation: CHAG, hydroxyapatite, pore size 260–600 μm; CHAP, hydroxyapatite, pore size 190–230 μm; TCP, tricalcium phosphate, pore size 100–300 μm. (From Ref. 87 with permission.)

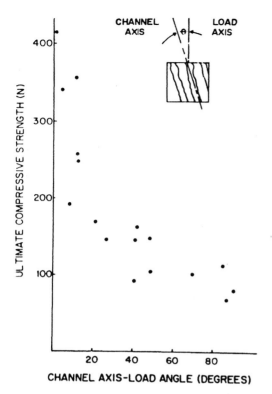

Figure 27 The relationship between longitudinal channel axis and ultimate compressive strength in a hydroxyapatite implant with ordered porosity. (From Ref. 93 with permission.)

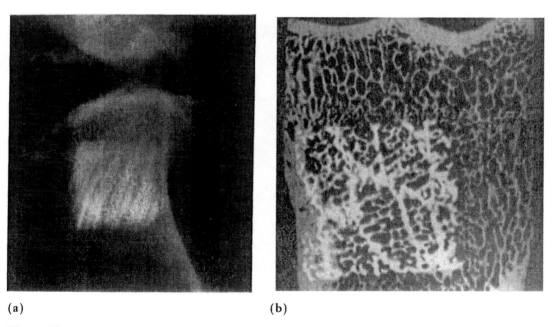

(a)   (b)

Figure 28 Incorporation of a coralline implant into the metaphysis of the tibia of the dog after 6 months. (From Ref. 86 with permission.)

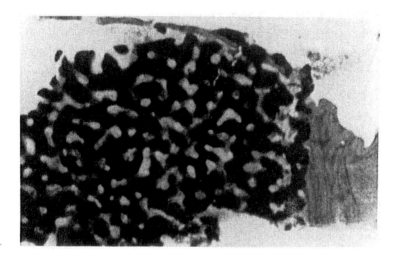

(a)

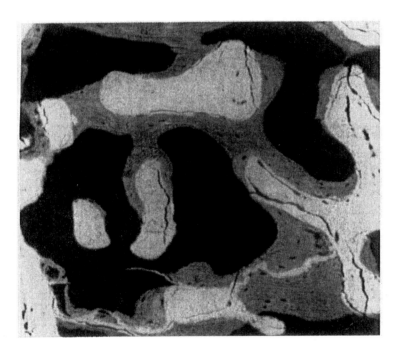

(b)

Figure 29   (a), Biopsy from human mandibular advancement; (b), backscatter scanning electron microscopic appearance of a section through the implant: white = implant, grey = new bone, and black = void space. (From Ref. 94 with permission.)

Table 8 Compressive Properties of Cancellous Bone Compared with Cancellous Autograft and Corraline Hydroxyapatite Implant (CHAG) 6 Months After Implantation

Materials	Average properties			No. of specimens tested	Ranges		
	Stiffness (N/cm)	Ultimate strength (N/cm^2)	Energy absorbed (N cm)		Stiffness (N/cm)	Ultimate strength (N/cm^2)	Energy absorbed (N cm)
Cancellous bone	7,950	754	93	6	14,760–3,750	1150–485	166.7–25.5
CHAG (load parallel to channel axis)	6,020	412	15.5	5	3,940–5,200	500–230	21.6–6.7
CHAG (load perpendicular to channel axis)	2,360	84	2.1	4	3,940–1,280	175–50	5.6–0.3
Cancellous graft at 6 months under dog tibial plateau	24,110	1519	232.4	6	36,301–7,160	2700–1000	609.6–93.6
CHAG graft at 6 months under dog tibial plateau	16,190	2488	389.7	6	6,960–750	3500–1730	514.4–160.5

Source: Ref. 95

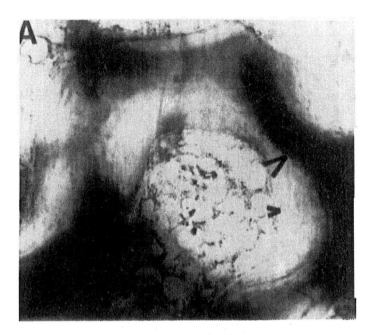

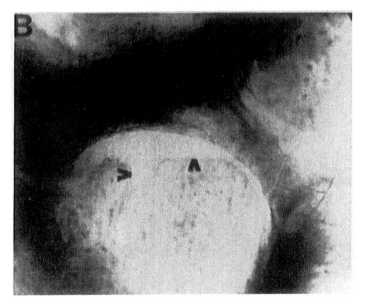

Figure 30   Bone ingrowth into porous coralline hydroxyapatite placed in the tibia of the rabbit at 24 weeks: (A) uncoated implant; (B) implant microcoated with poly(lactic) acid polymer. Black areas = hydroxyapatite and grey = new bone. Arrows in (A) indicate polymer coating. (From Ref. 98 with permission.)

reduces their strength. Also, the stiffness of ceramics is considerably greater than that of bone, Table 7. Compared to ceramics, the reduced brittleness and ability to absorb greater energy of impact in bone is due to its two-phase collagen/mineral structure. Therefore composites of hydroxyapatite and some other more flexible material, typically a polymer or collagen, have been explored. One example of a composite of this type is hydroxyapatite granules bound with atelocollagen (calf skin collagen treated with pepsin) [96]. This material does not have structural properties suitable for load bearing, nor does it maintain a pore structure, thus the collagen must be degraded before bone invasion can begin.

Alternatively, degradable polmers have been used either as a binder for HA granules [97] or as a coating on an implant [98]. Poly(lactic acid) coating of a porous HA implant of oriented porosity, similar to that shown in Fig. 24, has been found to increase its compressive strength, stiffness, and energy absorbed to failure, while still maintaining its internal pore structure. Bone ingrowth into this material was found to be slightly inhibited compared to implants without coatings because the coating partly occludes the pores of the implant. Bone grows to the coating, as shown in Fig. 30, but the coating must degrade before direct apposition of bone to the hydroxyapatite surfaces of the implant can take place (98).

VI. SUMMARY

Various biomaterials are available for use in orthopedic fracture surgery. Stainless steel will continue to be used, especially for implants requiring strength and ductility such as wires and screws, although titanium alloys have significant advantages in terms of biocompatability and resistance to corrosion. Adhesives have a potentially important role in repositioning of small, non-load-bearing fracture fragments, which are difficult to handle using conventional hardware; however, to be practical, an adhesive must be viscous enough to fill gaps and be able to bond to wet surfaces. Fibrin and viscous cyanoacrylate are two promising adhesive materials.

Degradable polymers are finding use in fracture fixation, with their main advantage being that no hardware removal is necessary at a later date. However, these materials have elastic moduli that are only about 10% of those of conventional metals; therefore, they should be considered mainly for low load bearing applications. Ceramics are used as bone fracture defect fillers. An appropriate pore size is required for adequate bone ingrowth, but increasing porosity decreases the strength of this very brittle material. However, bone ingrowth effectively reinforces the implant, improving its mechanical properties over time. Many of these materials, while not ideal in terms of meeting the requirements of the *in vivo* environment, offer important advantages and will find their place in fracture surgery.

REFERENCES

1. *Annual Book of Standards*, Sec. 13, Vol. 13.01, American Society for Testing and Materials, 1986, pp. 3–9.

2. Fraker, A. C., Corrosion of metallic implants and prosthetic devices, in: *Metals Handbook*, 9th ed, Vol. 13, *Corrosion*, ASM International, 1987.

3. Black, J., *Orthopedic Biomaterials in Research and Practise*, Churchill Livingstone, New York, 1988.

4. Pohler, O., and Straumann, F., Characteristics of the stainless steel ASIF/AO implants, in *ASIF/AO Basic Course Manual*, The Association for the Study of Internal Fixation, Davos, Switzerland.

5. Mears, D. C., *Materials and Orthopedic Surgery*, Williams and Wilkins, Baltimore, MD, 1979.

6. *Annual Book of Standards*, Sec. 13, Vol. 13.01, American Society for Testing and Materials, 1986, pp. 15-17.

7. French, H. G., Cook, S. D., and Haddad, R. J., Correlation of tissue reaction to corrosion in osteosynthetic devices, *J. Biomed. Mater. Res., 18*, 817, 1984.

8. Brunet, J., Sarkar, K., and Uhthoff, H. K., Ultrastructure of the fibrous tissue surrounding internal fixation devices, *Clin. Orthop., 208*, 84-94, 1986.

9. McNamara, A., and Williams, D. F., Enzyme histochemistry of the tissue response to pure metal implants, *J. Biomed. Mater. Res., 18*, 185-197, 1984.

10. Weber, S. C., and Chapman, M. W., Adhesives in orthopedic surgery: A review of the literature and *in vitro* bonding strengths of bone-bonding agents, *Clin. Orthop., 191*, 249-261, 1984.

11. Markoff, G., Quagliarello, J., Rosen, R. J., and Beckman, E. M., Uterine arteriovenous malformation successfully embolized with a liquid polymer, isobutyl 2-cyanoacrylate, *Am. J. Obstet. Gynecol., 155*, 659-660, 1986.

12. Barthelemy, C., Audigier, J. C., and Fraisse, H., A nontumoral esophagobronchial fistual managed by isobutyl-2-cyanoacrylate, *Endoscopy, 15*, 357-358, 1983.

13. Lobene, R. R., and Sharawy, A. M., The response of alveolar bone to cyanoacrylate tissue adhesives, *J. Periodontol., 39*, 150-156, 1968.

14. Bonette, G. H., Experimental fractures of the mandible, *J. Oral Surg., 27*, 568-574, 1969.

15. Corn, R. C., Corn, O., and Matsumoto, T., Osteosynthesis employing isobutyl-cyanoacrylate monomer, *Int. Surg., 57*, 483-487, 1972.

16. Hunter, K. M., Cyanoacrylate tissue adhesives in osseus repair, *Br. J. Oral Surg., 14*, 80-86, 1976.

17. Hampel, N. L., Pijanowski, G. J., and Johnson, R. G., Effects of isobutyl-2-cyanoacrylate on bone healing, *Am. J. Vet. Res., 47*, 1605-1609, 1986.

18. Brauer, G. M., Kumpula, J. W., Termini, D.J., and Davidson, K. M., Durability of the bond between bone and various 2-cyanoacrylates in an aqueous environment, *J. Biomed. Mater. Res., 13*, 593-606, 1979.

19. Harper, M. C., Stabilization of osteochondral fragments using limited placement of cyanoacrylate in rabbits, *Clin. Orthop., 231*, 272-276, 1988.

20. Spangler, H. P., Holle, J., et al., Die Verklebung experimenteller Leberverletzungen mittels hochkonzentriertem Fibrin, *Acta Chir. Aust., 7*, 89-93, 1975.

21. Spangler, H.P., Braun, F., et al., Die lokale Anwendung von Fibrinogen und Kollagen zur Blutstillung der Herzchirurgie, *Wein Med. Wochenschr., 126*, 86-89, 1976.

22. Stemberger, A., and Blumel, G., Fibrinogen-fibrin conversion and inhibition of fibrolysis, *Thorac. Cardiovasc. Surg., 30*, 209-214, 1982.

23. Lerner, R., and Binur, N., Current research review,: Current status of surgical adhesives, *J. Surg. Res., 48*, 165-181, 1990.

24. Bosch, P., Die Fibrinspongiosaplastik, Experimentalle Untersuchungen und Klinische Erfahrung, *Wien Klin. Wochenschr.* (Suppl.), *93*, 1, 1981.

25. Zilch, H., Animal experiments on cementing small osteochondral fragments, *Handchirurgie, 12*, 71-75, 1980.

26. Arbes, H., Bosch, P., Lintner, F., and Salzer, M., First clinical experience with heterologous

cancellous bone grafting combined with fibrin adhesive system, *Arch. Orthop. Trauma Surg.*, *98*, 183–188, 1981.

27. Bosch, P., Braun, F., and Spangler, H. P., Die Technik der Fibrinspongiosaplastik, *Arch. Orthop. Unfall-Chir., 90*, 63–75, 1977.

28. Zilch, H., Der Einfluss des Fibrinklebers auf die Revaskularisierung des Knochentransplantates, in *Fibrinkleber in Orthopadie und Traumatologie* (Cotta, H., and Braun, A., eds.), Georg Thieme Verlag, Stuttgart, 1982, pp. 62–64.

29. Bohler, N., Bosch, P., Sandbach, G., Eschberger, J., and Schmid, L., Experimentelle Erfahrungen, mit der Einklebung von Kortikaliszylindern, in *Fibrinkleber in Orthopadie und Traumatologie* (Cotta, H., and Braun, A., eds.), Georg Thieme Verlag, Stuttgart, 1982, pp. 68–70.

30. Rosen, H. B., Kohn, J., Leong, K., and Langer, R., Bioerodible polymers for controlled release systems, in *Controlled Release Systems: Fabrication Technology* (D. S. T. Hsieh, ed.), CRC Press, Boca Raton, FL, 1988, Vol. 2, Chap. 6.

31. Kulkarni, R.K., Moore, E.G., Hegyeli, A.F., and Leonard, F., Biodegradable poly(lactic acid) polymers, *J. Biomed. Mater. Res., 5*, 169–181, 1971.

32. Vert, M., Christel, P., Chabot, F., and Leray, J., Bioabsorbable plastic materials for bone surgery, in *Macromolecular Biomaterials* (G. W. Hastings, , and P. Ducheyne, eds.), CRC Press, Boca Raton, FL, 1984, Chap. 6.

33. Chu, C. C., An *in vitro* study of the effect of buffer on the degradation of poly(glycolic acid) sutures, *J. Biomed. Mater. Res., 15*, 19–27, 1981.

34. Smith, R., Oliver, C., and Williams, D.F., The enzymatic degradation of polymer *in vitro, J. Biomed. Mater. Res., 21*, 991–1003, 1987.

35. Brady, J.M., Cutright, D.E., Miller, R.A., Battistone, G. C., and Hunsuck, E.E., Resorption rate, route of elimination, and ultrastructure of the implant site of polylactic acid in the abdominal wall of the rat, *J. Biomed. Mater. Res., 7*, 155–166, 1973.

36. Gogolewski, S., Resorbable polymers for internal fixation, *AO/ASIF Dialogue, 3*(2), 6–8, 1990.

37. Wade, C. W. R., Hegyeli, A. F., and Kulkarni, R. K., Standards for *in vitro* and *in vivo* comparison and qualification of bioabsorbable polymers, *J. Test. Eval., 5*, 397–400, 1977.

38. Cutright, D. E., and Hunsuck, E. E., The repair of fractures of the orbital floor using biodegradable polylactic acid, *Oral Surg., 33*, 28–34, 1972.

39. Bostman, O., Hirvensalo, E., Makinen, J., and Rokkanen, P., Foreign-body reactions to fracture fixation implants of biodegradable synthetic polymers, *J. Bone Joint Surg., 72B*, 592–596, 1990.

40. Daniels, A. U., Taylor, M.S., Andriano, K.P., and Heller, J., Toxicity of absorbable polymers proposed for fracture fixation devices, *Trans 38th Orthop. Res. Soc., 17*, 88, 1992.

41. Miller, R. A., Brady, J. M., and Cutright, D.E., Degradation rates of oral resorbable implants (polylactates and polyglycolates): Rate modification with changes in PLA/PGA copolymer ratio, *J. Biomed. Mater. Res., 11*, 711–719, 1977

42. Chu, C. C., A comparison of the effect of pH on the biodegradation of two synthetic absorbable sutures, *Ann Surg., 195*, 51–59,1982.

43. Schakenraad, J. M., Nieuwenhuis, P., Molenaar, I., Helder, J., Dijkstra, P. J., and Feijen, J., *In vivo* and *in vitro* degradation of glycine/DL-lactic acid copolymers, *J. Biomed. Mater. Res., 23*, 1271–1288, 1989.

44. Daniels, A. U., Smutz, W. P., Andriano, K. P., Chang. M. K. O., and Heller, J., Dynamic environmental exposure testing of biodegradable polymers, *Trans. 15th Meeting Soc. Biomater., 12*, 74, 1989.

45. Heponen, V-P., Pohjonen, T., Vainionpaa, S., and Tormala, P., The effect of gamma-radiation on mechanical properties of biodegradable poly-L-lactide fibers, *Transactions of the 3rd World Biomaterials Congress*, Kyoto Japan, April 1988, p. 281.

46. Rozema, F. R., Bos, R. R. M., Boering, G., van Asten, J. A. A. M., Nijenhuis, A. J., and Pennings, A. J., The effects of different steam-sterilization programs on material properties of poly(L-lactide), *J. Appl. Biomater., 2*, 23–28, 1991.

47. Zimmerman, M., Parsons, J. R., and Alexander, H., The design and analysis of a laminated partially degradable composite bone plate for fracture fixation, *J. Biomed. Mater. Res., 21,* 345–361, 1987.

48. Leenslag, J. W., Gogolewski, S., and Pennings, A. J., Resorbable materials of poly(L-lactide) fibers produced by a dry spinning method, *J. Appl. Polym. Sci., 29,* 2829–2842, 1984.

49. Leenslag, J. W., Pennings, A. J., Bos, R. R. M., Rozema, F.R., and Boering, G., Resorbable materials of poly(L-lactide). VI. Plates and screws for internal fracture fixation, *Biomaterials, 8,* 70–73, 1987.

50. Tormalla, P., Vasneius, J., Vainionpaa, S., Laiho, J., Pohjonen, T., and Rokkanen, P., Ultra high strength absorbable self reinforced polyglycolide (SR-PGA) composite rods for internal fixation of bone fractures, *J. Biomed. Mater. Res., 25,* 1–22, 1991.

51. Anderson, P. A., Copenhaver, J.C., Tencer, A. F., and Clark, J. M., Response of cortical bone to controlled release of sodium fluoride: The effect of implant insertion site, *J. Orthop. Res., 9,* 890–901, 1991.

52. Guise, J. M., McCormack, A., Anderson, P.A., and Tencer, A. F., Effect of controlled release of sodium fluoride on trabecular bone, *J. Orthop. Res., 10,* 588–595, 1992.

53. Arm, D. M., and Tencer, A. F., *Controlled release of platelet derived growth factor,* presented at the 4th World Congress of Biomaterials, Berlin, Germany, 1992.

54. Prolo, D. J., and Rodrigo, J. J., Contemporary bone graft physiology and surgery, *Clin. Orthop., 200,* 322–342, 1985.

55. Friedlander, G. E., Current concepts review: Bone banking, *J. Bone Joint Surg., 64A,* 307–311, 1982.

56. Cowley, S. P., and Anderson, L.D., Hernias through donor sites for illiac-bone grafts, *J. Bone Joint Surg., 65A,* 1023–1025, 1983.

57. Blakemore, M. E., Fractures at cancellous bone graft donor sites, *Injury, 14,* 519–522, 1983.

58. Challis, J. H., Lyttle, J. A., and Stuart, A. E., Strangulated lumbar hernia and volvulus following removal of iliac crest bone graft, *Acta Orthop. Scand., 46,* 230–233, 1975.

59. Lotem, M., Maor, P., Haimoff, H., and Woloch, Y., Lumbar hernia at an iliac bone graft donor site, *Clin. Orthop., 80,* 130–132, 1971.

60. Escalas, F., and Dewald, R. L., Combined traumatic arteriovenus fistula and ureteral injury: A complication of iliac bone grafting, *J. Bone Joint Surg., 59A,* 270–271, 1977.

61. Younger, E. M., and Chapman, M. W., Morbidity at bone graft donor sites, *J. Orthop. Trauma, 3,* 192–195, 1989.

62. Damien, C. J., and Parsons, J. R., Bone graft and bone graft substitutes: A review of current technology and applications, *J. Appl. Biomater., 2,* 187–208, 1991.

63. Bright, R. W., and Burchardt, H., The biomechanical properties of preserved bone grafts, in *Osteochondral Allografts: Biology, Banking, and Clinical Applications* (G. E. Friedlander, H. J. Mankin, and K. W. Sell, eds.), Little, Brown, 1983, pp 241–247.

64. Kmender, A., Influence of preservation on some mechanical properties of human haversian bone, *Mater. Med. Pol., 8,* 13–17,1976.

65. Miller, E., Conrad III, E. U., Tencer, A. F., Mackenzie, A. P., and Strong, D. M., The biomechanical effects of freeze-drying and rehydration on human cortical allograft bone, *Clin. Orthop.* (in press, 1992).

66. Conrad III, E. U., Ericksen, D. P., Tencer, A. F., Strong, D. M., and Mackenzie, A. P., The effects of freeze drying and rehydration on cancellous bone, *Clin. Orthop.* (in press).

67. Mellonig, J. T., Bowers, G. M., and Cotton, W. R., Comparison of bone graft materials: Part II. New bone formation with autografts and allografts: A histological evaluation, *J. Periodontol., 52,* 297–302, 1981.

68. Oklund, S. A., Prolo, D. J., Gutierrez, R. V., and King, S. E., Quantitative comparisons of healing in cranial fresh autografts, frozen autografts, processed autografts, and allografts in canine skull defects, *Clin. Orthop., 205,* 269–291, 1986.

69. Burchardt, H., Jones, H., Glowczewskie, F., Rudner, C., Enneking, W. F., Freeze-

dried allograft segmental cortical-bone grafts in dogs, *J. Bone Joint Surg., 60A*, 1082–1090, 1978.

70. Buck, B. E., and Malinin, T. I., Bone transplantation and human immunodeficiency virus. An estimate of risk of acquired immunodeficiency syndrome (AIDS), *Clin. Orthop., 240*, 129–136, 1989.

71. Peltier, L. F., The use of plaster of Paris to fill defects in bone, *Clin. Orthop., 21*, 1–31, 1961.

72. Mackey, D., Varlet, A., and Debeaumont, D., Antibiotic loaded plaster of Paris pellets: An *in vitro* study of a possible method of load antibiotic therapy in bone infection, *Clin. Orthop., 167*, 263–268, 1982.

73. Bahn, S. L., Plaster: A bone substitute, *Oral Surg., Oral Med., Oral Pathol., 21*, 672–681, 1966.

74. Sanad, M. E. E., Combe, E. C., and Grant, A. A., The use of additives to improve the mechanical properties of gypsum products, *J. Dent. Res., 61*, 808–810, 1982.

75. Calhoun, N. R., Neiders, M. E., and Greene, Jr., G. W., Effects of plaster-of-paris implants in surgical defects of mandibular alveolar processes of dogs, *J. Oral Surg., 25*, 122–128, 1967.

76. Dahners, L. E., and Funderburk, C. H., Gentamicin-loaded plaster of Paris as a treatment of experimental osteomyelitis in rabbits, *Clin. Orthop., 219*, 278–282, 1987.

77. Yamazaki, Y., Oida, S., Akimoto, Y., and Shioda, S., Response of the mouse femoral muscle to an implant of bone morphogenic protein and plaster of Paris, *Clin. Orthop., 234*, 240–249, 1988.

78. deGroot, K., Klein, C. P. A. T., Wolke, J. G. C., and de Blieck-Hogervorst, J. M. A., Chemistry of calcium phosphate bioceramics, in *Handbook of Bioactive Ceramics*, Vol. 2 (T. Yamamuro, L. L. Hench, and J. Wilson, eds.), CRC Press, Boca Raton, FL, 1990, pp. 3–16.

79. Cameron, H. U., Macnaab, I., and Pilliar, R. M., Evaluation of a biodegradable ceramic, *J. Biomed. Mater. Res., 11*, 179–186, 1977.

80. Klein, C. A. P. T., Patka, P., and den Hollander, W., A comparison between hydroxylapatite and B-Whitlockite macroporous ceramics implanted in dog femurs, in *Handbook of Bioactive Ceramics*, Vol. 2, (T. Yamamuro, L. L. Hench, and J. Wilson, eds.), CRC Press, Boca Raton, FL, 1990, pp. 53–60.

81. Tracy, B. M., and Doremus, R. H., Direct electron microscopy studies of the bone–hydroxylapatite interface, *J. Biomed. Mater. Res., 18*, 719–726, 1984.

82. de Lange, G. L., The bone–hydroxylapatite interface, in *Handbook of Bioactive Ceramics*, Vol. 2 (T. Yamamuro, L. L. Hench, and J. Wilson, eds.), CRC Press, Boca Raton, FL, 1990, pp. 61–75.

83. Kitsugi, T., Yamamuro, T., Nakamura, T., Kokubo, T., Takagi, M., Shibuya, T., Takeuchi, H., and Ono, M., Bonding behavior between two bioactive ceramics *in vivo*, *J. Biomed. Mater. Res., 21*, 1109–1123, 1987.

84. Roy, D. M., and Linnehan, S. K., Hydroxyapatite formed from coral skeletal carbonate by hydrothermal exchange, *Nature, 247*, 220, 1974.

85. Holmes, R. E., Bone regeneration within a coralline hydroxyapatite implant, *Plast. Recon. Surg., 63*, 626–633, 1979.

86. Holmes, R. F., Bucholz, R. W., and Mooney, V., Porous hydroxyapatite as a bone graft substitute in metaphyseal defects, *J. Bone Joint Surg., 68A*, 904–911, 1986.

87. Shimazaki, K., and Mooney, V., Comparative study of porous hydroxyapatite and tricalcium phosphate as bone substitute, *J. Orthop. Res., 3*, 301–310, 1985.

88. Ito, K., and Ooi, Y., Osteogenic activity of synthetic hydroxylapatite with controlled texture — On the relationship of osteogenic quantity with sintering temperature and pore size, in *Handbook of Bioactive Ceramics*, Vol. 2 (T. Yamamuro, L. L. Hench, and J. Wilson, eds.), CRC Press, Boca Raton, FL, 1990, pp. 39–44.

89. Legros, R. Z., Parsons, J. R., Daculsi, G., Driessens, F., Lee, D., Liu, S. T., Metsger, S., Peterson, D., and Walker, M., Significance of the porosity and physical chemistry of calcium

phosphate ceramics,: Biodegradation–bioresorption, *Ann. NY Acad. Sci., 523*, 268–271, 1988.

90. Holmes, R. E., Bucholz, R. W., and Mooney, V., Porous hydroxyapatite as a bone graft substitute in diaphyseal defects: A histometric study, *J. Orthop. Res., 5*, 114–121, 1987.

91. de Putter, C., de Groot, K., and Sillevis Smitt, P. A. E., Transmucosal application of implants of dense hydroxylapatite in prosthetic dentistry, in *Ceramics in Surgery* (P. Vincenzini, ed.), Elsevier, Amsterdam, 1983.

92. Jarcho, M., Calcium phosphate ceramics as hard tissue prosthetics, *Clin. Orthop., 157*, 259–278, 1981.

93. Tencer, A. F., Mooney, V., Brown, K. L., and Silva, P. A., Compressive properties of polymer coated hydroxyapatite for bone grafting, *J. Biomed. Mater. Res., 19*, 957–969, 1985.

94. Holmes, R. E., Wardrop, R. W., and Wolford, L.M., Hydroxylapatite as a bone graft substitute in orthognathic surgery: Histologic and histometric findings, *J. Oral Maxillofac. Surg., 46*, 661–671, 1988.

95. Holmes, R. E., Mooney, V., Bucholz, R. W., and Tencer, A. F., A corraline hydroxyapatite bone graft substitute, *Clin. Orthop., 188*, 282–292, 1984.

96. Watanabe, M., Harada, K., Asahina, I., and Enomoto, S., Implantation of hydroxylapatite granules mixed with atelocollagen and bone inductive protein in rat skull defects, in *Handbook of Bioactive Ceramics*, Vol. 2 (T. Yamamuro, L. L. Hench, and J. Wilson, eds.), CRC Press, Boca Raton, FL, 1990, pp. 223–228.

97. Higashi, S., Yamamuro, T., Nakamura, T., Ikada, Y., Hyon, S-H., and Jamshidi, K., Polymer–hydroxyapatite composites for biodegradable bone fillers, *Biomaterials, 7*, 183–187, 1986.

98. Tencer, A. F., Woodard, P.L., Swenson, J., and Brown, K.L., Bone ingrowth into polymer coated porous synthetic coralline hydroxyapatite, *J. Orthop. Res., 5*, 275–282, 1987.

9
The Use of Biomaterials in Oral and Maxillofacial Surgery

A. Norman Cranin
The Brookdale Hospital Medical Center
Brooklyn, New York
and New York University College of Dentistry
New York, New York

I. INTRODUCTION

Alloplastic materials have been used in oral surgery since the days of the Egyptians. Twisted gold wire serving as implanted permucosal dental prostheses have been found by archeologists. Throughout the centuries, practitioners have attempted to replace lost teeth with biologic as well as alloplastic materials. During American revolutionary times, those at sea were subdued and their teeth extracted for use as transplants in the mouths of the more affluent. Because these teeth were untreated, their rejection was predictable on an antigenic basis. In more recent times, the antigenic potential of natural teeth used as homografts has been managed by treatments with x-radiation, glutaraldehyde, cryotherapy, and other forms of despeciation. With the advent of predictably behaved biomaterials in the mid-20th century, the need for implants of biologic origin (teeth, skin, bone, tendon) has diminished to some extent.

Although fascia lata has been of significant value in contributing to the animation of the palsied face, its harvesting involves the creation of a second surgical site. A synthetic substitute of established value, polytetrafluoroethylene (PTFE) membrane, has been demonstrated to function with competence. In regard to skin replacement therapy, no alloplast to date has been comparable to autogenous grafting. Bone grafting, practiced widely by oral and maxillofacial surgeons, delivers the best results with autogenous marrow grafts. A panoply of products, both synthetic and biologic, fail to offer the osteogenic capabilities of bone harvested from the patient. Bone morphogenic protein, a retrieved biologic, is said to be osteogenic [1]. No other products presently available can be termed anything more than osteoconductive fillers.

Such materials as chrome-cobalt-molybdenum alloy, aluminum oxides, commercially pure titanium and its alloys, hydroxyapatite, and a significant group of polymers have been produced in the forms of granules and blocks for augmentation and/or repair of oral and maxillofacial structures. A significant variety of dental implants made of these

265

same biocompatible materials, alone and in combination, are being produced in designs limited only by imagination, anatomy, and engineering skills.

The levels of performance reported by manufacturers, distributors, and users of these products challenge the highest percentages of success presented by those involved with bioprosthetic devices of all other kinds [2].

II. BIOMATERIALS

A. Metals

1. *Elements*

Tantalum.   Tantalum has been reported to be the most biocompatible of elements [3]. Since it cannot be cast, its applications are limited to wire drawn into pins (Fig. 1) and swaged into mortise forms (Figs. 2a, 2b).

Titanium.   Titanium, a commonly found metal, is available in commercially pure form and is highly biocompatible. Some rudimentary casting techniques have been introduced, but the majority of prostheses are machined or pressed into shape.

Although graft-forming mesh mortise forms are available (Fig. 3), the overwhelming number of products are dental implants of many shapes, configurations, and sizes (Fig. 4). In addition to the machine-finished surfaces of blade and root form implants, several products are available with irregular surfaces created by plasma spraying titanium (Fig. 5).

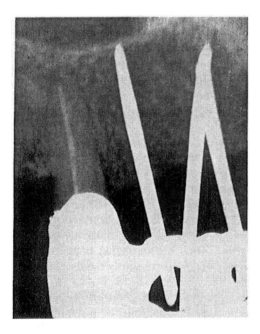

Figure 1   Tantalum wire drawn into pins are supporting a fixed prosthesis.

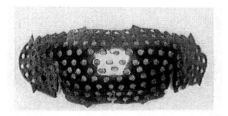

(a)

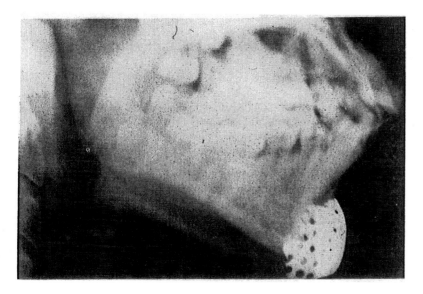

(b)

Figure 2   Tantalum can be swaged into mortise forms: (a), shaped into a chin prosthesis; (b), radiograph of the chin prosthesis illustrates proper placement.

2. Alloys

Titanium, Aluminum 6, Vanadium 4.   The alloy of titanium, aluminum 6, and vanadium 4 is considered to fall within the same range of biocompatibility as the element titanium. However, versatility is lent to the alloy in regard to strength and malleability. A number of dental implants are constructed of titanium alloy.

Chromium, Cobalt, Molybdenum.   The alloy of chromium, cobalt, and molybdenum is strong, not quite as biocompatible as titanium and its alloys, but very castable. Since many surgical prostheses and devices are fabricated using the lost wax technique, their shapes and configurations may be more complex and sophisticated than those made of the materials described in the paragraphs above (Figs. 6, 7a, 7b).

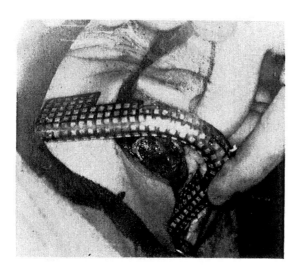

Figure 3   The titanium mortise-form mesh is being utilized in a mandibular reconstruction case. Its design permits placement of graft material within its interior.

Stainless Steel.   Stainless steel (316L ASTM, American Society for Testing and Materials) is an inexpensive, versatile, and very strong metal that may be cast or wrought into a wide variety of implantable devices of elaborate geometry (Figs. 8a, 8b). With the introduction of more biocompatible metals, use of stainless steel essentially has been abandoned. Its high level of reactivity in the saline environment and its responses to bending,

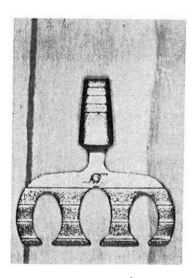

Figure 4   Titanium blade implants have many designs to accommodate the underlying anatomy.

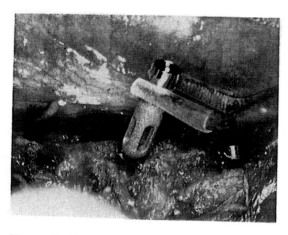

Figure 5 Titanium implants can be plasma sprayed with titanium oxide to increase the surface area for improved bone apposition.

cutting, and scratching, which often result in fatigue and stress fractures, have been significant causes for using alternate materials.

B. Ceramics

1. Aluminum Oxide

Aluminum oxide has played a long and reliable role in dental implantology. One of the earliest forms was introduced as synthetic sapphire almost 40 years ago [4]. Since that time, several forms of implants have been in use. They have been fabricated using the

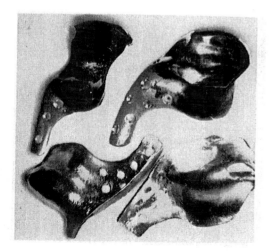

Figure 6 These cast chrome alloy implants have been designed as glenoid fossa replacements in temporomandibular arthroplasty.

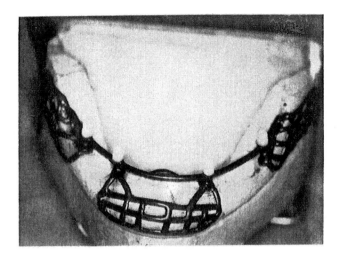

(a)

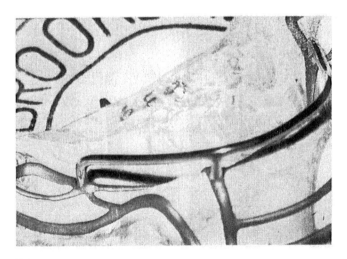

(b)

Figure 7   The lost wax technique: (a), after the implant is designed and waxed up, it is used to obtain a chrome alloy cast metal subperiosteal implant; (b), this cast subperiosteal implant is made with a strengthening Brookdale bar.

classic polycrystalline technique as free-standing root form implants [5] (Figs. 9a, 9b). The material is more bioinert than metals, but, because it lacks strength, the shapes tend to be bulky. In addition, single-crystal aluminum oxide blades and root forms have been cultured. These are extremely strong and have highly polished surfaces [6] (Fig. 10). Although popular in Japan, wide acceptance has not been perceived in the West.

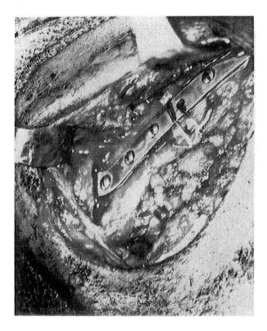

(a)

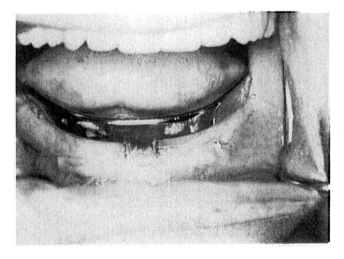

(b)

Figure 8 Stainless steel used as an implantable device: (a), a stainless steel fracture plate is used to reduce this mandibular fracture; (b), the stainless steel or titanium ramus frame implant has been quite successful in retaining mandibular denture prostheses.

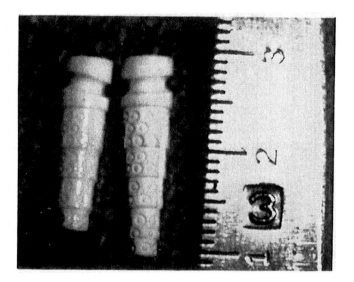

(a)

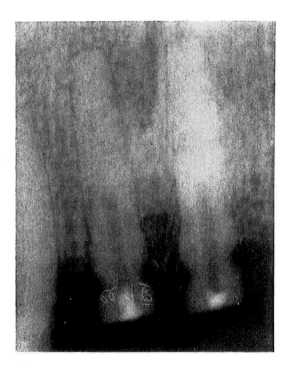

(b)

Figure 9   Aluminum oxide ceramic implants: (a), free-standing polycrystalline root form implants are bulky since the material lacks strength. They are ideal for immediate extraction sites. Osteointegration may be expected with these designs. (b), A radiograph of two polycrystalline implants in place shows successful bony integration.

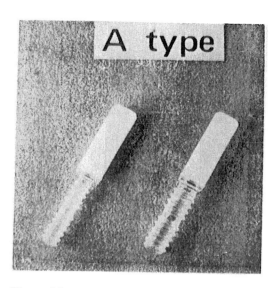

Figure 10   These single-crystal aluminum oxide root form implants are popular in Japan. They are fabricated by crystal culture.

2.   The Calcium Phosphates

Hydroxyapatite.   Hydroxyapatite is manufactured in a manner that can make it virtually indistinguishable from the biologic material it mimics. The number of ions of calcium in the compound will be responsible in inverse proportion to its level of solubility (Figs. 11a, 11b). It is available in block and particulate forms. The particles are manufactured in two sizes, 800 micrometers (μm) and 350 μm (20 and 40 mesh, respectively). Hydroxyapatite (HA) may be made as well by extracting the organic elements from coral. The resulting replaminoform porous geometry lends itself particularly well to encouraging bone ingrowth [7] (Fig. 12).

   HA particles have a tendency to migrate after their implantation. To minimize this complication, the material can be obtained in the form of beads strung to polylactic acid threads (PLA) or in a vehicle of plaster of paris, $Ca(SO)_4$ (Fig. 13). After setting in the biological environment, the position of the particles is maintained until invading fibrous tissue replaces the resorbed plaster (Figs. 14a, 14b).

Tricalcium Phosphate.   Tricalcium phosphate (TCP) is a resorbable form of hydroxyapatite and is used as an osteoconductive matrix after bone surgery. It is of particular benefit as a ridge maintenance device after dental extractions if implants are to be used subsequently since the nonresorbable forms prevent the preparation of accurate osteotomies.

C.   Polymers

1.   Polymethylmethacrylate

Polymethylmethacrylate (PMMA), when well cured by driving out all free monomer, is a biocompatible, strong, and easily fabricated material very suitable for maxillofacial prostheses such as chin and malar augmentative devices (Fig. 15). With the addition of

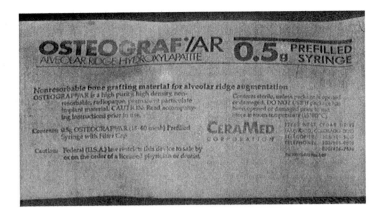

(a)

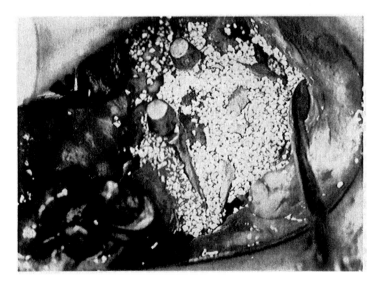

(b)

Figure 11 Hydroxyapatite ceramic: (a), is manufactured in particulate form and marketed in a syringe that is kept sterile by double bagging; (b), particles are being used to augment inaccuracies beneath a subperiosteal implant.

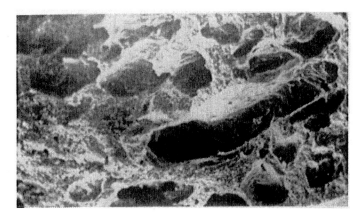

Figure 12 Replaminaform (coralline) porous geometry encourages bony ingrowth. The pores must be greater than 140 μm in diameter and of an interconnecting nature.

polyhydroxyethyl-methacrylate, a hydrophilic material, a satisfactory particulate copolymer has been created that functions in much the same manner as hydroxyapatite.

2. Silicone Rubber

Silicone rubber is made in block and sheet form and has been a compatible and reliable augmentative material, easily and accurately carved and cut at the operating table. It is used as an orbital floor prosthesis and has a demonstrated compliance in this role (Fig. 16).

In addition, chin and malar prominence augmentation may be performed using prefabricated as well as custom-carved prostheses (Figs. 17a, 17b).

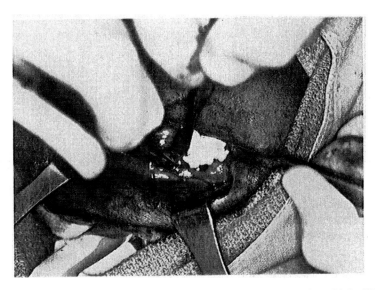

Figure 13 Hydroxyapatite particles in a plaster of paris vehicle (Hapset®) is convenient to use when the graft material is placed into sites that do not offer stable retention.

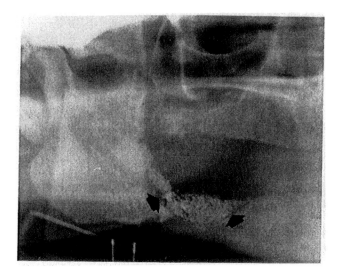

(a)

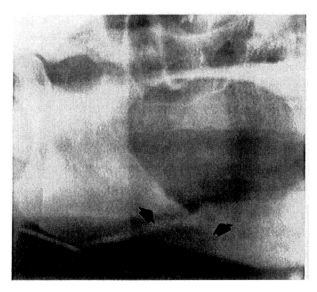

(b)

Figure 14   Use of hydroxyapatite in the biological environment: (a), a postoperative radiograph of a mandibular ridge augmented with hydroxylpatite reveals a successful graft and increased ridge height; (b), the mandibular ridge augmentation after a one-year follow-up shows a successful graft with bony ingrowth.

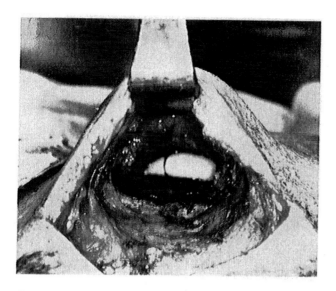

Figure 15 A polymethylmethacrylate chin augmentative device has been placed onto the symphysis of the mandible. Temporary fixation is achieved with several circummandibular sutures.

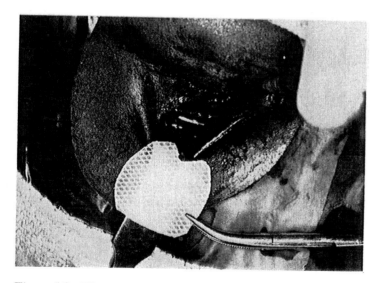

Figure 16 Silicone sheet prostheses are placed onto the floor of the orbit beneath the globe to treat blow-out fractures.

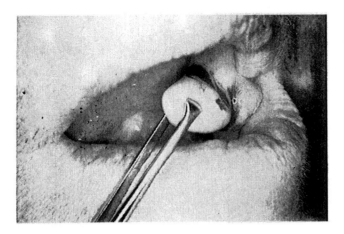

(a)

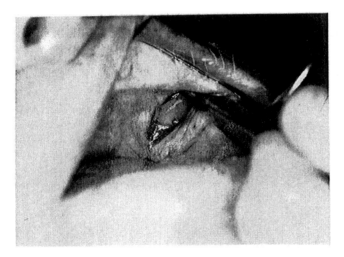

(b)

Figure 17 Malar prominence augmentation using a silicone rubber prosthesis: (a), an intraoral approach via a buccal mucosal incision is used; (b), the augmentation is in its proper position prior to suturing.

3. *Polytetrafluorethylene Teflon*

PTFE Teflon is available in sheet form, and has been used as an orbital floor prosthesis in the treatment of blow-out fractures (Figs. 18–20). Teflon is a constituent of Proplast, a porous implantable material available in block form that has been tailored for augmentation purposes. In addition, the material had been an integral part of a temporomandibular joint prosthesis recently withdrawn from the market. The material, though bioinert, failed to resist the compressive forces delivered by the mandible during function, and the resulting debris was responsible for a significant number of serious complications.

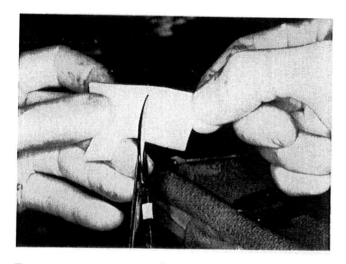

Figure 18 Polytetrafluoroethylene (PTFE) (Teflon) is available in sheet form. It may be cut to appropriate shapes and is valuable in treating orbital fractures.

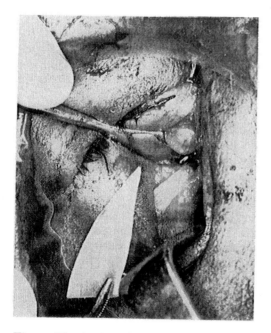

Figure 19 A properly cut polytetrafluoroethylene (PTFE) segment is fitted to treat an orbital blow-out fracture.

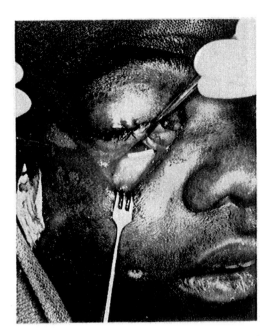

Figure 20   The polytetrafluoroethylene (PTFE) sheet is placed over the orbital floor prior to closure.

Another PTFE composite is Goretex®. This may be acquired in sheet form and is used successfully as a guided tissue augmentative membrane (GTAM). In such a function, the invagination of epithelium is discouraged during gingival healing after a grafting or implant procedure [8,9] (Figs. 21–23).

Millipore filter has, as a major component, PTFE. It is porous, often with 4-micron (μ) pores, and it has been suggested that it be used to line titanium fenestrated mortise prostheses prior to the placement of autogenous bone graft material within them (Fig. 24). Its presence permits the passage of fluids, but prohibits the mineralizing bone from creating cortical buds through the fenestrations that might make subsequent mortice form removal difficult.

4.   Polyethylene

Polyethylene polymer is manufactured in the form of tubes, sheets, and porous prefabricated augmentative prostheses. In these augmentative prostheses, it encourages the ingrowth of fibrous connective tissue that anchors it reliably into position. The sheets may be used as orbital floor implants and the tubes have served successfully as stents for vestibular plastics and to anchor transdermal sutures (Figs. 25–27).

5.   Polylactic Acid/Polyglycolic Acid

Polylactic acid/polyglycolic acid (PLA/PGA) are hydrolyzable polymers manufactured in the form of sutures and woven mesh. The PLA is more rapidly resorbed and, with the addition of the PGA, additional time *in situ* is made possible and greater strength becomes available. The mesh is used as a GTAM; a benefit not presented by the non-

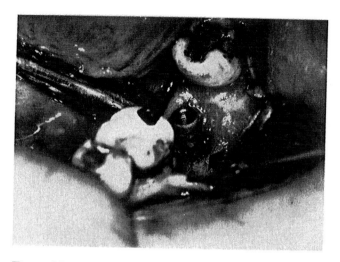

Figure 21   A bony defect surrounding the cervix of a dental implant is present. Such defects are termed *saucerization*.

resorbable Goretex, which requires a second operation for its removal, is its dissolution after serving its role in the guidance of epithelium (Figs. 28–30).

6.   Collagen

Collagen is a biologic polymer available in the form of sheets, plugs, and a spun flocculent for use as a coagulant and resorbable material in postextraction sites, antral commu-

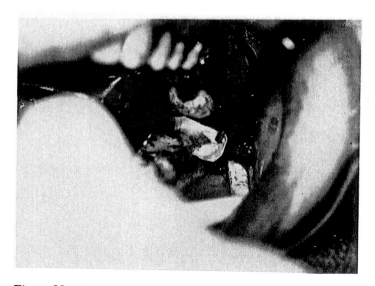

Figure 22   A polytetrafluoroethylene (PTFE) (Goretex) membrane is placed over the defect after grafting so that bony ingrowth may be encouraged.

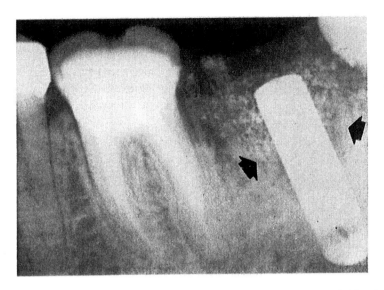

Figure 23   A postoperative radiograph shows the graft material in place and of good density.

nications, and other osseous defects. It offers a matrix over which the mucosa may be sutured (Figs. 31a–d).

D.   Composites

The materials listed in the sections above may be employed as well in the form of composites.

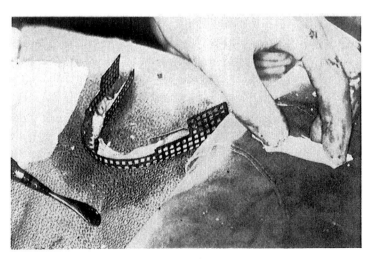

Figure 24   Millipore filter material is utilized to line a titanium mortise prosthesis that will be used in mandibular reconstruction.

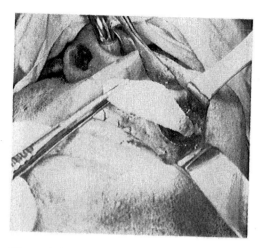

Figure 25   Porous polyethylene is placed through an oral incision into a maxillary defect.

1. Metal-Ceramic Composites

Metal-ceramic implant devices are the most frequently used combination of materials. Hydroxyapatite has been applied to titanium and titanium alloy infrastructures using plasma spray techniques (Figs. 32, 33). The projected benefits are a more highly compatible surface, an increased amount of surface area, and firmer interfacial bonding [10]. Recent problems have been cited regarding delamination of the ceramic coatings. With the loss of the HA, subsequent implant failure has been the usual result. Upon removal

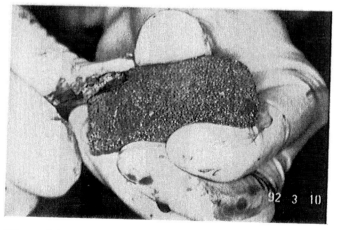

Figure 26   The polyethylene, after being soaked in the patient's blood, requires reshaping to fit more accurately into the host site.

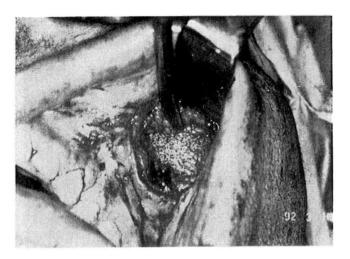

Figure 27   The implant fits well prior to closure of the surgical site.

of such implants, the HA coating has been shown on occasion to remain attached to the bony walls of the host site (Fig. 34).

2.   Ceramic-Polymer Composites

For ceramic-polymer composites, calcium hydroxide has been applied to the surfaces of polymethylmethacrylate beads. These have been used in the same manner as hydroxyapatite particles as an osteoconductive matrix to be placed in defects after bone surgery.

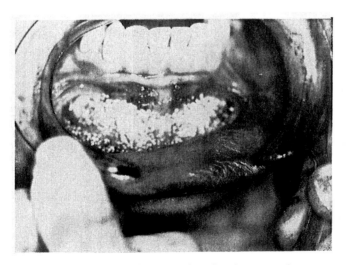

Figure 28   Polymethylmethacrylate beads are used to augment the chin after autogenous bone harvesting was completed.

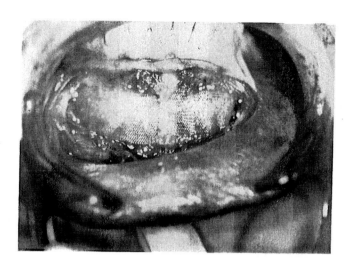

Figure 29   Polyglactic (Vicryl®) mesh membrane is placed over the chin graft to assist in holding the graft material in place, as well as to discourage epithelial downgrowth into the site.

3. Polymer-Carbon Composites

Polymer-carbon composites have been used in porous forms as cosmetic plumpers in plastic and maxillofacial surgery and as components of prostheses for temporomandibular joint replacement. In the role of prostheses components, because of the forces delivered by the masticatory apparatus to the temporal base, the porous composite has been shown to lose structural integrity. The resultant debris, after its dissemination, became responsible for a significant spectrum of complications. The material, though biocompatible, was selected inappropriately for the function planned for it [11].

III.   DEVICES

A.   Dental Implants

Dental implant prostheses occupy a significant and growing position in the realm of oral rehabilitation. They are of different designs and gain retention in a number of ways based on design, material, or a combination of these. All dental implants share a common nomenclature: *infrastructure*, the portion designed to acquire retention; *abutment*, the portion that serves as a prosthetic retainer; and *cervix*, the highly polished, constricted portion connecting the two (Figs. 35–37). They are stabilized by either bone, periosteum, or fibrous connective tissue. Such implants, when in a state of satisfactory health, acquire a hemidesmosomal adherent gingival cuff that acts as a deterrent to incursions of detritus and endotoxin-producing organisms [12].

1. Subperiosteal Implants

Subperiosteal implant prostheses, introduced in the United States in 1947, have been used with consistent success. There have been very few changes in technique or design over the years. Subperiosteal implants have been shown to be successful for as long as 40 years.

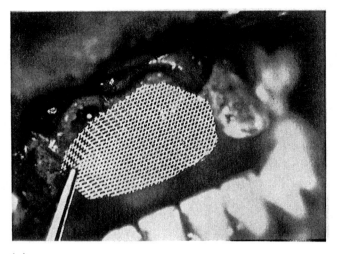

(a)

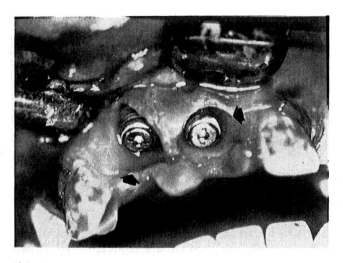

(b)

Figure 30   Vicryl mesh membrane for use as an epithelial guidance device: (a), it is cut to size and is to be placed over a graft material; (b), bony discrepancies are present after the extraction of teeth and the immediate placement of implants into their alveoli; (c), the defects are grafted with demineralized allograft bone; (d), the mesh membrane is then placed over the grafted areas, and the site is ready to be sutured.

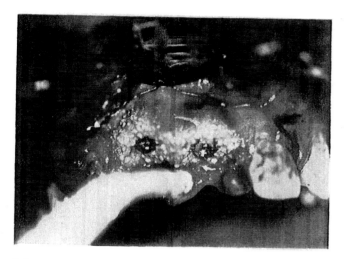

(c)

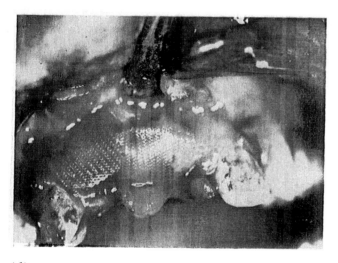

(d)

They consist of a meshlike infrastructure that fits on the maxillary or mandibular bone in a saddlelike fashion and to which are attached permucosal abutments that serve as retentive devices for prostheses.

Subperiosteal implants may be unilateral, bilateral, or complete, depending on the location of remaining teeth, if any. They may be fabricated by the lost wax casting technique using titanium for smaller designs and chrome alloy for larger devices. In order to produce a model of the bony surfaces of the jaw, a direct impression is made in a first-stage surgical operation (Fig. 38). More recently, computerized tomography (CT) scanning has enabled engineers to produce computer-aided design/computer-aided manufacturing (CAD/CAM) models on which the casting may be made [13,14] (Fig. 39).

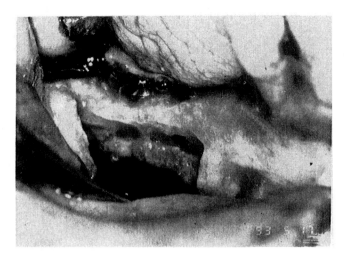

(a)

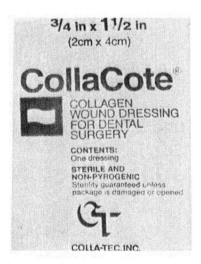

(b)

Figure 31   The use of collagen as a biologic polymer: (a), the inferior alveolar nerve is exposed from the lateral border of the mandible; (b), collagen CollaCote® wound dressing is packaged in sheet form; (c), the CollaCote dressing is cut and placed into position over the nerve after implant placement in the position formerly occupied by the neurovascular bundle; (d), the collagen dressing has absorbed blood and achieves an appropriate shape prior to closure.

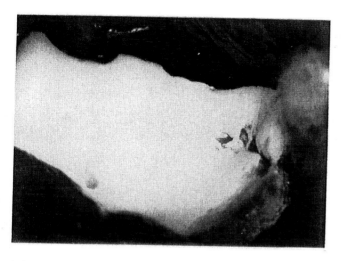

(c)

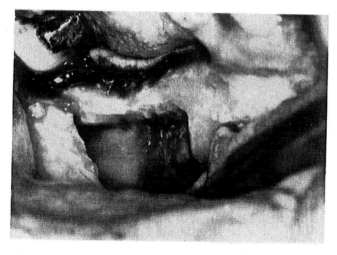

(d)

Designs have become more encompassing in the past decade, thereby permitting a distribution of occlusal forces over greater areas of bone. With the introduction of the Brookdale bar in 1973, rigidity was added to these implants, thereby granting them stability and longevity [15] (Figs. 40–43). The bar also permitted the fabrication of a tripodal design that avoided surgical exposure of the dehiscent mandibular nerve and spared patients the problems of dysesthesia of the mental branch, which supplies sensation to the lower lip and chin (Fig. 44). Both removable and fixed prostheses have been employed in conjunction with subperiosteal implants (Fig. 45).

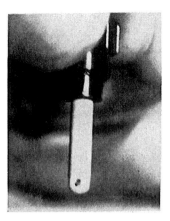

Figure 32 A hydroxyapatite-coated root form implant acquires a surface that offers an osteophylic environment to the host site.

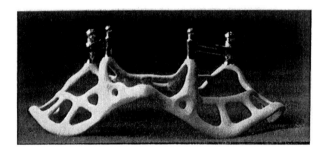

Figure 33 Subperiosteal implants coated with hydroxyapatite (HA) also are available.

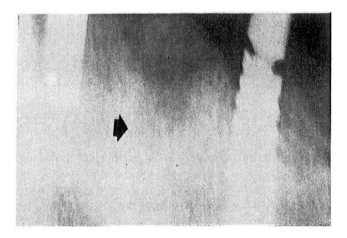

Figure 34 Hydroxyapatite (HA) delamination from its substrate does occur; in this radiograph, the hydroxyapatite-bone interface is evident after implant removal.

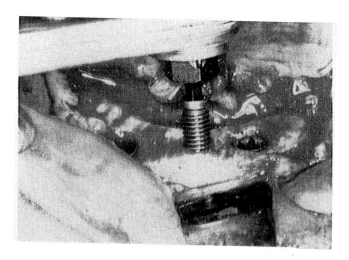

Figure 35 A titanium root form is being rotated into position. Note the threaded infrastructure and polished cervix.

2. Endosteal Implants

Endosteal implants have become the most popular types of dental implants in recent decades [16]. There are two major designs, the blade and the root form. Each has an infrastructure that is placed within the medullary cavity of bone and attached to it, either fixed or detachable, in a permucosal prosthetic abutment.

Blade Implants. Blade implants were introduced in 1967 [17] and are made of titanium. They are thin in outline and gain their retention by being placed in a narrow osteotomy cut into the alveolar ridge. Fenestrations in the blade permit bone to grow through them

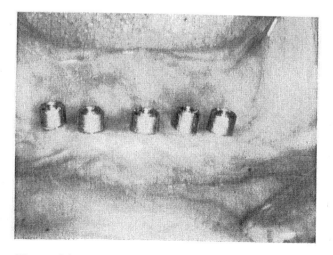

Figure 36 These titanium endosteal implants have become osseointegrated and the fixed-detachable (removable) abutments are in place.

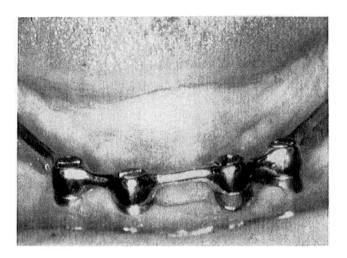

Figure 37 A precision-made bar is secured over the abutments with titanium screws and will aid in retaining a lower denture.

and anchor the implant. There are many designs and a great variety of dimensions of blades. They are used generally as abutments for fixed prostheses (Figs. 46–48).

The relationship that blade infrastructures maintain with their host sites has been referred to as fibroösseous integration [18,19]. This phenomenon demonstrates a fibrous connective tissue sling supporting the blade infrastructure. As occlusal forces are delivered to the abutment, forces are transmitted to the fibers attached to the adjacent bony

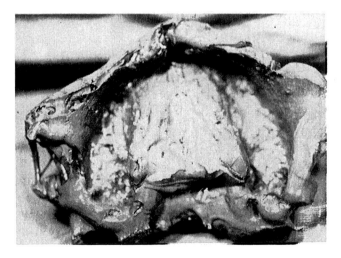

Figure 38 A polysulfide maxillary bone impression is made for the cast fabrication of a subperiosteal implant.

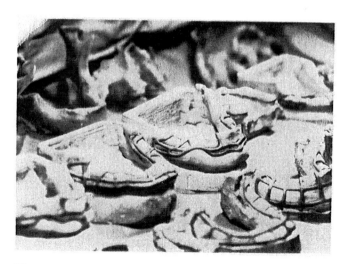

Figure 39 Direct bony impressions of bone (front of photo) and computer-aided design/computer-aided manufacturing (CAD/CAM) (rear of photo) casts are two techniques that can be used to fabricate subperiosteal implants.

walls. These tension forces are said to keep the bone in a state of dynamic remineralization [20] (Figs. 49, 50).

The prognosis for blade implants is not as reliable or predictable as for root forms.

Root Form Implants.   Root form implants have the general appearance of dental roots and are made of titanium or titanium-vanadium-aluminum alloy, sometimes coated with

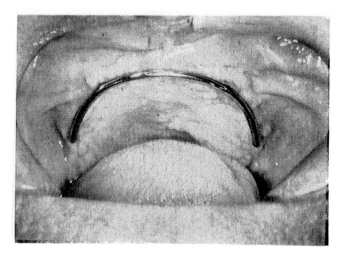

Figure 40   The subperiosteal implant with a polished Brookdale bar has proven to be a successful implant.

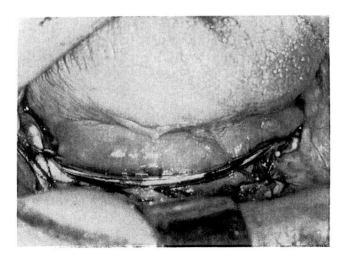

Figure 41   The Brookdale bar's 3-millimeter (mm) clearance allows for proper hygiene of the subperiosteal implant.

hydroxyapatite. They are manufactured in diameters from 3.15 mm to 5.5 mm and in lengths from 7 mm to 18 mm (Figs. 51, 52). Their abutments most frequently are detachable, which requires a second minor operative procedure for their placement. In addition to these most widely used threaded or smooth-sided press-fit implants are the less popular aluminum oxide implants made in Germany (polycrystalline) and Japan (single crystal).

The operative procedures required to insert root form implants (which are available sterile in a variety of innovative package designs) involve exposing the host bone and

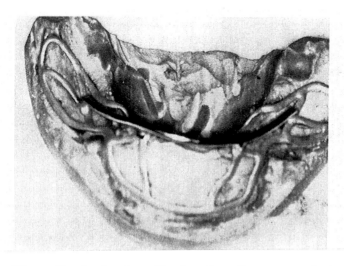

Figure 42   A subperiosteal implant fits well over a cast obtained by a direct bony impression.

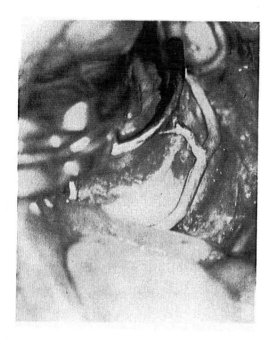

Figure 43 The intimate contact of the implant over bone is illustrated.

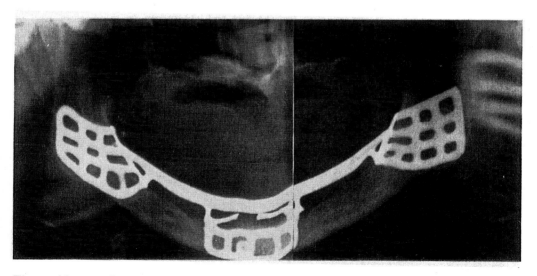

Figure 44 A radiograph illustrates the tripodal design that has added to the success of the subperiosteal implant.

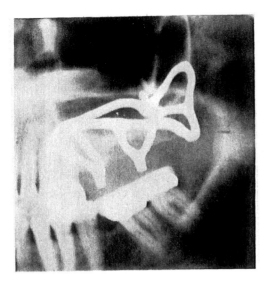

Figure 45   Radiograph of the unilateral subperiosteal implant shows a successful implant in place.

preparing it by drilling and/or tapping to receive the implant infrastructure (Figs. 53, 54). These are then screwed or gently malleted into the prepared sites (Fig. 55). After a period of maturation (three months for the mandible, six months for maxillae), the infrastructures are exposed and permucosal abutments screwed into their hollow, threaded interiors (Figs. 56, 57). Attached to these abutments, using a number of imaginative engineering devices, are functional and esthetic prostheses (Fig. 58).

When a state of osseointegration is achieved (which occurs in most cases and is described as direct bone contact at the light microscopic level) (Fig. 59) [21]. An excellent prognosis with very slight host site deterioration, over many years, has been reported [22,23].

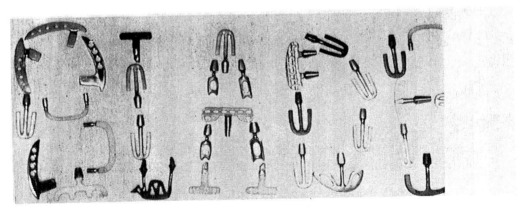

Figure 46   Many blade implant designs have been fabricated to fit within the anatomical confines of the oral cavity.

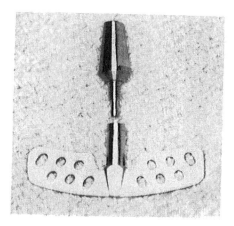

Figure 47   The titanium blade with a polished collar and abutment have functioned well for many years.

Other Endosseous Designs.   Other endosseous designs include transmandibular implants, endodontic stabilizers, and ramus frames. Each of these requires special instrumentation and insertion techniques (Figs. 60, 61).

B.   Skeletal Implants

1.   *Reparative*

Chrome Alloy and Titanium Plates and Screws.   Chrome alloy and titanium plates and screws in myriad sizes and shapes are in use to fix fractured facial bones and to stabilize bone segments after orthognathic surgery. Most of these plates and screws are permitted

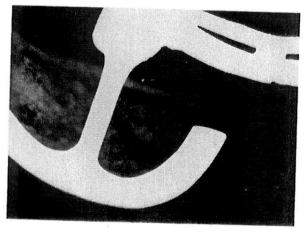

Figure 48   A radiograph of an anchor blade implant shows its success in supporting a fixed prosthesis in the mandible.

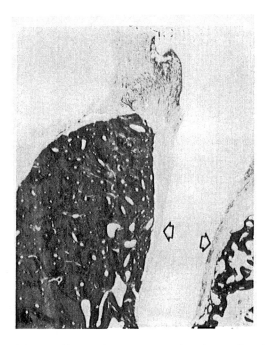

Figure 49 A fibrous connective tissue sling is present in this histologic specimen that used to contain a blade implant.

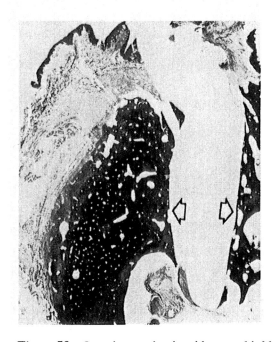

Figure 50 Osseointegration is evident on this blade histologic specimen.

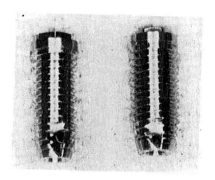

Figure 51   Titanium root form implants are usually of the threaded- or screw-type design.

to remain in place after their terms of active use have been completed (usually six to eight weeks) (Figs. 62, 63).

Pins and Rods.   Pins and rods, both smooth and threaded, have been used for osteosynthesis. These are made of stainless steel and require removal after healing. Most are percutaneous and some support extraskeletal fixation devices (Fig. 64).

Teflon and Silicone Rubber Sheets.   Sheets of Teflon and silicone rubber are used as orbital floor prostheses in cases of blow-out fractures. They provide a smooth and compliant surface on which the globe can rest and function.

Bone Grafting Materials and Guided Tissue Augmentation Membranes.   Sheets of polylactic/polyglycolic acid (PGA/PLA) mesh and Teflon composite are used as epithelium retardants and GTAMs in periodontal and oroantral repairs. They are placed with and

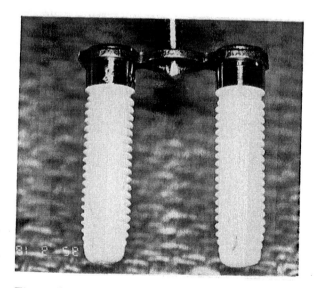

Figure 52   Hydroxyapatite-coated root form implants can be designed as press-fit types, but hydroxyapatite-coated threaded implants are also available.

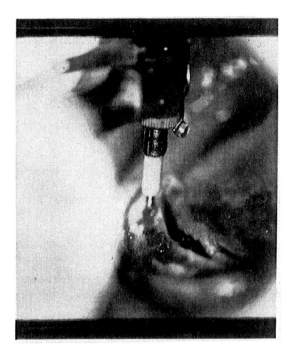

Figure 53 Osteotomies are cut into the mandible to a specific size so that endosteal implants can be placed.

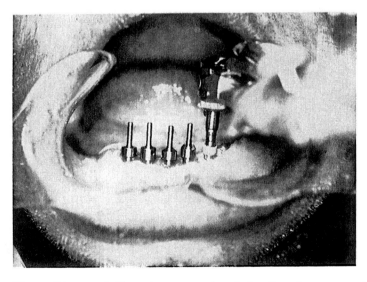

Figure 54 Parallelling pins are used to help align the osteotomies so that the occlusal forces transmitted from the final prosthesis to the bone will be distributed properly.

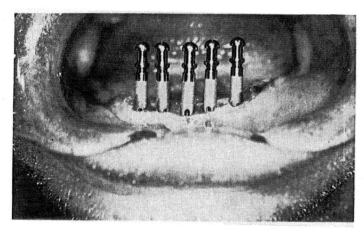

Figure 55   Five titanium plasma sprayed implants are placed into their osteotomy sites.

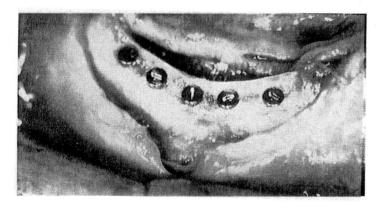

Figure 56   The implants placed properly and in good alignment.

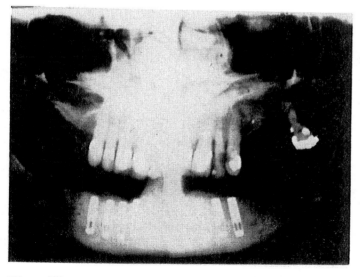

Figure 57   Radiograph illustrating that the implants are parallel to one another.

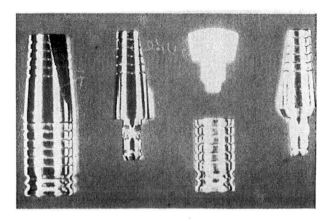

Figure 58   Many permucosal abutment designs, sizes, and angles are available to be placed into implants.

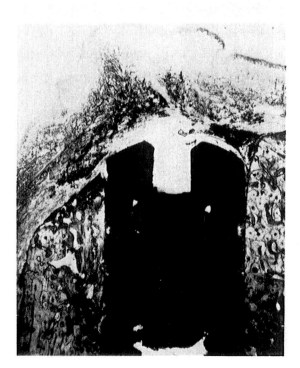

Figure 59   Osseointegration is defined by a bony interface between the implant and the bone at the light microscopic level.

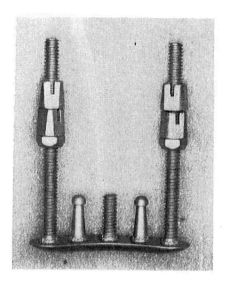

Figure 60 A transosteal implant can be placed into the anterior area of the mandible via a submandibular skin approach.

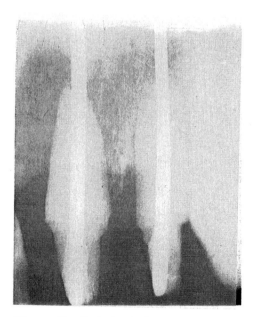

Figure 61 Endodontic implant stabilizers can be used to anchor teeth into the bone via entry through their root canals.

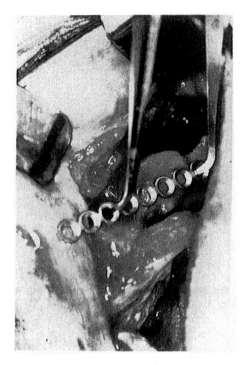

Figure 62   Titanium fracture plates have been used to reduce fractures with great success.

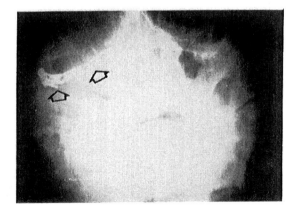

Figure 63   Radiograph showing that an orbital fracture plate can be used to treat a fracture of the orbital rim.

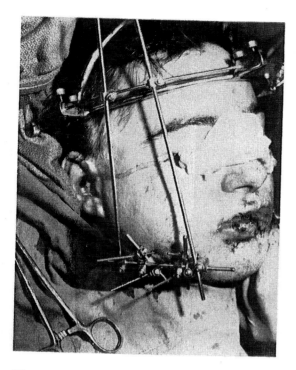

Figure 64 Stainless steel extraskeletal fixation devices are utilized to reduce multiple facial skeleton fractures.

without bone grafting materials such as hydroxyapatite and freeze-dried bone beneath the epithelial flaps prior to suturing.

Stainless Steel Wire.   Stainless steel wire remains an important biomaterial for purposes of osteosynthesis as well as to secure dental prostheses temporarily.

2. Augmentative/Cosmetic Implants

Polymethylmethacrylate, silicone rubber, and composite preformed prostheses are in use as malar and chin implants. In order to place such devices, a surgical pocket must be made subperiosteally. Upon healing, the reattachment of the periosteum stabilizes the implant. Over the years, bone resorption has been demonstrated beneath some of these implants.

Recently, porous polyethylene preformed prostheses have been inserted in cases of hemifacial microsomia and for other situations of asymmetry. These prostheses are light, have good morphologic integrity, may be altered with a scalpel at the operating table, and encourage connective tissue ingrowth for anchorage.

REFERENCES

1. Likist, M.R., Lietze, A., Mizutani, H., et al. A bovine low molecular weight bone morphogenic protein (BMP) fraction. *Clin. Orthop.*, 162:272, 1982.
2. Rizzo, A. (editor). Proceeding of the consensus development conference on dental implants. *J. Dent. Educ.*, 52:678, 1988.

3. Formiggini, M. Proteste dentaria a mezzo di infibularone directta endoalvolare. *Revista Italians di Stomatologia*, March 1974.

4. Sandhaus, S. Noveaux aspects de l'implantologie, *Compte Rendu des Jouneés Implantaires de Lausanne Med. Hygiene*, 2:17–21, 1965.

5. Ahngawa, Y., Hashimoto, M., Kando, N., Satomi, K., Takata, T., and Tsuru, H. Initial bone-implant interface of submergible, and supramergible endosseous single crystal sapphire implants. *J. Prosth. Dentistry*, 55(1):96–99, 1986.

6. Steflik, D.E., Kath, D.C., and McKinney, R.V. Human clinical trials of the single crystal sapphire endosteal implant. *J. Oral Implantology*, 13:39–53, 1986.

7. Jarcho, M. Calcium phosphate ceramic as hard tissue prosthesis. *Clin. Orthop. Res.*, 157: 259–278, 1981.

8. Becker, W., and Becker, B.E. Guided tissue regeneration for implants placed into extraction sockets and for implant dehiscences: Surgical techniques and case reports. *Int. J. Periodont. & Rest. Dent.*, 10:377–391, 1990.

9. Becker, W., Becker, B., Prichard, J., Cafferse, R., and Rosenberg, E. Report for treated Cl III and Cl II furcations and vertical osseous defects. *Int. J. Periodont. & Rest. Dent.*, 3:9–23, 1988.

10. Lemons, J.E. Hydroxylapatite coatings. *Clin. Orthop. Rel. Res.*, 235:220, 1988.

11. Souder, W., and Paffenbarger, G.C. Physical Properties of Dental Material. National Bureau of Standards Circular C433, U.S. Government Printing Office, Washington, DC, 1942.

12. James, R.A., and Schultz, R.L. Hemidesmosones and the adhesion of junctional epithelial cells to metal implants. *J. Oral Impl.*, 4(3):294–302, 1974.

13. Golec, T.S. CAD-CAM multiplanar diagnostic imaging for subperiosteal implants. *Dent. Clin. North Amer.*, 30:85–95, 1986.

14. Truit, H.P., James, R., and Bayne, P. Non-invasive technique for mandibular subperiosteal implants—A preliminary report. *J. Prosth. Dent.*, 55:497, 1986.

15. Cranin, A.N., Rabkin, M.F., Silverbrand, H., and Sher, J. The Brookdale bar subperiosteal implant (abstract). *Trans. Fourth Annual Meeting, Society of Biomaterials*, 2:7, 1978.

16. National Institute of Health Consensus Development Conference Statement on Dental Implants. *J. Dent. Educ.*, 52:824–827, 1988.

17. Linkow, L.I. The blade-vent—A new dimension in endosseous implantology. *Dent. Concepts*, 11:3–12, 1968.

18. Weiss, C.M. A comparative analysis of fibroosteal integration and other variables that affect long term bone maintenance around dental implants. *J. Oral Implantology*, 13:467, 1987.

19. Vagder, T.I., and Fung, J.Y. Comparative photoelastic stress analysis of four blade type endosteal implants. *J. Oral Implantology*, 3(2):257–269, 1979.

20. Suetsugi, T., Kitah, M., and Murakami, Y. Stress analysis of blade implant—Mechanical properties of implant materials and stress distribution. *J. Oral Implantology*, 8(3):393–410, 1979.

21. Branemark, P.I., Hansson, B.O., Adele, R., Breine, V., and Lindstrom, V. *Osseointegrated Implants in the Treatment of the Edentulous Jaw*, Almquist and Niksell Int., Stockholm, Sweden, 1977.

22. Adell, R., Lockholm, M., Rockler, B., and Branemark, P.I. A 15 year study of osseointegrated implants in the treatment of the edentulous jaw. *J. Oral Surg.*, 6:387–416, 1981.

23. Albrektsson, T., Dahl, E., Enborn, L., et al. Osseointegrated oral implants. A Swedish multicenter study of 8139 conservatively inserted Nobelpharma implants. *J. Periodontics*, 59(5):287–296, 1988.

10
Biodegradable Materials in Joint Replacement Arthroplasty

Stanley L. Kampner
University of California Medical Center
San Francisco, California

I. INTRODUCTION

It can be argued that the single largest contribution in orthopedics toward improvement of the incapacitated adult over the past 30 years has been prosthetic joint replacement arthroplasty. Prior to the 1960s, the arthritic, destroyed joint was primarily salvaged with extraarticular procedures, intraarticular debridements, and crude hemiprosthetic and total joint replacement arthroplasty devices that afforded inconsistent and limited success (Figs. 1a, 1b).

Charnley and McKee in the 1960s, with improved designs regarding actual fixation of hip implants to bone with acrylic cement (Fig. 2), changed the total concept of treatment for the arthritic joint with total joint prosthetic replacement arthroplasty utilizing metal alloy and polymeric materials [18,51]. This allowed individuals who were totally sedentary as a result of long-standing destroyed arthritic joints to become pain free and improve their overall function.

A primary conceptual improvement change and reason for clinical success was securing fixation of the prosthetic device to the bone into which it was implanted. Previously, the devices were merely seated into bone with limited fixation; after a short period of time, they frequently became grossly loose. Following fixation of implants to bone utilizing polymethylmethacrylate cement, every implant became essentially "custom made" for the bone into which they were implanted and thus "part of the bone" (Fig. 3).

II. FIXATION METHODS

Cement fixation of these implants did give excellent short-term results; however, in the younger, heavier, and more active individual, greater stresses were applied to the replaced joint, resulting in breakdown of this mechanical bonding between bone, cement, and

307

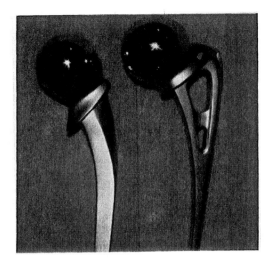

(a)

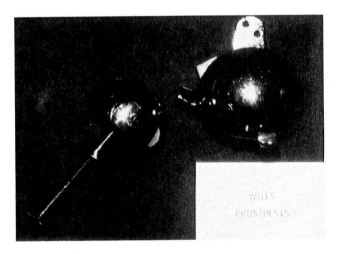

(b)

Figure 1   Joint repair prior to the 1960s: (*a*), Thompson and Austin–Moore femoral hemiarthroplasty components to replace only the diseased femoral head side of the hip joint without any secure anchorage to bone other than a simple interference type fit into the medullary canal; (*b*), a crude total hip prosthetic replacement arthroplasty fabricated from stainless steel to be anchored to bone by mechanical means designed by Dr. Phillip Wiles in 1938.

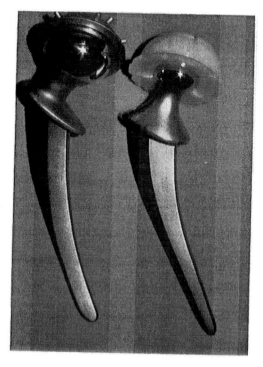

Figure 2 Charnley and McKee total hip prosthetic replacement implants designed to be anchored to bone with acrylic cement when replacing the destroyed acetabular and femoral side of the hip joint.

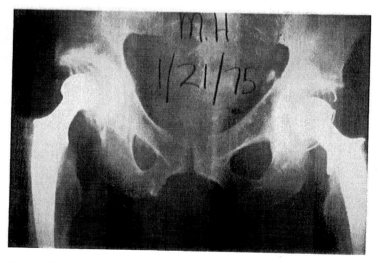

Figure 3 X-ray of bilateral total hip prosthetic replacement arthroplasties with the acetabular and femoral components "custom made" to fit and anchored to bone with the radiopaque methylmethacrylate cement anchoring the implant to bone.

implant [25]. The acrylic cement not infrequently fractured and/or became loose at its bone-cement-implant interface (Fig. 4), thereby placing the device into a category similar to implanted devices prior to use of cement fixation, in which the implant was not securely fixed to the bone, resulting in pain. This indicated a failure of the procedure as the result, with total joint revision often being required.

As a consequence of increasing numbers of failures with cemented devices, alternate methods of fixation of the implant to bone were sought. One of these alternatives, which is currently the state of the art in implant fixation in joint replacement arthroplasty, allows for a more physiologic fixation consisting of biologic attachment. This is obtained by coating the surface of the implant with a porous material to allow bony ingrowth into the definitive implant under the proper conditions (Fig. 5). This would hold the implanted device by a biological fixation rather than by an interposed material fixation between implant and bone (Fig. 6). Since it is the patient's tissue that has grown into the implant, the device actually becomes a permanent part of the bone of the patient, thus theoretically obviating the problem of implant loosening. This was hoped to be the optimal "final" solution to joint replacement arthroplasty, precluding any future failure of a "holding" material (e.g., polymethylmethacrylate cement) and subsequent loosening of the implant fixation to bone.

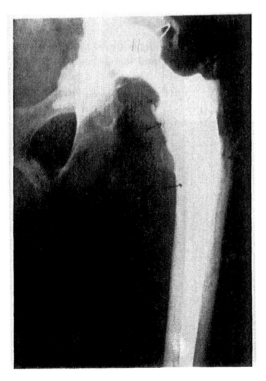

Figure 4   X-ray of total hip prosthetic replacement arthroplasty showing radiolucency at the interface between bone and the radiopaque acrylic cement, indicative of loosening.

III. FIXATION PROBLEMS

There still exist, however, other problems when an implant is fixed to bone, whether it is fixed by acrylic cement or by tissue ingrowth. One is the problem of abnormal stress transference across the joint implant to the respective bone. The most ideal stress transference of load across the joint to the bone would obviously be to try to approach the normal anatomic and physiological situation. To accomplish this, one would not only use an implant material with the mechanical properties and characteristics similar to bone, but also design an implant that would only replace the destroyed arthritic joint's surface. This would, therefore, place a minimal amount of implant material within the bone.

Currently, this is most difficult to do successfully with most joints since porous coated implants require immediate rigid fixation for a minimum time period of at least 6 to 12 weeks to allow sufficient bone to grow into the device to hold it securely [15,26,65]. If the device is not held rigidly, micromotion will occur at the implant-bone interface, resulting in a fibrous tissue ingrowth, in contrast to the more stable, securely fixed, bony ingrowth (Fig. 7).

The most common current method of holding the implant device rigidly in the bone is by incorporating a stem on the device that "press fits" into the intramedullary cavity of the bone. This interference or press fit into the shaft of the bone does hold the device rigidly to allow a satisfactory bone ingrowth for secure fixation, as well as creates the desired proper anatomical placement of the implant in a reproducible manner.

The trade-off of this design is that loading of the bone is now no longer physiologic. Instead of being loaded primarily at the proximal end of the bone near the joint surface as in the normal situation, the bone becomes loaded more distally in the shaft where the implant stem device is adjacent to the bone [54]. The result is an abnormal transference of stress bypassing or unloading the proximal end of the bone, with a subsequent resorption of that bone as the bone remodels with time (Fig. 8) [28,50,74]. The bone, in essence, has been "stress shielded" by the stem placed down the bony shaft.

With larger-diameter stems currently being implanted to afford greater initial rigid fixation for bony attachment, proximal bone resorption appears more frequently and to a greater extent than seen with cemented devices. Animal studies with multiple different implanted devices have shown extreme proximal bone resorption in which much of the bone "melted away" as a result of stress shielding [11,70] (Fig. 9).

One can only presume that this extent of bony resorption continues to take place in the human, albeit at a slower pace. This bone resorption creates a weakness of bone in that area over a period of years, thus creating the potential for fracture or complete disappearance of the bone that was previously holding the implant securely. The bone now becomes "the weak link" in the system, replacing the potential for acrylic cement failing in cemented joint replacements. The result is the same regardless of cemented or cementless arthroplasties, with loosening of the implant within the bone and with all the consequences described above to occur in such a state.

Another problem not infrequently seen in cemented implants that was hoped to be obviated with cementless devices was the occasional extensive osteolysis found throughout all areas of the bone into which the stem was implanted (Fig. 10). These areas of osteolysis were felt to be the result of an extreme histiocytic foreign-body reaction (Fig. 11), theorized to be secondary to fractured particulate polymethylmethacrylate cement and thus attributed to "cement disease" [24,35,44].

This problem of osteolysis seen with cemented devices has not only been similarly

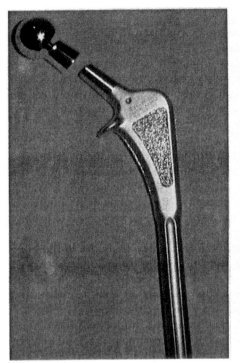

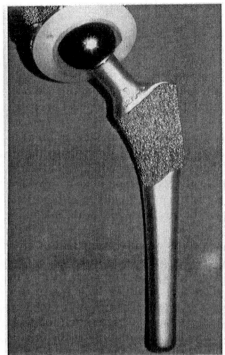

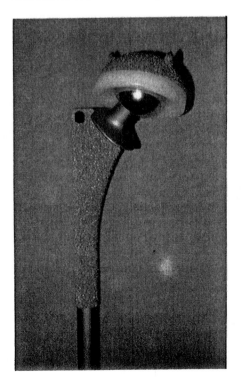

seen with porous, coated, uncemented implants, but it has appeared at least as frequently, with equal involvement, and earlier in the postoperative course (Fig. 12). This "cementless disease" was felt to be secondary to a histiocytic foreign-body reaction to particulate polyethylene from wear of the high-density polyethylene-bearing surface and/or particulate metal alloy, whether cobalt-chromium or composed of titanium 6, aluminum 4, and vanadium [14,33,36,40,47,48,58].

A more appropriate term for this osteolytic phenomena would be *particulate disease* since this can result from any submicron wear particles if these are present in sufficient numbers. In terms of reaction to metal alloy submicron particles, it has been hypothesized to result from fretting secondary to the micromotion occurring at the implant-bone interface [1,4,14,37,39,53,58]. It has similarly been shown, both in animal studies and clinically, that motion does occur between the screws affording fixation of acetabular and tibial plate components, occasionally even resulting in fracture of the screws [21,40].

Aside from the pathologic effect on the bone into which these devices were implanted, not infrequently the clinical result was less than desired and, in some cases, less optimal than seen with cemented total joint replacement arthroplasty. The most notable exception seen with cementless devices was thigh pain following total hip replacement arthroplasty [3,16,21,29,31,63,64,73]. The exact cause of this was uncertain. This pain appeared to be mechanical in nature and was usually associated with initiating ambulation, whether arising from a chair, ascending stairs, or the like. This has been hypothesized as resulting from inadequate fixation and sizing of the distal stem into the long bone, where there is micromotion taking place distally at the stem-bone interface [27,44]; the corollary hypothesis is that it results from "too tight" a fit of stem to bone, which results in a high "stress riser" about the bone at the abrupt change of high elastic modulus to a lower elastic modulus [27,46,60].

The problems, therefore, previously seen with cemented devices, and appearing to be obviated with use of cementless devices, were similarly seen with cementless devices. In fact, in some respects, the solution of utilizing cementless stemmed devices appeared to exacerbate some of the problems seen with cemented devices and now became the problem.

In any event, it appears that the most optimal surgical procedure for a destroyed, arthritic joint, aside from "regrowing new cartilage," is implant replacement of those destroyed surfaces securely attached directly to bone with minimal or no stem about the implant. This would accomplish the most ideal biomechanical solution from the standpoint of physiologic transference of stresses across the joint to the bone, as well as potentially avoid other unwanted problems and sequelae associated with fixed stems.

IV. SOLUTIONS TO FIXATION PROBLEMS

Although composite polymeric materials approaching the elastic modulus of bone presently being developed [34,45,46,69] may be an improvement over the stiffer metal alloy stems, it would be highly impractical, if not impossible, to have available an inventory of composite material stems approaching the broad spectrum of bone quality and elastic modulus seen with individual patients, who vary from male to female and from young to

---

Figure 5   Different total hip prosthetic replacement porous coated designs for interference fit, allowing for biological tissue ingrowth to anchor the implant to bone, ideally, by bony ingrowth.

(a)

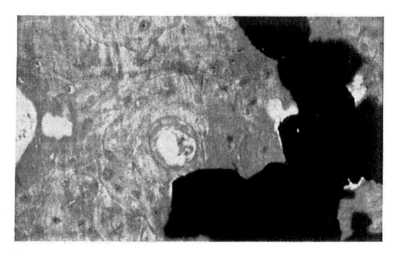

(b)

Figure 6 Photomicrograph showing (a) mature bone ingrowth into the porous material and (b) a three-dimensional interlock fixation of the implant to the bone into which it is implanted.

middle age to elderly. Even assuming the availability of such an inventory, the lower elastic modulus and thus increased bending and repetitive flexing of the stem would hypothetically result in increased motion about the implant within bone, thereby resulting in a less stable fibrous interface fixation, in contrast to the more stable bony fixation. This has been observed in the laboratory [12,38,45,56,69,74].

Assuming the requirement of some type of stem or screw fixation to correctly align

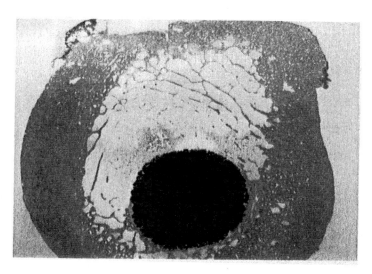

Figure 7   Photomicrograph of a transverse section taken through a porous coated stem within the femur showing an inadequately sized and fixed implant, resulting in poor fixation with fibrous tissue ingrowth only.

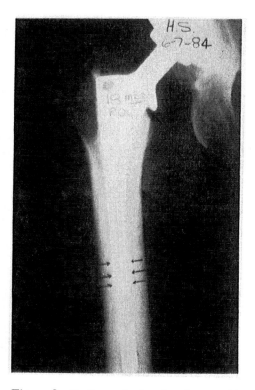

Figure 8   Radiograph showing decreased bone mineralization about the entire proximal portion of the femur, with bone resorption about the femoral calcar along with bony thickening about the distal femoral aspect adjacent to the distal porous coating, consistent with stress shielding proximally and loading distally.

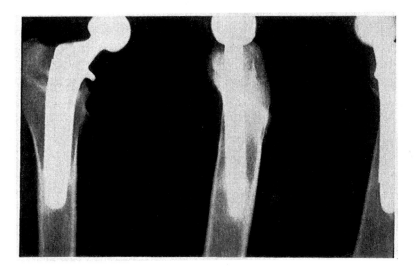

(a)

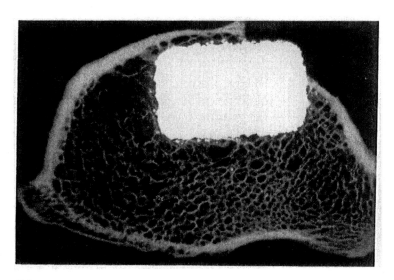

(b)

Figure 9 Radiographs showing extreme bone resorption about the proximal femur in (a) a dog model in which the femoral component and a total hip prosthetic replacement arthroplasty stress shielded the proximal bone over a six-month period (b). (Courtesy Jorge Galante, M.D.)

and adequately anchor the implant while bone ingrowth is occurring about the porous coated implant, the most ideal mechanical solution, from the standpoint of physiologic transference of stresses across the joint to the bone, would be to have the stem "disappear" once its function has been accomplished (Fig. 13). This would similarly avoid micromotion of the implant within bone with resultant fretting and potential osteolysis as

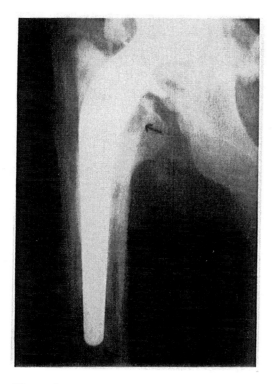

Figure 10 Radiograph showing extensive osteolysis of the femur with a cemented femoral component.

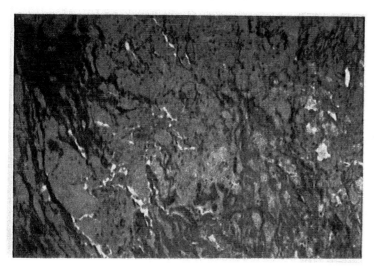

Figure 11 Photomicrograph showing sheets of macrophages in reaction to foreign particulate matter.

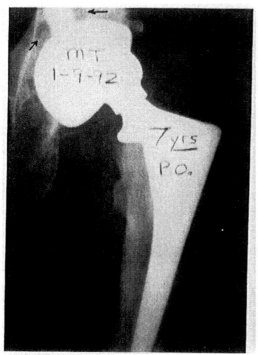

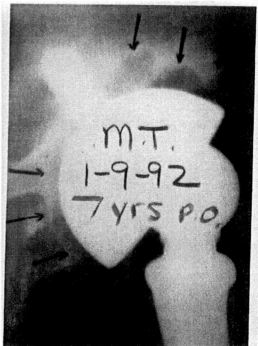

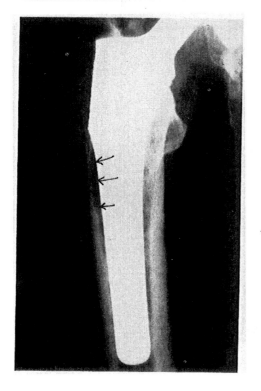

well as avoid fracture of fixation screws, among other potential problems. This could be accomplished by designing an implant for which the stem consists of a biodegradable resorbable material and the proximal definitive implant, adjacent to the replaced joint, is made of a permanent nonresorbable material, such as the presently available metal alloys. The stem would continue its function to align the implant into bone properly and reproducibly and anchor it rigidly into its appropriate position for the sufficient period of time required for bony ingrowth to occur. Once ingrowth has occurred and the implant proximally is directly fixed to the bone into which it is implanted, the function of the stem is no longer required. It then not only becomes superfluous, but becomes potentially detrimental to the overall bone physiology, as noted above. The resorption of the materials can be engineered to take place at any predetermined time period (i.e., 6 weeks, 8 weeks, 12 weeks, 6 months, 1 year, etc.), depending on the particular joint or bone involved and how long a period is deemed necessary before there is adequate fixation of the implant.

Following resorption of the stem, the most ideal concept would be a resurface-type design in which the remaining permanent portion of the implant device in the bone is only that portion closest to the joint surface (Fig. 14). The biomechanical end result is that the bone holding the implanted device is stressed primarily adjacent to the joint surface, as is seen in the normal physiologic situation. There will be, therefore, a more normal transference of stresses to the bone and no unloading of stresses on the bone immediately beneath the implant surface. In essence, the stressed bone will be as close to normal as possible, unaware that a prosthetic joint has been implanted. In such a situation, all the advantages of the stem remain, while all the disadvantages are obviated. With resorption of the stem, any potential for micromotion of implant within bone, as well as fretting, is negated and the potential for thigh pain should similarly be negated. In the cases of acetabular and tibial plate components transfixed with biodegradable screws following attachment to bone, the screws slowly resorb, thus precluding any potential for fracture or fretting.

Such an implantable device, by definition, would be a composite modular structure composed of at least two components. The component comprising the articulating bearing surface is made of a permanent, nonresorbable material (e.g., metal alloy, ceramic, carbon, polymer, etc.). The porous coating to allow bony ingrowth for implant fixation is applied only to this portion, along with ideally coating this with a calcium-phosphate material such as hydroxyapatite, tricalcium phosphate, or combinations of such to enhance and speed the process of bony ingrowth attachment. Biomechanically, this stresses the bone only in the area adjacent to the implant surface, which, physiologically, is the closest to the normal situation conceivable.

The stem portion of the implant could be fabricated from a variety of biodegradable, resorbable materials, including polylactic acid, polyglycolic acid, polylactic acid/polyglycolic acid copolymers, polyetheretherketone (PEEK), polyorthoester, and polycarbonate

---

Figure 12 Radiograph showing extensive osteolysis present about the femur and acetabulum adjacent to uncemented components as a result of an extreme histiocytic foreign-body reaction. Note the asymmetry about the femoral head component within the acetabular component as the result of abnormal polyethylene wear of the acetabular component, probably resulting in the osteolysis present in the superior aspect of the acetabulum.

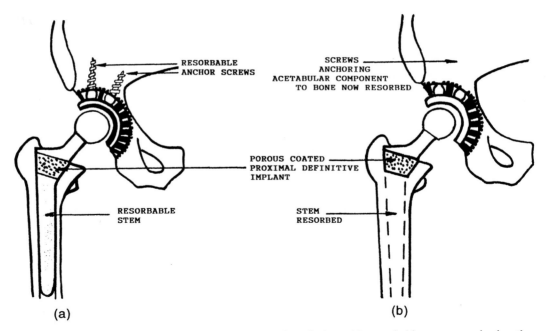

Figure 13 (a) Total hip prosthetic replacement implant design with resorbable screws anchoring the acetabular component and a resorbable femoral stem fixed to the definitive proximal articulating component, thereby affording secure anchorage to the bone during the period of bony ingrowth (b) into the proximal definitive component.

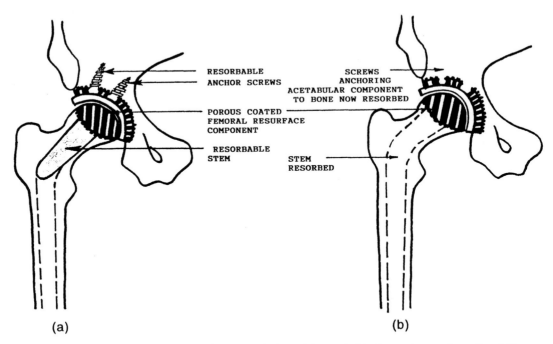

Figure 14 (a) Resurface total hip replacement design with resorbable femoral stem degrading following a sufficient time period to allow for adequate bony ingrowth (b) to fix the proximal articular resurface definitive component.

[9,19,20,23,34,43,49,52,71]. The amount of stem portion would vary according to the joint and bone involved. It could consist of a major amount of the total implant device in some joints, whereas in other joints the stem portion may make up a small percentage of the total device. This concept of using a resorbable stem on the implant device could be utilized for any and all joints of the body, typically including the hip, knee, shoulder, elbow, wrist, finger joints, ankle, and toe joints. It could also conceivably be utilized in complex reconstructive cases of head and facial implants, as well as for dental implants.

Already existing and presently being implanted in humans are resorbable pins, rods, and screws for small-fracture fixation [8,13,22,57,59]. These are primarily fabricated from materials currently used as resorbable sutures, including homopolymers of polylactic acid and polyglycolic acid, various copolymers of polyglycolic acid and polylactic acid, and polydioxanone.

One primary problem with resorbable fixation devices thus far has been premature loss of mechanical strength characteristics, which begins prior to gross macroscopic degradation [52,68,71]. The degradation process occurs principally through hydrolysis of these polymers and, to a lesser extent, through nonspecific enzymatic action [9,10,61,66]. The rates of degradation vary, depending on the material, molecular weight, crystallinity, thermal history, and geometry of the implant. It has been shown that the principal route of ultimate elimination is respiration, with minimal excretion in the urine and feces [9,30]. Multiple studies have shown that these polymeric materials are completely absorbable within bone and, as the degradation proceeds, bone is deposited on and within, eventually replacing the implant [9,10,22].

The property characteristics of the initial and retained strengths of these rods and screws can be improved. The device could be fabricated as a composite by introduction of fibers of the same or different materials [19,42,61,68], thus reinforcing the polymeric matrix. Hydrolytic degradation and premature loss of required mechanical characteristics can be delayed by applying various coatings, including cyanoacrylate, polydioxanone, polyhydroxybutyrate, or polylactide to the implant [67,72,75]. Unfortunately, while these coatings have been shown to delay the loss of strength characteristics of fiber-reinforced polyglycolic acid rods *in vitro*, this has not been the case *in vivo*.

There has been clinical use of these resorbable polymeric materials in the form of small nails, screws, and rods to fix small fractures and intraarticular osteochondral fragments [5,8,13,17,19,57,59]. Most of these implant materials have been fabricated from polyglycolic acid, polylactic acid, polyglycolic/polylactic acid copolymer, and polydioxanone. These have been successful in conditions for which retained strength of the biodegradable polymer for extended periods is not required. The results in these cases have been compromised in that a significant percentage went on to develop a sterile abscess about the implant site [6,7,17,62].

Histologic analysis of that sterile abscess fluid showed a typical foreign-body reaction with predominantly inflammatory mononuclear cells and many giant cells [6,62,66]. This suggests a lymphocyte-mediated immunological reaction against the implant. This is probably related to the relatively rapid degradation of the implant in a small superficial area (e.g., ankle, elbow, etc.) that is not entirely resorbed, thereby overwhelming the local cellular environment and resulting in an immunologic foreign-body-type reaction. Typically, fluctuance develops at the implant site at an average of 12 weeks postoperatively, with either spontaneous or surgical drainage producing a sterile exudate containing liquid remnants of the degrading implants [6,9]. Following this, the drainage subsides within 3 weeks, with the final clinical and radiographic result being unaffected [6].

Table 1   Mechanical Properties of Injection-Molded Poly-L-Lactic Acid

	Strength (MPa)	Modulus (GPa)	Elongation at yield (%)
Tensile	70	3.7	8
Flexural	118	4	
Shear	62		

Even though the clinical result is ultimately unaffected, this complication is clearly not representative of the ideal biodegradable implant. Either the implant cannot be utilized in a superficial area of the body such as the ankle or elbow, in which the surrounding soft tissues and cellular structures will not be overwhelmed by the particulate fragments of the degrading implant, or the resorbable implant material must degrade much slower, thereby being compatible with the normal resorptive capacities of the local cellular environment so that there is no local foreign-body immune response.

Unless this relatively rapid degradation of material and thus concurrent loss of mechanical strength characteristics can be overcome, certainly there is no place for a bioresorbable implant stem in total joint replacement, for which significant load and stresses are applied to that implant. The implant will not only fail from a mechanical perspective, but there will also be the potential for a particulate foreign-body immune response within the bone and therefore the potential for osteolysis, as presently seen with both cemented and cementless joint replacement implants.

Different orthopedic implant companies have developed a high molecular weight, high strength poly-L-lactic acid (PLLA) polymer that does appear to have the property characteristics for such an optimal bioresorbable implant, at least for securing anchoring devices to bone (e.g., for acetabular components in total hip arthroplasty and tibial plate components in total knee arthroplasty) while bony attachment is occurring [41]. The PLLA typically has an average molecular weight above 700,000. The mechanical properties appear to be excellent, with a tensile strength at yield of 73 megapascal (MPa), a flexural strength of 118 MPa, the modulus of elasticity at 4 gigapascal (GPa), the elongation at yield at 5%, and the sheer strength at 62 MPa (Table 1) [41]. The PLLA implants retain more than 80% of the initial tensile strength for up to 12 months, with this strength-stable period decreasing to 9 months after gamma radiated for sterilization purposes (1.5 megarads [Mrads]) [41]. The strength retention for ethylene oxide sterilization is similar to that for the 1.5-Mrad-treated PLLA. In contrast to retention of the optimal mechanical strength characteristics, the molecular weight does exhibit a steady decrease from the beginning and, in approximately six months, loses more than 50% (Fig. 15) [41].

The structural characteristics of this PLLA material do appear to be adequate for fabrication of large-diameter screws to anchor joint replacement implants such as hemispherical acetabular components in hip replacement arthroplasty and tibial plate components in total knee prosthetic replacement arthroplasty (Fig. 16). These biodegradable screws of the high molecular weight PLLA polymer have been utilized to fix porous coated acetabular components in a canine model (Fig. 17) [2,49,55]. All dogs had an uneventful recovery. Contact radiographs of the harvested acetabular specimens taken at the time of sacrifice showed no radiolucent lines or other evidence of implant loosening.

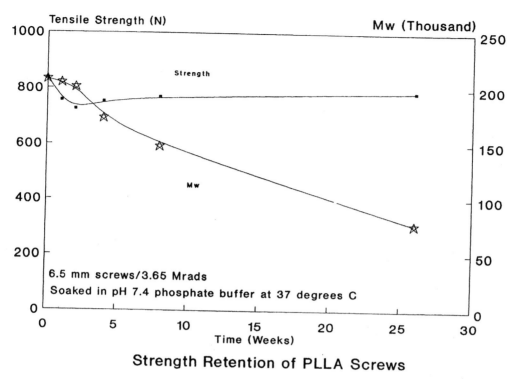

Strength Retention of PLLA Screws

Figure 15 Strength retention of 6.5-mm diameter poly-L-lactic acid (PLLA) polymeric screws showing the rapid decrease in the molecular weight of the material to more than 50% of its original molecular weight by 25 weeks, but retaining most of the strength characteristics.

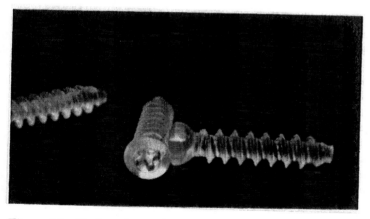

Figure 16 Biodegradable poly-L-lactic acid (PLLA) 6.5-mm-diameter screws used to fix the acetabular component in total hip replacement arthroplasty.

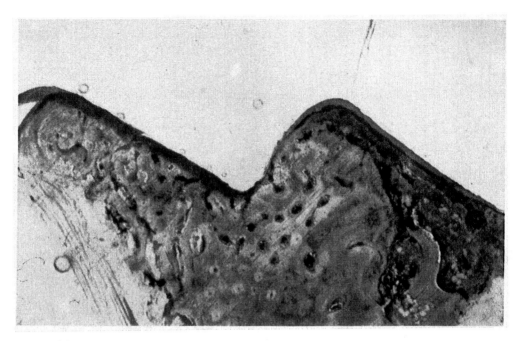

Figure 17   Photomicrograph of hematoxylin-eosin-stained undecalcified sections of poly-L-lactic acid (PLLA) screw through a titanium alloy acetabular cup in a canine total hip replacement 12 weeks after implantation. There is intimate bone apposition adjacent to the PLLA screw as well as ingrowth into the porous surface of the acetabular component. No resorption of the PLLA screw has occurred 12 weeks after implantation. (Courtesy Harry Rubash, M.D.)

There was noted radiographic voids where the biodegradable screws had been placed and, most important, there appeared to be normal bone immediately adjacent to the screws. There were no osteolytic areas or any other evidence of bone resorption about the region adjacent to the screws.

Similar biodegradable screws have been utilized clinically in the human to fix the acetabular component to the pelvis in total hip replacement arthroplasty by Herberts, Malchau, and Karrholm in Sweden, with similar excellent short-term results [32]. Again, as in the canine studies, radiographs showed only a void where the 6.5-mm-diameter screws had transfixed the acetabular component to the pelvis, with no evidence of osteolysis or foreign-body reaction adjacent to the screws.

In no case, in either the canine or human study, has there been any development of fluid or drainage from the hip, as had been noted in prior studies fixing small fractures using different polymeric materials with a more rapid biodegradation. This difference may be related to the combination of the slower degradation of the higher molecular weight PLLA polymer and the bone into which it is implanted, where the degradation products are sufficiently phagocytized and metabolized by the local cells. This adequate degradation process, therefore, would not overwhelm the local cellular environment, resulting in a foreign-body immunologic reaction and production of an exudate of liquid remnants of the degrading polymeric implant.

Aside from the currently existing bioresorbable screws to anchor joint replacement

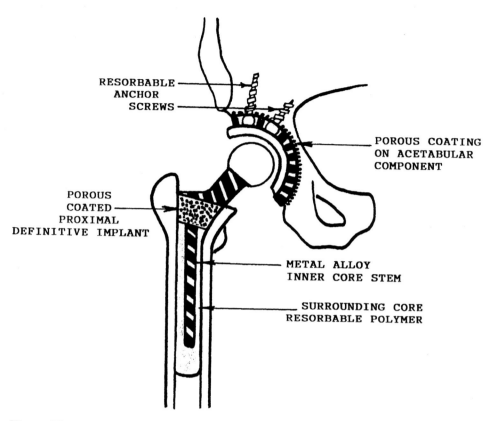

Figure 18 Total hip replacement composite design consisting of a small-diameter inner core of metal alloy, extending from the definitive permanent articulating bearing surface component and surrounded by the resorbable polymer. Initially, this would be an exact interference fit affording secure stable fixation while bony ingrowth is taking place about the proximal porous coated segment. The inner-core metal alloy would increase the mechanical strength characteristics required for a load-bearing stem, such as in the hip.

surface implants, orthopedic and material companies are presently developing composite polymeric materials that either approach or do have the structural characteristics that would allow fabrication of a stemmed device to be implanted intramedullarly and connected to a nonresorbable articulating surface component in a load-bearing situation such as with total hip or total knee replacement arthroplasty. With the stem being totally resorbable following bony attachment to the definitive porous coated permanent articulating bearing component, the ultimate result becomes the ideal for joint replacement arthroplasty in that there remains only the presence of a resurfacing-type implant or a minimum of implant material within bone. All the previously noted clinical residuals, sequelae, and complications seen with current joint replacement would now be theoretically obviated or entirely negated.

At this stage, however, with the totally resorbable polymers not proven to have the property structural characteristics for a load-bearing stem, it remains possible to utilize resorbable polymers for a more limited goal. This could be achieved by utilizing a compa-

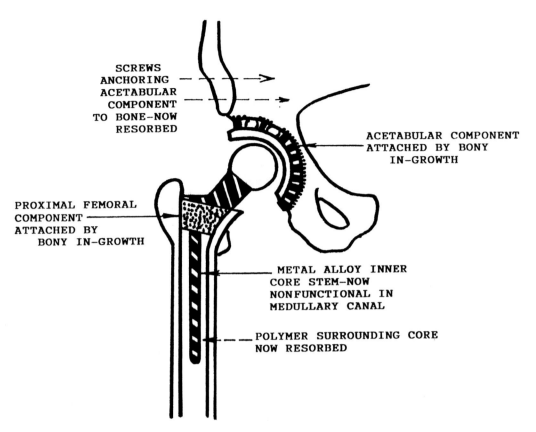

Figure 19 The outside surrounding polymeric sleeve is completely degraded and resorbed, leaving only the small metal alloy inner-core-diameter stem, which is essentially free floating within the femoral intermedullary canal and thus nonfunctioning.

rable high molecular weight PLLA polymer to fabricate the currently bioresorbable screws. To increase the mechanical strength characteristics required for a load-bearing stem such as in the hip or knee, a composite modular structure could be made utilizing a small-diameter inner core of metal alloy extending from the definitive permanent articulating bearing surface component surrounded by a sleeve fabricated of the resorbable polymer. Initially, this would give secure rigid anchorage of the stemmed component with an interference fit, exactly as the current state of the art in prosthetic joint replacement arthroplasty (Fig. 18).

After an optimal period of time elapses for sufficient bony attachment to occur about the proximal permanent porous coated articulating bearing component, the polymer surrounding the metal alloy core begins to degrade slowly and ultimately totally disappears (Fig. 19). The result is that there is now only a small-diameter stem in the medullary cavity of the bone, thereby obviating (and, it is hoped, negating entirely) the previously mentioned problems seen with current stemmed devices. Even though there is a small-diameter stem within the medullary cavity, there is no load taking place through that stem, which now becomes nonfunctional and, theoretically, the bone is unaware that any stem is actually present. The bone only knows that there is an implant present near the articulating surface of the joint being replaced and where the only stresses are being transferred from implant to bone. If this is the case, the current problem seen with stemmed devices or distal loading of the bone, with resultant proximal bone resorption (such as seen in hip replacement arthroplasty as well as thigh pain, whether it be from implant micromotion taking place within the bone or just a mismatch in the elastic modulus between implant and bone) is now negated. Similarly, with the remaining small-diameter stem being entirely free within the bony medullary cavity, there is no longer any potential for fretting, which could potentially cause osteolysis resulting from particulate metal alloy submicron fragments initiating any foreign-body immune response.

Ultimately, the goal is for no remaining stem within the bone utilizing a totally resorbable polymeric stem. The end result then will be (the potential goal in every surgical procedure on an arthritic joint) to replace only the articular surface that is destroyed and to leave behind within the body a minimal amount of implant material required for pain relief and a successful joint replacement.

REFERENCES

1. Alexander, J. W.; Noble, P. C.; and Kamaric, E. The Effect of Ion-Implantation on the Fretting of Titanium Implant in Bone. Presented at 37th Annual Meeting, Orthopaedic Research Society, March 5, 1991, Anaheim, CA.
2. Anderson, G.; Greis, P.; and Rubash, H.: Biodegradable Screw Fixation of the Acetabular Component in a Canine Total Hip Replacement Model. Personal communication, 1991.
3. Barrack, R. L.; Jasty M.; Bragdon, D.; Haire, T.; and Harris, W. H. Thigh Pain Despite Bone In-Growth Into Uncemented Femoral Stems. *J. Bone Joint Surg.*, 74-B:507–510, 1992.
4. Bennett, N. E.; Wang, J. T.; Manning, C. A.; and Goldring, S. R. Activation of Human Monocyte/Macrophages and Fibroblasts by Metal Particles; Release of Products with Bone Resorbing Activities. Presented at 37th Annual Meeting, Orthopaedic Research Society, March 5, 1991, Anaheim, CA.
5. Bostman, O.; Hirvensalo, E.; Vaininopaa, S.; Makela, A.; Vihtonen, K.; Tormala, P.; and Rokkenen, P. Ankle Fractures Treated Using Biodegradable Internal Fixation. *Clin. Orthop.*, 238:195–203, 1989.
6. Bostman, O.; Hirvensalo, E.; Makinen, J.; and Rokkanen, P. Foreign-Body Reactions to Fracture Fixation Implants of Biodegradable Synthetic Polymers. *J. Bone Joint Surg.*, 72-B: 592–595, July 1990.
7. Bostman, O.; Paivarinta, U.; Partio, E.; Vasenius. J.; Manninen. M.; and Rokkanen, P. Degradation and Tissue Replacement of an Absorbable Polyglycolide Screw in the Fixation of Rabbit Femoral Osteotomies. *J. Bone Joint Surg.*, 74-A:1021–1031, August 1992.
8. Bostman, O.; Vainionpaa, S.; Hirvensalo, E.; Makela, A.; Vihtomen, K.; Tormala, P.; and Rokkanen, P. Biodegradable Internal Fixation for Malleolar Fractures. A Prospective Randomized Trial. *J. Bone Joint Surg.*, 69-B:615–619, 1987.
9. Bostman, O. M. Current Concepts Review Absorbable Implants for the Fixation of Fractures. *J. Bone Joint Surg.*, 73-A:148–153, January 1991.
10. Brady, J. M.; Cutright, D. E.; Miller, R. A.; Battistone, G. C.; and Hunsuck, E. E. Resorption Rate, Root of Elimination, and Ultra-Structure of the Implant Site of Polylactic Acid in the Abdominal Wall of the Rat. *J. Biomed. Mater. Res.*, 7:155–166, 1973.
11. Bragdon, R.; Jasty, M.; Russotti, G.; Cargill, E.; Harrigan, T. P.; and Harris, W. H. Stress Related Bone Loss Around Proximally Porous Coated Canine Femoral Components. Presented at Annual Meeting of the Society for Biomaterials, April 28, 1989, Lake Buena Vista, FL.

12. Bragdon, C. R.; Jasty, M.; Lowenstein, J. D.; and Burke, D. W.: The Histology of Bone In-Growth at the Implant/Bone Interface Under Known Amounts of Micromotion. Presented at 39th Annual Meeting Orthopaedic Research Society, February 18, 1993, San Francisco, CA.

13. Bucholz, R. W.; Henley, M. B.; and Henry, S. L. Biosorbable Screw Fixation of Ankle Fractures. Presented at 60th Annual Meeting, American Academy of Orthopaedic Surgeons, February 20, 1993, San Francisco, CA.

14. Buly R. L.; Huo, M. H.; Salvati, E.; Brien, W.; and Bansal, M. Titanium Wear Debris in Failed Cemented Total Hip Arthroplasty. *J. Arthroplasty*, 7:315–323, September 1992.

15. Cameron, H. U.; Pilliar, R. M.; and Macnab, I. The Effect of Movement on the Bonding of Porous Metal to Bone. *J. Biomed. Mater. Res.*, 7:301–311, 1973.

16. Campbell, A. C. L.; Rorabeck, C. H.; Bourre, R. B.; and Chess, Nott, L. Thigh Pain After Cementless Hip Arthroplasty: Annoyance or Ill Omen. *J. Bone Joint Surg.*, 74-8:63–66, 1992.

17. Casteleyn, P. P.; Handelberg, F.; and Haentjens, P. Biogradable Rods Versus Kirschner Wire Fixation of Wrist Fractures. *J. Bone Joint Surg.*, 74-8:858–861, November 1992.

18. Charnley, J. The Long-Term Results of Low-Friction Arthroplasty of the Hip Performed as a Primary Intervention. *J. Bone Joint Surg.*, 54-B:61–70, August 1972.

19. Christel, P.; Chabot, F.; Leray, J. L.; Morin, C.; and Vert, M. Biodegradable Composites for Internal Fixation. In *Biomaterials 1980*, edited by G. D. Winter, D. F. Gibbons, and Hanns Plenk, Jr., Wiley, New York, 1982, pp. 271–280.

20. Cohn, D.; and Younes, H. Biodegradable PEO/PLA Block Co-Polymers. *J. Biomed. Mat. Res.*, 22:993–1009, 1988.

21. Collier, P.; Dorr, L. D.; Jacobs, J. J.; Li, W.; Moreland, J. R.; and Whiteside, L. A. A Symposium: Mechanisms of Material and Design-Related Implant Failure. *Orthopaedic Review*, September 1991, Supplement.

22. Cutright, D. E.; and Hunsuck, E. E. The Repair of Fractures of the Orbital Floor Using Biodegradable Polylactic Acid. *Oral Surg.*, 33:28–34, 1972.

23. Daniels, A. U.; Chang, M. K. O.; Andrano, K. P.; and Heller, J. Toxicity and Mechanical Properties of a Degradable Polyorthoester. Presented at 15th Annual Meeting Society for Biomaterials, April 29, 1989, Lake Buena Vista, FL.

24. Dannenmaier, W. C.; Haynes, D. W.; and Nelson, C. L. Granulomatous Reaction and Cystic Bony Destruction Associated with High-Wear Weight in a Total Knee Prosthesis. *Clin. Orthop.*, 198:224–229, 1985.

25. Dorr, L. D.; Takei, G. K.; and Conaty, J. P. Total Hip Arthroplasties in Patients Less than 45 Years Old. *J. Bone Joint Surg.*, 65-A:474–479, 1983.

26. Ducheyne, P.; De Meester, P.; Aernoudt, E.; Materns, M.; and Mulier, J. C. Influence of Functional Dynamic Loading on Bone In-Growth into Surface Pores of Orthopaedic Implants. *J. Biomed. Mater. Res.*, 11:811–838, 1977.

27. Engh, C. A.; Bobyn, J. D.; and Glassman, A. H. Porous-Coated Hip Replacement—The Factors Governing Bone In-Growth, Stress Shielding, and Clinical Results. *J. Bone Joint Surg.*, 69-B:45–55, January 1987.

28. Eng. C. A.; McGovern, T. F.; Bobyn, J. D.; and Harris, W. H. Quantitative Evaluation of Periprosthetic Bone Remodeling After Cementless Total Hip Arthroplasty. *J. Bone Joint Surg.*, 74-A:1009–1020, August 1992.

29. Galante, J. O.; Lemons, J.; Spector, M.; Wilson, P. D., Jr.; and Wright, T M. Review—The Biologic Effects of Implant Materials. *J. Orthop. Res.*, 9:760–775, 1991.

30. Gogolewski, S.; and Pennings, A. J.: Resorbable Materials of Poly (L-Lactide). *Colloid and Polymer Sci.*, 261:477–484, 1983.

31. Heekin, R. D.; Callaghan, J. J.; Hopkinson, W. J.; Savory, C.G.; and Xenos, J. S. The Porous-Coated Anatomic Total Hip Prosthesis, Inserted Without Cement. *J. Bone Joint Surg.*, 75-A:77–91, January 1993.

32. Herberts, P.; Malchau, H.; and Karrholm, J. The Evaluation of Bioabsorbable Screws in

Acetabular Cup Fixation Stereo-Photogrammetric Analysis, A Controlled Study. Presented at 40th Annual Meeting Orthopaedic Research Society, February 15, 1994, New Orleans, LA.

33. Jacobs, J. J.; Galante, J. O.; Glant, T.; Kienapfel, H.; Sumner, D. R.; and Urban, R. Femoral Endosteal Lysis in Titanium-Base Alloy Cementless Total Hip Replacement. Presented at 58th Annual Meeting, American Academy of Orthopaedic Surgeons, March 9, 1991, Anaheim, CA.

34. Jasty, M.; Bragdon, C. R.; Maloney, W. J.; Mulroy, R.; Haire, T.; Crowninshield, R. D.; and Harris, W. H. Bone Ingrowth into a Low Modulus Composite Plastic Porous Coated Canine Femoral Component. *J. Arthroplasty*, 7:253–259, September 1992.

35. Jasty, M. J.; Floyd, W. E., III; Schiller, A. L.; Golding, S. R.; and Harris, W. H. Localized Osteolysis In Stable Non-Septic Total Hip Replacement. *J. Bone Joint Surg.*, 68-A:912–916, 1986.

36. Jasty, M.; Haire, T.; and Tanzer, M. Femoral Osteolysis: A Generic Problem with Cementless and Cemented Components. Presented at 58th Annual Meeting, American Academy of Orthopaedic Surgeons, March 9, 1991, Anaheim, CA.

37. Kim, K. J.; Greis, P.; Wilson, S. C.; D'Antonio, J. A.; McClain, E. J.; and Rubash, H. E. Histological and Biochemical Comparison of Membranes from Titanium, Cobalt-Chromium, and Non-Polyethylene Hip Prosthesis. Presented at 37th Annual Meeting, Orthopaedic Research Society, March 5, 1991, Anaheim, CA.

38. Kuiper, J. H.; and Huiskes, R. Finite Element Simulation of Dynamic Micro-Motion at the Interface of Bone and Prosthesis. Presented at 39th Annual Meeting, Orthopaedic Research Society, February 18, 1993, San Francisco, CA.

39. Langkamer, V. G.; Case, C. P.; Heap, P.; Taylor, A.; Collins, C.; Pearse, M.; and Solomon, L. Systemic Distribution of Wear Debris After Hip Replacement. *J. Bone Joint Surg.*, 74-B: 831–839, November 1992.

40. Lewis, P. L.; Bourne, R. B.; Rorabeck, C.H.; and Veale, G. A. Screw Osteolysis: A Sign of Impending Failure of Cementless Knee Replacements. Presented at 60th Annual Meeting, American Academy of Orthopaedic Surgeons, February 20, 1993, San Francisco, CA.

41. Lin, S.; Krebs, S.; Parr, J.; and Crowninshield, R. Poly (L-Lactide Acid) Orthopaedic Fixation Devices. Presented at 17th Annual Meeting, Society for Biomaterials, May 3, 1991, Scottsdale, AZ.

42. Lin, S. T.; Krebs, S. L.; La Course, W. C.; and Kumar, B. Bioabsorbable Glass Fibers. Presented at Fourth World Biomaterials Congress, April 24, 1992, Berlin.

43. Lin, S.; Krebs, S.; and Kohn, J. Characterization of a New Degradable Polycarbonate. Presented at 17th Annual Meeting, Society for Biomaterials, May 3, 1991, Scottsdale, AZ.

44. Linder, L.; Lindberg, L.; and Carlsson, A. Aseptic Loosening of Hip Prosthesis – A Histologic and Enzyme Histochemical Study. *Clin. Orthop.*, 175:93–104, May 1983.

45. Magee, F. P.; Weinstein, A.M.; Longo, J. A.; et al. A Canine Composite Femoral Stem: An *In Vivo* Study. *Clin. Orthop.*, 235:237–252, 1988.

46. Maistrelli, G. L.; Fornasier, V.; Binnington, A.; McKenzie, K.; Sessa, V.; and Harrington, I. Effect of Stem Modulus in a Total Hip Arthroplasty Model. *J. Bone Joint Surg.*, 73-B:43–46, January 1991.

47. Maloney, W. J.; Callaghan, J.; and Galante, J. O. Cementless Disease Around Stable Cementless Femoral Components: A New Entity. Presented at 58th Annual Meeting, American Academy of Orthopaedic Surgeons, March 9, 1991, Anaheim, CA.

48. Maloney, W. J.; Jasty, M.; Harris, W. H.; Galante, J. O.; and Callaghan, J. J. Endosteal Erosion in Association with Stable Uncemented Femoral Components. *J. Bone Joint Surg.*, 72-A:1025–1034, August 1990.

49. Matsusue, U.; Yamamuro, T.; Oka, M.; Shikinami, Y.; Hyon, S.-H.; and Ikada, Y. Bioabsorbable High Strength Poly (L-Lactide) Screw. Presented at Fourth World Biomaterials Congress, April 24, 1992, Berlin.

50. McGovern, T. F.; Bobyn, J. D.; Mortimer, E. S.; Engh, C.; and Harris, W. H. Bone Mineral Content in the Proximal Femur Following Cementless Total Hip Arthroplasty. Presented at Implant Retrieval Symposium of the Society for Biomaterials, September 17, 1992, St. Charles, IL.

51. Mc Kee, G. K. Development of Total Prosthetic Replacement. *Clin. Orthop.*, 72:103–115, 1970.

52. Miller, R. A.; Brady, J. M.; and Cutright, D. E.: Degradation Rates of Oral Resorbable Implants (Polylactates and Polyglycolates): Rate Modification with Changes in PLA/PGA Co-Polymer Ratios. *J. Biomed. Mater. Res.*, 11:711–719, 1977.

53. Molnar, G. M.; Jacobs, J. J.; Erhardt, P.; Urban, R. M.; Glant, T. T.; and Galante, J. O. Particulate Titanium Induced Bone Resorption in Organ Culture. Presented at 37th Annual Meeting, Orthopaedic Research Society, March 5, 1991, Anaheim, CA.

54. O'Connor, D.; Jasty, M.; Sedlacek, R. C.; Harris. W.; and Engh, C. Direct Measurement of Femoral Bone Strains After Years of Service of AML Femoral Components. Presented at Implant Retrieval Symposium of the Society for Biomaterials, September 17, 1992, St. Charles, IL.

55. Otsuka, N. Y.; Binnington, A. G.; Davey, J. R.; and Fornasier, V. L. Fixation with Biodegradable Devices of Acetabular Components in a Canine Model. Presented at 60th Annual Meeting, American Academy of Orthopaedic Surgeons, February 22, 1993, San Francisco, CA.

56. Otani, T.; Whiteside, L. A.; and White, S. E. Strain Distribution in the Proximal Femur with Flexible Composite and Metallic Femoral Components Under Axial and Torsional Loads. *J. Biomed. Mater. Res.*, 27:575–587, May 1993.

57. Partio, E. K.; Hirvensalo, E.; Partio, E.; Pelttari, S.; Jukkala, K.; Bostman, O.; Hanninen, A.; Tormala, P.; and Rokkanen, P. Totally Absorbable Screws in the Fixation of Talocrural Arthrodesis and Subtalar Arthrodesis. Presented at Fourth World Biomaterials Congress, April 24, 1992, Berlin.

58. Peters, P. C.; Engh, G. A.; and Dwyer, K. A. Aggressive Endosteal Erosion in Cementless Total Knee Arthroplasty: A Radiographic, Implant and Histologic Analysis. Presented at 37th Annual Meeting, Orthopaedic Research Society, March 5, 1991, Anaheim, CA.

59. Pihlajamaki, J.; Bostman, O.; Hirvensalo, E.; Tormala, P.; and Rokkanen, P. Absorbable Pins of Self-Reinforced Poly-L-Lactic Acid for Fixation of Fractures and Osteotomies. *J. Bone Joint Surg.*, 74-B:853–857, November 1992.

60. Pilliar, R. M.; Cameron, H. U.; Welsh, R. P.; and Binnington, A. G. Radiographic and Morphologic Studies of Load-Bearing Porous-Surfaced Structured Implants. *Clin. Orthop.*, 156:249–259, 1981.

61. Rokkanen, P.; Majola, A.; Vasenius, J.; and Vainionpaa, S. Strength Retention of Self-Reinforced Polyglycolide (SR-PGA) and SR-Polylactic Acid (PLA) Composite Rods *In-Vitro* and *In-Vivo. Acta Orthop. Scandinavica*, Supplement 235:51, 1990.

62. Santavirta, S.; Konttinen, Y. T.; Saito, T.; Gronblad, M.; Partio, E..; Kemppinen, P.; and Rokkanen, P. Immune Response to Polyglycolic Acid Implants. *J. Bone Joint Surg.*, 72-B: 597–600, July 1990.

63. Skinner, H. B. Isoelasticity and Total Hip Arthroplasty. *Orthopedics*, 14:323–328, 1991.

64. Skinner, H.B.; and Curlin, F. J. Decreased Pain with Lower Flexural Rigidity of Uncemented Femoral Prosthesis. *Orthopedics*, 13:1223–1228, 1990.

65. Spector, M. Factors Augmenting or Inhibiting Biologic Fixation. In *The HIP, Proceedings of the 14th Open Meeting of the HIP Society*, edited by R. A. Brand, C. V. Mosby, St. Louis, 1987, p. 219.

66. Suganuma, J.; and Alexander, H. Biological Response of Intramedullary Bone to Poly-L-Lactic Acid. *J. Applied Biomat.*, 4:13–27, 1993.

67. Tormala, P.; Vainionpaa, S.; Kilpikari, J.; and Rokkanen, P. The Effects of Fiber-

Reinforcement and Gold Plating on the Flexural and Tensile Strength of PGA/PLA Co-Polymer Materials *In-Vitro. Biomaterials*, 8:42–45, 1987.

68. Tormala, P.; Vasenius, J.; Vainionpaa, S.; Laiho, J.; Pohjonen, T.; and Rokkanen, P. Ultra-High-Strength Absorbable Self-Reinforced Polyglycolide (SR-PGA) Composite Rods for Internal Fixation of Bone Fractures: *In-Vitro* and *In-Vivo* Study. *J. Biomed. Mater. Res.*, 25:1–22, 1991.

69. Tullos, H. S.; McCaskill, B. L.; Dickey, R.; and Davidson, J. Total Hip Arthroplasty with a Low-Modulus Porous-Coated Femoral Component. *J. Bone Joint Surg.*, 66-A:888–898. 1984.

70. Turner, T. M.; Sumner, D. R.; Urban, R. M.; Rivero, D. P.; and Galante, J. O. A Comparative Study of Porous Coatings in a Weight-bearing Total Hip Arthroplasty Model. *J. Bone Joint Surg.*, 68-A:1396–1409, 1986.

71. Vainionpaa, S.; Vihtonen, K.; Mero, M.; Patiala, H.; Rokkanen, P.; Kilpikari, J.; and Tormala, P. Fixation of Experimental Osteotomies of the Distal Femurs of Rabbits with Biodegradable Material. *Arch. Orthop. and Traumat. Surg.*, 106:1–4, 1986.

72. Vasenius, J.; Vainionpaa, S.; Vihtonen, K.; Mero, M.; Mikkola, J.; Rokkanen, P.; and Tormala, P. Biodegradable Self-Reinforced Polyglycolide (SR-PGA) Composite Rods Coated with Slowly Biodegradable Polymers for Fracture Fixation: Strength and Strength Retention *In-Vitro* and *In-Vivo. Clin. Materials*, 4:307–317, 1989.

73. Vresilovic, E. J.; Hozack, W.; Booth, R. E.; and Rothman, R. H. The Incidence of Thigh Pain After Uncemented Femoral Prosthesis as a Function of Femoral Stem Size. Presented at 38th Annual Meeting, Orthopedic Research Society, February 18, 1992, Washington, DC.

74. Weinans, H.; Huiskes, R; and Grootenboer, H. J. Effects of Material Properties of Femoral Hip Components on Bone Remodeling. *J. Orthop. Res.*, 10:845–853, 1992.

75. Zimmerman, M.; Parsons, J. R.; and Alexander, H. The Design and Analysis of a Laminated Partially Degradable Composite Bone Plate for Fracture Fixation. *J. Biomed. Mater. Res.: Applied Biomaterials*, 21:345–361, 1987.

11

Development of Phosphate-Microfiber-Reinforced Poly(Orthoester) for Absorbable Orthopedic Fixation Devices

Kirk P. Andriano and A. U. Daniels
University of Utah School of Medicine
Salt Lake City, Utah

Jorge Heller
APS Research Institute
Redwood City, California

I. INTRODUCTION

Metallic implant devices have been used for bone fracture fixation for many years. These devices align bone fragments, bring their surfaces into close proximity, and control the relative motion of the bone fragments so that union can take place. However, load sharing between the device and bone is in proportion to device and bone structural stiffness. Complete healing of the bone requires normal loads and is therefore prevented as long as the device is present and bears part of the load usually borne by the bone [1–3]. Also, sudden removal of the device can leave the bone temporarily weak and subject to refracture. On the other hand, some device structural stiffness is necessary to limit bone motion at the fracture site since gross motion is known to result in nonunion.

Consequently, replacing a metallic fracture-fixation device with a bioabsorbable polymer or composite device that has an appropriate combination of initial strength and stiffness, biocompatibility (sterilizability and low toxicity), and capability for intraoperative reshaping (where needed) is of considerable interest since subsequent absorption has two very important advantages. First, as absorption reduces the device cross section and/or the material's elastic modulus, the load is gradually transferred to the healing bone. Second, because the device eventually will be completely absorbed, surgical removal is not necessary for complete bone healing.

Recent reviews of candidate polymers and composites for use in absorbable fracture-fixation devices have focused on synthetic poly(alpha-hydroxy acid) polymers such as poly(lactic acid) (PLA), poly(glycolic acid) (PGA), and their copolymers [4,5]. These polymers are hydrophilic in nature, and polymer samples with large volume-to-surface ratios degrade via a bulk hydrolysis mechanism that is much more complex than once thought, and strongly influenced by polymer morphology [6–9]. One inherent characteristic of semicrystalline absorbable poly(alpha-hydroxy acids) is heterogeneous degradation resulting from the existence of two phases. The amorphous regions of the polymer tend to hydrolyze at a higher rate than the higher density crystalline regions, resulting in a material that loses its mechanical strength at a rate faster than it loses mass.

Animal and human clinical studies of absorbable polymeric materials proposed for fracture-fixation devices have identified potential problems for devices made from PLA and PGA. Canine experiments have shown resorption of intramedullary bone against poly(L-lactic acid) (PLLA) surfaces once mass loss from the implant commences [10]. *In vivo* studies have identified birefringent crystals in the deep inguinal lymph nodes of goats after 2-years implantation of transcortical plugs containing PLLA and hydroxyapatite. These birefringent crystals are thought to be PLLA since no calcium or phosphate ions were found in the lymph nodes [11].

In human reconstructive surgery, the occurrence of sinus formation through local nonbacterial inflammatory reactions with considerable tissue swelling weeks or months after implantation has been reported for PGA devices [12]. Review reports of these inflammatory lesions describe the characteristics of a nonspecific foreign-body reaction that often necessitates aspiration or a second surgery [12–16]. Also, similar problems with the crystalline degradation products of PLLA used for zygomatic fracture repair have occurred 2 to 3 years after implantation [17]. Presumably, the greater hydrolytic degradation rate in the interior of large implants (2–20 grams [g]) as compared with the surface results in release of large amounts of acidic degradation products once the implant surface is breached [6–8]. This may exceed local tissue clearance capabilities when end-stage degradation of the implant (mass loss) is reached [10,18].

Totally absorbable composites have been fabricated using absorbable polymers reinforced with higher strength absorbable organic polymer fibers of PGA or PLA [19–21]. When compared with the unreinforced polymer, these "self-reinforced" glycolide and lactide composites show large increases in strength but only modest increases in stiffness since the fibers are organic in nature. PLA matrix composites reinforced with continuous, absorbable, calcium-phosphate-based glass fibers show large increases in both strength and rigidity [22,23]. But, unfortunately, composites of this type made to date lose strength rapidly after short-term exposure to an aqueous physiological environment, indicating a water-sensitive fiber-matrix interface, but do retain a greater proportion of their stiffness. Reinforcement of absorbable polymers with short nonabsorbable fibers (i.e., carbon fibers) may result in better retention of mechanical strength after aqueous exposure [24], but fiber residue could result in an inflammatory response and mechanical irritation if fibers enter the joint space.

A hydrophobic absorbable polymer that undergoes limited hydration so that hydrolysis occurs mainly at the surface of the polymer, releasing near-neutral pH degradation products gradually over time, has not been evaluated for fabrication of composites for absorbable orthopedic fixation devices. This chapter describes a first effort to create a completely absorbable composite implant material, using a poly(orthoester) (POE) reinforced with absorbable, randomly oriented, calcium-sodium-metaphosphate (CSM) microfibers (Table 1). Such a composite could be used in devices for low-load mechanical stabilization of hard or soft tissues. An initial design goal was to produce a benignly absorbable composite material with mechanical properties similar to bone that would retain the majority of these properties for the initial healing period of bone, approximately 4 to 6 weeks.

Table 1   Physical Properties of CSM Microfiber

Property	Value
Form	
Particle shape	Fibrillar
Texture	Soft
Dimensional	
Density, g/cc	2.86
Fiber diameter, microns	1 to 5
Aspect Ratio	20 to 30
BET surface area, m^2/g	1.0 to 1.8
Mechanical	
Tensile strength, GPa	2.55
Tensile modulus, GPa	124
Mohs hardness	3.7 to 4.3
Thermal	
Stability	Melts at 749°C
Heat capacity, cal/g-k	0.19
Linear expansion, inches/°C	
Longitudinal	0.5×10^{-5}
Transverse	1.1×10^{-5}
Miscellaneous	
Oil absorption, g/100g	350 to 380
Moisture pickup, %	1.1 (82% relative humidity)

Source: Adapted from Ref. 32

II.   POLY(ORTHOESTER) POLYMERS

A.   Polymer Background, Synthesis, and Degradation

Poly(orthoesters) are a family of synthetic absorbable polymers that have been under development for medical applications for a number of years [25]. This family of highly hydrophobic absorbable polymers is completely amorphous [26]. Hydrolytic degradation of the bulk polymer occurs predominantly by surface hydrolysis [27], in contrast to the bulk hydrolysis of more hydrophilic PGAs and PLAs. POEs have been successfully used as erodible matrices for delivery of therapeutic agents [25]. Polymer hydrolysis rates can be accelerated by adding acidic excipients to the bulk polymer or retarded by adding basic excipients [23]. Hydrolysis rates also increase with decreasing molecular weight (MW) [29].

The synthesis of POEs has been described previously [30], and is shown in Fig. 1. Briefly, the rigid diol *trans*-cyclohexanedimethanol and the flexible diol 1,6-hexanediol in the desired ratio are added to tetrahydrofuran, and the mixture is stirred until all solids dissolve. A solution of the diketene acetal 3,9-bis(ethylidene 2,4,8,10-tetraoxaspiro [5,5] undecane) is then added, and the polymerization is initiated by the addition of a catalytic amount of *p*-tolulenesulfonic acid dissolved in tetrahyrofuran. After the initial exotherm subsides, the mixture is stirred for about two hours (h), and polymer is isolated by precipitation into a large excess of methanol containing a small amount of triethylamine stabilizer, followed by filtration and vacuum drying at 60°C for 24 hours. Polymers

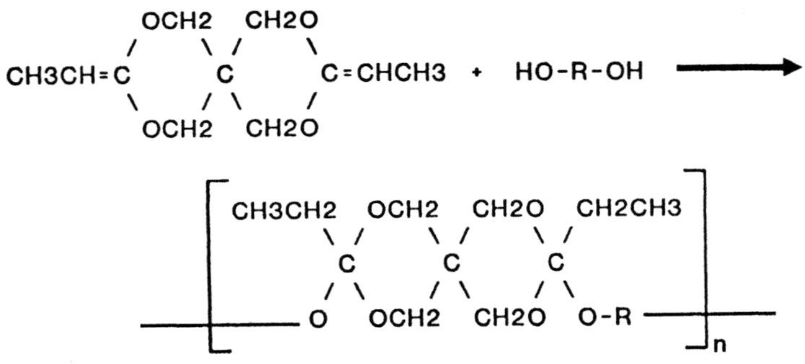

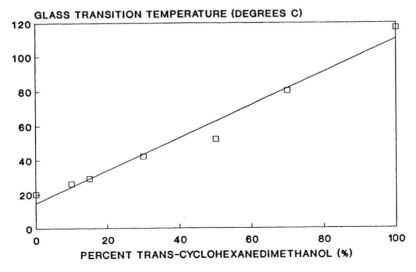

Figure 1   Synthesis of poly(orthoester).

prepared by this procedure typically have molecular weights in the 80–100-kilodalton (kDa) range. By giving special attention to exact stoichiometry and using very pure (>99.5%) reagents, molecular weights in excess of 180 kDa have been achieved. Lower molecular weight materials (20–30 kDa) can be prepared by slightly skewing the stoichiometry.

Polymers with a wide range in glass transition temperature T_g can be synthesized by varying the ratio of rigid to flexible diols (Fig. 2). However, the effect of T_g on elastic modulus is modest for POEs reported here since the T_g is well above room temperature and the service temperature for implants (i.e., 37°C).

When bulk POE of the type described above is exposed to an aqueous environment, the polymer undergoes an initial hydrolysis of the orthoester linkages to yield a mixture of the diols used in the synthesis and the mono- and dipropionates of pentaerythritol.

Figure 2   Effect of different molar ratios of *trans*-cyclohexanedimethanol and 1,6-hexanediol on the glass transition temperature of poly(orthoester).

These mono- and diesters eventually hydrolyze to pentaerythritol and propionic acid (Fig. 3) [31].

Even though orthoester linkages are much more labile than the ester linkages, the polymer is highly hydrophobic, so that initial hydrolysis is largely confined to the outer surface of a polymer specimen. Therefore, degradation of this polymer may not generate acidic products rapidly at the implantation site, provided that the water-soluble, low molecular weight products can diffuse away. This could be a significant advantage over the bulk hydrolysis of poly(alpha-hydroxy acids), which hydrolyze directly to yield large amounts of acidic compounds, both soluble and insoluble, when end-stage degradation is reached.

Another advantage of poly(orthoesters) over PGA and PLLA may be their morphology. For these completely amorphous polymers, T_g could be an important design factor for customization of bioabsorbable composites. If the T_g of the matrix is maintained above physiological temperature (37°C), the composite will remain rigid after fabrication. If the composite is briefly heated to a temperature above the T_g, it could be custom formed into any desired shape and subsequently cooled below the T_g, where it would maintain the new shape and be dimensionally stable. This could be useful for intraoperative reshaping when needed.

B. Polymer Characterization and Fabrication

POEs having 60:40 and 90:10 molar ratios of *trans*-cyclohexanedimethanol and 1,6-hexanediol, respectively, were used in this work. As an aid in developing processing conditions for this family of polymers, the rheological and thermal properties of 60:40 POE (MW = 86,000) and 90:10 POE (MW = 73,000) polymers were determined. Dynamic rheometry was used to determine the viscoelastic properties of the polymer samples in their melt phases. In addition, differential scanning calorimetry (DSC) was used to confirm the reported glass transition temperatures of the polymer samples and their propensities for thermal degradation above their T_g's.

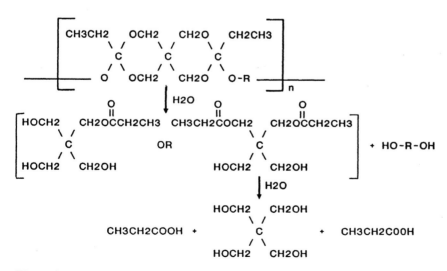

Figure 3 Hydrolytic degradation of poly(orthoester).

For the 90:10 POE, DSC scans revealed a T_g of about 98°C, with the polymer showing some degree of thermal degradation when heated above 180°C in air. Rheological scans indicated viscosity of the melt behaved normally between 110°C and 180°C. Within this temperature range, melt viscosity of the polymer was rather high, 10^4 to 10^6 poise, at low shear rates. For the 60:40 POE, DSC scans indicated a T_g of about 70°C, with the polymer showing some thermal degradation at 130°C. Rheological scans for this polymer indicated the melt behaves normally between 85°C and 155°C. Melt viscosity was also between 10^4 and 10^6 poise.

Since poly(orthoesters) are completely amorphous polymers and therefore relatively viscous, it is best to use polymers having molecular weights of less than 100 kD for hot compression molding. Polymer melt viscosities are a function of polymer molecular weight. As the DSC data indicate, both 60:40 and 90:10 POEs possess thermal degradation temperatures averaging some 70°C above each polymer's T_g when heated in air. This represents a rather narrow processing temperature range. In addition, as indicated by the rheology data, both POEs possess rather high melt viscosities near their thermal degradation temperatures, suggesting melt processing of these polymers by extrusion or injection molding could be difficult. However, a recent report on the physical and mechanical properties of absorbable polymers suggests degradation temperatures of POEs can be extended to over 300°C when heated in an inert atmosphere (nitrogen) [32]. Higher processing temperatures should lower POE melt viscosity, thereby aiding polymer processing by extrusion or injection molding.

For specimen fabrication, quantities of both the 60:40 and 90:10 POE polymers were reduced to coarse powders having a maximum particle diameter of less than 250 microns. This was accomplished by milling the polymer at room temperature in open air and passing the material through a 40-mesh screen.

Test specimens of 60:40 and 90:10 POE (38.1 × 12.7 × 1.6 millimeters [mm]) were prepared by hot compression molding for biocompatibility and *in vitro* hydrolysis testing. Using a hydraulic press with heated and water-cooled platens, 0.9 gram (g) of powdered polymer was hot pressed in a dual-plunger stainless steel die in air 115°C for 60:40 POE and 120°C for 90:10 POE at 4000 pounds per square inch (psi) for 5 minutes. Polymer specimens were then cooled to ambient temperature while maintaining pressure at 4000 psi.

C. Polymer *In Vitro* Degradation Studies

1. *Effect of pH Exposure*

To determine if pH had any effect on the hydrolytic degradation rate of bulk POE, 12 specimens of molded 60:40 POE were placed into vials filled with Tris-buffered saline (20 mM [millimolar] Tris/150 mM NaCl) at pH 7.4, sealed, and placed into a water bath at 37°C. Another 12 60:40 POE specimens were placed in vials along with Tris-buffered saline at pH 5.0 and maintained at 37°C. Of these, 3 specimens were removed at 1, 3, 6, and 12 weeks from each pH solution and tested to failure in three-point bending, according to American Society for Testing and Materials (ASTM) Standard D 790-81 Method 1 [33].

The effects of exposure to Tris-buffered saline pH 5.0 and pH 7.4 at 37°C are shown in Fig. 4. Initial flexural yield strength of 60:40 POE was 65.2 ± 0.8 megapascal (MPa) (mean ± standard deviation [SD]) and the initial modulus of elasticity was 1.58 ± 0.02

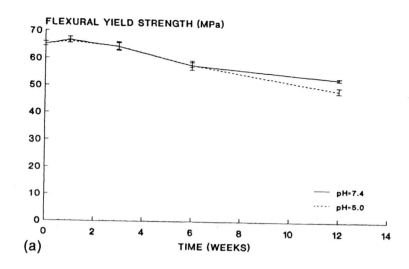

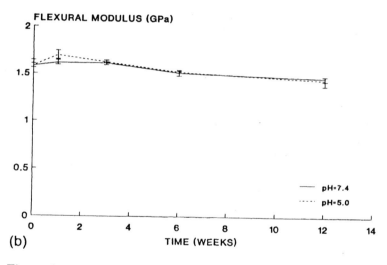

Figure 4 Effects of saline pH at 37°C *in vitro* on mechanical properties of hot-molded 60:40 poly(orthoester) (POE): (*a*), flexural yield strength (megapascal, MPa) (mean ± standard deviation, SD); (*b*), flexural modulus (gigapascal, GPa) (mean ± SD).

gigapascal (GPa). POE retained approximately 80% of its initial flexural yield strength and 92% of its initial modulus of elasticity after 12 weeks *in vitro* exposure (pH 7.4). The final values for strength and stiffness were 50.9 ± 0.5 MPa and 1.45 ± 0.05 GPa, respectively.

Statistical analysis of variance and covariance for the two pHs showed no significant difference ($p < 0.05$) in the rate of degradation of mechanical properties:

$$\text{Strength:} \quad F(1,26) = 3.7270, \quad p = 0.056$$
$$\text{Modulus:} \quad F(1,26) = 0.9112, \quad p = 0.394$$

This seems extraordinary at first, since incorporation of as little as 0.1 weight percent of an acidic excipient such as suberic acid into the polymer results in complete erosion of the polymer in a pH 7.4 buffer in as little as one day. Clearly, the insensitivity of the polymer to an external acidic environment is due to the high initial hydrophobicity of the polymer [25]. This makes the acid-sensitive orthoester linkages virtually inaccessible to the external acid. The lack of change of mechanical properties was further supported by weight loss data, showing virtually no weight loss at pH 7.4 and only minimal weight loss at pH 5.0 in 12 weeks (Fig. 5).

2. *Exposure to* In Vitro *Mechanical Loads*

To determine the effect of *in vitro* exposure and mechanical loads on degradation of POE's mechanical properties, several *in vitro* mechanical loading studies were performed.

Experimental details and fixture design have been described elsewhere [34]. Briefly, 18 molded 60:40 POE specimens were exposed to intermittent cyclic loading in aerated Tris-buffered saline (pH 7.4) at 37°C. The specimens were immersed continually, but only loaded for 630 cycles at 1 hertz (Hz) per day to simulate the activity of a sedentary postsurgical patient. This value was calculated from the time spent walking for a sedentary adult multiplied by an average cadence [35,36]. The load was 8.0 newtons. This corresponded to a stress in the outer regions of the specimen of 10% of the initial flexural yield strength of the POE polymer. Specimens were turned over every day so that both sides of the specimens were exposed to both tensile and compressive loads and to avoid adding the effects of creep to the experiment. Three specimens were removed at 2, 4, 8, 16, 32, and 40 days and tested in three-point bending to detect changes in stress-strain behavior.

To determine the effects of a constant load on degradation rate, 18 specimens were subjected to a static load of 3.6 newtons while exposed to Tris-buffered saline at body temperature. This corresponded to a stress in the outer regions of the specimen of 2% of the initial flexural yield strength of 60:40 POE. Of the specimens, 3 were removed at 2, 4, 8, 16, 32, and 40 days and tested in the same manner as the above-mentioned specimens.

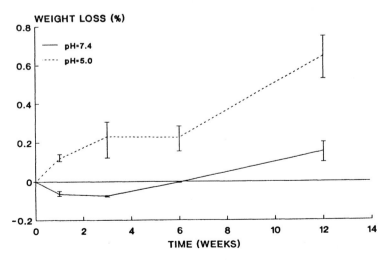

Figure 5   Percent weight loss of hot-molded 60:40 poly(orthoester) (POE) after *in vitro* exposure to saline at pH 5.0 and pH 7.4 at 37°C.

Finally, to determine to what extent loading augments the effect of the chemical environment on degradation rate, nine unloaded specimens were immersed in Tris-buffered saline at physiological pH and temperature. Three specimens were removed and tested at 7, 21, 42 days.

Results of cyclic, static, and unloaded exposure of 60:40 POE specimens to Tris-buffered saline at body temperature and pH are shown in Fig. 6. A combination of both exposure to Tris-buffered saline and intermittent cyclic loading decreased the initial

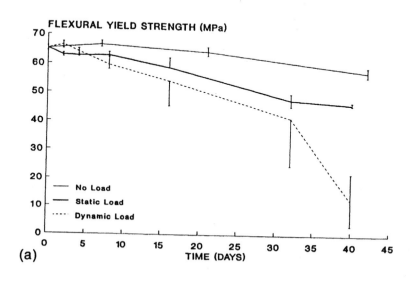

(a)

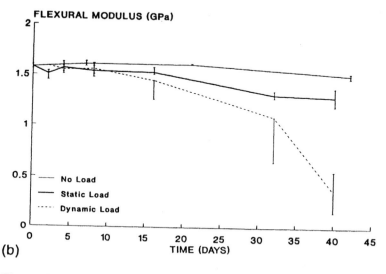

(b)

Figure 6   Comparison of *in vitro* mechanical loading conditions on mechanical properties of hot-molded poly(orthoester) (POE) specimens immersed in aerated pH 7.4 Tris-buffered saline at 37°C: (*a*), flexural yield strength (megapascal, MPa) (mean ± standard deviation, SD); (*b*), flexural modulus (gigapascal, GPa) (mean ± SD).

flexural strength and modulus by 75% after 40 days. The final flexural yield strength was 12.6 ± 9.3 MPa and the flexural modulus of elasticity was 0.37 ± 0.2 GPa.

For the static-loading exposures, strength decreased by 29% and stiffness by 20% after 40 days. The final flexural yield strength was 46.3 ± 0.6 MPa and the flexural modulus of elasticity was 1.51 ± 0.09 GPa.

For the unloaded exposures, both strength and stiffness decreased by less than 10% after 42 days. The final flexural yield strength was 57.6 ± 1.7 MPa and the flexural modulus of elasticity was 1.51 ± 0.03 GPa.

For data grouped according to type of load (no load, static, and cyclic), strength and modulus for all load conditions decreased in a linear fashion (Fig. 6). Flexural yield strength decreased significantly with exposure time for no-load, static-load, and cyclic-load conditions. Modulus of elasticity decreased significantly with exposure time for all three load conditions (Table 2).

Analysis of variance indicated that the change in slope of flexural strength as a function of time differed significantly among the three loading groups, $F(4,48) = 26.611$, $p < 0.000001$. In addition, the change in slope of the modulus of elasticity as a function of time also differed significantly among no load, static load, and cyclic loads, $F(4,48) = 22.186$, $p < 0.000001$.

Data for the pH exposure study were obtained using specimens that were kept immersed in Tris-buffered saline in the absence of any mechanical load. Although no-load degradation studies are typical for bioabsorbable polymers and composites, they are not representative of actual use in mechanical stabilization of tissues. A real device is exposed to either a quasi-static load or, more likely, to a markedly dynamic load. The experiments reported here involved subjecting specimens to such loads during exposure. Loads were either static or dynamic and applied in four-point bending as reported elsewhere [34].

The data indicated that mechanical properties of specimens subjected to intermittent cyclic loading decreased at a significantly more rapid rate than specimens subjected to no-load or static-load conditions. The increase in degradation rate with mechanical loading is likely due to the opening up of microscopic cracks when the surface of a specimen is in tension. These microscopic cracks then provide a path for water to penetrate into the device, which allows polymer hydrolysis to take place with consequent deterioration of mechanical properties.

This hypothesis is likely since cyclic loading of 60:40 POE specimens in air for 25,200

Table 2   Linear Regression Equations

	Flexural yield strength versus time	
No load:	$S_b = -0.2084\,(T) + 67.21$,	$r = 0.8890, p < 0.0001$
Static load:	$S_b = -0.4919\,(T) + 65.23$,	$r = 0.9623, p < 0.00001$
Cyclic load:	$S_b = -1.1727\,(T) + 69.91$,	$r = 0.9017, p < 0.00001$
	Flexural modulus of elasticity versus time	
No load:	$E_b = -0.0020\,(T) + 1.614$,	$r = 0.6851, p < 0.0140$
Static load:	$E_b = -0.0069\,(T) + 1.567$,	$r = 0.8673, p < 0.00001$
Cyclic load:	$E_b = -0.0264\,(T) + 1.699$,	$r = 0.8494, p < 0.00001$

S_b = flexural yield strength, E_b = flexural modulus of elasticity, T = time

cycles at 1 Hz, the same number of cycles as for the 42-day intermittent cyclic loading exposures, showed no significant decrease in flexural strength or modulus [34]. This suggests the effects of hydrolytic exposure and mechanical loading are synergistic on the degradation of POE mechanical properties.

III. CALCIUM-SODIUM-METAPHOSPHATE MICROFIBERS

A. Microfiber Description and Preparation

Calcium-sodium-metaphosphate mineral microfibers were developed as a nontoxic replacement for asbestos, but the material has not been used commercially as yet (Monsanto Chemical Co., St. Louis, MO). This degradable and bioabsorbable microfiber is a crystalline, inorganic polymer of metaphosphate with a negative charge that is balanced by calcium and sodium ions (Fig. 7) [37,38]. The fiber exhibits an effective aspect ratio of 60:1 because of its fibrillated ends, and potentially can be used with a wide range of coupling agents for reinforcing thermoplastic and thermosetting polymers [37].

CSM microfibers are manufactured from pure elemental phosphorus using oxygen, sodium carbonate, and lime [37]. The microfibers cover a wide range of lengths and diameters, from submicrons to hundreds of microns, depending on the type and degree of comminution to which the material is exposed. These crystalline microfibers possess the tensile strength and stiffness of Kevlar, 2.6 GPa and 124 GPa, respectively [37]. Table 1 lists additional physical properties of CSM microfibers.

The surface of the CSM microfibers is slightly acidic. This is due to chain-end hydrolysis of the inorganic polymer, resulting in a small quantity of surface acidic products. This resulting free hydrogen can react with the methoxy groups of commercially available silane coupling agents to form silanol bonds between the inorganic fiber surface and the coupling agent [39], resulting in a polysiloxane film.

Since an acid fiber surface will catalyze hydrolysis of POEs, the fibber surface was made basic by treating it with a diamine-silane, (N,beta-aminoethyl-gamma-amino-propyl-trimethoxysilane; Z-6020, Dow Corning, Midland, MI). This was accomplished in the following manner. To 100 ml of a 0.3% solution of silane coupling agent in methanol was added 15 g of CSM microfibers, which was stirred until a slurry was formed. The slurry was then filtered and the residue dried in a convection oven at 90–100°C for 3.5 hours. After cooling to room temperature, the treated microfibers were sieved through a 40-mesh sieve, washed with excess methanol to remove any unbonded coupling agent, and finally dried in a convection oven at 90–100°C for 1 hour.

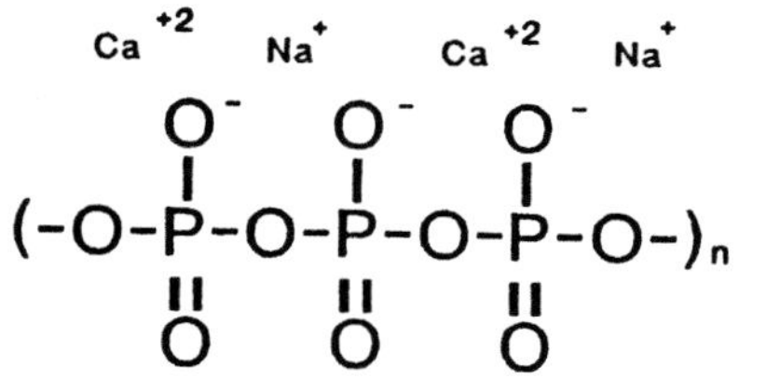

$$\text{Ca}^{+2} \quad \text{Na}^{+} \quad \text{Ca}^{+2} \quad \text{Na}^{+}$$

$$(-O-\underset{\underset{O}{\overset{\overset{O^-}{|}}{\|}}{P}-O-\underset{\underset{O}{\overset{\overset{O^-}{|}}{\|}}{P}-O-\underset{\underset{O}{\overset{\overset{O^-}{|}}{\|}}{P}-O-)_n$$

Figure 7 Chemical structure of polymetaphosphate inorganic polymeric backbone chain. The polymetaphosphate polymers lie next to each other in planes, with cations in the spaces in between and ionically bonded to the polymer.

B. Microfiber Characterization

The hydrolytic degradation of polymetaphosphate fibers in the body is a two-stage process. First, when exposed to an aqueous media, polymer chains at the fiber surface dissolve; second, these dissolved polymer chains then undergo chain-end hydrolysis, yielding metaphosphate, which is removed by normal metabolic pathways [14].

In order to quantify both CSM microfiber degradation due to dissolved polymer chains at the microfiber surface and water resistance of the polysiloxane film barrier, two degradation studies were performed. First, 50 milligrams (mg) of untreated CSM microfiber samples were placed into vials containing 20 ml of normal saline, while another set of microfiber samples was placed in vials containing 20 ml of distilled water. The sample-filled vials were sealed and placed in a shaker bath and maintained at a temperature of 37°C. Microfiber samples immersed in normal saline and distilled water were removed at 1, 2, 4, and 7 weeks and dried in a vacuum oven at 50°C for 48 hours. The remaining fibrous residue was weighed using a standard laboratory analytical balance and any change in weight was recorded.

Second, the amount of coupling agent actually placed onto the microfibers can be semiquantitatively determined by titration of a microfiber slurry in water, provided the coupling agent has acidic or basic functional groups [39]. To determine if a polysiloxane film barrier would prevent early surface dissolution of the microfiber, 2.5 grams of CSM microfibers pretreated with diamine-silane were boiled in 100 ml of deionized water for 1 hour. The slurry was then filtered and dried at 90–100°C for 1 hour.

Titration of a 2% slurry of the treated microfibers in deionized water (weight/weight) using 0.001 N sulfuric acid was performed until pH 4 was reached. Similar titrations were performed with CSM microfibers treated with diamine-silane and untreated microfibers, followed by comparison of the titration curves. The greater the volume of sulfuric acid needed to reach pH 4, the greater the number of basic sites on the fiber surface was, hence the greater the amount of coupling agent on the microfiber surface. This was used as a semiquantitative indicator for determining if the polysiloxane film barrier was intact after boiling the diamine-silane-treated fibers for 1 hour in water.

Results of the microfiber dissolution study are shown Fig. 8. The CSM microfibers lost about 10% of their mass after 7 weeks of exposure to distilled water and lost 15% in normal saline at 37°C.

CSM microfibers may degrade somewhat more rapidly *in vivo* than *in vitro*. Phosphatase enzymes are reported to increase the hydrolytic decomposition rate of polymetaphosphate by a factor of about 10^6 [40]. Solubility of CSM microfibers exposed to a media of epithelial cells showed a two-to-threefold increase and a sevenfold increase in solubility for media containing lung alveolar macrophages [38].

Results of acid titration of 2% CSM microfiber slurries in deionized water with 0.001 normal (N) sulfuric acid are shown Fig. 9. To reach a pH of 4.0 for microfibers treated with diamine-silane coupling agent, 22 ml of acid was required, while 10 ml of acid was needed for fibers subjected to boiling water, compared with 5 ml of acid for untreated microfibers. Results suggest that the chemical bond between the polysiloxane film and the CSM microfiber surface resists hydrolysis, even after being subjected to boiling water for one hour. This resistance should help prevent early dissolution of the microfibers.

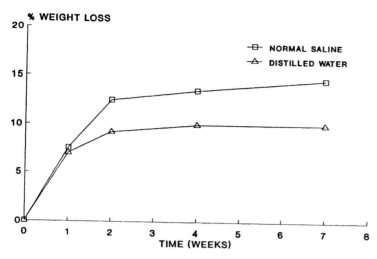

Figure 8 Percent weight loss of calcium-sodium-metaphosphate (CSM) microfibers after *in vitro* exposure at 37°C to distilled water and normal saline.

IV. BIOCOMPATIBILITY TESTING

A. Acute Cytotoxicity of Component Materials

Acute cytotoxicity of 60:40 POE, 90:10 POE, CSM microfibers, and silane-treated CSM microfibers was evaluated by standard tissue culture agar overlay assay [41] using the direct cell contact method and L929 mouse fibroblast cells.

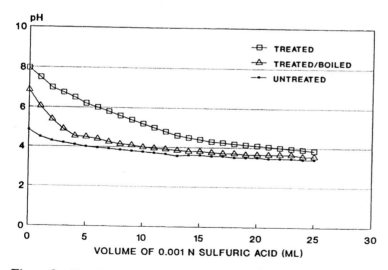

Figure 9 Titration of 2% calcium-sodium-metaphosphate (CSM) microfiber slurries using 0.001 normal (N) sulfuric acid.

After sterilization with ethylene oxide, appropriate amounts of each test material were aseptically placed onto separate agar, along with positive and negative controls (natural black rubber and polyethylene, respectively). Triplicate samples and controls were incubated at 37°C for 24 h. Neutral red was added for 2 to 3 h. The cells were then evaluated using an inverted microscope.

Results were scored by adding the area of decoloration (zone index) and the area of lysis (lysis index). The final score was recorded as the response index, which is the ratio of zone index to lysis index.

The 60:40 and 90:10 POE, untreated CSM fibers, and CSM fibers treated with the diamine-silane coupling agent were acutely noncytotoxic. Responses were comparable to negative controls (Table 3). This agrees with other acute toxicity testing [42,43], which describe 60:40 and 90:10 poly(orthoester) and untreated CSM microfibers as acutely nontoxic in United States Pharmacopeia tests for systemic, intracutaneous, and intramuscular implant toxicity.

Although the preliminary data showing a lack of acute toxicity of poly(orthoesters) and calcium-sodium-metaphosphate microfibers are very promising, the question of long-term toxicity cannot be answered until composite implant studies in animals have been carried out to complete absorption of the implant. There is a preliminary report on the histological evaluation of CSM/POE composites in a rabbit model with promising results. Unfortunately, the study was terminated before complete absorption of the implant [42]. This has also been a failing of many animal studies of the past involving PLA and PGA implants.

Table 3   Results of Standard Tissue Culture Agar Overlay Response Index Equal to Zone Index/ Lysis Index for Direct Test

Sample	Replicate 1	Replicate 2	Replicate 3	Average
+ Control	2.0/5.0[a]	2.0/5.0	2.0/5.0	2.0/5.0
− Control	0.0/0.0	0.0/0.0	0.0/0.0	0.0/0.0
60:40 POE	0.0/0.0	0.0/0.0	0.0/0.0	0.0/0.0
Results: Noncytotoxic				
+ Control	2.0/5.0	2.0/5.0	2.0/5.0	2.0/5.0
− Control	0.0/0.0	0.0/0.0	0.0/0.0	0.0/0.0
90:10 POE	0.0/0.0	0.0/0.0	0.0/0.0	0.0/0.0
Results: Noncytotoxic				
+ Control	2.0/5.0	2.0/5.0	2.0/5.0	2.0/5.0
− Control	0.0/0.0	0.0/0.0	0.0/0.0	0.0/0.0
CSM fibers (untreated)	0.0/0.0	0.0/0.0	0.0/0.0	0.0/0.0
Results: Noncytotoxic				
+ Control	2.0/5.0	2.0/5.0	2.0/5.0	2.0/5.0
− Control	0.0/0.0	0.0/0.0	0.0/0.0	0.0/0.0
CSM fibers (treated)	0.0/0.0	0.0/0.0	0.0/0.0	0.0/0.0
Results: Noncytotoxic				

[a]Zone/lysis

B. Toxicity of Accumulated Polymer Degradation Products

As mentioned above, one of the main concerns for use of poly(alpha-hydroxy acid) polymer implants for fracture fixation is the potential for adverse tissue reactions due to accumulation of acidic degradation products. This complication seems likely to occur since, as suggested in animal studies by Spenelhauer et al. [44], a high rate of noninfectious inflammatory response was associated with intermediate molecular weight degradation products of poly(alpha-hydroxy acids). The high rate of sterile inflammatory response occurred when PLA copolymer weight average molecular weight fell below 20,000 daltons. Use of a higher initial molecular weight PLA copolymer delayed, but did not eliminate, the inflammatory response.

To investigate this problem, a comparison study was performed to determine the acute toxicity of accumulated hydrolytic degradation products of 60:40 poly(orthoester) and commercially available implant grades of poly(glycolic acid) and of two different molecular weights of poly(L-lactic acid). PGA (Medisorb 100PGA) was obtained from Du Pont, as well as a low molecular weight PLLA (Medisorb 100L), while a high molecular weight PLLA (BP-0600 PLA) was obtained from Birmingham Polymers.

Samples about 2-mm thick and weighing 0.25 g were fabricated by hot compression molding at recommended temperatures and then sterilized with ethylene oxide. Once sterilized, samples of each material were tested for ethylene oxide residuals and sterility. All samples tested sterile and had residual levels well below maximum acceptable levels. The highest level of ethylene oxide was 10.2 parts per million (ppm), and the most stringent Food and Drug Administration (FDA) guideline for implants is 25 ppm.

For each polymer, 15 samples were placed in individual sterile glass vials containing 10 ml of sterile distilled water to simulate implantation in a confined space. Another 15 samples were placed in vials containing 10 ml of sterile Tris buffer (0.05 M). Samples were incubated at 37°C for 10 days and 4, 8, 12, and 16 weeks. At each time interval, 3 samples of each incubation solution and each polymer were evaluated. Similarly, hot-molded positive controls (polyethylene containing 40% by weight *trans*-cinnamic acid) and negative controls (pure polyethylene) were also tested for toxicity at 10 days.

For each incubation solution, pH and toxicity were measured, and for each partially-degraded polymer specimen, dry weight and inherent viscosity (to detect change in molecular weight) were determined. Incubation solution toxicity was measured using the bacterial bioluminescence acute toxicity assay [45]. The toxicity assay is accomplished by monitoring the bacterial light output of a test vial containing *Photobacterium phosphoreum*, before and at 5 and 15 minutes after sample addition, against a simultaneous negative control [45]. Toxicity is proportional to relative light loss in the test sample against the negative control. A remaining light reading of 50% or less is considered toxic. Results of various biomaterials in this test parallel those for other acute toxicity tests. However, this test is more rapid, quantitative, and somewhat more sensitive [45]. Water solutions much below pH 4 or above pH 10 generally also produce a toxic response in this test [46].

The 10-day negative controls were uniformly nontoxic, and the positive controls were uniformly toxic. The PGA incubation solutions were toxic after 10 days for both distilled water and Tris-buffered water (Table 4). In addition, the lower molecular weight PLLA incubation solutions in water were toxic at 4 weeks. None of the incubation solutions for the higher molecular weight PLLA and POE were toxic at 16 weeks.

For PGA, acidity of the water solutions increased rapidly to below pH 3, and pH for

Table 4 Data for Final Exposures and First Toxic Exposures (Mean ± SD)

16-week data	Polymer		Incubation solution	
Material and exp. media	Mass loss (%)	Final viscosity (% of original)	pH	Remaining light (%)
PGA (W)	64.85 ± 0.63	18.7 ± 2.4	2.49 ± 0.06	0.0 ± 0.00
PGA (T)	63.38 ± 0.66	25.9 ± 2.8	2.85 ± 0.04	0.0 ± 0.00
PLA-LW (W)	4.69 ± 1.36	47.0 ± 1.7	3.03 ± 0.04	0.0 ± 0.00
PLA-LW (T)	3.62 ± 0.09	48.7 ± 2.6	6.80 ± 0.02	82.1 ± 2.88
PLA-HW (W)	−0.05 ± 0.01	79.5 ± 3.4	7.30 ± 0.06	96.2 ± 6.32
PLA-HW (T)	−0.10 ± 0.05	77.0 ± 4.6	7.72 ± 0.02	88.4 ± 6.24
POE (W)	1.29 ± 0.12	95.4 ± 1.6	6.56 ± 0.05	57.2 ± 7.95
POE (T)	1.58 ± 1.61	89.3 ± 8.3	7.75 ± 0.05	68.4 ± 6.69
First Toxic Data				
PGA (W), 10 day	3.25 ± 0.30	35.4 ± 6.7	2.81 ± 0.05	0.00 ± 0.00
PGA (T), 10 day	3.46 ± 0.40	29.3 ± 3.3	5.50 ± 1.25	0.00 ± 0.00
PLA-LW (W), 4 week	0.47 ± 0.57	87.9 ± 3.6	3.57 ± 0.13	7.16 ± 10.1

W = sterile distilled water, T = sterile tris buffer, LW = low molecular weight, HW = high molecular weight

the low molecular weight PLLA fell more slowly to the same range. The pH of the other water solutions remained well above 6 during the entire 16 weeks. For the Tris buffer incubation solutions with PGA present, pH fell rapidly to about 5 and then 3. By 12 weeks, the pH with the low molecular weight PLLA present had decreased to below 7. It remained above 7 for all other polymers in Tris buffer.

Weight loss for all polymers was below 5% at 16 weeks, except for PGA, which was 64%. Inherent viscosity, change in molecular weight, at 16 weeks was greatest in PGA exposures, with 18.7% of the original viscosity in water and 25.9% in Tris buffer. In contrast, POE exposures showed the smallest decrease, with 95.4% of the original viscosity in water and 89.3% in Tris buffer.

Rapid weight loss for PGA explains the extreme drop in pH and resultant toxicity. The difference in onset of toxicity for the two PLLAs was most likely due to the difference in molecular weight and corresponding rate of degradation [47]. Weight loss for the high molecular weight PLLA was less than for POE, but change in inherent viscosity was greater than for POE. This suggests that poly(orthoesters) do indeed degrade initially by surface hydrolysis and erosion rather than by bulk hydrolysis as the data show for PGA and PLLA. For POE, the slow release of nearly pH-neutral degradation products gradually over time could reduce complications reported for large PGA fracture-fixation devices [18–22].

V. COMPOSITE FABRICATION VARIABLES

The initial mechanical properties and *in vitro* cyclic loading studies suggest POE alone would be an inadequate material for large fracture-fixation devices for long bone fixation of the femur or tibia. Since successful fracture fixation has been reported for absorbable materials that have mechanical properties similar to cortical bone [4], this suggests POEs may be useful as matrix polymers in fiber-reinforced polymer composites for fracture-fixation devices. Reinforcement of POE with randomly oriented CSM microfibers would increase initial mechanical properties, and composites of POE would show superior load-carrying capacity. Also, the random nature of microfiber reinforcement would yield an isotropic composite material with uniform mechanical properties under different loading conditions: tension, compression, bending, and torsion. This could be an important advantage over anisotropic self-reinforced lactide and glycolide composites that become progressively weaker in torsion as fiber orientation is increased in the axis of orientation with increasing draw ratio.

A. Composite Fabrication

Composite specimens measuring 38.1 × 12.7 × 1.60 mm were prepared in the following manner. First, 90:10 POE was reduced to a granular form (particle diameter less than 250 microns) by milling the polymer at room temperature in open air and using material that passed through a 40-mesh screen. Microfiber and polymer were combined by dry mixing in air. CSM microfibers were placed into a narrow bottle (diameter of 5 cm and length of 15 cm) fitted with a stirring rod assembly. Milled polymer was sprinkled into the bottle while blending the microfibers with the impeller of the stirring rod. After final addition of the polymer, blending was maintained for 15 minutes at low to medium speed (10–30 revolutions per minute [rpm]).

Test specimens were prepared by hot compression molding in air of an appropriate amount of dry-mixed composite in a three-piece stainless steel die at selected temperatures (20°C to 100°C) above the T_g and a pressure of 2700 psi for 5 minutes using a hydraulic press with heated and water-cooled platens. Composite specimens were then cooled to ambient temperature while maintaining the pressure at 2700 psi.

B. Microfiber Loading

To determine the effect of microfiber loading on initial mechanical properties, CSM/POE composites were fabricated from CSM microfibers treated with the diamine-silane coupling agent and 90:10 POE at 170–175°C. Microfiber loading was 0%, 10%, 20%, 30%, 40%, and 50% by volume. Two composite specimens at each microfiber load were tested to failure in three-point bending to determine flexural yield strength and stiffness.

Composite specimens fabricated at microfiber loads of 30% or less by volume were uniform in appearance. Those with higher microfiber loads showed some inconsistency in wetting out of the microfiber surface by the polymer as observed by visual inspection. Flexural modulus increased in a linear fashion with increasing fiber content for the entire composition range studied ($r^2 = 0.9962$). Maximum increase in stiffness (525%) was observed at $V_f = 50\%$ (mean strength = 103 MPa and mean modulus = 9.4 GPa). Flexural yield strength also increased with increasing fiber content, peaking at $V_f = 40\%$, then declining thereafter. Maximum increase in strength (77%) was observed as $V_f = 40\%$ (mean strength = 115 MPa and mean modulus = 8.2 GPa) (Fig. 10).

C. Pressing Temperature

To determine what effect pressing temperature would have on initial flexural mechanical properties, CSM/POE composite specimens were fabricated from 30 volume percent

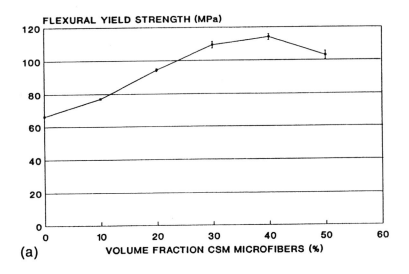

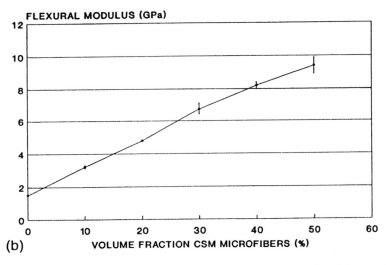

Figure 10 Microfiber loading of diamine-silane-treated calcium-sodium-metaphosphate/poly (orthoester) (CSM/POE) composites: (*a*), flexural yield strength (megapascal, MPa) (mean ± standard deviation, SD); (*b*), flexural modulus (gigapascal, GPa) (mean ± SD).

CSM microfibers treated with the diamine-silane coupling agent and 90:10 POE. Specimens were fabricated at pressing temperatures of 120°C, 170°C, 185°C, and 200°C. Initial flexural yield strength and flexural modulus were determined in three-point bending.

Figure 11 shows the effects of increased fabrication temperature on the initial mechanical properties of composites constructed with diamine-silane-treated microfibers (V_f = 30%). As fabrication temperatures were increased, composite flexural yield strength and modulus continued to increase until the temperature reached 185°C. With an addi-

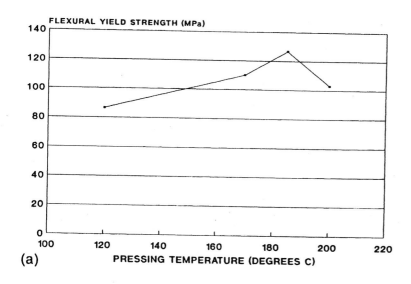

(a)

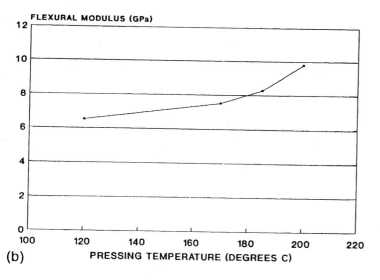

(b)

Figure 11 Effect of pressing temperature on diamine-silane-treated calcium-sodium-metaphosphate/poly(orthoester) (CSM/POE) composite initial mechanical properties: (*a*), flexural yield strength (megapascal, MPa); (*b*), flexural modulus (gigapascal, GPa).

tional increase in temperature, strength declined, while modulus continued to increase. When compared with unreinforced 90:10 POE, increase in flexural strength of the composite at 185°C was 95% (127 MPa) and flexural modulus was 453% (8.3 GPa).

Rather narrow temperature processing windows and high melt viscosities near their respective thermal degradation temperatures are possessed by 60:40 and 90:10 POEs. These limitations may have resulted in composites with incomplete wetting between the microfiber, which has a high surface area (1.0–1.8 square meters per gram [m^2/g]), and the matrix polymer. Mechanical properties of CSM/90:10 POE composites improved with increasing fabrication temperature, suggesting improved wetting was achieved. Unfortunately, at temperatures above 185°C, strength decreased, probably due to thermal degradation of the polymer. As mentioned above, the thermal degradation temperature of POEs can be extended to over 300°C when heated in an inert atmosphere such as nitrogen [32]. This should improve microfiber wetting and significantly improve initial mechanical properties of the composite material. However, such studies have not yet been carried out.

D. Wet Strength Retention Studies

The rapid strength loss of absorbable poly(lactic acid) composites fabricated with absorbable calcium-phosphate-based glass fibers is due to the disruption of the polymer/fiber interface by water [38], and not due to polymer chain degradation of either the polymer or reinforcing fibers. As fluids diffuse into the polymer or wick along the fiber/fiber interfaces, the polymer/fiber interface is compromised and the fibers lose their reinforcing effect. Since absorbable phosphate fibers degrade first through surface dissolution [14], the adhesion between the fiber and the polymer matrix is broken once water molecules reach the interface. To see if an outer polymer coating would slow the loss of composite strength and stiffness by retarding the influx of fluids, a comparison study was performed.

The first group of composite test specimens was prepared by hot compression molding of 1.27 g of dry-mixed 90:10 POE polymer and untreated CSM microfibers (V_f = 30%) and pressed at 180°C to 185°C. Additional specimens were prepared by the same method using CSM microfibers treated with the diamine-silane coupling agent. Half of these CSM/POE composite specimens was encapsulated in pure 60:40 POE by hot pressing the POE around the test specimens.

Composite test specimens were machined to 36.5 × 11.1 × 1.00 mm. Milled 60:40 POE (rather than 90:10 POE) was used to encapsulate the composite specimens because of its lower glass transition temperature. Of the 60:40 POE, one-fifth gram was placed in the cavity of a rectangular stainless steel mold (38.1 × 12.7 mm). Gentle tapping on the sides of the mold helped to distribute the powdered polymer evenly at the bottom of the mold. A composite test specimen was very carefully placed on top of the powdered polymer and centered. On top of the test specimen was placed one-quarter of a gram of milled 60:40 POE. Again, gentle tapping on the sides of the mold evenly distributed the powdered polymer. The upper plunger of the mold was then fitted in place and the polymer/composite system was further processed by hot compression molding at 115–120°C for 5 minutes at 2700 psi. Encapsulated composite specimens were cooled to ambient temperature while maintaining pressure at 2700 psi.

Reproducibility of the encapsulation procedure was excellent, resulting in a uniform coating of polymer for all specimens fabricated. Examination of specimen cross sections by light microscopy revealed the coating procedure left approximately a 300-micron thick coating of polymer on the test specimens that appeared free of voids and cracks.

Initial flexural yield strength and modulus were measured using three-point bending. Specimens for *in vitro* degradation tests were immersed in Tris-buffered saline (200 mM Tris and 150 mM NaCl), pH 7.4 at 37°C. Three composite specimens were tested to failure in three-point bending at various time periods up to 6 weeks.

For comparison, Fig. 12 shows the initial mean flexural mechanical properties of 90:10 POE (strength = 65 MPa and modulus = 1.5 GPa) and composites fabricated with

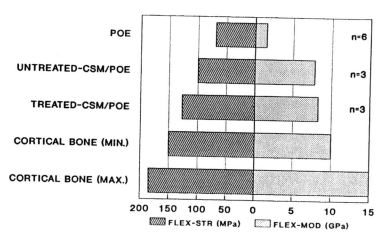

Figure 12 Comparison of flexural mechanical properties for poly(orthoester) (POE), composites of untreated calcium-sodium-metaphosphate/poly(orthoester) (CSM/POE), treated CSM/POE, and the minimum and maximum reported literature values for cortical bone.

untreated CSM microfibers (strength = 100 MPa and modulus = 7.8 GPa) and treated CSM microfibers (strength = 125 MPa and modulus = 8.3 GPa). Composite specimens with diamine-silane-treated CSM microfibers possessed flexural strength and stiffness similar to reported literature values of cortical bone (strength = 150–185 MPa and modulus = 10–15 GPa) [48,49].

POE-coated composite specimens after 4 weeks immersion in the Tris-buffered saline showed no obvious signs of delamination or degradation by visual inspection. Figure 13 shows percent retention of mean flexural yield strength and modulus after *in vitro* exposure.

Because surface acidity of the CSM microfibers accelerates hydrolysis of the acid-sensitive poly(orthoester), the microfiber surface was made basic by treating it with a diamine-silane coupling agent. When compared to untreated microfibers, use of the silane coupling agent modestly improved initial mechanical properties of the composite and markedly improved wet strength resistance after *in vitro* exposure to Tris-buffered saline.

An outer polymer coating of hot-pressed 60:40 POE sufficiently retarded influx of water to further slow the degradation of the polymer/fiber interface. The coated composite material retained 70% of its strength and stiffness for 4 weeks. For comparison, there is a report of poly(DL-lactic acid) composites reinforced with continuous calcium-metaphosphate glass fibers and coated with hot films of poly(ϵ-caprolactone) to act as a water barrier [50]. When exposed to physiological saline, these coated composites retained about 50% of their flexural modulus after 4-weeks exposure. The ability of poly(orthoester) to act as a superior water barrier when compared to poly(ϵ-caprolactone) may be due to the more hydrophobic nature of the polymer.

VI. CONCLUSIONS

Bioabsorbable composites based upon hydrophobic amorphous thermoplastic matrices offer potential advantages over those of semicrystalline thermoplastic poly(alpha-hydroxy acids). The single-phase morphology yields hydrolytic degradation in which

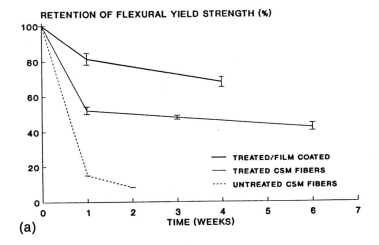

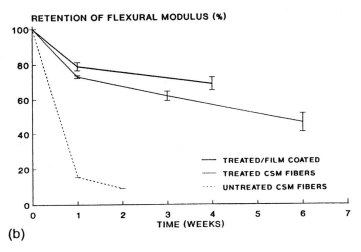

Figure 13 Percent retention of mechanical properties after *in vitro* exposure to Tris-buffered saline, pH 7.4 at 37°C: (*a*), flexural yield strength (megapascal, MPa) (mean ± standard deviation, SD); (*b*), flexural modulus (gigapascal, GPa) (mean ± SD).

strength loss more closely matches mass loss. The slow surface release of nearly pH-neutral degradation products gradually over time during the implant life-span will be less of a burden on local tissue clearance capability. This could be a real advantage in fracture fixation.

Absorbable amorphous thermoplastic poly(orthoesters) based on two diols (*trans*-cyclohexanedimethanol and 1,6-hexanediol) and a diketene acetal (3,9-bis ethylidene 2,4,8,10-tetraoxaspiro [5,5] undecane) have been synthesized. The polymer is more hydrophobic in comparison to poly(alpha-hydroxy acid) polymers such as PGA and PLLA, and hot-molded bulk samples undergo initial surface hydrolysis. The pH of accumulated degradation products in a limited quantity of exposure media is nearly pH neutral and less toxic in comparison to the accumulated acidic degradation products of PGA and PLLA as determined by the bacterial bioluminescence acute toxicity test. However, the initial mechanical properties and *in vitro* mechanical loading studies show POE alone to be a possibly inadequate material for fracture-fixation devices for long bone fixation. Reinforcement of POE with absorbable fibers may be necessary for the use of POE in mechanical stabilization of hard tissues.

Totally absorbable composite systems have been fabricated using randomly oriented, crystalline microfibers of calcium-sodium-metaphosphate for isotropic reinforcement. CSM/90:10 POE composites prepared with diamine-silane-treated microfibers have initial mechanical properties similar to cortical bone. The composite is deformable at temperatures above the polymer's T_g (98°C), but is rigid at body temperature (37°C); this could prove to be a unique and very useful property for certain orthopedic applications. The component materials show no acute cytotoxicity as determined by tissue culture agar overlay. A hot-molded 60:40 POE coating slows loss of composite strength and stiffness enough to suggest that this composite material is a viable candidate for further consideration for fabrication of low-load bone and soft tissue fixation devices.

ACKNOWLEDGMENTS

Support was provided by Technology and Ventures Division, Baxter Health Care, Incorporated, Irvine, California; Osteotech, Incorporated, Shrewsbury, New Jersey; by SRI International, Menlo Park, California; and the Orthopedic Bioengineering Laboratory at the University of Utah School of Medicine, Salt Lake City, Utah.

REFERENCES

1. Bradley, G.W., G.B. McKeena, H.K. Dunn, A.U. Daniels, and W.O. Statton, Effects of flexural rigidity of plates on bone healing. *J. Bone Jt. Surg.*, 61A(6):866–872 (1979).
2. Terjesen, T., and K. Apalest, The influence of different degrees of stiffness of fixation plates on experimental bone healing. *J. Ortho. Res.*, 6:293–299 (1988).
3. Woo, S.L.-Y., W.H. Akeson, R.D. Coutts, L. Rutherford, D. Doty, G.F. Jemmott, and D.A. Akeson, A comparison of cortical bone atrophy secondary to fixation with plates with large differences in bending stiffness. *J. Bone Jt. Surg.*, 15A:190–195 (1976).
4. Daniels, A.U., M.K.O. Chang, K.P. Andriano, and J. Heller, Mechanical properties of biodegradable polymers and composites proposed for internal fixation of bone. *J. Appl. Biomater.*, 1:57–78 (1990).
5. Gogolewski, S., Resorbable polymers for internal fixation. *Clin. Mater.*, 10:13–20 (1992).
6. Li, S., H. Garreau, and M. Vert, Structure-property relationships in the case of the degradation of massive aliphatic poly(alpha-hydroxy acids) in aqueous media, Part 1: Poly(DL-lactic acid). *J. Mater. Sci.: Mater. Med.*, 1:123–130 (1990).
7. Li, S., H. Garreau, and M. Vert, Structure-property relationships in the case of the degradation of massive poly(alpha-hydroxy acids) in aqueous media, Part 2: Degradation of lactide-glycolide copolymers: PLA37.5GA25 and PLA75GA. *J. Mater. Sci.: Mater. Med.*, 1:131–139 (1990).
8. Li, S., H. Garreau, and M. Vert, Structure-property relationships in the case of the degradation of massive poly(alpha-hydroxy acids) in aqueous media, Part 3: Influence of morphology on poly(L-lactic acid). *J. Mater. Sci.: Mater. Med.*, 1:198–206 (1990).
9. Therin, M., P. Christel, S. Li, H. Garreau, and M. Vert, *In vivo* degradation of massive poly(alpha-hydroxy acids): Validation of *in vitro*. *Biomaterials*, 13:594–600 (1992).

10. Suganuma, J., and H. Alexander, Biological response of intramedullary bone to poly-L-lactic acid. *J. Appl. Biomater.*, 4:12–27 (1993).

11. Verheyen, C.C.P.M., J.R. de Wijn, C.V. van Blitterswijk, P.M. Rozing, and K. de Groot, Examination of efferent lymph nodes after two years transcortical implantation of poly(L-lactide) containing plugs: A case report. *J. Biomed. Mater. Res.*, 27:1115–1118 (1993).

12. Böstman, O., Intense granulomatous inflammatory lesions associated with absorbable internal fixation devices made of polyglycolide in ankle fractures. *Clin. Orthop.*, 178–199 (1992).

13. Böstman, O., Foreign-body reactions to fracture fixation implants of biodegradable synthetic polymers. *J. Bone Jt. Surg.* [*Br.*], 72-B:592–596 (1990).

14. Böstman, O., Osteolytic changes accompanying degradation of absorbable fracture fixation implants. *J. Bone Jt. Surg.* [*Br.*], 73-B:679–682 (1991).

15. Böstman, O., E. Partio, E. Hirvensalo, and P. Rokkanen, Foreign-body reactions to polyglycolide screws. Observation in 24/216 malleolar fracture cases. *Acta Ortho. Scand.*, 63:173–176 (1992).

16. Böstman, O., Current concepts review absorbable implants for the fixation of fractures. *J. Bone Jt. Surg.*, 73A:148–153 (1991).

17. Rozema, R.M., R.R.M. Bos, G. Boering, C.J.P. Schoots, W.C. de Bruijn, A.J. Nijenhuis, and A.J. Pennings, Late tissue response to bone-plates and screws of poly(L-lactide) used for fixation of zygomatic fractures. *Trans. Ninth Europ. Conf. on Biomater.*, 9:154 (1991).

18. Laurencin, C., C. Morris, H. Pierri-Jacques, E. Schwartz, and L. Zou, The development of bone-bioerodible polymer composites for skeletal tissue regeneration: Studies of initial cell adhesion. *Trans. Ortho. Res. Soc.*, 36:183 (1990).

19. Törmälä, P., J. Vasenius, S. Vainionpää, J. Laiho, T. Pohjonen, and P. Rokkanen, Ultra-high-strength absorbable self-reinforced polyglycolide (SR-PGA) composite rods for internal fixation of bone fragments: *In vitro* and *in vivo* study. *J. Biomed. Mater. Res.*, 25:1–22 (1991).

20. Matsusue, Y., T. Yamauro, M. Oka, Y. Shikinami, S.-H. Hyon, and Y. Ikada, *In vitro* and *in vivo* studies on bioabsorbable ultra-high-strength poly(L-lactide) rods. *J. Biomed. Mater. Res.*, 26:1553–1567 (1992).

21. Tunc, D., and B. Jadhav, Development of absorbable, ultra high strength poly(lactides). *Polymer Science Technology, Progress in Biomedical Polymers*, 39:239–248 (1990).

22. Casper, R.L., B.S. Kelley, R.L. Dunn, A.G. Potter, and D.N. Ellis, Fiber-reinforced absorbable composite for orthopedic surgery. *Polym. Mater. Sci. Eng.*, 53:497–501 (1985).

23. Kelley, B.S., R.L. Dunn, and R.A. Casper, Totally resorbable high-strength composite material. *Polymer Science Technology, Advances in Biomedical Polymers*, 35:75–85 (1987).

24. Zimmerman, M., J.R. Parson, and H. Alexander, The design and analysis of a laminated partially degradable composite bone plate for fracture fixation. *J. Biomed. Mater. Res.: Appl. Biomater.*, 21(A3):345–361 (1987).

25. Heller, J., Poly(ortho esters). *Advances in Polymer Sciences*, 107:43–92 (1993).

26. Heller, J., D.W.H. Penhale, B.K. Fritzinger, and S.Y. Ng, Controlled release of contraceptive agents from poly(ortho esters). *Cont. Del. Sys.*, 4:43–53 (1983).

27. Heller, J., and K. Himmelstein, Poly(ortho esters) biodegradable polymer systems. *Methods of Enzymol.*, 112:422–436 (1985).

28. Heller, J., Control of polymer erosion by the use of excipients. In *Polymers in Medicine II*, E. Chielini, P. Giusti, C. Migliaresi, and L. Nicolais, eds. New York: Plenum Press, pp. 357–368 (1986).

29. Andriano, K.P., A.U. Daniels, and J. Heller, Characterization of poly(ortho ester) films for use as surgical implants. *Trans. Ortho. Res. Soc.*, 17(1):89 (1992).

30. Ng, S.Y., D.W.H. Penhale, and J. Heller, Poly(ortho esters) by the addition of diols to a diketene acetal. *Macromol. Synth.*, 11:23–26 (1992).

31. Heller, J., S.Y. Ng, D.W.H. Penhale, B.K. Fritzinger, L.M. Sanders, R.A. Burns, A.G.

Gaymon, and S.S. Bhosale, The use of poly(ortho esters) for the controlled release of 5-fluoracil and a LHRH analogue. *J. Cont. Rel.*, 6:217–224 (1987).

32. Engelberg, I., and J. Kohn, Physics-mechanical properties of degradable polymers used in medical applications: A comparative study. *Biomaterials*, 12:291–304 (1991).

33. American Society for Testing and Materials, *ASTM D 790-81*. Standard test methods for flexural properties of unreinforced and reinforced plastics and electrical insulating materials. Philadelphia: American Society for Testing and Materials (1981).

34. Smutz, W.P., A.U., Daniels, K.P. Andriano, E.P. France, and J. Heller, Mechanical test methodology for environmental exposure testing of biodegradable polymers. *J. Appl. Biomater.*, 2:13–22 (1991).

35. Cochran, G.V.B., *A Primer of Orthopedic Biomechanics*. New York: Church Livingstone (1982).

36. Schoenborn, C.A., Health habits of U.S. adults. *Public Health Reports*, 101(6):571–580 (1986).

37. B. Monzyk, Phosphate fiber: A unique reinforcement. *Plast. Compound.*, 42–46 (September–October 1986).

38. Nair, R.S., *In vitro* and *in vivo* toxicity and biodegradation studies of phosphate fiber. Presented at the Society of Automotive Engineers, Atlantic City, NJ, October 1986.

39. Plueddemann, E.P., *Silane Coupling Agents*. New York: Plenum Press (1982).

40. Van Wazer, J.R., Phosphorus and Its Compounds. New York: Wiley Interscience (1958).

41. Autian, J., Toxicological evaluation of biomaterials: Primary acute toxicity screening program. *Artif. Org.*, 1:53–60 (1977).

42. Andriano, K.P., A.U. Daniels, W.P. Smutz, R.W.B. Wyatt, and J. Heller, Preliminary biocompatibility screening of several biodegradable phosphate fiber reinforced polymers. *J. Appl. Biomater.*, 4:1–12 (1993).

43. Daniels, A.U., M.O.K. Chang, K.P. Andriano, and J. Heller, Toxicity and mechanical properties of a degradable poly(ortho ester). *Trans. Soc. Biomater.*, 12:235 (1989).

44. Spenelhauer, G., M. Vert, J.P. Benoit, and A. Boddaert, *In vitro* and *in vivo* degradation of poly(D,L-lactide/glycolide) type microspheres made by solvent evaporation method. *Biomaterials*, 7:557–563 (1939).

45. Burton, S.A., R.V. Peterson, S.N. Dickman, and J.R. Nelson, Comparison of *in vitro* bacterial bioluminescence and tissue culture bioassays and *in vivo* tests for evaluating acute toxicity. *J. Biomed. Mater. Res.*, 20:827–838 (1986).

46. Daniels, A.U., K.P. Andriano, B.A. Felix, and E.A. Hamber, The effect of pH and buffer solutions on the bacterial bioluminescence test for acute toxicity. *Trans. Soc. Biomater.*, 14: 110 (1991).

47. Pistner, H., D. Bendix, J. Muhling, and J. Reuther, Poly(L-lactide): A long-term degradation study *in vivo*. Part III. Analytical characterization. *Biomaterials*, 14:291–298 (1993).

48. Evans, F.G., *Mechanical Properties of Bone*. St. Louis: Charles J. Thomas (1973).

49. Reiley, D.T., The mechanical properties of cortical bone. *J. Bone Jt. Surg.*, 56A:1001–1022 (1974).

50. Kelley, B.S., R.L. Dunn, T.E. Jackson, A.G. Potter, and D.N. Ellis, Assessment of strength loss in biodegradable composites. *Proc. Third World Biomaterials Congress*, 471 (1988).

12
Fiber-Reinforced Composite Biomaterials for Orthopedic Implant Applications

Robert A. Latour, Jr.
Clemson University
Clemson, South Carolina

I. INTRODUCTION

Synthetic biomaterials are used in a wide variety of orthopedic implant applications to augment and/or replace components of the musculoskeletal system. For any implant material and application, two equally important aspects must be considered: the ability of the material to carry out its intended function (chemically, physically, and mechanically), and the response of the body to the presence of the implant (both locally and systemically). The important aspects of structural orthopedic biomaterials' behavior are primarily the properties of ultimate strength, fatigue strength, stiffness, wear, and durability. The important aspects of biologic response to implant materials include local and systemic inflammatory responses (physiologic biocompatibility) and the response of the skeleton to altered stress/strain fields surrounding the implant (mechanical biocompatibility).

Metals, polymers, and ceramics are the materials most commonly used today in orthopedic implant applications. While the use of these material systems can be considered to be very successful overall, there remain many applications in which their performance, in terms of either material behavior or biologic response, is suboptimal.

While surgical-grade metals, metal alloys, and ceramics possess high strength and excellent mechanical property retention *in vivo*, in many applications their approximately 10-fold higher modulus compared with cortical bone causes stress-shielding-induced bone resorption, potentially contributing to implant failure or bone fracture [1,2]. The loss of bone in the proximal femur due to the use of rigid metallic femoral components in hip joint arthroplasty can be particularly problematic for cases requiring revision surgery as the remaining bone stock may be insufficient to support the new femoral stem properly [3–5]. In temporary implant applications, such as in the case of fracture fixation, metallic implants often must be removed following bony union, requiring a second surgery and the risk of associated complications.

359

Polymeric materials exhibit material properties obviously very different from ceramics and metals. These materials are more compliant than cortical bone, have insufficient strength for high-load-bearing applications, and are susceptible to fatigue failure and dramatic changes in geometry over time due to cold flow or creep. Polymers are therefore limited to use in relatively low-level load-bearing applications. For example, relatively recently, absorbable polymeric biomaterials have been developed for fracture fixation. However, because of low strength, devices made from these materials are limited to only very low load-bearing applications.

As well stated in the old axiom "necessity is the mother of invention," the material limitations of metals, ceramics, and polymers have led to the development of fiber-reinforced polymer (FRP) composite biomaterials as a relatively new class of biomaterial for the treatment of musculoskeletal problems in ways that cannot be accomplished with conventional materials.

II. FIBER-REINFORCED POLYMER COMPOSITES IN ORTHOPEDIC APPLICATIONS

A. Overview

Fiber-reinforced polymer composites can be designed to possess a wide range of elastic moduli and strengths, ranging from those of bulk polymer to structural metal alloys. Because of this flexibility, composite materials possess great potential for development as structural orthopedic implant materials that are potentially strong and rigid enough to provide skeletal structural support, while being compliant enough to minimize stress shielding in the surrounding bone tissue. In addition to the use of FRP composites as an alternative to metallic implants, fiber reinforcement has also been investigated as a means of improving the mechanical properties of bulk polymers for various orthopedic implant applications. Bulk polymeric materials used in load-bearing orthopedic applications are placed under high stresses relative to their ultimate properties, often resulting in component failure due to wear, creep, and fracture [6–8]. Fiber reinforcement of polymers, therefore, presents a potential method of improving properties of fracture, creep, and wear resistance, thus reducing the incidence of implant failure.

FRP materials are being considered for orthopedic use primarily in four areas of application. As a potential improvement over metal implants, FRP composites are being considered for use as fracture-fixation devices and as femoral components for total hip arthroplasty (THA). As a means of improving mechanical properties of present-day polymeric biomaterials, fiber reinforcement has been investigated to improve the performance of polymethylmethacrylate (PMMA) bone cement and ultra-high molecular weight polyethylene (UHMWPE) articulation components. The following paragraphs summarize the use of FRP composite materials in each of these areas.

B. Fracture Fixation

Skeletal fractures often require surgical intervention to realign and stabilize the bone fragments to enable the normal healing processes to occur. One of the most commonly used methods of internal fixation is fracture-fixation plating. Internal fracture-fixation plates currently in clinical use are primarily made of high-strength, corrosion-resistant, 316L-grade stainless steel. These plates provide very rigid fixation to the fracture site. However, because plate modulus is approximately 10 times that of cortical bone (stainless

steel = 200 gigapascal [GPa], cortical bone = 18 GPa), a high degree of stress shielding, and subsequent osteoporosis, can occur in the cortical bone beneath the plate
[2,9,10].

Stress analysis has shown that the use of these high modulus plates can result in a
45% decrease in stress in the cortical bone beneath the plate [2]. *In vivo* studies in dogs
have shown the occurrence of cortical thinning and increased porosity beneath rigid
fixation plates applied to femoral fractures, with the degree of cortical thinning and
porosity increasing even as late as 9 to 12 months postoperation [10]. The clinical significance of plate-induced osteoporosis is the weakening of bone at the fracture site, which
can increase the incidence of refracture following plate removal [10-12]. This contributes
to the need for plate removal following fracture healing, after which the fracture site
must be protected for several months in order to allow the bone at the fracture site to
undergo proper remodeling to achieve its original strength [2].

A widely restated misconception concerning plate-induced stress shielding is that
stress shielding would be prevented if the modulus (longitudinal) of a fracture-fixation
plate was made to be equivalent to cortical bone. In actuality, however, the simple fact
that a plate coupled to a bone will carry some of the applied load, and thus the bone will
not carry the full load, indicates that some level of stress shielding will occur whenever a
fracture-fixation plate is fastened to a bone. In this situation, the degree of stress shielding
will decrease proportionately to the decrease in plate modulus; however, it will not be
zero until the plate stiffness actually decreases to zero. This statement is supported by the
following simplified mechanical analysis and the illustration in Fig. 1.

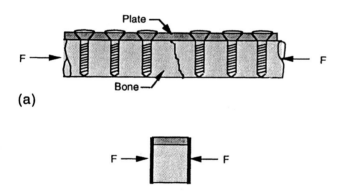

(a)

(b)

Figure 1   Stress shielding: (*a*), illustration of a fracture-fixation plate fixing a long bone fracture;
(*b*), illustration of the middle segment under axial loading with assumption that bone/plate construct deforms such that plane cross sections remain plane after deformation. Because the plate will
always carry a portion of the applied load, the plate will always partially stress shield the underlying
bone. Stress shielding will decrease as a continuous function that is proportional to plate modulus,
and will not be eliminated unless the plate modulus equals zero. An "isoelastic" plate with axial
modulus equal to cortical bone is therefore not a special, or even necessarily a desirable, condition,
but rather only one condition on a continuously varying relationship between plate induced stress
shielding and plate stiffness. Composite plates provide ability to tailor plate stiffnesses to a much
greater extent than with macroscopically homogeneous isotropic materials like metals.

If an applied load F is shared between the bone and plate with the force carried in each component expressed as the average stress times its cross-sectional area, then force balance requires

$$F = F_b + F_p = \sigma_b A_b + \sigma_p A_p \tag{1}$$

where

σ = stress
A = cross-sectional area, and
b and p = the bone and plate, respectively.

Based upon the simplifying assumption that plane sections remain plane after the application of load F, the longitudinal strain in the plate must be equal to the longitudinal strain in the bone. Therefore, assuming a condition of uniaxial stress,

$$\epsilon = \frac{\sigma_b}{E_b} = \frac{\sigma_p}{E_p}; \quad or \quad \sigma_p = \frac{E_p}{E_b}\sigma_b \tag{2}$$

Substituting Eq. 2 into Eq. 1 and rearranging,

$$F = \sigma_b A_b + \frac{E_p}{E_b}\frac{A_p}{A_b}\sigma_b A_b = \sigma_b A_b\left[1 + \frac{E_p}{E_b}\frac{A_p}{A_b}\right];$$

$$\sigma_b = \frac{F}{A_b}\left[\frac{E_b A_b}{E_b A_b + E_p A_p}\right] = (\sigma_b)_n\left[\frac{E_b A_b}{E_b A_b + E_p A_p}\right] \tag{3}$$

where $(\sigma_b)_n$ stands for the normal level of stress carried by the bone segment when no plate is present. Equation 3 therefore represents the stress level in the bone when the plate is present as a function of the normal stress level in the bone and the stiffnesses (EA) of the plate and bone. Equation 3 can be rearranged to express the percent stress shielding as a ratio of the change in normal stress in the bone divided by the normal stress level:

$$\% \text{ stress shielding} = \left(1 - \frac{\sigma_b}{(\sigma_b)_n}\right) \times 100\% = \left[1 - \frac{E_b A_b}{E_b A_b + E_p A_p}\right] \times 100\% \quad or$$

$$\% \text{ stress shielding} = \left[\frac{E_p A_p}{E_b A_b + E_p A_p}\right] \times 100\% \tag{4}$$

Thus, as indicated in Equation 4, whenever a plate is applied to bone, some degree of stress shielding will occur. Also, it must be understood that the degree of stress shielding is dependent upon the relative plate stiffness, and is just as dependent upon the plate cross-sectional area (geometric property) as it is upon the plate longitudinal modulus (material property). Therefore, the only condition in which no stress shielding will occur is when either the plate modulus or cross-sectional area is equal to zero or, in other words, when a plate is not present at all. The concept of the development of low modulus fracture-fixation plates to address stress shielding is valid in terms of decreasing stress shielding; however, plates to address stress shielding are valid in terms of decreasing stress shielding, but not in terms of totally preventing stress shielding. As evident by Eq. 4, the relationship between percent stress shielding and plate stiffness is a continuous function that does not exhibit any local maximum or minimum points. Thus, the concept of designing a fracture-fixation plate to possess the identical longitudinal elastic modulus of cortical bone will not represent some ideal or special condition for the avoidance of stress shielding, as is often misstated in the literature, but rather only represents one point on a continuous function between stress shielding and implant stiffness. In the design of compliant fracture-fixation plates to avoid stress shielding, the optimum design will be determined by finding the level of stiffness that will induce the least amount of stress shielding to the underlying bone while providing sufficient stiffness for fracture stability.

While plate-induced stress shielding is a concern and contributes to fracture site weakening due to bone resorption, other factors, such as plate-induced disruption to the periosteal blood circulation and the presence of screw holes, also contribute to the weakening of bone at a fracture site. Thus, even if plate-induced stress shielding could be completely avoided, the fracture site would still require protection following plate removal to enable the bone to remodel and regain normal strength levels.

The ideal situation for fracture fixation, although not yet realized for high-load-bearing conditions, would be to develop an implant that can initially impose the necessary degree of fracture stabilization to promote rapid fracture union, and then gradually and biocompatibly absorb into the body, allowing for controlled stress transfer to the healed fracture and gradual transitioning of the bone toward its normal state following fracture healing. This would promote rapid fracture union while eliminating the occurrence of bone resorption due to postunion stress shielding [2,9,10] and, more importantly, would also eliminate the need of a second operation for plate removal following complete healing at the fracture site [13].

Figure 2a illustrates the ideal situation for a fracture-fixation device in which the implant stiffness decreases over time proportionately to the amount of stiffness that the healing fracture recovers. This same illustration is often wrongly portrayed as the ideal situation for implant strength versus bone strength as a function of time. This again is a misconception as it would certainly be more advantageous for the implant strength to remain at a maximum level for at least as long as it takes for the fractured bone to regain full strength. This situation is illustrated in Fig. 2b. As composite materials can be potentially designed with more flexibility to control strength and stiffness separately compared with homogeneous materials, it may be useful to at least indicate the true ideal

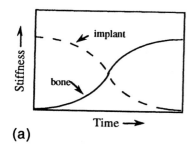

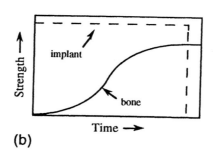

(a)   (b)

Figure 2 Illustration of the ideal situation for design of a fracture-fixation device: (*a*), to provide adequate stability, the plate should be initially stiff, and then decrease in stiffness with time as bone heals and stiffens in order to transfer applied load to bone (i.e., prevent stress shielding); (*b*), implant strength does not cause stress shielding, and the stronger the implant, the better the protection against bone refracture will be. Therefore, ideally, the implant should maintain at least a minimum level of strength sufficient to prevent implant failure in all patients and not lose strength until the fractured bone fully regains its normal strength and stiffness level. Ideally, there is no benefit for implant strength to decrease with time prior to complete healing of the fractured bone.

case of maintaining implant strength as high and as long as possible to prevent *in vivo* fatigue fracture.

In efforts to develop internal fracture fixation more closely approaching this idealized condition compared with that achieved by the use of metallic plates, researchers have been investigating the use of FRP composite materials. Designs have included absorbable plates using bioabsorbable matrix and fibers [13], with the goal of providing initial rigid fracture fixation without the need for implant retrieval and low modulus, nonabsorbable, short-fiber, molded plates [2,14], and continuous-fiber FRP laminated plates with various ply orientations and percentage of fiber fill [9,11,15–17] designed to minimize stress shielding. The nonabsorbable plates, however, still have the significant drawback of the need for a second surgical procedure for implant retrieval.

The most widely used materials for absorbable fracture-fixation devices are those that were initially developed for absorbable sutures and made from alpha-polyesters: polyglycolic acid (PGA), polylactic acid (PLA), and polyparadioxanone (PDS) [18]. In 1962, a braided PGA material was first developed by American Cyanamid (Wayne, NJ). This material was commercialized as Dexon® in 1970 [19–21]. A few years later, in 1975, a copolymer of PGA/PLA was developed and marketed as an absorbable suture called Vicryl® [19]. Since this time, a great worldwide effort has been undertaken for the extension of this technology toward the development of absorbable devices for fracture-fixation devices [19].

The first use of PGA polymer for fracture-fixation devices was suggested by Schmitt and Polistina [22]. Some of the first reported uses of absorbable polymers for fracture-fixation devices were conducted in 1971 by Kulkarni et al. [23] and Getter et al. [24], who investigated the use of PLA rods, screws, and plates to treat mandibular fractures in dogs. From these studies, it was quickly realized that one of the primary limitations/problems of these materials was their lack of strength. This then led to numerous attempts to strengthen absorbable polymers through the use of fiber reinforcement. Christel et al. are apparently the first to report the use of fully absorbable composites (1980) with PGA fiber reinforced PLA plates for fracture fixation [25]. Numerous investigation followed and by 1990, over 40 different formulations of absorbable polymers, copolymers, and their composites were developed for fracture fixation. By 1990, two of these formulations were commercially available in the form of pins for cancellous bone fixation. These were made from self-reinforced (SR) PGA (BioFix®, Bioscience Ltd., Tampere, Finland), and PDS (Orthosorb®, Johnson & Johnson, Raynham, MA). Other companies are developing PLA-based absorbable fracture-fixation devices [21].

A brief description of some of the most commonly investigated absorbable polymers and fibers is presented next and their chemical formulas are presented in Table 1. PGA is the simplest linear aliphatic polyester of the absorbable polymers. PGA has a very high degree of crystallinity and was used for the development of the first synthetic absorbable suture. PGA is very hydrophilic, and rapidly hydrolyzes in the presence of water. PLA is the second most common semicrystalline absorbable polymer. PLA has a more hydrophobic character than PGA due to substitution of a methyl group in place of a hydrogen atom. PLA is a chiral molecule; it has two stereoisomeric forms, termed poly(L-lactic acid) (PLLA) and poly(D-lactic acid) (PDLA).

These two isomers are also sometimes combined as a copolymer of alternating mers of PLLA and PDLA acids (PDLLA). PLLA and PDLA are semicrystalline, while the copolymer PDLLA is amorphous due to the interference in molecular packing caused by

Table 1 Chemical Structures for Several Biodegradable Polymers

Polymer	Chemical structure
Polyglycolic acid	$(-O-CH_2-\overset{\displaystyle O}{\overset{\|}{C}}-)_n$
Polylactic acid	$(-O-\overset{\displaystyle CH_3}{\underset{\|}{C}H}-\overset{\displaystyle O}{\overset{\|}{C}}-)_n$
Poly-p-dioxanone	$(-O-(CH_2)_2-CH_2-O-CH_2-\overset{\displaystyle O}{\overset{\|}{C}}-)_n$
Poly-ε-caprolactone	$(-O-(CH_2)_5-\overset{\displaystyle O}{\overset{\|}{C}}-)_n$
Polyorthoester	
Poly-β-hydroxybutyrate	$(-\overset{\displaystyle O}{\overset{\|}{C}}-CH_2-\overset{\displaystyle CH_3}{\underset{\|}{C}H}-O-)_n$
Poly-β-hydroxyvalerate	$(-\overset{\displaystyle O}{\overset{\|}{C}}-CH_2-\overset{\displaystyle CH_2CH_3}{\underset{\|}{C}H}-O-)_n$
Poly-DTH-iminocarbonate	

the alternating isomers in the molecular structure. PLLA is the most commonly used type of PLA and has a significantly reduced rate of hydrolysis compared with PGA.

Copolymers of PGA/PLA are also often utilized. In these copolymers, the presence of PLLA significantly reduces the crystallinity of PGA to the point at which a 50:50 copolymer of PGA/PLA typically degrades in hydrous environments more rapidly than does pure PGA.

The third absorbable polymer borrowed from absorbable suture technology (the first two being PGA and PLA) for fracture-fixation application is poly-p-dioxanone (PDS) [26]. Interestingly, being creatures of habit, the acronym PDS is still widely used with this material for fracture-fixation device development even though it stands for Poly-Dioxanone Suture. Two other absorbable polymers closely related and also often paired as copolymers are poly-β-hydroxybutyrate (PHB) and poly-β-hydroxyvalerate (PHV). Other less widely used absorbable polymers being developed as potential absorbable composite matrix materials for the development orthopedic implant devices are poly-ε-caprolactone (PCL), poly-orthoester (POE), and tyrosine-dipeptide-derived polycarbonates (i.e., poly-DTH-iminocarbonate). These materials degrade more slowly than PGA, PLA, and PDS polymers, making them more attractive as polymer matrix materials for the development of fully absorbable composite materials for load-bearing fracture-fixation applications [21,27,28].

Several types of absorbable reinforcements have been investigated as a potential means of strengthening and stiffening absorbable polymers to enable their use to be extended into load-bearing fracture-fixation applications. Self-reinforced (SR) polymer composites have been made either by sintering absorbable suture fibers together or by the mechanical deformation of spherulitic crystalline structure. This has been investigated with PGA, PLAs, PDS, PHB, and several of their various copolymers [22,29,30]. One of the primary drawbacks to polymeric fibers is their very low compressive strength. Absorbable ceramic fibers and particulate reinforcements have therefore also been investigated. These include calcium phosphate glasses [31–37], bioglasses [38], and hydroxyapatite [38].

Reinforced polymer matrix composites have been produced from a very wide assortment of the above-listed reinforcements, polymers, and copolymers. Numerous *in vitro* and *in vivo* studies have been undertaken in attempts to investigate and understand better the mechanical degradation behavior and controlling variables of these composites. Degradation and absorption of these materials is generally considered to be by hydrolysis of the polymer chains by absorbed water. Water first must diffuse into the material and causes swelling due to the disruption of intermolecular bonding (van der Waals forces) within the material, thus "loosening" the internal structure. In the polyester family of materials, water is believed to cleave covalent bonds of the polyester groups within the polymer chains by hydrolysis, leading to decreased molecular weight and subsequent mass and strength loss of the material.

In addition to hydrolysis, comparison between *in vitro* and *in vivo* studies of the effect of exposure to physiologic saline versus subcutaneous and intramedullary *in vivo* environments suggests that *in vivo* degradation rates may be faster [39,40]. This may be due to enzymatic activity *in vivo* [41,42], or possibly be only due to the more dynamic nature of the *in vivo* environment involving assisted transport of water and degradation products by convection and mechanical loading/agitation of the material [43].

Absorption rates can be controlled by the chemical composition, structure, and processing of the polymer. Molecular weight distribution, cross-link density, and degree of crystallinity are key factors that are known to influence absorption rates, although there are many more variables that have a significant influence upon their behavior.

As is typical with the development of many types of new materials, the influence of many variables upon material performance makes it very difficult to make direct comparisons among the many studies reported in the literature. This condition is true for the absorbable polymers by themselves, and is further acerbated by the additional factors introduced with the use of fiber reinforcement to fabricate absorbable composites. Some of the many variables known to influence behavior are listed in Table 2.

In addition to these variables, other attempts have been made to control the degradation rate by the use of surface coatings [44,45] and siloxane coupling agents for fiber/matrix adhesion [36,37]. A relatively recent and very thorough literature search on the mechanical durability studies for absorbable polymers and composites has been reported by Daniels et al. [42]. Therefore, instead of reiterating this vast amount of data in this overview of absorbable composite materials, readers are referred to this source and others for particular mechanical durability results [19,22,29,30,34–48].

Table 2 Factors Influencing Degradation Behavior of Implant Devices Manufactured from Biodegradable Polymers

Material	Processing	Implant design	Environment	Surgical
Chemical composition	Temperature	Size	Storage conditions (temperature, moisture content, oxidation, aging)	Surgical team's skill
Average molecular weight	Pressure	Shape	Sterilization method (ethylene oxide, irradiation)	Implant handling
Molecular weight distribution	Cooling rates	Volume/surface area	Implant preparation (cutting, thermoforming)	Patient care
Percent crystallinity	Flow fields during molding		Implantation site	Patient physiology
Additives (i.e., monomer, oligomers, catalyst, pigments, plasticizers, antioxidants)	Machining			
Molecular and phase orientation				
Reinforcement volume fraction, aspect ratio, orientation, coupling agents				
Void volume				
Matrix and reinforcement anisotropic strengths, moduli, Poisson's ratios				
Matrix/reinforcement interface and/or interphase strength				
Residual stresses (expansion coefficient differences)				
Moisture diffusion coefficients				
Properties of degradation products				

367

Despite the considerable effort in developing absorbable materials for fracture fixation, the goal of producing absorbable composite materials with sufficient strengths, moduli, and durability to enable their use for anything but the fixation of non-load-bearing cancellous bone fractures and osteotomies still remains elusive. One of the primary problems cited that remains to be overcome is the development of sufficiently long-term hydrolytically stable interfacial bonding between the fiber and matrix [13,30,36–38]. This is a very difficult problem as the fiber/matrix interface is a high energy area of the material, which is often bonded by dipole-dipole or hydrogen-type van der Waals bonding with a high affinity for the highly polar water molecules. Thus, even in nonabsorbable composites, the interface is an area of the material readily susceptible to hydrolytic degradation [49–51].

In addition to this, with the use of absorbable fibers, obviously, as soon as the first layer of atoms/ions/molecules is hydrolyzed on the fiber surface, the fiber and matrix will become chemically debonded. This situation is similar to the problem initially encountered in the development of glass-fiber-reinforced thermoset composite materials for the marine industry for boat hull applications. In this situation, the problem was solved by the development of silane-based coupling agents, which are believed to form hydrolytically stable (at least in an equilibrium sense) covalent bonding between the fiber and matrix and shield the fiber from hydrolytic attack [52]. Although silane-based coupling agents have been investigated as a means of delaying the degradation of absorbable composite materials, it is apparent that the coupling agents utilized have not been able to protect the interface from rapid hydrolysis.

It therefore is perhaps necessary that a new class of coupling agents must be developed specifically for this application. If such biocompatible coupling agents can be engineered, it is foreseeable that someday all temporary implant devices may be manufactured from fully absorbable composite materials, and retrieval operations for device removal would only be undertaken to address cases of device failure, nonunion, or infection.

Of all the absorbable polymers, PGA and PLLA have been most widely studied in terms of mechanical durability and biocompatibility. Biocompatibility studies in tissue culture and in both subcutaneous and intramedullary sites in *in vivo* studies in laboratory animals have indicated that these materials apparently induce only mild, nonspecific inflammatory responses, and can be generally considered to create an acceptable biologic response [19,41,53]. However, as described below, clinical studies in human patients have revealed biocompatibility problems with these materials involving aseptic sinus tract formation in a substantial percentage of patients [54].

Although the number of investigations presenting research results with absorbable composite materials is too large to cover in detail, several interesting studies are addressed here. Zimmerman, Parsons, and Alexander have reported on a partially absorbable composite laminate plate using continuous carbon fiber with a PLA matrix [55]. Although possessing relatively high modulus and strength when dry (one-half the modulus of stainless steel and equal annealed flexural strength), this composite material was found to lose over 50% of its flexure modulus after only four weeks of saline immersion. *In vivo* experiments evaluating this plate design for femoral osteotomy fixation in a canine model resulted in hypertrophic nonunion in all four animals; following 10 weeks of implantation time, the plates were found to be extremely flexible due to extensive delamination of the laminate plies.

Several other investigation teams have reported on the clinical use of self-reinforced absorbable polymer composites in the form of pins, rods, and screws in low-load-bearing applications for the fixation of cancellous bone fractures and osteotomies [18,22,54,56–59]. Results with these materials have been very favorable, aside from the complication of aseptic sinus formation in approximately 6–9% of the cases. Sinus formation was found to occur similarly to the development of stitch sinus formation associated with the use of internal bioabsorbable suture materials made from these same polymeric materials. In patients exhibiting sinus formation, the implants were found to induce nonspecific foreign-body reactions with abundant foreign-body giant cells; however, in some cases, this response was also found in patients exhibiting an uneventful clinical course. Sinus formation is believed to occur as a result of the degradation products from the implant temporarily overwhelming the local tissue's ability to clear them. This was believed to occur in patients representing the tail end of a continuous spectrum of biologic responses to the implant within the patient population. Sinus formation was found to occur after bony union in all cases without any apparent complication to the healed fracture. These patients all completed asymptomatic recovery.

Thus, while bioabsorbable FRP composites have not yet been developed that are able to retain their mechanical integrity sufficiently long for usage in high-load-bearing applications, these materials have been shown to be effective for fracture management in low-load-bearing applications in which the implant primarily functions to hold bony segments in position until union is achieved. In such cases, substantial savings in time, cost, and surgical complications are provided by eliminating the need for retrieval surgery. While this application has been relatively successful, the problems of polymer degradation product clearance with these relatively small implants raises serious concern whether these same materials can be used in higher-load-bearing applications requiring larger implant designs, such as in large fracture-fixation plates and intramedullary nails. For these applications, more slowly absorbing polymeric biomaterials may have to be developed to avoid polymer degradation product clearance problems. Because tissue clearance ability should be proportional to vascularity, biocompatibility of these materials can be expected to be location dependent, as has been experienced clinically, with orthopedic applications likely being more problematic than use of the same materials in soft tissues with a much greater vascular and lymphatic system drainage for degradation products.

Low stiffness, nonabsorbable FRP composite materials have been investigated for use in high-load-bearing applications with the objective of reducing stress shielding in the surrounding bone [60–62]. Gillett et al. reported on the testing of a short-fiber-reinforced composite material (carbon fiber/nylon 6-10) for fracture fixation of midshaft femoral fractures in a canine model [2]. The composite was made with 30 weight percent (wt%) chopped fiber and possessed a flexural strength equivalent to cortical bone, and a flexural modulus about one-half that of bone. In this study, rapid fracture union was established with the plates. The plates were removed following a 16-week implantation period and mechanically tested to evaluate residual strength and stiffness. This revealed a 20% loss of plate flexural strength and 30% loss of flexural stiffness due to implantation.

Brown et al. have also investigated the use of 30 wt% chopped composite reinforced with carbon fiber (CF) to fabricate fracture-fixation plates using three different matrix materials: polysulfone (PSF), polybutylene terephthalate (PBT), and polyetheretherketone (PEEK) [14,63]. Samples were fabricated and then immersed in physiologic saline for a three-week period, followed by mechanical testing for flexural strength and fracture toughness evaluation. In the dry condition, the flexural strength of the PSF, PBT, and

PEEK plates were found to be 178, 168, and 272 MPa, respectively, and the fracture toughness was measured to be 5.6, 4.7, and 7.4 MPa·m$^{1/2}$, respectively. The reinforced PSF and PBT composites each lost approximately 15% of flexural strength and 11% of fracture toughness following saline immersion, while the PEEK strength and toughness was not significantly different from the dry control condition. Thus, of these materials, CF/PEEK was determined to be the best candidate of the three composite systems in terms of mechanical performance for use as a nonabsorbable bone plate for fracture fixation. Clinical trials with short FRP composites remain to be conducted to determine if these materials are mechanically suitable for high-load-bearing fracture-fixation applications, with insufficient fatigue strength being a possible limitation.

Continuous fiber-reinforced polymer composites can be made with mechanical strength much greater than short-fiber composites, and are most likely the best candidates for successful development of nonabsorbable intermediate modulus, high strength fracture fixation plates. Woo et al. reported on a study involving a 55 volume percent (vol%) carbon-fiber-reinforced polymethylmethacrylate (CF/PMMA) composite laminate with alternating ±35° plies for use in fracture fixation of radii in dogs [17]. The composite fracture plates were reported to possess a modulus 10% of that of stainless steel, with a flexural strength about 50% of that of equally sized stainless steel plates. Fracture healing was reported to be equivalent, if not superior, to that achieved with stainless steel plates. Following only 16 weeks of implantation, however, plate flexural strength was found to be decreased by 40%, raising the question of whether the *in vivo* fatigue strength of this plate design would be adequate for load-bearing fracture fixation in humans.

Ekstrand et al. also investigated the dry-versus-wet mechanical behavior of a CF/PMMA composite [62]. The flexural strength was measured for samples exposed to either a 37°C dry environment or immersion in 37°C distilled water for periods up to three months. In agreement with Woo et al.'s findings, this material again exhibited a significant drop in strength following wet environment conditioning. Fracture surfaces were evaluated by scanning electron microscopy (SEM) for each sample group. Fractographic analysis of the samples suggested that the drop in mechanical strength was due to the degradation of the interfacial bond strength by hydrolysis.

Another continuous fiber composite plate made with carbon fiber and epoxy has been reported [11,16]. This plate was based upon a $[0/+45/0/-45]_s$ laminate design [62]. This design provided a high strength composite plate with ultimate flexural strength reported to be 10% greater than the yield strength of a similarly sized stainless steel plate, and with the fatigue strength at two million fully reversed fatigue cycles reported to be 67% greater than the stainless steel plate. Composite plate fatigue failure occurred by delamination versus catastrophic failure. Even with these exceptional properties, Bradley reported that veterinary and clinical trials revealed that the composite plates were operating at the borderline of acceptable strength and rigidity [16].

In a 20-patient clinical trial of these plates, midshaft tibial fractures were plated with two different plate designs. For the first plate design used with seven patients, three of the seven patients complained of severe aching pain, presumed to be due to insufficient rigidity of the plate, which allowed excessive motion at the fracture site. A second design with increased stiffness performed more satisfactorily. The two types of plates were mechanically tested to compare their bending stiffnesses to those for standard stainless steel plates.

Results showed that the first and second plate designs had 43% and 53% of the stiffness of an AO stainless steel DCP plate, respectively. Tibial fractures were found to heal satisfactorily with both types of composite plate. The results of this clinical trial indicate that, while intermediate modulus plates may be advantageous to reduce stress shielding in the surrounding bone and may result in fracture healing equal to that achieved by rigid plates, the degree of allowable plate compliance (and thus the degree of prevention of stress shielding) will be dictated by patient comfort. Thus, the encouraging results with extremely flexible plates in canine studies may not be representative of a situation that will be tolerable in human patients because of severe fracture site pain induced by compliant fixation and subsequent excessive motion at the fracture site.

This situation presents somewhat of a 'catch 22' situation for the development of nonabsorbable, relatively compliant, FRP fracture-fixation devices. The incentive for the development of these implants is that of reducing stress shielding in the surrounding bone following fracture union. It is quite possible, however, that, in order to reduce stress shielding significantly, the rigidity of the implant must be reduced to such an extent that patient discomfort will prohibit its use under high-load-bearing conditions. Thus, the implants may only be suited for use in fracture fixation for the upper extremities and other relatively low-load-bearing areas of the body compared with long bones of the lower extremities. However, because these areas are not highly load bearing, the problem of stress shielding is no longer relevant or relevant only to a relatively small degree. This question remains to be answered by further investigations.

C. Femoral Components for Total Hip Arthroplasty

When disease or trauma require the replacement of the hip joint, the femoral neck and head are removed and an artificial hip joint femoral component is implanted in their place. Femoral components are presently made from high-strength, corrosion-resistant metal alloys of stainless steel, cobalt chromium, and titanium. Current designs of the femoral component incorporate a long tapering stem to fit down the femoral canal and is used to secure the implant to the femur. Fixation of the stem within the canal is achieved by using PMMA bone cement as a grouting agent or by press fitting a canal-filling textured or porous-surfaced component within the intramedullary space. Cemented metallic femoral components are considered to have approximately 90% survivability at 10 years postimplantation, with implant failure generally due to cement breakdown and subsequent loosening.

This understanding has led to the development of the porous ingrowth concept as a means of achieving fixation without the use of bone cement, thus ideally creating a more durable implant. However, because of the greater cross-sectional area necessary to fill the intramedullary space, these designs result in implants with much greater stiffness compared with the cemented stems. Thus, while the problems due to cement breakdown have been avoided, problems associated with proximal stress shielding and subsequent bone resorption have developed in their place. Thus, one problem has been traded for another problem of potentially equal magnitude, with clinical results of one system not being overwhelmingly superior to those of the other [63].

The occurrence of the stress shielding phenomena in hip joint arthroplasty can be appreciated by considering load transfer through the hip joint in a normal joint (see Figs. 3a and 3b). In the normal hip joint, load is transferred from the joint articular surface to the femoral head, through the femoral neck and metaphysis, and then to the femoral shaft. This results in a relatively high stress environment throughout the proximal femur by load transmission of the full joint load directly down the axis of the neck and femur.

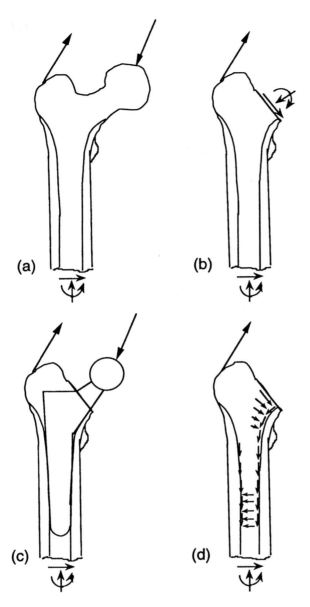

Figure 3   Illustration of the biomechanics of the transfer of hip joint load to the proximal femur. Each diagram illustrates the same abductor muscle force proximally and resultant shaft forces and moments distally, but show different loading situations for the transfer of joint load to the femur: (a), normal femur with joint applied to femoral head; (b), normal femur illustrating that applied joint load is transfered down the neck and must be fully supported by the base of the femoral neck and the calcar region; (c), femur with hip joint femoral component in place showing joint load acting on femoral head and the stem fixed within the femoral canal; (d), illustration depicting the nonphysiologic manner in which joint load is transferred to the femur by the femoral component. As with the fracture fixation plate, some degree of stress shielding will always be present with a femoral component, but will tend to decrease in the proximal femur as stem bending stiffness decreases. Thus, an "isoelastic" stem does not represent a unique case that will eliminate stress shielding, but rather only one point on a plot relating stem stiffness to proximal stress distribution.

When a stiff metal stem is inserted into the femoral canal to replace a diseased joint, much of the joint load is transferred directly to the femoral shaft by way of the stem, thus bypassing the metaphysis region of the proximal femur (see Figs. 3c and 3d). As a means of providing a cementless implant system for hip arthroplasty that does not induce a high level of stress shielding in the proximal femur and thus potentially providing a more durable artificial hip joint, low-stiffness FRP composite femoral components are being investigated.

FRP components can be made to be canal filling with axial and bending stiffnesses much less than similarly sized metal components, while potentially having sufficient fatigue strength for long-term use in this relatively high-load application. Because FRP composite stems are able to be produced with a much reduced stiffness, they are able to deform under applied load to a much greater extent than their metallic counterparts. Deformation of the femoral component allows a greater amount of the joint load to be transferred to the proximal femur, thus reducing the occurrence of stress-shielding-induced bone resorption in this area. As with the use of composite materials for the design of fracture-fixation devices, the literature abounds with statements that wrongly suggest that, if a femoral component is designed with a modulus equivalent to bone, then the problem of stress shielding would be completely alleviated. This is the concept behind the development of the so-called isoelastic hip joint prosthesis [64].

However, as indicated in Fig. 3, the mechanism of load transfer in an artificial hip joint is extremely nonphysiologic, and will always result in some degree of stress shielding in the proximal femur. In addition, stiffness of the implant is the important parameter to be addressed and is a function of both elastic modulus and geometry (cross-sectional area for axial stiffness and moment of inertia for bending stiffness). The more compliant the femoral component, the more it will deform under applied joint load, and thus higher loads will be applied to the proximal femur. However, due to the nonphysiologic mechanism of joint load transfer, some degree of stress shielding will occur, and matching the modulus of the stem material to that of cortical bone will not result in a unique and special situation, but rather only one point in a continuous relationship between stem material modulus and stress shielding given a set component geometry. As with fracture-fixation plates, concern also exists whether polymer matrix composite femoral components can be developed to possess adequate fatigue strength for this high-load application, especially in the rather aggressive physiologic environment.

Ainsworth, Tarr, and Claes have reported on the development of a composite hip stem using continuous carbon-fiber-reinforced polysulfone [1]. They reported that the ultimate and saline-immersed fatigue strengths of this design are equal to or greater than presently used designs made of titanium and cobalt alloys, while possessing a modulus of elasticity only 50% of that for titanium alloy and only 25% of that for cobalt alloy. They also studied the change in the stress field occurring in the proximal femur following implantation of femoral components using strain-gaged canine femurs. Upon the application of load, the composite component resulted in a strain distribution along the proximal femur more closely matching that of the normal (non-implant-containing) femur than did the stiffer metal alloy stems, thus suggesting lower degrees of stress shielding with the low stiffness stem.

Magee et al. reported upon an *in vivo* study of more than two years of another carbon-fiber-reinforced polysulfone (CF/PSF) composite femoral component composed of a uniaxial fiber core with an outer layer of bidirectional braided CF/PSF and a thin outer coating of pure polysulfone. The results of this study were also encouraging. The cortical thickness and density of the bone surrounding the implant were found to be unchanged compared with the contralateral control side (no implant), even after more than two years postoperation. In addition to this, the density of the cancellous bone in the metaphyseal area of the femur was found to increase in response to the implant. This is in direct contrast with results from other studies with stiff, porous-surface metal femoral components that have shown adverse bone remodeling and bone resorption even after only six-months postoperation [66].

Magee et al. concluded that the more compliant stem provided sufficient proximal stress transfer to result in constructive bone remodeling. This condition is considered highly beneficial as it serves to provide additional support to the implant. Unfortunately, this paper did not provide a comparison of the composite prosthesis with a metallic stem of equivalent geometry as a control. Therefore, it cannot be stated whether the beneficial results were due to component modulus or were only due to implant design geometry relative to the canine femur. Although mechanical testing of the composite stems was not reported in this paper, no visible evidence of delamination or microfracture was found upon retrieval, and no implant was reported to have failed *in vivo* up to 38-months postoperation in this study.

While the concept of lower modulus FRP femoral components providing an implant system with longer *in vivo* service life and lower rates of complication is very attractive and conceptually feasible, many development problems must be expected, as with any new material system and design. These will need to be addressed before the composite femoral components can be considered for widespread clinical use. Problems include how to fabricate stems economically from FRP composite, how to fix the implant adequately within the intramedullary canal, how the surrounding tissue will respond to the potential release of polymer and carbon-fiber particulate wear debris that may be generated from the implant if it abrades against the surrounding bone, and how to evaluate stem mechanical behavior mechanically (experimentally and analytically) to determine if fatigue resistance is sufficient for this relatively high-load application.

FRP composite stems are anisotropic components that must withstand complex and dynamic three-dimensional (3-D) loading for more than 15 years in the *in vivo* environment. These conditions greatly complicate the design of these components. Composite laminate theory has been primarily developed under assumptions of thin-plate-type geometry under in-plane loading conditions with out-of-plane stresses equal to zero. Thus, design and analysis can only be properly conducted by detailed, fully three-dimensional analyses such as with the use of 3-D finite-element models. The required thickness of a canal-filling FRP composite femoral component for THA dictates that the stem must contain upward of 120 plies. In order to model such thick composite laminated structures accurately, state-of-the-art sophisticated computers must be used, such as the former National Computer System's Cray supercomputer in Urbana, Illinois. Also, because of the multitude of possible ply layups that can be considered in the design of an FRP femoral stem (assuming a laminated design) and the fact that stem boundary conditions will be a function of the mode of implant fixation and the properties of the surrounding femur, implant design and optimization are very difficult problems requiring complex analytical modeling.

In addition to the difficulties in design and analysis of an FRP composite stem, there are also concerns about the long-term durability of FRP composite materials *in vivo* due to environmental degradation. Latour and Black [51,52] and Latour, Black, and Miller [67] have studied the behavior of the fiber/matrix interfacial bond in a CF/PSF composite, comparing dry strength with that following saturation in physiologic saline and inflammatory exudate. Results showed a 40% loss in ultimate bond strength following either saline or exudate saturation, and a fatigue life following saturation of only about 80,000 cycles under a peak stress level of only 15% of the dry bond strength level. Further studies by Meyer and Latour have demonstrated that CF/PEEK FRP composite material combinations may provide more durable interfacial bonding following long-term exposure in 37°C physiologic saline [68].

Spector et al. have reported similar findings in coupon tests of CF/PSF and CF/PEEK using a proprietary layup comparing dry versus saline-saturated samples [62]. Their results found that CF/PSF lost 45% and 44% of ultimate compressive and flexural strength, respectively. The CF/PEEK composite, however, was found to be more durable with only a 10% and 2% loss in ultimate compressive and flexure strength, respectively, following saturation. Contrary to these results, a subsequent study reported by Overland et al. found that CF/PSF laminates exhibited no significant loss in shear strength following simulated *in vivo* exposure, perhaps indicating that differences in laminate processing techniques may have a very significant effect on the environmental durability of these materials [69].

The excellent property retention of CF/PEEK laminates has further been documented in studies currently being conducted by the author and coworkers at Clemson University Department of Bioengineering, with little to no reduction in compressive, tensile, and shear strengths and modulus occurring up to 5000 hours of exposure in 95°C physiologic saline [70–72].

Biocompatibility of carbon fiber, polysulfone, and polyetheretherketone have been investigated in both *in vitro* and *in vivo* studies [61,73–75]. *In vitro* cell culture test results have shown excellent cellular biocompatibility of these materials, and *in vivo* tests in animal models have shown these materials to exhibit a nonspecific foreign-body response similar to that found with polymeric implant materials currently in use.

Clinical trials to evaluate the first generation of CF/PSF hip stems began in January 1990 (Silhouette Composite Hip Program, Biomet, Limited, Bridgend, South Glamorgan, United Kingdom). However, these trials have reportedly been discontinued due to problems of stem fracture *in vivo*. Thus, while the application for FRP composites as an orthopedic implant material is promising, at the present time much research remains to be conducted before they can be considered safe for widespread clinical use.

D. Reinforced Bone Cement

Polymethylmethacrylate (PMMA) is used as a bone cement for implant fixation in total joint arthroplasties, and is mixed and polymerized intraoperatively by the surgical team just prior to the time of application. The bone cement essentially consists of prepolymerized PMMA powder that is mixed with methylmethacrylate liquid monomer. Barium sulphate is also typically included in the powder to provide a measure of radiopacity to enable the cement mantle to be visible in radiographs. PMMA is particularly useful as a bone cement because of its relatively low-temperature *in situ* cure. This allows it to be mixed intraoperatively and pressurized within the bone cavity while still in a relatively viscous state during the early stages of polymerization.

Following the insertion of cement, the implant is pressed in position while the viscosity of the cement is still relatively low. This enables the cement to conform readily to both the bony architecture of the implant site and the contour of the implant to ensure intimate contact with minimal gap formation. The cement is then allowed to cure, which provides rapid, rigid fixation.

The use of PMMA bone cement for femoral component fixation has generally been very successful for periods of time of 10 to 15 years. PMMA, however, is a relatively brittle polymer and is susceptible to fatigue fracture *in vivo*. This has been associated with aseptic loosening of implants and the subsequent need for revision surgery [8,76,77].

Several investigators have evaluated fiber-reinforced bone cement (PMMA) with short fibers of carbon [8,76,78], polyaramid [76,79,80], stainless steel [81], titanium [82], ultra-high molecular weight polyethylene [83,84], and PMMA (self-reinforcement) [85] in order to improve its mechanical behavior. Results have shown that the addition of about 7 wt% or less of short reinforcing fibers (<1 centimeter [cm] in length) can result in about a 30% increase in ultimate tensile and compressive strength, 100% increase in modulus, and 75% increase in impact fracture toughness over bulk bone cement [78,80,82,83].

Fatigue tests under controlled load have shown that the incorporation of reinforcing fibers can increase the fatigue crack growth resistance by an order of magnitude over unreinforced cement [8]. Fractographic studies have shown that the increase in strength and toughness is primarily controlled by the behavior of the fiber/matrix interfacial bond [78,81]. The processes of interfacial debonding and fiber pull-out during fracture provide means of energy absorption and crack deflection that are not present in the bulk PMMA. These factors combine to decrease the overall notch sensitivity of the reinforced cement.

The problems associated with the use of fiber-reinforced PMMA are the difficulties in obtaining good fiber wetting and distribution within the polymer [79] and the decreased intrusion properties of the resulting bone cement [8,78]. In one study, Pourdeyhimi et al. reported that mixing problems actually resulted in a decreased flexural strength and modulus of polyaramid-reinforced bone cement [79]. The decrease in strength and modulus was associated with poor fiber distribution, poor fiber/matrix contact, and high void content within the cement.

The incorporation of fibers into the cement during the curing process has also been demonstrated to decrease the ability of the cement to flow into small orifices. Because of this, there is concern whether the reinforced cement will be able to intrude sufficiently into bony trabeculae to provide the necessary level of mechanical interlock to support the prosthesis [8,78]. Difficulties in PMMA mixing and intrusion increase in magnitude as the percent of fiber volume increases, and thus limits the amount of fiber reinforcement that can be incorporated in bone cement to improve its overall performance. This remains an active and important area of research, especially with the revived interest in PMMA fixation over the past five years due to problems associated with biological fixation via bony ingrowth.

E.   Reinforced Ultra-High Molecular Weight Polyethylene

Ultra-high molecular weight polyethylene (UHMWPE) is used as a low friction articulation surface in total joint arthroplasties. Although this material has proven to function very well in this application, it does experience wear, creep, and fracture *in vivo*, which can eventually lead to component failure. In addition to these mechanical problems, polyethylene wear debris is currently a very great concern in joint replacement due to adverse tissue reactions that have been associated with bone resorption and subsequent loss of implant fixation [6–8].

In an attempt to improve the mechanical properties of bulk UHMWPE and decrease wear debris, short-carbon-fiber-reinforced UHMWPE (CF/PE) articulation components have been evaluated in both clinical and analytical studies. Test samples taken from a commercially available CF/PE total knee tibial condyle component showed a fiber content of about 10 wt% randomly oriented within the UHMWPE matrix, with the carbon fibers being about 3 mm in length [8]. While the component manufacturer initially claimed that increased fatigue and creep resistance and decreased wear were achieved by the CF/PE composite material, subsequent independent research was unable to support these claims [86].

Several studies have reported that tensile fatigue tests comparing samples taken from the tibial condyles of total knee articulation components have shown the CF/PE material to possess about an order of magnitude higher fatigue crack growth rate than the bulk UHMWPE [6–8]. Fractographic studies revealed a brittle fracture surface with the composite as opposed to ductile failure with the bulk UHMWPE. The fracture surfaces of the composite showed little evidence of fiber fracture, with bare fibers protruding along the fracture surface indicative of low interfacial bond strength. The lower fatigue resistance of the composite material has been primarily attributed to low interfacial bond strength between the carbon fiber and UHMWPE. The combination of low bond strength and high matrix ductility was found to create a situation in which the fibers were unable to reinforce the matrix and instead acted as multiple stress concentration sites distributed throughout the material for the rapid initiation and propagation of fatigue cracks.

Latour and Meyer investigated interfacial bond strength between a high-strength carbon fiber and UHMWPE in physiologic saline using a single-fiber pull-out test technique to obtain a quantitative measure of CF/PE interfacial bond strength [87]. The ultimate bond strength was measured to be only 4.5 MPa, compared with a theoretical maximum achievable bond strength of 40 MPa based upon the ultimate tensile strength of UHMWPE. This finding agrees with the qualitative description of the CF/UHMWPE fracture surfaces implicating low interfacial bonding as a reason for poor material performance [6–8].

McKellop et al. reported upon the wear properties of bulk UHMWPE and CF/PE articulated against surgical-grade metal alloys and also found the composite to be inferior to the unreinforced material [86]. Wear rates with the CF/PE were found to be 1.8 to 8.6 times greater than the plain UHMWPE material. The increased wear could be associated with third-body wear resulting from broken pieces of the carbon fibers dislodged from the composite surface during the test.

While the fatigue crack growth and wear rates were found to be increased with the addition of carbon fibers to the UHMWPE, creep deformation was found to be reduced for a given loading condition. Unfortunately, due to the increased modulus of the CF/UHMWPE material, higher contact stresses may occur at the articulation surface in applications such as a total knee arthroplasty. The presence of the higher contact stresses will tend to increase the creep rate and thus may counteract the possible benefit of the composite material in this area [6,7].

Clinical trials with CF/UHMWPE tibial condyle components have substantiated the analytical studies, with no benefit being realized by the composite material compared with components made from plain UHMWPE [7,88]; this application has thus been discontinued. While CF has been determined not to be a viable candidate material for the reinforcement of UHMWPE to improve its performance as an articulation surface, other reinforcements that are tougher than CF and that bond well to UHMWPE may still have potential; this research area should not be totally abandoned because of the poor outcome of one attempt at matrix reinforcement.

III. SUMMARY

FRP composite materials have been shown to possess significant potential for use in orthopedic applications as both a structural material that is more biomechanically compatible with bone (thus reducing the adverse effects of stress shielding) and a means of potentially improving the mechanical properties of polymer presently used in bulk form. As demonstrated by the results of CF/PE, however, mechanical properties are not always improved through fiber reinforcement. In addition to this, the mechanical properties of many FRP composite material combinations (nonabsorbable) have been demonstrated to be degraded in physiologic environments.

These realizations serve to emphasize the complexities involved in designing composite materials and the importance of understanding the underlying factors that govern their mechanical behavior. These factors must be understood and applied in the process of material selection and component design in order to satisfy the demands of each specified application. Only then will the full potential of this class of materials be realized, enabling reliable composite materials to be designed and produced that are superior to materials currently in clinical use today in terms of both patient care and medical cost.

REFERENCES

1. Ainsworth, R.D., Tarr, R.R., and Claes, L., Methodology for the development of a composite materials hip replacement implant, *First International Conf. — Composites in Bio-Medical Engineering*, 23/1–7 (1985).
2. Gillett, N., Brown, S.A., Dumbleton, R.P., and Pool, R.P., The use of short carbon fiber reinforced thermoplastic plates for fracture fixation, *Biomaterials*, 6:113–121 (1985).
3. Callaghan, J.J., Total hip arthroplasty. A clinical perspective, *Clin. Orthop.*, 276:33–40 (1992).
4. Dorr, L.D., Luckett, M., and Conaty, J.P., Total hip arthroplasty in patients younger than 45 years, *Clin. Orthop.*, 260:215–219 (1990).
5. Engh, C.A., and Bobyn, J.D., The influence of stem size and extent of porous coating on femoral bone resorption after primary cementless hip arthroplasty, *Clin. Orthop.*, 231:7–28 (1988).
6. Connelly, G.M., Rimnac, C.M., Wright, T.M., Hertzsberg, R.W., and Manson, J.A., Fatigue crack propagation behavior of ultrahigh molecular weight polyethylene, *J. Orthop. Res.*, 2:119–125 (1984).
7. Wright, T.M., and Bartel, D.L., Carbon fiber-reinforced UHMWPE for total joint replacement components, *First International Conf. — Composites in Bio-Medical Engineering*, 21/1–21/4 (1985).
8. Wright, T.M., Connelly, G.M., Rimnac, C.M., Hertzberg, R.W., and Burstein, A.H., Carbon fiber reinforcement of polymeric materials for total joint arthroplasty. In *Biomaterial and Biomechanics 1983* (P. Ducheyne, G. Van der Perre, and A.E. Aubert, Eds.), pp. 67–72, Elsivier Sci. Publ. B.V., Amsterdam (1984).
9. Tayton, K., Johnson-Nurse, C., McKibbon, B., Bradley, J., and Hastings, G., The use of semi-rigid-carbon-fiber-reinforced plastic plates for fixation of human fractures: Results of preliminary trials, *J. Bone and Joint Surg.*, 64-B:105–111 (1982).
10. Woo, S. L.-Y., Akeson, W.H., Coutts, R.D., Rutherford, L., Doty, D., Jemmott, G.F., and

Amiel, D., A comparison of cortical bone atrophy secondary to fixation with plates with large differences in bending stiffness, *J. Bone and Joint Surg.*, 58-A:190–195 (1976).

11. Bradley, J.S., Hastings, G.W., and Johnson-Nurse, C., Carbon fiber reinforced epoxy as a high strength, low modulus material for internal fixation plates, *Biomaterials*, 1:38–40 (1980).

12. Hastings, G.W., and Thanh Thuy, N.G.T., Biomechanically compatible materials: Carbon fibre reinforced plastics. In *Biocomparability of Implant Materials* (D. Williams, Ed.), Pitman Publ. Corp., New York, pp. 128–133 (1976).

13. Kelley, B.S., Dunn, R.L., Jackson, T.E., Potter, A.G., and Ellis, D.N., Jr., Assessment of strength loss in biodegradable composites, *Trans. Society for Biomaterials*, 11:471 (1988).

14. Brown, S.A., Hastings, R.S., Mason, J.J., and Moet, A., Characterization of short-fiber reinforced thermoplastics for fracture fixation devices, *Biomaterials*, 11:541–547 (1990).

15. Akeson, W.H., Woo, S.L.-Y., Coutts, R.D., Matthews, J.V., Gonsalves, M., and Amiel, D., Quantitative histological evaluation of early fracture healing of cortical bones immobilized by stainless steel and composite plates, *Calcif. Tissue Res.*, 19:27–37 (1975).

16. Bradley, J.S., Cautionary note on the strength of materials for internal fixation devices, *Biomaterials*, 2:124 (1981).

17. Woo, S.L.-Y., Akeson, W.H., Levenetz, B., Coutts, R.D., and Matthews, J.V., Potential application of graphite fiber and methyl methacrylate resin composites as internal fracture fixation plates, *J. Biomed. Mater. Res.*, 8:321–338 (1974).

18. Bostmari, O.M., Current concepts review. Absorbable implants for the fixation of fractures, *J. Bone and Joint Surg.*, 73A:148–153 (1991).

19. Raiha, J.E., Biodegradable implants as intramedullary nails. A survey of recent studies and an introduction to their use, *Clinical Materials*, 10:35–39 (1992).

20. Frazza, E.J., and Schmitt, E.E., A new absorbable suture, *J. Biomed. Mater. Res. Symp.*, 1: 43–58 (1971).

21. Pulapura, S., and Kohn, J., Trends in the development of bioresorbable polymers for medical applications, *J. Biomaterials Applications*, 6:216–250 (1992).

22. Schmitt, E.E., and Polistina, R.A., Polyglycolic acid prothetic devices, U.S. Patent 3,463,158 (1969).

23. Kulkarni, R.K., Moore, E.G., Hegyeli, A.F., and Leonard, F., Biodegradable poly(lactic acid)polymers, *J. Biomed. Mater. Res.*, 5:169–181 (1971).

24. Getter, L., Cutright, D.E., Bhaskar, S.N., and Augsburg, J.-K., A biodegradable interosseous appliance in the treatment of mandibular fractures, *J. Oral. Surg.*, 30:344–348 (1972).

25. Christel, P., Chabot, F., Lray, J.L., Morin, C., and Vert, M., Biodegradable composite for internal fixation. In *Biomaterials 1980* (G.D. Winter, D.F. Gibbon, and H. Plenck, Eds.), pp. 271–280, John Wiley and Sons, New York (1982).

26. Hofmann, G.O., Biodegradable implants in orthopaedic surgery—A review on the state-of-the-art, *Clinical Materials*, 10:75–80 (1992).

27. Engelberg, I., and Kohn, J., Physico-mechanical properties of degradable polymers used in medical applications: A comparative study, *Biomaterials*, 12:292–304 (1991).

28. Knowles, J.C., Mahmud, F.A., and Hastings, G.W., Piezoelectric characteristics of a polyhydroxybutyrate-based composite, *Clinical Materials*, 8:155–158 (1991).

29. Törmälä, P., Vasenius, J., Vainionpää, S., Laiho, J., Pohjonen, T., and Rokkanen, P., Ultra-high-strength absorbable self-reinforced polyglycolide (SR-PGA) composite rods for internal fixation of bone fractures: *In vitro* and *in vivo* study, *J. Biomed. Mater. Res.*, 25:122 (1991).

30. Vainionpää, S., Kilpikari, J., Laiho, J., Helevirta, P., Rokkanen, P., and Törmälä, P., Strength and strength retention in vitro, of absorbable, self-reinforced polyglycolide (PGA) rods for fracture fixation, *Biomaterials*, 8:46–48 (1987).

31. Zimmerman, M., Guastavino, T., Parsons, J.R., Alexander, H., and Linn, S., The *in-vivo*

biocompatibility and *in-vivo* degradation of absorbable glass fiber reinforced composites, *Trans. Society for Biomaterials*, 9:165 (1986).

32. Lin, T.C., Totally absorbable fiber reinforced composites for internal fracture fixation devices, *Trans. Society for Biomaterials*, 9:166 (1986).

33. Kelley, B.S., Dunn, R.L., Battistone, G.C., Casper, R.A., Vincent, J.W., and Boronski, R.A., Totally resorbable, high-strength, glass/ceramic fibers for strengthening and reinforcing biodegradable composites, *Trans. Society for Biomaterials*, 9:167 (1986).

34. Kelley, B.S., Dunn, R.L., and Casper, R.A., Totally resorbable high-strength composite material. In *Advances in Biomedical Polymers* (C.G. Gebelein, Ed.), pp. 77–85, Plenum Press, New York (1987).

35. Andriano, K.P., Daniels, A.U., Smutz, W.P., and Wyatt, W.B., Preliminary biocompatibility screening of several biodegradable phosphate fiber reinforced polymers, *J. Applied Biomaterials*, 4:1–12 (1993).

36. Andriano, K.P., and Daniels, A.U., Effectiveness of silane treatment on absorbable microfibers, *J. Applied Biomaterials*, 3:191–195 (1992).

37. Andriano, K.P., Daniels, A.U., and Heller, J., Biocompatibility and mechanical properties of a totally absorbable composite material for orthopaedic fixation devices, *J. Applied Biomaterials*, 3:197–206 (1992).

38. Knowles, J.C., Hastings, G.W., Ohta, H., Niwa, S., and Boeree, N., Development of a degradable composite for orthopaedic use: *In vivo* biomechanical and histological evaluation of two bioactive degradable composites based on the polyhydroxybutyrate polymer, *Biomaterials*, 13:491–496 (1992).

39. Vasenius, J., Vainionpää, S., Vihtonen, K., Mäkelä, A., Rokkanen, P., Mero, M., and Törmälä, P., Comparison of *in vitro* hydrolysis, subcutaneous and intramedullary implantation to evaluate the strength retention of absorbable osteosynthesis implants, *Biomaterials*, 11:501–504 (1990).

40. Matsusue, Y., Yamamuro, T., Oka, M., Shikinami, Y., Hyon, S.-H., and Ikada, Y., *In vitro* and *in vivo* studies on bioabsorbable ultra-high-strength poly(L-lactide) rods, *J. Biomed. Mater. Res.*, 26:1553–1567 (1992).

41. Schakenread, J.M., Hardonk, M.J., Feijen, J., Molenaar, I., and Nieuwenhuis, P., Enzymatic activity toward poly(L-lactic acid) implants, *J. Biomed. Mater. Res.*, 24:529–545 (1990).

42. Daniels, A.U., Chang, M.K.O., Andriano, K.P., and Heller, J., Mechanical properties of biodegradable polymers and composites proposed for internal fixation of bone, *J. Applied Biomaterials*, 1:57–78 (1990).

43. Smutz, W.P., Daniels, A.U., Andriano, K.P., France, E.P., and Heller, J., Mechanical test methodology for environmental exposure testing of biodegradable polymers, *J. Applied Biomaterials*, 2:13–22 (1991).

44. Vasenius, J., Vainionpää, S., Vihtonen, K., Mero, M., Mäkelä, A., Törmälä, P., and Rokkanen, P., A histomorphologic study on self-reinforced polyglycolide (SR-PGA) osteosynthesis implants coated with slowly absorbable polymers, *J. Biomed. Mater. Res.*, 24:1615–1635 (1990).

45. Törmälä, P., Vainionpää, S., Kilpilari, J., and Rokkanen, P., The effects of fibre reinforcement and gold plating on the flexural and tensile strength of PGA/PLA copolymer materials, *in vitro*, *Biomaterials*, 8:42–45 (1987).

46. Babayan, A.M., Pilliar, R.M., and Grnypas, M.D., Resorbable short-fibre reinforced composites for fracture fixation, *Trans. Society for Biomaterials*, 15:245 (1992).

47. Schakenraad, J.M., Nieuwenhuis, P., Molenaar, I., Helder, J., Dijkstra, P.J., and Feijen, J., *In vivo* and *in vitro* degradation of glycine/DL-lactic acid polymers, *J. Biomed. Mater. Res.*, 23:1271–1288 (1989).

48. Claes, L.E., Mechanical characterization of biodegradable implants, *Clinical Materials*, 10:41–46 (1992).

49. Latour, R.A., Jr., Black, J., and Miller, B., Fracture mechanisms of the fiber/matrix interfacial bond in fiber reinforced polymer composites, *Surface and Interface Analysis*, 17:477–484 (1991).
50. Latour, R.A., Jr., and Black, J., Development of FRP composite structural biomaterials: Ultimate strength of the fiber/matrix interfacial bond in simulated *in vivo* environments, *J. Biomed. Mater. Res.*, 26:593–606 (1992).
51. Latour, R.A., Jr., and Black, J., Development of FRP composite structural biomaterials: Fatigue strength of the fiber/matrix interfacial bond in simulated *in vivo* environments, *J. Biomed. Mater. Res.*, 27:1281–1291 (1993).
52. Plueddemann, E.P., *Silane Coupling Agents*, 2nd Ed., Plenum Press, New York, 1991.
53. Santavirta, S., Konttinen, Y.T., Saito, T., Gronblad, M., Partio, E., Kemppinen, P., and Rokkanen, P., Immune response to polyglycolic acid implants, *J. Bone and Joint Surg.*, 72B: 597–600 (1990).
54. Böstman, O., Hirvensalo, E., Mäkinen, J., and Rokkanen, P., Foreign-body reactions to fracture fixation implants of biodegradable synthetic polymers, *J. Bone and Joint Surg.*, 72-B:592–596 (1990).
55. Zimmerman, M., Parsons, J.R., and Alexander, H., The design and analysis of a laminated partially degradable composite bone plate for fracture fixation, *J. Biomed. Mater. Res.: Applied Biomater.*, 21.A3:345–361 (1987).
56. Partio, E.K., Böstman, O., Vainionpää, S., Patiala, H., Hirvensalo, E., Vihtonen, K., Törmälä, P., and Rokkanen, P., The treatment of cancellous bone fractures with biodegradable screws, *Acta Orthop. Scand.*, Supplement 227, 59:18 (1988).
57. Rokkanen, P., Böstman, O., Hirvensalo, E., Vainionpää, S., and Törmälä, P., Three years audit of biodegradable osteofixation in orthopedic surgery, *Acta Orthop. Scand.*, Supplement 227, 59:18–19 (1988).
58. Törmälä, P., Vainionpää, S., Pellinen, M., Heponen, V.-P., Laiho, J., Tamminaki, M., Mikkola, J., and Rokkanen, P., Totally biodegradable polymeric self-reinforced (SR) rods and screws for fixation of bone fractures, *Trans. Society for Biomaterials*, 11:501 (1988).
59. Mäkelä, E.A., Böstman, O., Kekomäki, M., Södergärd, J., Vainio, J., Törmälä, P., and Rokkanen, P., Biodegradable fixation of distal humeral physeal fractures, *Clin. Orthop.*, 283: 237–243 (1992).
60. Ekstrand, K., Ruyter, I.E., and Wellendorf, H., Carbon/graphite fiber reinforced poly (methyl methacrylate): Properties under dry and wet conditions, *J. Biomed. Mater. Res.*, 21: 1065–1080 (1987).
61. Wenz, L.M., Merritt, K., Brown, S.A., and Moet, A., *In vitro* biocompatibility of polyether-etherketone and polysulfone composites, *J. Biomed. Mater. Res.*, 24:207–215 (1990).
62. Spector, M., Cheal, E.J., Jamison, R.D., Alter, S., Madsen, N., Strait, L., Maharaj, G., Gavins, A., Reilly, D.T., and Sledge, C.B., Composite materials for hip replacement prostheses, *Advanced Materials: Looking Ahead to the 21st Century*, 22:1119–1130 (1990).
63. Cheal, E.J., Spector, M., and Hayes, W.C., Role of loads and prosthesis material properties on the mechanics of the proximal femur after total hip arthroplasty, *J. Orthop. Res.*, 10:405–422 (1992).
64. Morscher, E., Mathys, R., and Hench, H.R., Iso-elastic endoprosthesis—A new conception in artificial joint replacement, In *Advances in Artificial Hip and Knee Joint Technology-Engineering in Medicine*, Vol. 2 (M. Schaldach and D. Hohmann, Eds.), p. 402, Springer, Berlin (1976).
65. Magee, F.P., Weinstein, A.M., Longo, J.A., Koeneman, J.B., and Yapp, R.A., A canine composite femoral stem: An *in vivo* study, *Clin. Orthop.*, 235:237–252 (1988).
66. Sumner, D.R., Turner, T.M., Urban, R.M., Galante, J.O., Experimental studies of bone remodeling in total hip arthroplasty, *Clin. Orthop.*, 276:83–90 (1992).
67. Latour, R.A., Jr., Black, J., and Miller, B., Interfacial bond degradation of carbon fiber-polysulfone thermoplastic composite in simulated *in vivo* environments, *Trans. Society for Biomaterials*, 13:69 (1990).

68. Meyer, M.R., and Latour, R.A., Jr., Long-term durability of interfacial bonding in carbon fiber/polyetheretherketone and carbon fiber/polysulfone composites following exposure to simulated physiologic saline, *Trans. Society for Biomaterials*, 16:15 (1993).

69. Overland, M.K., Clayden, N.J., Everall, N.J., Koeneman, J.B., and Magee, F.P., Effect of long-term *in-vivo/in-vitro* environmental exposure on the shear strength of polysulfone/carbon fiber composites, *Trans. Society for Biomaterials*, 16:14 (1993).

70. D'Ariano, M.D., Latour, R.A., Jr., Kennedy, J.M., Schutte, H.D., Jr., and Friedman, R.J., Long term shear strength durability of CF/PEEK composite in physiologic saline, *Trans. Society for Biomaterials*, 17:184 (1994).

71. Zhang, C., Latour, R.A., Jr., Kennedy, J.M., Schutte, H.D., Jr., and Friedman, R.J., Long term compressive strength durability of carbon fiber reinforced PEEK composite in physiologic saline, *Trans. Society for Biomaterials*, 17:160 (1994).

72. Klett, L.B., Kennedy, J.M., and Latour, R.A., Jr., Effects of long term saline exposure on the tensile properties of carbon fiber reinforced polyetheretherketone (PEEK), Carbon '94, International Conference on Carbon, Granada, Spain, July 4–8, 1994.

73. Adams, D., and Williams, D.F., The response of bone to carbon-carbon composites, *Biomaterials*, 5:59–64 (1984).

74. Jockisch, K.A., Brown, S.A., Bauer, T.W., and Merritt, K., Biological response to chopped-carbon-fiber-reinforced peek, *J. Biomed. Mater. Res.*, 26:133–146 (1992).

75. Tayton, K., Phillips, G., and Ralis, Z., Long-term effects of carbon fiber on soft tissues, *J. Bone and Joint Surg.*, 64-B:112–114 (1982).

76. Saha, S., and Pal, S., Improvement of mechanical properties of acrylic bone cement by fiber reinforcement, *J. Biomech.*, 17:467–478 (1984).

77. Weber, F.A., and Charnley, J., A radiologic study of fractures of acrylic cement in relation to the stem of a femoral head prosthesis, *J. Bone and Joint Surg.*, 57-B:297–301 (1975).

78. Pilliar, R.M., Blackwell, R., Macnab, I., and Cameron, H.U., Carbon fiber-reinforced bone cement in orthopaedic surgery, *J. Biomed. Mater. Res.*, 10:893–906 (1976).

79. Pourdeyhimi, B., Robinson, H.H., IV, Schwartz, P., and Wagner, H.D., Fracture toughness of K29/poly(methyl methacrylate) composite materials for surgical applications, *Annals of Biomed. Engr.*, 14:277–294 (1986).

80. Wright, T.M., and Trent, P.S., Mechanical properties of aramid fibre-reinforced acrylic bone cement, *J. Mater. Sci. Letts.*, 14:503–505 (1979).

81. Fishbane, B.M., and Pond, R.B., Sr., Stainless steel fiber reinforcement of polymethylmethacrylate, *Clin. Orthop. & Rel. Res.*, 128:194–199 (1977).

82. Topoleski, L.D.T., Ducheyne, P., and Cockler, J.M., The fracture toughness of titanium-fiber-reinforced bone cement, *J. Biomed. Mater. Res.*, 26:1599–1617 (1992).

83. Poureyhimi, B., and Wagner, H.D., Elastic and ultimate properties of acrylic bone cement reinforced with ultra-high-molecular-weight polyethylene fibers, *J. Biomed. Mater. Res.*, 23:63–80 (1989).

84. Wagner, H.D., and Cohn, D., Use of high-performance polyethylene fibres as a reinforcing phase in poly(methylmethacrylate) bone cement, *Biomaterials*, 10:139–141 (1989).

85. Buckley, C.A., Lautenschlager, E.P., and Gilbert, J.L., High strength PMMA fibers for use in a self-reinforced acrylic cement: Fiber Tensile properties and composite toughness, *Trans. Society for Biomaterials*, 14:45 (1991).

86. McKellop, H., Clarke, I., Markolf, K., and Amstutz, H., Friction and wear properties of polymer, metal, and ceramic prosthetic joint materials evaluated on a multichannel screening device, *J. Biomed. Mater. Res.*, 15:619–653 (1981).

87. Latour, F.A., Jr., and Meyer, M.R., Fiber reinforcement of ultrahigh molecular weight polyethylene, *Trans. Society for Biomaterials*, 14:285 (1991).

88. Rosenthall, L., Radiophosphate visualization of the foreign body reaction to wear debris from total knee prosthesis, *J. Nuclear Medicine*, 28:915–917 (1987).

13

The Morphological Patterns of Organization of Synthetic Filamentous Prostheses in Reconstructive Orthopedic Surgery

David G. Mendes and Jochanan H. Boss
Bnai Zion Medical Center
Haifa, Israel

I. INTRODUCTION

The surgical reconstruction of injured, torn, diseased, or otherwise lost ligaments and tendons poses a therapeutic dilemma for the orthopedic surgeon. Insight gleaned from clinical practice and morphological analysis of retrieved specimens is hardly encouraging. Unless surgically treated, torn ligaments and tendons heal by formation of scar tissue, biochemical, biomechanical, and morphological properties of which differ from those of normal collagenous tissue [1]. Initial results of diverse surgical interventions are commonly satisfactory, but failures are all too often met in the long run. The operative options span a wide spectrum, ranging from suturing techniques, replacement with autogeneic and allogeneic grafts or reconstituted collagenous implants, to substitution with synthetic filamentous prostheses. A discussion of the pros and cons of each of these modalities is beyond the intended scope here. Suffice it to say that, after reconstructive surgery employing synthetic biomaterials, recovery is rapid, another of the patient's structures is not weakened, and functionality does not depend on tissular remodeling of the transplanted graft.

Such a seemingly gentle surgical approach as suturing of a torn ligament or tendon leads to remodeling such that the original anatomical and histological configuration is not restored. This is especially true after the repair of the intraarticular ligaments. Long-term follow-up evaluation has not justified the hope that anatomic repositioning of a residual ligament results in morphological and functional reconstitution [2]. As early as 1916,

383

Jones asserted that stitching was futile because the ensuing cicatricial tissue sets a limit to the reparative capabilities of ligaments [3]. Since similar or more pronounced remodeling takes place within patellar tendon autografts substituting for the anterior cruciate ligament (ACL), the constructs may elongate or fail under low forces [4].

When morphologically evaluating the results of reconstructive surgery, the location of the repaired structure has to be taken into account. Spontaneous healing processes of extra-articular ligaments and tendons exceed and apparently also overtake those of intraarticular ligaments [5]. This difference in the healing proficiency is reflected in the greater expression of procollagen type I messenger ribonucleic acid (mRNA) in a lacerated medial collateral ligament than in an injured ACL [6]. The intra-articular ligament is invested by the synovial membrane, is bathed in the synovial fluid, and partly depends for its nourishment on vessels originating at the bony attachments. It is unknown to what extent the different reparative potentials pivot on dissimilar vascular and interstitial sustenance, the synovial fluid environs, unlike biomechanical properties or a combination of these. Be this as it may, the morphological reaction patterns being in essence of a similar disposition, the results of both intra- and extraarticular operations are dealt with in this chapter.

Synthetic filamentous constructs possess a simple configuration that does injustice to the complicated architectonics of the native structures they are planned to replace. The smallest units of the natural ligaments and tendons are the *microbundles*. They are composed of densely packed and broad collagenous fibers and are separated from each other by a loosely textured and well-vascularized areolar fibrous tissue, which makes some mutual movements feasible. The microbundles are bound into *macrobundles*, which are also separated from one another by areolar tissue. Anatomically, the macrobundles form the functional units of the ligaments and tendons.

Because of its special clinical concern, studies have focused on the anatomy of the human ACL. Significantly, the anteromedial, intermediate, and posterolateral compound macrobundles resist anterior subluxation in flexion and extension. The changes of the fiber lengths during knee flexion and extension suggest that the isometric point is located anterior and superior to the femoral origin of the intermediate bundle. However, since the ligament originates from a relatively large area of the bone, it is impossible for most of the fibers to be isometric [7]. The fibers pass directly from the femur to the tibia or take a spiral path around the axis of the ligament [8]. Because of the relative rotations of the attachments, the fibers become twisted on themselves as the knee flexes [9]. With the knee at 90° flexion, the posterior fibers slacken and leave the anterior fibers to resist anterior tibial glide. Because they pass close to the anteromedial bundle, the so-called over-the-top implants tighten in flexion. Since there are no isometric bundles, in fact, considerable length changes are inevitable within artificial filamentous substitutes [7,10].

Implantation of tendon auto- and allografts instead of ligaments and tendons has been popularized in recent years. This technique nearly takes for granted that ligaments and tendons, being uniformly shaped, are mutually interchangeable. This is far from the truth. Distinctive ligaments and tendons are not only anatomically and histologically unlike one another and, to a certain extent, differ biochemically from each other, but their morphological and chemical characteristics alter throughout their length. Illustratively, when compared with the patellar tendon, the ACL is richer in cells, glycosaminoglycans, collagen type III, and fibronectin [11–14]. When planning to give back prosthetically what has been lost, it should not be overlooked that twisting of the ACL is resisted by a combination of capsular shearing and slanting, collateral ligament action, as well as joint surface and meniscal geometry [10,15]. These recently realized facts may hamper reconstructive surgery using grafts. How much more so do they hinder the substitution of ligaments and tendons with synthetic prostheses? It is hardly conceivable that advancement and sophistication in the fabrication of synthetic devices will, in the near future, hand the surgeon an implement so accomplished that, when exchanging for the native structure, its tissular organization will result in the formation of a *neoligament* or *neotendon*.

By way of introduction, these anatomophysiological data have been dwelt upon in some length because they reasonably explain why present-day artificial implants cannot restore all the potentials of native ligaments and tendons. The operative endeavors, the principles of which are beyond the scope of this chapter [16], and the chosen prostheses are compromises at best. In conferring some elasticity to the prosthesis, braiding of artificial filaments reduces the disruptive effects of linear impact stresses. Contemplating the biological behavior of implants, synthetic filamentous devices withstand the immediate postoperative loads because secure fixation to the bone is accomplished with proper techniques [17].

Morphological studies are impeded by scant data about the appearances of implants that have successfully functioned for many months, and preferably years, samples being mostly retrieved after one complication or another has been clinically recognized. Identical tissular responses and organizational patterns are evinced in specimens obtained from patients with failed prostheses and from animals with successfully functioning prostheses. Therefore, it is conditionally justified to assume, in keeping with custom, that the morphological perspective learned from the analysis of clinical cases reflects what actually happens, obviously except for the deviant appearances of explicitly anomalous implants.

II. CARBON FILAMENTOUS PROSTHESES

Biocompatibility and noncarcinogenicity, coupled with the ability to sustain tissue growth, are the rationale for the utilization of filamentous carbon as a synthetic substitute [18–21]. The optimistic notion that tissular organization of implanted carbon filaments leads to an innervated composite [22], the tensile strength of which approaches that of natural ligaments and tendons, has turned out to be unfounded [23].

To increase stability and elasticity, the implants are coated in one way or another [18], expecting the investing tissues to regenerate a functionally effective substitute prior to rupture of the carbon filaments [24]. Orthopedic surgeons are cognizant of the superior functional results and healing tendency of substituted extra-articular ligaments and tendons when matched with their intra-articular counterparts. Notwithstanding the essentially similar morphological patterns of organization at both sites, the ingrowing collagenous tissue is more luxurious, better oriented, and less inflamed in the extra-articular location.

Chronic and recurrent knee instability, an unstable prosthetic situation, and revision arthroplasty have been the indications for reconstruction of the ACL with a carbon prosthesis [25]. Though no longer in fashion, a review of the organizational pattern of filamentous carbon implants is worthwhile because important biological principles have been deduced from the study of retrieved samples. Despite a high tensile strength, the brittleness of the carbon filaments in bending necessitated the withdrawal of this prosthesis from clinical practice. Regardless of the excellent early functional results and patients' satisfaction with their reconstructed ACL, rupture of the implants next to the femoral or tibial exit and often unacceptably severe detritic synovitis are the expected outcome of the cumulative effect of breakage of individual carbon filaments during daily activities. Indeed, the occasional patient with a well-functioning joint insisted on removal of the prosthesis because unbearable synovitic pain, not knee instability, made life miserable.

A. Experimental Studies in Animals

Filamentous carbon tows and braids have been studied experimentally in dogs for the replacement of ligaments and tendons [26]. The individual filament is 8–10 micrometers (μm) in diameter and has a tensile breaking load of 0.15 newton (N). The unidirectional longitudinal tow is composed of 40,000 filaments. Its ultimate tensile strength is 600 N. Coating with biodegradable gelatin makes the tow more resilient and protects it during surgery. The braid, interwoven at 43°, consists of 11 strands, each of which accommodates 3000 filaments. Its ultimate tensile strength is 610 N. It is coated with a 2–4-μm thick layer of absorbable collagen.

Since not all filaments simultaneously reach their maximum length, the failure strength of the prosthesis represents the sum total of the failures of the fibrils at different points in time. The implants have been formerly anchored to cortical bone by expanding rivets made of carbon filaments embedded in polysulfone matrix [27]. The rivets occasionally loosen in the wake of bone resorption (in clinical practice), so the technique has been modified such that the implants are passed through 4.5-millimeters (mm) wide bony tunnels prior to their cortical anchorage. Thus, immediate firm and long-term secure fixation is achieved.

Long-lasting fixation is enhanced by biological attachment, Sharpey-like fibers fastening the tissue-ingrown prosthesis to its bony bed [28]. For the reconstruction of the ACL, the bony edges at the exits from the femoral and tibial tunnels are rounded off and the intra-articular portion of the implant is ensheathed in a pedicled synovial sleeve in order to encourage tissular ingrowth and minimize the effects of shear forces, which are responsible for the formation of wear particles.

The reconstructed calcaneal tendons of rabbits regain their normal strength after six months [29]. One year after surgery, there are no significant differences in the tensile strength of dogs' tendons reconstructed with tows or braids. After a year, the average tensile strength of operated dogs' quadriceps tendons is 372 N (i.e., 88% of normal) and 225 N after replacement with carbon filamentous implants and approximation (but otherwise unrepaired), respectively. The reduced tensile strength of the tissue-ingrown, grossly wavy looking implant is related to physical factors. First, tissular ingrowth progresses during limb activity, proceeds at irregular steps, and evolves as the filaments are in varying states of tension and relaxation. When tested for tensile strength, not all the filaments simultaneously reach their full length. Second, the energy partly dissipates as shear forces on tensioning. Significantly, failure of the reconstructed tendons consistently occurs at either one of the host-implant junctions. Inspection of the tows and braids after removal of the investing fibrous capsules, immediately or following digestion of the on- and ingrowing connective tissue, does not reveal fragmentation of the carbon filaments. Correspondingly, there is no loss of tensile strength of the recovered prostheses.

The diameter of the tows and braids increases about threefold after one year of implantation consequent to ample tissular growth. Fibrous tissue thoroughly permeates the breadth and length of the prostheses. Some small groups of centrally located filaments are unorganized and encased within sleeves of fibrous tissue even several years postoperatively [30]. Otherwise, each filament is surrounded by concentrically layered histiocytes, fibroblasts, and connective tissue fibers. This stereotypical organizational pattern of the carbon filaments is referred to as the evolvement of *composite units* (Fig. 1).

The newly synthesized collagen and reticulin fibers of and in between the composite units are oriented parallel to the longitudinal axes of the filaments, which evidently conduct the direction of fiber production by the proliferating fibroblasts. Contrasting with the abundance of collagen and reticulin fibers, elastic fibers are conspicuous by their absence. Mono- and polykaryonic macrophages, admixed with some lymphocytes and rare plasma cells, are closely associated with some filaments.

This granulomatous reaction varies in extent from one region of the implant to another. Scanning electron microscopically, the fibroblasts and connective tissue fibers are seen to cohere intimately to the carbon filaments. Transmission electron microscopically, some tiny fragments of carbon are found to have been ingested by the mono- and polykaryonic macrophages. Because macrophages, reticulin fibers, and blood vessels abound in replacements retrieved a year postoperatively, the differentiating connective tissue is comparatively immature and the reactive as well as reparative processes continue for at least many months.

The carbon filaments, being stronger than the collagen fibers, primarily provide the tensile strength of the tissue-ingrown prosthesis. The on- and ingrowing fibrous tissue gives the organized implant some degree of elasticity and protects the filaments against shear stresses. When the implant tightens under tensile forces, the fibrous tissue is

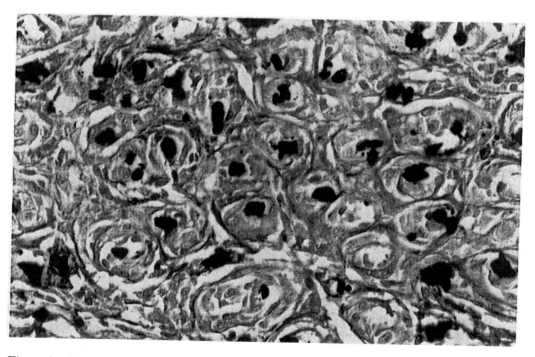

Figure 1   Composite units. Cross section of an animal's extra-articular ligament substituted by a carbon filamentous prosthesis. Each filament is concentrically surrounded by cells (histiocytes and fibroblasts) and collagen fibers. A network of loosely textured connective tissue is present in between the composite units (Masson's stain, ×400).

squeezed in between the filaments. The collagen fibers closely cohere, but poorly adhere to the carbon filaments. Consequently, when sufficient tensile force is applied to the carbon component of retrieved samples, the filaments slide out of their investing connective tissue and yield centrally empty composite units. Comparably, the filaments and their encircling tissue are once in a while seen, on scanning electron micrographs, to be dissociated from each other by empty spaces.

Joint immobilization adversely affects the articular and para-articular apparatus. The effects of continuous passive motion (CPM) has been studied in rabbits with medial collateral ligaments that have been replaced by carbon filamentous braids. Though there are no discernible differences in the extent of tissular ingrowth and inflammatory response, the failure load is higher and the implant stiffness is greater in the CPM-treated than the control animals. However, in as much as more bone and less fibrous tissue penetrate in between the implant and its bony bed within the intraosseous tunnels, the bone-ligament complex is stronger when the stifles are exercised by CPM. Whereas the severed and repositioned ligament fails in its midsubstance, the carbon filamentous substitute of CPM-treated rabbits is as strong as its natural counterpart and fails, as do native ligaments, at its insertion site [31]. The beneficial effects of CPM are related to the empirically recognized motion-induced betterment of fibrous tissue synthesis, organization, and alignment [1,32]. There is a 17°–30° loss of flexion in patients with knees immobilized after ligamentous reconstructions [33].

B. Filamentous Carbon and Absorbable Polymer Composite

The filamentous carbon and absorbable polymer composite combines the advantages of permanent and scaffold replacements [34]. It consists of 10,000 carbon filaments coated with polylactic acid (PLA) or PLA-poly-ϵ-caprolactone copolymer. It has been used to replace the proximal third of the Achilles tendon of rabbits. Tissular ingrowth begins after the first postoperative week. By three months, the carbon filaments are spread apart by abundant and highly cellular fibrous tissue with scant inflammatory and granulomatous changes. The filaments are pulled out of the anastomotic site after the second postoperative week. On the other hand, failure at tension occurs at an average force of 340 N by rupture through the gastrocnemius muscle after the fourth week, both the mechanism and force at failure being similar to those witnessed in the contralateral normal limb. Similarly, the mechanical properties of dogs' patellar tendons reconstructed with absorbable polymer-coated carbon filaments are like those of their unoperated counterparts. The central region of the implants is composed of collagen fibers surrounding the carbon filaments and is akin to the corresponding zone of the normal patellar tendon [35].

C. Tendon Replacement in Patients

The organizational pattern of and the tissular ingrowth into tendon replacements of patients are essentially identical to those of carbon filamentous tows and braids implanted in animals. Contingent on the ample ingrowth of fibrous tissue, the diameter of the implants increases three- to fourfold by 12–18 postoperative months. Some carbon filaments are encased within the composite units, which are now and then cellular but are more often hyalinized.

As perceived on scanning electron microphotographs, two cell types cling to the filaments. The relatively small, round, and smooth cells are macrophages [36]. The relatively large fusiform or stellate fibroblasts spread their processes out along the filaments, giving the impression that they crawl on the carbon strands. The fibroblasts and fibrocytes as well as the abundantly produced collagen and reticulin fibers are oriented parallel to the longitudinal axes of the carbon filaments [28]. In well-organized prostheses, retrieved after having adequately functioned for several years, the filamentous component is relatively rarefied because of the absolute predominance of the collagenous tissue (Fig. 2). Still, mono- and polykaryonic macrophages accompanied by some lymphocytes focally infiltrate even the best-organized prostheses.

The scenery of macrophagic infiltration and fibroblastic proliferation persisting for many a year implies that the perpetual presence of the undigestible foreign body provokes an indefinitely ongoing reactive process. Hence, it is inconceivable that carbon filamentous prostheses, though well organized and incorporated in their environs, may ever attain the histological picture of a normal ligament or tendon. Moreover, the tiny carbon detritic fragments littering the tissues within and without the implants provoke a granulomatous response, expressed by the infiltration of mono- and polykaryonic macrophages admixed with some lymphocytes, plasma cells, neutrophils, and eosinophils. This inflammatory and granulomatous reaction cannot but exert untoward effects on the tissular attributes of the replacement (see Section II.F for more information).

Irregularly shaped, elongated, and optically empty spaces occasionally occur in between well-organized bundles of carbon filaments. The spaces are lined by large and

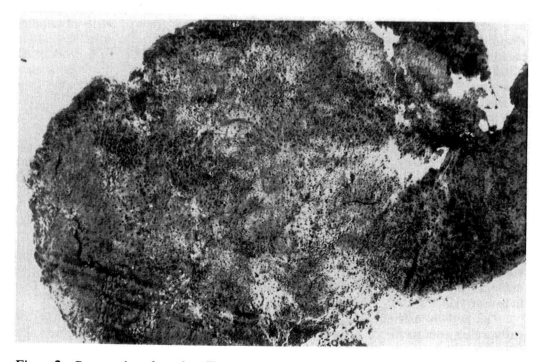

Figure 2   Cross section of a carbon filamentous prosthesis that replaced a patient's Achilles tendon for many years. The filaments are spread apart and make up a small portion of the construct, most of which is composed of collagen fibers. Plastic-embedded specimen stained by von Kossa's technique (×8).

cytoplasm-rich cuboidal cells, which rest on a thin fibrous plate [28]. Being reminiscent of synovial cysts, their evolvement is referred to as *synovial metaplasia* and derives from micromotion focally affecting a mechanically disrupted connective tissue [37,38]. This synovial metaplasia evinces the effects of movements between segments of the organized implant.

The occurrence of small foci of coagulative necrosis, albeit infrequently, in the midst of well-organized prostheses suggests the effects of a persisting and noxious agent [39]. Probably because of the collapse of the formerly present supportive tissue, the carbon filaments are closely packed in such necrotic areas. It has been suggested that the necrosis is caused by circulatory impediment consequent to relative motion and compressive forces of the carbon filaments during activities [28].

The low shear strength of the carbon filaments obviates knot tying. The filament breaks when knots are cinched. Reliable methods have had to be devised for the soft-tissue fixation of the implants. Unless special precautions are taken, slippage of the carbon filaments occurs at the anastomotic sites [40].

D. The Significance of the Filamentous Carbon Prosthesis in the Context of Reconstructive Surgery

When the filamentous carbon prosthesis was first introduced into clinical medicine for reconstructive surgery and concurrently studied in experimental animals, the biologically challenging question was posed as to whether it would function as a permanent implant or a temporary scaffold for tissular ingrowth [41–44]. The analysis of retrieved samples clearly shows that mesenchymal cells easily and amply populate the interfilamentous territories, where they multiply and differentiate into fibroblasts. The newly synthesized collagen fibers display, polarization optically, crimp and noncrimp compositional patterns in different regions of the organized implant [45]. It stands to reason that load sharing by the artificial and biological fibers occurs when tensile forces are applied to the construct. This decidedly is in accordance with the initially encouraging clinical results reported by many investigators [41,43–48].

The morphological features of the organized prosthesis, as summarized above, negates the contention that a neoligament or neotendon ensues in the wake of tissular ingrowth. Notwithstanding claims to the contrary [41,43,49], ligamentous and tendinous replacements do not acquire the histological characteristics of their innate counterparts. In view of the short life span of the monocytes and other leukocytes [36], it is self-evident that the continuing recruitment of the inflammatory cells lasts for a long time, probably for the duration of the service of the implant. Besides the ongoing inflammatory-granulomatous response, the uniqueness of the composite units, within which the spatial disposition of the collagen and reticulin fibers and the high cellularity constitute the organizational hallmark, sets aside the organized carbon filamentous prosthesis as a case in its own right.

The initially offered conundrum is more than of academic interest. Whether the carbon filaments perform as a permanent prosthesis or a temporary scaffold for tissular ingrowth will determine their performance. The tensile strength of a permanent versus a temporary replacement is established by the properties of the carbon filaments versus those of the collagen fibers. The load-extension curves of organized tows and braids, retrieved one year after implantation in the stead of the dogs' quadriceps tendon, approximate those of the normal tendons, respectively yielding at 370 N and 420 N in the load-to-failure tests [50]. By the way, these results favorably compare with the tensile strength of severed but unrepaired tendons (i.e., gap healing by scar formation), which yield at about 225 N.

Though the tensile strength of the organized filamentous carbon prosthesis is almost 90% of that of dogs' native quadriceps tendons, it is less than 60% of that of the fresh tows (670 N) and braids (610 N). These discrepancies cannot be attributed to the gradual load takeover by the newly formed collagen (and reticulin) fibers and concomitant failure or fragmentation of the carbon filaments [27]. Enzymatic digestion of the fibrous tissue of organized implants discloses negligible fragmentation and lack of deterioration in the physical properties of the carbon filaments (inasmuch as failure has occurred, in such experiments, at loads averaging 680 N).

Paradoxically at first sight, the relative weakness of the organized prosthesis is related to the stiffness of the carbon filaments: neither *in vivo* nor *in vitro* does it reach its theoretical strength because merely a small portion of all the filaments (estimated at 10–15%) reaches full length and carry load at any one time [51]. Moreover, a functionally substantial part of the organized implant is occupied by cells (whether fibroblasts, fibrocytes, macrophages, or leukocytes), which are ineffective as far as the tensile strength is concerned. In comparison with the healthy tendon and ligament, which (being poor in cells, vessels, and reticulin fibers) intrinsically consist of the load-carrying collagen fibers, only a portion of the tissue-ingrown prosthesis is functionally sharing the applied loads. Evidently, tensile forces acting upon the organized implant are resisted by the stiff carbon filaments, whereas the connective tissue fibers, being concealed by the shielding effect of the carbon filamentous component, do not add much strength to the construct. Indeed, because of sliding of the carbon filaments within their investing cellular-fibrous sheaths, disruption of the composite units occurs at low loads of 30–85 N [52]. The fibrous tissue contributes toward the integrity of the implant by protecting the filaments from shear stresses and, surrounding each filament with a concentric tissular shell, by providing some string effect or elasticity under load. In conclusion, inasmuch as the collagen fibers do not confer much supplementary tensile strength, the filamentous carbon prosthesis performs as a permanent implant.

E. Anterior Cruciate Ligament Replacement in Patients

The clinical results of ACL replacements with carbon filamentous prostheses of one type or another are reportedly fair to excellent in the first postoperative years, particularly in patients operated on in the immediate posttraumatic stage [33]. The high incidence of late complications (e.g., rupture at the exit from the osseous tunnel or in the midsubstance and detritic synovitis) has bestowed disrepute on this reconstructive modality. The tissular reaction patterns occurring in human ACL replacements are similar to those in animals inasmuch as the formation of composite units and lush collagenous tissue expresses the organized stereotype.

The thickening and discoloration (by deposited carbon debris) of the joint capsule, as seen at retrieval of failed implants, reflects the histologically ascertained detritic synovitis, which is of clinical relevance since it may cause intractable and excruciating pain. Histologically, the inner aspect of the joint capsule is covered by chronically inflamed, hypervascular, and hypertrophic villi, which are lined by hyperplastic synoviocytes. The inflamed and fibrotic villi and underlying tissue contain myriad giant-celled granulomas, which hold countless, less than 5-μm long, carbon particles. Small foci of necrosis are sometimes found in the superficial zone. Infrequent clustered hemosiderin-laden macro-phages suggest past hemorrhagic events. Thus, there is no credence to the viewpoint that spread of carbon filaments or fragments thereof in the joint cavity is without clinically harmful consequences [53,54]. Corroborated experimentally, intra-articularly injected carbon microparticles are taken up by subsynovial phagocytes and provoke a granuloma-tous inflammation [18].

The granulomatous response, mono- and polykaryonic macrophages abutting the carbon filaments, persists within the intra-articular and intraosseous portions of the implants for months and years (Fig. 3). Indeed, it is still evident in samples of patients who were operated on 10 or more years prior to harvesting the failed prosthesis. Usually, mature, densely textured, and at times hyalinized collagen fibers, which are well aligned with respect to the carbon filaments, make up most of the ingrown tissue; they are more prominent at the perimeter of the implant. The fibrous tissue is loosely textured and imbibed with glycosaminoglycans where focally clustered leukocytes randomly infiltrate the organized implant. Focally, groups of crowded carbon filaments are devoid of in-grown tissue. Whereas composite units sporadically occur or are absent in samples ob-tained many years postoperatively, the overall cellularity is independent of the time factor such that segments rich in fibroblasts and poor in collagen fibers, indicative of prolifera-tive activity, are found many years after the implantation. These findings vary in extent

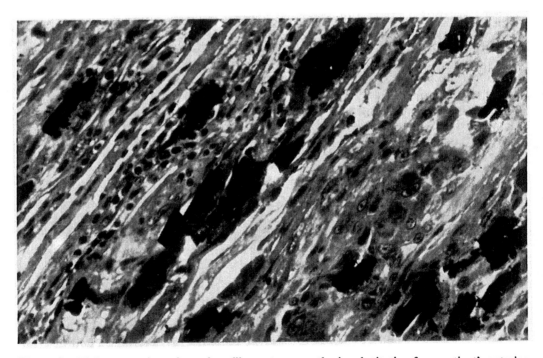

Figure 3 High-power view of a carbon filamentous prosthesis substituting for a patient's anterior cruciate ligament for over 10 years. There is a florid mono- and polykaryonic macrophagic response in relation to the filaments. The fibrous tissue is focally infiltrated by lymphocytes. Plastic-embedded specimen stained by von Kossa's technique (×400).

not only from one patient to another, but also from one segment of an implant to another [33,45,55].

The composite units disappear with time, and the bulk of carbon filaments per surface area rarefies in comparison with the luxuriously produced collagen fibers. That focally persisting delicate collagen fibers display a noncrimp pattern signifies their lack of waviness. This is not surprising because noncrimp collagen fibers are encountered in diverse filamentous implants, a phenomenon ascribed to varying localized tensile forces, which unevenly act on the collagen fibers [56]. The predominating broad collagen fibers disclose a high amplitude and low frequency crimp pattern (Fig. 4) of the healthy ACL. Though normally structured and well-aligned collagen fibers prevail, the histological features of the natural ligament are not attained. The carbon filaments having stimulated the formation of a simplified connective tissue, the appearances are more akin to scar tissue than to a healthy ligament.

Electron microscopically, the carbon filaments are accompanied by histiocytes and fibroblasts. That the cytoplasm of the latter is studded with distended cisternae of the rough endoplasmic reticulum evinces continual synthetic activity for the duration of the service of the prosthesis. Some flocculent and stringy proteoglycans are in close spatial relation to the fibroblasts and collagen fibrils. The macrophages hold vacuoles, lipid droplets, and various inclusions. While tiny carbon fragments are rarely scattered in between the collagen fibrils, a few larger ones turn up in the phagocytic vacuoles of the macrophages. Such small amounts of carbon breakdown particles in the interstitium and phagocytes denote a lack of excessive disintegration of the filaments [57]. Untoward effects of the carbon shreds on the environs are not recognizable, but the phagocytosis of the larger particles is expectedly associated with release of lysosomal enzymes and mediators of inflammation, which likely contribute to the ongoing inflammation.

The organizational patterns of the intra-articular and intraosseous portions of the carbon filamentous implants are identical. Yet, the interposition, in most cases, of a thick granulomatous and cicatrizing interfacial membrane (IM) in between the organized implant and the surrounding bony shell of the femoral and tibial tunnels lends something special to the intraosseous location [58]. The outstanding rigidity and mechanical strength of the carbon filaments provide satisfactory function in the longitudinal axis, but their inordinate brittleness limits the bending and torque functions. The synovial fluid and para-articular tissues are burdened with extra- and intracellular carbon particles [53,59]. Breakdown of filaments also takes place within the intraosseous tunnels, in which the implants are subjected to shear stresses during activities of the knee joint. Particulate carbon, when deposited at the bone-implant interface, prompts a foreign-body granulomatous response that results in the formation of the functionally detrimental IM.

Unlike ACL replacement with a patellar tendon autograft [60], carbon (as well as other synthetic) filamentous prostheses do not induce the development of an enthesislike junction (i.e., anchorage of the organized implant to the bone via a complex of collagen fibers, fibrocartilage, calcified fibrocartilage, and bone complex). The biofunctionality of the prosthesis is consequently dependent on mechanical (rivets, screws, etc.) rather than biological fixation to the bone. The IM is anchored to the implant by the ingrowing tissue and to the bone via Sharpey-like fibers. The progressive increase in strength of this fastening mechanism with time [61] coincides with a shift in the mode of failure of rabbits' medial collateral ligaments replaced with carbon filamentous implants, which fail

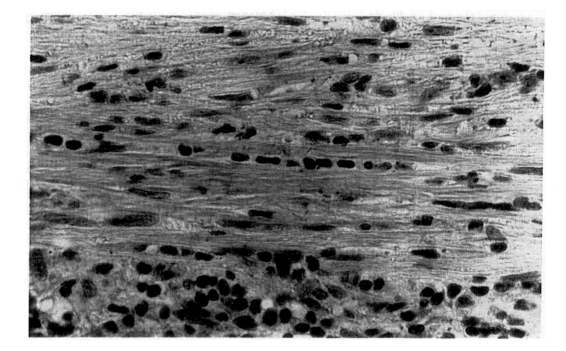

(a)

(b)

Figure 4 After many years' replacement of a patient's anterior cruciate ligament by a carbon filamentous prosthesis, well-oriented and broad collagen fibers constitute most of the construct: (a), there is small focal inflammatory infiltrate consisting of lymphocytes and histiocytes; (b), under polarized light, the bundled collagen fibers exhibit a high amplitude and low frequency crimp pattern. Plastic embedded specimen stained by Movat's technique (×200).

at the bone-prosthesis junction and in the midsubstance after the 4th and 12th postoperative week, respectively [62].

As true for other intraosseous devices, osseointegration of carbon filaments does not ensue unless interfacial motion is evaded [63]. Indeed, in rare instances, when an ACL replacement is retrieved for an indication other than knee instability, woven-fibered bony trabeculae are seen growing into the perimeter of the implant and firmly link the bony shell and prosthesis with each other [64]. Success of implantation surgery notably depends on achieving initial stability of the prosthesis in its environment, be it soft or hard tissue [65,66]. The appraisal of the osseointegrated carbon filaments proves that the knee joint can be stabilized with synthetic filamentous devices.

Satisfactory clinical results have been reported in patients whose ACL has been replaced with a double-armed uniaxial tow composed of 10,000 carbon filaments coated with PLA-poly-ε-caprolactone copolymer. Arthroscopical biopsies, taken during the 27-month follow-up, disclose ample ingrowth of well-vascularized collagenous tissue [67].

F. The Chemical Composition of the Ingrowing Fibrous Tissue

Chemically, the hydroxyproline content (reflecting the ingrowing fibrous tissue) of well-organized carbon filamentous braids, which have replaced pigs' ACLs for 16 weeks, is less than 60% of that of the animals' native ligament. The initially high ratio of dry-to-wet weight normalizes with time, purportedly corresponding to the "maturation" of the ingrowing fibrous tissue. The large amounts of DNA and RNA accord with the histologically observed heightened fibroblastic proliferation in such implants [68].

The everlasting inflammatory and granulomatous reactions and the scarlike features of organized carbon filamentous prostheses raise serious doubts about the normality of the synthesized collagen. It has been repeatedly verified in humans and experimental animals as well as *in vitro* that carbon filaments awaken the mesenchymal cells to produce structurally and tinctorially normal collagen fibers [26,28,41–43,45,49,50,69–71]. However, a clear-cut predominance of Type III over Type I collagen is detected by biochemical and immunohistochemical analyses of the fibrous tissue of properly organized implants, which have replaced patients' ACLs for many years [57]. Thus, the unequivocally established immaturity of the ingrowing fibrous tissue and ongoing collagen synthesis [72,73] correlate with the abundantly present fibroblasts. Contrasting with the unadulterated ligament, in which fibrocytes and Type I collagen constitute the main building blocks, the fibrous tissue of the carbon-filament-induced "neoligament," which is foremost composed of fibroblasts and Type III collagen, holds the nature of a young scar tissue. Moreover, since Type IV (and/or Type V) collagen is also recovered from the implants, signaling heightened cellular metabolic activity, the fibrous tissue of the carbon filamentous prosthesis has the biochemical qualities of a hypertrophic scar [73]. Given the sturdy environmental conditions in the joint cavity [74], it is unlikely that nutritional impediment is causally related to the inadequacy of the newly synthesized collagen. Mediatory substances of inflammation profoundly affect the functional potential of the fibroblasts, therefore the unrelenting inflammatory and granulomatous reaction evoked by the foreign filaments may be responsible for the production of the scar-tissue-type collagen [57].

Fibroblasts, which migrate into damaged areas, secrete fibronectin, proteoglycans, and large amounts of Type III collagen, which lessen by the end of the proliferative phase of wound healing and further decrease with scar maturation [75–77]. The biochemical profile of the fibrous tissue of the inveterate organized carbon filamentous implant conforms to the early phases of scar tissue formation. This contrasts with the "ligamentiza-tion" of rabbits' patellar tendon autografts, in which the amount of Type III collagen reaches its peak by the 6th postimplantation week and decreases to that of the normal ACL by the 30th postoperative week [78].

G.   Comments

The functional results of the augmented repair of damaged or ruptured patellar, quadri-ceps, and Achilles tendons as well as collateral ligaments with carbon filamentous pros-theses are generally good. In fact, implants replacing patients' collateral ligaments are capable of carrying substantial cyclic tensile loads during walking [55,79]. On the other hand, ACL replacements ordinarily function for just some years prior to their excision being mandated by one complication or another. An altogether negativistic attitude to the technique [80] thwarts the experience of those surgeons whose patients are still satisfied with their prostheses 15 or so years after the operation.

Rupture of the implant refers to an abrupt catastrophic failure, which either gradu-ally evolves in the wake of a sequentially increasing number of broken filaments or fails suddenly when the implant snaps in its entirety. Fragmentation pertains to the breakage of individual filaments. More commonly occurring in the knee joint than in the extra-articular locations, it may be so extensive as to bring about chronic or recurrent joint effusions and painful synovitis [81].

H.   Meniscal and Lumbar Fascial Reconstructions

Digressing from the main theme, carbon filaments have been evaluated for the repair of structures other than ligaments and tendons. For instance, defects of rabbits' menisci, bridged by bundled filaments, are overgrown by well-oriented fibrous tissue, which in-cludes fibrocartilaginous islands, while scar tissue formation ensues when continuity is reestablished with a synovial flap [82]. Woven filamentous patches induce the formation of ordered fibrous tissue [83]. Following their insertion into a defect of the rabbits' lumbar fascia, fibrous healing is observed as early as the fifth postoperative week. The rupture strength of the tissular ingrown implant, which increases with time, is greater than that of the collagenous tissue filling defects treated with a Dacron mesh [84].

III.   POLYMERIC FILAMENTOUS PROSTHESES FOR THE RECONSTRUCTION OF THE ANTERIOR CRUCIATE LIGAMENT

The biological effects of diverse polymeric filaments differ from one another. For exam-ple, polypropylene induces a florid foreign-body granulomatous response, sometimes accompanied by neutrophilic infiltration, but little tissular ingrowth [85]. The highly biocompatible and biomechanically stronger polyester (Dacron) makes up a salutary scaffold for the penetration of fibrous tissue [85–87]. Not having gained much popularity in experimental medicine and clinical practice, the Marlex, Teflon, nylon, and Aramide prosthetic ACL replacements are merely mentioned here for the sake of completeness [87–91].

A.   Polyester Prostheses

The polyester (Dacron) implant for the replacement of rabbits' ACLs is made from 5000 filaments, measuring 15 μm in diameter. Its breaking strength of 430 N is similar to that of the natural ligament (415 N). Importantly, and in contrast to comparable carbon filamentous replacements, the polyester substitutes do not suffer loss of strength for a service period of nine months. Histologically, the polyester filaments are spaced out by an adequately ingrowing fibrous tissue, the collagen fibers of which are mostly aligned in parallel to the intact polyester filaments (i.e., in the direction of loading). The collagen fibers closely adhere to the filaments, some of which are set apart from one another by 1.5-μm thick partitions of collagen fibrils. Pools of interstitial fluid, which likely facilitate interfilamentous movements, focally collect in between the filaments [86]. The accompanying giant-celled granulomatous response is within the expected range for nonresorbable polymeric filaments [91]. The intra-articular portion is enveloped by a layer of fibrous tissue, which thickens with time and is covered by a synovial-like lining. The bony anchorage, however, is ineffective because osteogenesis does not occur within the intraosseous tunnels such that the implants are separated from and attached to the bony shell by an investing layer of fibrous tissue [92].

The polyester tow replacing the sheep's ACL is reportedly devoid of ingrowing tissue during an observation period of up to 9 months [86]. In the rabbit, on the other hand, the pattern of tissular organization of the filamentous polyester prosthesis, proceeding as it does from an encapsulating fibrous tissular sheath at 12 weeks to a fully ingrown implant by 36 weeks, is characteristic of comparatively biocompatible biomaterials [93]. Still, the ingrowth is so slow that it does not get to the central area of the intra-articular midzone of the implant by 9 months. The Dacron-polyglycolic acid (PGA) braid accommodates a space-occupying biodegradable component and a nondegradable supporting scaffold. Inserted into the canine knee, it displays limited tissular ingrowth and reduced size (due to degradation of the PGA) after one year. When it is protected intra-articularly by a synovial sleeve, abundant fibrous ingrowth occasions a twofold increase in its size and bony trabeculae interdigitate with the filaments within the intraosseous tunnels. It is reasoned that the supporting Dacron scaffold shields the ingrowing tissue from the effects of linear stresses during the maturational process and improves the bony anchorage [94].

Though satisfactory experimental and clinical results have been reported after reconstruction of the ACL with Dacron prostheses [94–99], reoperations for implant failure are not an uncommon necessity [100]. A closer look at the outcome brings to light a high incidence of synovitis, partial or complete rupture, instability, and decreased range of motion. While stability of the knee is maintained for the first two postoperative years after implantation of the knitted double-velour Stryker–Meadox prosthesis, half of all patients present with either a ruptured or an elongated implant during the third to fifth year. As a rule, early rupture occurs at the exit from a bony tunnel and is related to tension concentration and frictional forces at this site. Late ruptures mostly take place within the midsubstance of a frayed implant, many filaments of which have broken. When elongation is the cause of joint instability, the lax prosthesis (with but few broken filaments) pursues a winding intra-articular course [101].

Patients' and rabbits' retrieved specimens essentially display similar organizational patterns. There are histological signs of maturation of the ingrowing fibrous tissue. However, except for the localities of the exit from the bony tunnels, in which fibrous tissue is copious, the overall amount of collagen fibers is meager. The polyester filaments and their wear particles provoke a giant-celled granulomatous response in the implant itself and in the synovial membrane; freely floating breakdown products are detected in joint effusions [101–104]. As in the experimental model, the bony anchorage is feeble in as much as the perimeter of patients' implants is separated from the bony shell by a fibrous IM. In view of the superb resistance of Dacron to fatigue, the insinuating synovial fluid, permeating fibrous tissue, infiltrating inflammatory cells, and evolving granulation tissue appear to adversely affect the mechanical properties of the polyester filaments [105,106].

B.   Polytetrafluoroethylene Prosthesis

The expanded polytetrafluoroethylene (ePTFE, Gore-Tex) filamentous prosthesis is intended to perform as a permanent replacement. Initially fixated to the bone with screws, it is anticipated that ingrowth of osseous and fibrous tissues into the highly porous microstructure will secure a firm bony anchorage [107]. In the canine model, bony trabeculae interdigitate with the PTFE filaments in the femoral and tibial tunnels [108]. The high ultimate tensile strength (5300 N) and porosity, allowing for ample tissular ingrowth [109,110], promise long-lasting success [109,110]. While breakage of ePTFE implants is uncommon in some authors' experiences, other investigators' patients have presented with a 10% incidence of attenuation or rupture of the prosthesis within the first postoperative year [111,112]. The clinical results are disappointing and the expectations have not been met because of frequent detritic synovitis consequent to partial or complete rupture of the ePTFE strands, impingement-related cold flow, and bone resorption secondary to abrasion against the lateral notch wall [113,114].

The Gore-Tex ACL prosthesis consists of several strands that are wound into loops. Each strand is about 0.6 mm in diameter and is made of filaments with a porosity of 75–85 volume percent (vol%) air; 60-μm long filamentous segments connect dense PTFE notches with one another. The tissular penetration into the prosthesis proceeds haphazardly; regions in which the filaments are surrounded by fibrous tissue still alternate with unorganized territories several months to years after implantation. The ingrowth of tissue is notably poor within the intraosseous portion of the implant. The somewhat better organized intra-articular portion is covered by a synovial-like lining. The ingrowing fibrous tissue is infiltrated by mono- and polykaryonic macrophages admixed with some mono- and polymorphonuclear leukocytes. The fibroblasts and collagen fibers are oriented parallel to the longitudinal axes of the filaments. Many small PTFE particles are phagocytosed by the macrophages. When the inflammatory-granulomatous response is especially harsh, cellular debris is scattered throughout and the collagen fibers and PTFE filaments do not interdigitate with each other [115,116].

At the ultrastructural level, the newly formed collagen fibers and some capillaries contact, but never insert into, the PTFE filaments. Where fibrous tissue is luxuriant, collagen fibers surround single filaments in an arcadelike fashion, creating a perpendicularly interdigitating filamentous-tissular network. Where fibrous tissue is flimsy, collagen fibers hardly interdigitate with the filaments, large segments of which are sequestered within polykaryonic macrophages. The interdigitating complex of collagen fiber and PTFE filament being of ostensible functional importance in resisting the stresses, its focal absence predictably weakens the construct [115].

The bulk of the implant within the intraosseous tunnels is in contact with fibrocartilage or bone. Osseointegration of the ePTFE prosthesis is a matter of practical and theoretical interest. Bony tissue grows in between PTFE strands whenever there is a quiescent IM, but defaults to emerge at locales with an inflammatory-granulomatous IM. Since interfacial micromotion actuates bone resorption and fends off osseointegration, it follows that the prostheses are initially well fixated but segmentally lose contact with the bone at sites of inflammatory-granulomatous reactivity. Inasmuch as the PTFE is an inert biomaterial, the harmful interfacial situation is plausibly related to detrimental mechanical factors, implant shape, implant microstructure, or generation of excessive wear particles [115–118].

C. Leeds–Keio Scaffold

The Leeds–Keio (LK) scaffold is a tubular-shaped, open-weave fabric made of slightly twisted terylene filaments that have a diameter of 8–12 μm. Following its insertion through the femoral and tibial tunnels, it is held in place with bony plugs and staples. In the experimental animal, the LK scaffold is ingrown by connective tissue within a few months of its implantation, but the collagen fibers are improperly oriented with respect to the artificial filaments. Tissular ingrowth progresses with time, the bundles are enwrapped by ample fibrous tissue, and the individual filaments are surrounded by collagenous tissue after the sixth month. There is no osteogenesis in the intraosseous tunnels and the implant is separated from the bony shell by a progressively thickening fibrous sleeve. Sufficient incorporation of the bony plugs and tissular ingrowth account for the increment of the ultimate strength of 850 N of the fresh device to 2600 N of the ingrown scaffold after 17 months [92,119,120].

In the well-organized LK scaffold, even in those specimens which were retrieved from patients with a clinically failed prosthesis, the newly formed fibrous tissue makes up two-thirds of the cross section. The outer aspect consists of a synovial-like membrane. The extraneous fibrous tissue consists of thick type I collagen fibers, which are aligned parallel to the prosthesis and are intermixed with some elastic fibers. The lumen of the implant and the interfilamentous interstices are occupied by loosely textured, delicately fibered, and nonoriented fibrous tissue. An abundance of fibroblasts attests to heightened synthetic activity many months postoperatively. A mono- and polykaryonic macrophagic response is sparse. The organizational pattern indicates that the tissular ingrown LK prosthesis (at least its fibrous circumference) is adequately equipped to transfer and has definitely carried the load [121].

The proplast prosthetic ligament stent deserves mere reference in the present context and the interested reader is referred to the relevant literature [122,123].

D. Carbon and (Nonresorbable) Polymeric Filamentous Composite

The rationale of the utilization of the "Westminster composite prosthesis" is the protection of a carbon filamentous core by a polymeric sleeve, which is composed of an open network of polyester filaments. It is applied as such or as an augmentation device for the reconstruction of intra- and extra-articular ligaments. Replacing the ACL, partial or complete rupture of the implant is experienced by a minority of patients within a few years of the operation. A mildly inflamed synovial-like membrane encloses the intra-articular part of the prosthesis and overlays a thick covering of fibrous tissue, in which are scattered foreign-body granulomas provoked by the littering carbon and polyester particles. When the implants are passed through a drill hole in the lateral femoral condyle, they tend to break at the prosthesis-bone interface. That most implants remain intact when they are routed over the top reiterates the significance of proper techniques in the success of reconstructive surgery. The conception of the Westminster prosthesis is prudent in that the polyester coating provides containment of the carbon filaments, guards against their fragmentation, and concurrently engenders mechanical reinforcement by tissular ingrowth [124,125].

E. Polymeric Implant with Augmented Autograft

Scientific thinking not being restrained by the law of the excluded middle, bringing into union the advantages of an auto- or allograft and an artificial prosthesis is viewed optimistically. Theoretically, the strong polymeric filaments carry the load and protect the weak, necrotic, and avascular graft from elongation and disruption in the immediate postoperative period until the processes of revascularization, cellular repopulation, fibroblastic proliferation, production of collagen fibers, and remodeling eventuate in the formation of a functionally competent neoligament [17]. The realization of this premise is contingent on multifarious factors, as yet incompletely understood, such as the quantity and quality of collagen fibers produced in the presence of a foreign body that, unless resorbable, is committed to elicit a host response persisting for the lifetimes of the patient and prosthesis.

The so-called ligament-augmentation device (LAD) technique, accomplished by enclosing polypropylene filaments within a patellar or semitendinosus tendon autograft, has gained popularity in the reconstruction of the cruciate ligament. The composite is introduced into the joint through a tibial tunnel and fixed over the top of the femoral condyle with staples [126]. Early ingrowth of fibrous tissue in between the individual filaments is attended by a giant-celled granulomatous reaction. The interfilamentous fibrous tissue increases in amount with time. In human samples retrieved some years postoperatively, the grafted tendon exhibits variable cellularity, degenerative changes, and disorganized fibrous tissue. Within the intraosseous tunnel of the sheep, the fibrous IM sequentially differentiates from fibrocartilage at the two-month interval to an enthesislike bone-implant junction after six months. With the regressive alterations being pronounced in the intra-articular portion of the replacement and an enthesislike junction evolving in patients as well, failure of the organized implant as a rule takes place in the midsubstance of the composite [90,92].

On the practical side, salutary results are attained with the LAD operation in the treatment of posterior cruciate ligament injuries. The synthetic filaments adequately maintain the tibia in the reduced position for as long as it takes the body's reparative processes to build up the collagenous framework of a neoligament [127]. Extensive ingrowth of fibrous tissue coincides with a scarce granulomatous response [104].

A foreign-body-induced granulomatous detritic synovitis is a purportedly rare occurrence in patients with an LAD-augmented ACL replacement because the polypropylene filaments are concealed, so to speak, under the grafted autogeneic tissue [128]. Synovitis soon manifests itself during the first six postoperative months in many patients (25%), but its incidence declines thereafter and is belatedly diagnosed in close to 5% of the patients, whose LAD is found to be abraded, ruptured, or impinging on the intercondylar notch. In most cases, phagocytosed polypropylene breakdown particles are seen in the polykaryonic macrophages of the granulomatous tissue. In cases without discernible particles in the chronically inflamed synovial membrane, the etiology of the synovitis is elusive [128–130].

F. High Tensile Polyethylene Filamentous Prosthesis

With the high tensile polyethylene filamentous (HTPEF) prosthesis having newly been introduced into clinical practice, experimental data are mainly accessible. These authors have studied a single retrieved human specimen and its organizational pattern is ascertained to be identical to that of goats' implants. However, whereas foreign-body granulomas generated by wear particles in the environs of the implant are virtually nonexistent in animals' samples obtained during an observation period of one year, they pervade the patient's periprosthetic fibrous tissue. The following description is based on what has been learned from the analysis of the experimental model.

The HTPEF prosthesis is comprised of elliptical, 15–25-μm thick polyethylene (PE) filaments, which are of 150 denier. For implantation in the goat's stifle, the filaments are braided, in shoelacelike fashion, to a thickness of 2 mm. The prostheses have an average ultimate tensile strength of 1240 N and an average elongation to failure of 16%. They lose 57% of their strength (UTS-537 N) following 10^7 cycles of loading at 4 N and withstand 9×10^6 cycles of loading at 8 N prior to failure. The average ultimate tensile strength and elongation to failure are unchanged (1210 N and 16%, respectively) after subcutaneous implantation for three months.

Designed as a permanent replacement of the goat's ACL, the prosthesis is inserted through femoral and tibial tunnels and fixed with PE corks and staples to the cortices. The pattern of tissular organization does not modify after the third postoperative month. The implants are encircled by a thick layer of fibrous tissue, but the bulk of the implant is poorly organized. The rare fibrocytes and histiocytes and the proteinaceous material, which occupy the interfilamentous spaces, make up 10% or less of the volume. The fibrous layer investing the intra-articular portion of the implant is covered by a synovial-like lining. Thin, obliquely oriented fibrous tracks link the encircling fibrous tissue at irregular intervals with a thick central fibrous band (Fig. 5).

The collagen fibers of the investing and central fibrous tissue run along the direction of the implant and thus in the direction of the load. At the outer and inner perimeters of the prosthesis, an interfacial giant-celled granulomatous tissue invades in between the PE filaments (Fig. 6) and makes up 50–60% of the volume at these sites. It merges with the investing fibrous layer and central fibrous band. Consequent to the unfolding of the central fibrous band and less so because of the development of the oblique fibrous tracks and tissular ingrowth, the cross section of the implant enlarges by about 50%. Within the intraosseous tunnels, the thick fibrous IM is anchored via Sharpey-like fibers to a shell of compact bone, akin to a neocortex.

Osteoclastic activity at the bony aspect facing the implant and osteoblastic activity and osteoid seams on the opposite aspect evince ongoing bone remodeling and accord with an increase of about 50% of the diameter of the femoral and tibial tunnels [131,132]. This tendency of the bone to undergo resorption at the side facing an insert and accretion on the opposite surface is a universal biological phenomenon in implantology and portends unruly biochemical, biomechanical, or both effects of the implant on the subjacent osseous tissue [133].

Biomechanical tests have disclosed that the goat's natural ACL has greater stiffness and a lower hysteresis than the explanted HTPEF prostheses. In the tear tests performed under displacement control, the load increases without load drop until at least 540 N (range, 540–1120 N), when damage of the explants is first noticed. Two failure modes of the operated stifles are evident *in vitro*. In the minority of cases, prosthetic failure happens within the substance of the prosthesis at low loads ($F_{max} = 15$ N, i.e., 10–15% of the unused HTPEF braids). Fixation failure takes place in the majority of cases; the artificial ligaments are pulled out of the femoral or tibial tunnels at loads and displacements of 140–620 N and 11–13 mm, respectively. The failure loads of the HTPEF braids removed from the stifles after loss of the bony anchorage remain in the range from 530 to 1250 N [134].

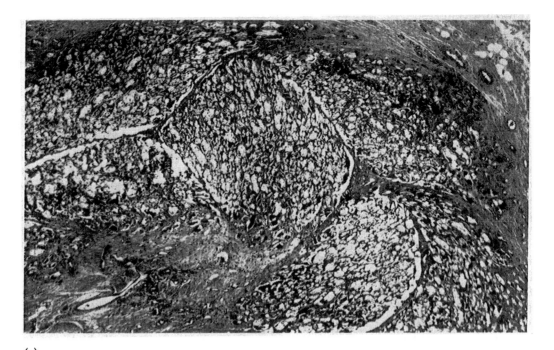

(a)

(b)

Figure 5 Cross section of the intra-articular portion of a high tensile polyethylene fiber braid replacing a goat's anterior cruciate ligament for one year: (a), the poorly organized filamentous bundles are separated from each other by oblique fibrous tracks, which link the thick fibrous central band with the investing fibrous layer; (b), and these features are advantageously elucidated when viewed under polarized light. Rare polymeric filaments are noted to have been incorporated within the central fibrous band. Plastic-embedded specimen stained by von Kossa's technique (×40).

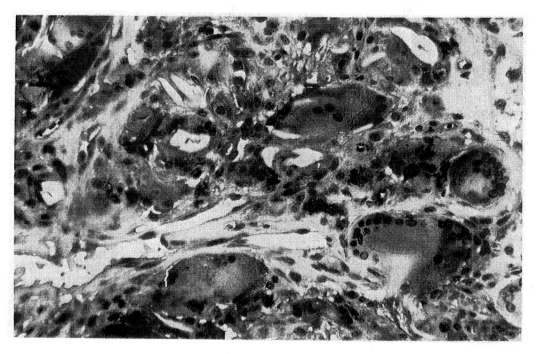

Figure 6 High power view of Fig. 5 displaying the interfacial granulomatous zone interposed at the inner and outer perimeters of the bulk of the implant. Well-vascularized granulation tissue invades the interfilamentous interstices. Polykaryonic macrophages contain or abut upon the polymeric filaments. Plastic-embedded specimen stained by von Kossa's technique (×200).

In summary, notwithstanding the satisfactory clinical results and the facts that the goats behave normally and their stifles are stable for at least a year after ACL replacement by the HTPEF braid, the morphological and biomechanical evaluations disclose inadequate tissular ingrowth and anchorage. Inasmuch as the polyethylene as such is biocompatible [135], biomechanical factors should be implicated in the failure of tissular organization and fixation. With the HTPEF braid physically fixated to the outer cortical bone of the femur and tibia and thus functioning as both a spiral and a string, interfacial motion during loading cycles is a foregone outcome. There is a large body of clinical and experimental evidence to attest to the bone-resorbing effects of interfacial movements [136]. Indeed, nonloaded HTPEF braids, inserted horizontally in the upper tibial metaphysis, are invested by thinner IMs and are properly ingrown by tissue. Still, when compared with the extremely subtle investing fibrous capsule and the luxurious tissular ingrowth observed in subcutaneously implanted HTPEF braids, the conclusion is inevitable that, some, as yet imponderable, stamina are particular to the osseous environment [134].

IV. CONCLUSIONS AND COMMENTS

The extra-articular replacement of ligaments and tendons by carbon filamentous prostheses induces the formation of functionally efficacious and morphologically properly organized and collagenized substitutes. The low-grade chronic inflammation and granulomatous reactions, which go on for many years and predictably persist lifelong, appear to be quantitatively inconsequential. The newly formed collagen and reticulin fibers are guided in the direction of the carbon filaments, the amount of fibrous tissue within the implant is substantial in comparison with the number of the filaments, and the inflammatory-granulomatous response is relatively mild. The well-aligned fibrous tissue does, in fact, impart to the replacements the alluded histological attributes of a *neoligament* and a *neotendon*.

Even though there is no flawless anatomomicroscopical restoration of the natural motif (as described in Section I), the failure to structurally duplicate a healthy ligament or tendon may not be the critically crucial issue in assuring functional potency. In that the fibrous tissue in the implant adapts to its physiological role, growing stronger with time, flexible carbon filamentous devices have an advantage over other prosthetic replacements [43]. There are different biomechanical, functional, nutritional, and circulatory conditions in the extra- and intra-articular locations. The availability of undifferentiated, pluripotential mesenchymal cells is unequal as well [33].

Not surprisingly, therefore, the *extra-articular replacements* are clinically proficient and optimally organized when compared with the *intra-articular replacements*, in which the omnipresent and substantial inflammatory-granulomatous reaction and the poorly reconstructive vigor commonly result in a catastrophic clinical outcome. All things being equal, the implantation site undoubtedly plays a pivotal role in the host's reactivity to carbon filaments [137].

The coalition of a single-bundled or braided configuration of filamentous prostheses with the actuated fibrous tissue cannot assume the complex functional adroitness of native ligaments and tendons. It is hoped that the manufacture of more sophisticated implants embodying, for instance, a multibundled artificial ligament will, in the not too distant future, promote the ingrowing fibroblasts to assemble a more physiologically built ligament and tendon [138].

Does suturing a synovial sleeve to the intra-articular portion of the implant [139] guarantee a more successful result of ACL replacements? There is no ready answer short of stating that uncovered filamentous implants become, at least in the experimental animal, invested by a robust, synovial-like membrane within a comparatively short time interval. The on- and ingrowing tissue protects the alloplastic material at sites of high mechanical stress, reduces internal friction between the filaments, and lessens internal abrasion. The engrafted synovial membrane permits the diffusion of nutritional ingredients and growth-promoting factors from the synovial fluid into the implant and, by restraining the permeation of hyaluronic acid, safeguards the nascent fibrous tissue against the fibrolytic activity of the joint fluid [94]. The price paid for these benevolent rewards is the deterioration of at least some mechanical properties of the prosthesis [96].

The sutured synovial sleeve does not prevent detritic synovitis. This bothersome complication will continue to aggrieve the patients and frustrate the surgeons. In a canine model in which diverse implants (polyether urethane urea, polyethylene, polyethylene terephthalate, and ePTFE) have been used to replace the ACL, the omnipresent structural alterations of the devices have been documented as early as the sixth postoperative week. Detritic synovitis is ubiquitous, with small intracellular and large extracellular polymeric particles accumulating in all synovial membranes. Importantly, particles are also incorporated, albeit rarely, in the joint cartilage and meniscus and migrate to the regional lymph nodes. Abnormal motion of the femoral and tibial cartilage against one another, compounded by the deterioration of the implants, results in damage to the articular surfaces [140].

This is a pessimistic perspective of ACL reconstructive surgery. Extrapolations from experimental to clinical medicine are notoriously fraught with misunderstandings, but detritic synovitis is indubitably commonplace in synovial biopsies of patients with failed synthetic ACL replacements. It behooves bioengineers and materials scientists to search for biomaterials that are resilient but resist abrasive forces.

Though at the boundary of the theme, experimentation with completely biodegradable prostheses may be worth undertaking. Pioneering research is being conducted. For instance, rabbits' Achilles tendons have been partially replaced with poly(2-hydroxymethylmethacrylate)-poly(caprolactone) blend hydrogel matrix reinforced with polylactide fibers. The stress-strain behaviors of the prosthesis and natural tendon are similar at the early parts of straining. The composite is an effective load transmitter. It is incorporated into the residual tendon without an inflammatory response and is replaced by fibrous tissue where these biomaterials have been resorbed [141].

That carbon debris from juxta-articular implantations migrates into the synovial membrane, in which it evokes a granulomatous detritic synovitis [53], throws doubt on the wisdom of resorting to carbon filamentous prostheses even in the retrosynovial placements. Good sense emphatically denies any role to carbon filamentous implants in intra- and juxta-articular reconstructive surgery [86,142].

Having granted that what fails is not necessarily germane to what succeeds, meaningful insight is gained from the analysis of specimens retrieved from patients with deteriorated carbon filamentous ACL replacements. The processes of tissular ingrowth into the interfilamentous interstices, the succeeding fibroblastic proliferation and differentiation, and the attendant synthesis of collagen and reticulin fibers as well as the accompanying granulomatous reaction are essentially similar to each other after implantation of carbon and polymeric prostheses. Given that the interior milieu within synthetic (nonresorbable) filamentous prostheses are of a similar nature (ignoring for the moment the different chemical compositions of diverse implants), universal rules may, conditionally, govern the organizational phenomena.

The histologically and tinctorially acceptable (by classical criteria) maturation of the collagen fibers of the organized carbon filamentous prosthesis has turned out to be deceptive. Fibroblasts and type III collagen dominate the scene many years after implantation; *the phenotypic profile of the organized implant is that of a "young" and immature scar tissue.* Particulate carbon being nonresorbable and the inept maturation of the collagen fibers being causally related to the foreign-body-induced inflammatory-granulomatous response, the fibrous tissue is apt never to attain the distinctive attributes of the natural ligament. In the case that this is a cogent argument, the reconstruction of ligaments and tendons with nonresorbable artificial filamentous implants is a priori doomed not to realize the hoped-for normal collagenization.

This would not be the researchers' first disenchant in their quest for a faultless substitute. In the 1970s, when Jenkins advocated the applicability of carbon implants, he visualized a *temporary scaffold* serving to arouse the growth of fibrous tissue and to secure the conduit of the collagen fibers [143]. He did not err in expecting the carbon filaments to support propagation of fibroblasts and alignment of the collagen fibers. However, he misread the genuine performance of the implant, which has been ascertained to act the role of a *permanent substitute.* Since the tensile strength of the organized prosthesis is determined by the cooperative strength of the carbon filaments and the fibrous tissue [68], deterioration of the implant and defective functionality of the collagen fibers synergistically lead to prosthetic failure.

The collagen fibers are aligned in the direction of the longitudinal axis of the carbon or polymeric filaments. This functional orientation is indicative of load bearing and highlights the quintessence of resorting to suitably engineered devices with fitting strength and stiffness [86]. Configurations that do not encourage tissular ingrowth are subject to fatigue, abrasion, debris generation, creep elongation, and anchorage failure [144]. Filamentous implants, which are inadequately strengthened by healthy collagenous tissue, perform as any other permanent orthopedic device.

In the face of the verified mechanical properties of our unused prostheses that satisfy the requirements on theoretical grounds, one has to account for the high incidence of complications to which ACL reconstructions are prone. Regardless of the high tensile strength, which exceeds the demand, the extended bending forces through an untold number of cycles are greater than the implants can tolerate. While abrasion at the bony edges, intercondylar notch, and osteophytes as well as cracking weaken the implant, the magnitude of the contribution of biochemical degradation and creep has yet to be ascertained [116]. These mechanisms, plausibly performing in concert, culminate in prosthetic failure and detritic synovitis. Early success of ACL reconstruction with any of the synthetic devices is commonplace, but material fatigue, fretting, and wear most often lead to disaster. The writing on the wall is clear: intra-articular synthetic prostheses may cause osteoarthritis rather than prevent it [145].

When biomechanically testing explanted stifles, ACL reconstructions typically give out within the femoral or tibial tunnel. Since synthetic filaments are encased by a concentrically arrayed fibrous IM in the intraosseous tunnels, the bone-implant junction does not conform to an enthesis, which optimally distributes the tensile forces acting on the ligaments. The fibrous IM accounts for the biomechanically feeble attachment to the bone, poor absorption and distribution of forces, as well as susceptibility to damage of the bone and implant from excessive strain [92]. Because they are fixated to the bone by means of staples, screws, or rivets, artificial ligaments are stress shielded within the bony tunnels and an enthesislike junction cannot evolve in the absence of mechanical stress [114]. Restoring a physiologically genuine biomechanical situation in reconstructive surgery is fundamental [115]. Whereas the fibrous tissue induced by artificial filaments by themselves links with the bone via the functionally insufficient IM, the bone-implant bond is reestablished via an enthesislike junction after reconstruction of the ACL with polypropylene filaments internalized within tendon autografts [90,92].

Ligamentization implies adaptation of tendon grafts to the new milieu of the knee joint. In being remodeled, the grafts come to be akin to the histologically and biochemically native ACL rather than to the tissue of the donor site [78]. Such adaptive processes do not materialize after substitution of the ACL by synthetic filaments. Notwithstanding the luxurious fibroblastic proliferation and collagen synthesis in the interstices of filamentous prostheses, the spatial orientation and compositional properties of the collagenous tissue, which is formed anew in the implants, are dictated by the mechanics and non-self-attributes of the artificial filaments rather than by the functional exigencies of the joint.

The present-day prostheses by and of themselves, as well as by the fragments they release, elicit an inflammatory-granulomatous response that, in synergy with biomechanical factors, impedes the healing processes so that the artificial filaments, fibroblasts, collagen and reticulin fibers, granulation tissue, inflammatory infiltrates, and regressively altered or necrotic tissue make up a hybrid. Until such time as bioengineers and materials scientists overcome the defiant and unruly effects of synthetic filaments, prosthetic and biological replacements will vie with each other, though currently the latter appear to have gained the upper hand. Ratner rightly maintains that our biomaterials have been "developed based on a trial-and-error optimization approach rather than being engineered to produce the desired interfacial reaction". The record of the synthetic filaments clearly illustrates Ratner's dictum that future biomaterials "instead of fighting biology" should be designed to "smoothly integrate into living systems" [146].

ACKNOWLEDGMENT

The authors gratefully acknowledge the American Chapter of the Bnai–Zion Fraternal Organization, the German-Israeli Foundation (GIF) for Scientific Research and Development, the Directorate of Research and Development of the Israeli Ministry of Defense, and the Federmann House, Ltd. for their generous support of the laboratory of bone pathology, the research of the Center for Implant Surgery and the Association of Patients with Implanted Joints.

REFERENCES

1. Frank, C., Woo, S. L. Y., Amiel, D., Harwood, F., Gomez, M., and Akeson, W. Medial collateral ligament healing. A multidisciplinary assessment in rabbits. *Am. J. Sports Med.* 1983; 11:379–389.
2. Feagin, J. A., Curl, W. W. Isolated tear of the anterior cruciate ligament. Five year follow-up study. *Am. J. Sports Med.* 1976; 4:95–102.
3. Jones, R. Disabilities of the knee joint. *Brit. Med. J.* 1916; 2:169–183.
4. Kennedy, J. C., Roth, J.H., Mendenhall, H. V., and Sanford, J. B. Intraarticular replacement of the anterior cruciate ligament deficient knee. *Am. J. Sports Med.* 1980; 8:1–8.
5. Lyon, R. M., Akeson, W. H., Amiel, D., Kitabayashi, L. R., and Woo, S. L. Y. Ultrastructural differences between the cells of the medial collateral and anterior cruciate ligaments. *Clin. Orthop.* 1991; 272:279–286.
6. Wiig, M. E., Amiel, D., Ivarsson, M., Nagineni, C. N., Wallace, C. D., and Arfors, K. E. Type I procollagen gene expression in normal and early healing of the medial collateral and anterior cruciate ligaments in rabbits: An *in situ* hybridization study. *J. Orthop. Res.* 1991; 9:374–382.
7. Amis, A. A., and Dawkins, G. P. C. Functional anatomy of the anterior cruciate ligament. Fibre bundle actions related to ligament replacements and injury. *J. Bone Joint Surg.* 1991; 73B:260–267.
8. Arnoczky, S. P. Anatomy of the anterior cruciate ligament. *Clin. Orthop.* 1983; 172:19–25.
9. Hefzy, M. S., and Grood, E. S. Sensitivity of insertion locations on length pattern of anterior cruciate ligament fibers. *J. Biomech. Eng.* 1986; 108:73–82.
10. Amis, A. A. Anterior cruciate ligament replacement: Knee stability and effects of implants. *J. Bone Joint Surg.* 1989; 71B:819–824.
11. Amiel, D., Frank, C., Harwood, F. L., Fronek, J., and Akeson, W. H. Tendons and ligaments: A morphological and biochemical comparison. *J. Orthop. Res.* 1984; 1:257–265.
12. Amiel, D., Foulk, R. A., Harwood, F. L., and Akeson, W. H. Quantitative assessment by competitive ELISA of fibronectin (Fn) in tendons and ligaments. *Matrix* 1989; 9:421–427.
13. Vogel, K. G., Oerdoeeg, A., Pogany, G., and Olah, J. Proteoglycans in the compressed region of human tibialis posterior tendon and in ligaments. *J. Orthop. Res.* 1993; 11:68–77.
14. Kleiner, J. B., Amiel, D., Roux, R. D., and Akeson, W. H. Origin of replacement cells for the anterior cruciate ligament autograft. *J. Orthop. Res.* 1986; 4:466–474.

15. Noyes, F. R., Grood, E. S., Butler, D. L., and Paulos, L. E. Clinical biomechanics of the knee: Ligament restraints and functional stability. *AAOS Symposium 1978.* C. V. Mosby Co., St. Louis, 1980, pp. 1–35.

16. Wroble, R. R., and Brand, R. A. Paradoxes in the history of the anterior cruciate ligament. *Clin. Orthop.* 1990; 259:183–191.

17. Johnson, R. J., Beynnon, B. D., Nicols, C. E., and Renstrom, P. A. F. H. The treatment of injuries of the anterior cruciate ligament. *J. Bone Joint Surg.* 1992; 74A:140–151.

18. Wolter, D. Biocompatibility of carbon fibre and carbon fibre microparticles. *Aktuel Prob. Chir. Orthop.* 1983; 26:28–36.

19. Alexander, H., Weiss, A. B., and Parsons, J. R. Absorbable polymer-filamentous carbon composites — A new class of tissue scaffolding materials. *Aktuel Prob. Chir. Orthop.* 1983; 26:78–91.

20. Neugebauer, R., and Claes, L. The biological reaction of the tissues to carbon fibre ligament prosthesis in sheep knees. *Aktuel Prob. Chir. Orthop.* 1983; 26:96–100.

21. Strover, A. E., and Firer, P. The use of carbon fiber implants in anterior cruciate ligament surgery. *Clin. Orthop.* 1985; 196:88–98.

22. Kramer, B., and King, R. E. The histological appearance of carbon fiber implants and neoligaments in man. *S. Afr. Med. J.* 1983; 63:1130115.

23. Maekisalo, S., Skuttnabb, K., Holmstroem, T., Groenblad, M., and Paavolinen, P. Reconstruction of the anterior cruciate ligament with carbon fiber. An experimental study on pigs. *Am. J. Sports. Med.* 1988; 16:589–593.

24. Wolter, D., Burri, C., Fitzer, E., Helbing, G., Mueller, A., and Rueter A. Der alloplastische Ersatz des medialen Knieseitenbandes mit Kohlenstofffasern beim Schaf. *Unfallheilkunde* 1978; 81:390–403.

25. Mendes, D. G., Gottfried, Y., Grishkan, A., Angel, D., and Boss, J. H. Histology of carbon fibers reconstruction. *Proc 29th Ann Meeting Orthop Res Soc* 1983; 187.

26. Mendes, D. G., Iusim, M., Angel, D., Rotem, A., Roffman, M., Grishkan, A. Mordochovich, D., and Boss, J. H. Histologic pattern and biomechanical properties of the carbon fibre-augmented ligament and tendon. A laboratory and clinical study. *Clin. Orthop.* 1985; 196:51–60.

27. Strover, A. E. Technical advances in the reconstruction of knee ligaments using carbon fibers. In *Alloplastic Ligament Replacement*, C. Burri and L. Claes, Eds., Hans Huber, Bern, 1983, pp. 127–134.

28. Mendes, D. G., Angel, D., Grishkan, A. and Boss, J. H. Histological response to carbon fibre. *J. Bone Joint Surg.* 1985; 67B:645–649.

29. Amis, A. A., Campbell, J. R., and Miller, J. H. Strength of carbon and polyester fibre tendon replacements: Variation after operation in rabbits. *J. Bone Joint Surg.* 1985; 67B:829–834.

30. Forster, I. W., and Shuttleworth, A. Tissue reaction to intraarticular carbon fibre implants in the knee. *J. Bone Joint Surg.* 1984; 66B:282–288.

31. Zarnett, R., Velazquez, R., and Salter, R. B. The effect of continuous passive motion on knee ligament reconstruction with carbon fibre. An experimental investigation. *J. Bone Joint Surg.* 1991; 73B:47–52.

32. Salter, R. B., Simmonds, D. F., Malcolm, B. W., Rumble, E. J., Macmichael, D., and Clements, N. D. The biological effect of continuous passive motion on the healing of full-thickness defects in articular cartilage. An experimental investigation in rabbits. *J. Bone Joint Surg.* 1980; 62A:1232–1235.

33. Leyshon, R. L., Channon, G. M., Jenkins, D. H. R., and Ralis, Z. A. Flexible carbon fibre in late ligamentous reconstruction for instability in the knee. *J. Bone Joint Surg.* 1984; 66B:196–200.

34. Alexander, H., Weiss, A. B., and Parsons, J. R. Ligament repair and reconstruction with an absorbable polymer coated carbon fiber stent. *J. Orthop. Surg. Tech.* 1987; 3:1–14.

35. Alexander, H., Parsons, J. R., Strauchler, I. D., Corcoran, S. F., Gona, O., and Mayott, C. W. Canine patellar tendon replacement with a polylactic acid polymer-filamentous carbon tissue scaffold. *Orthop. Rev.* 1981; 10:41–51.

36. Adams, D. O. The granulomatous inflammatory response: A review. *Am. J. Path.* 1976; 84: 164–191.

37. Gonzalez, J. G., Ghiselli, R. W., and Santa Cruz, D. J. Synovial metaplasia of the skin. *Am. J. Surg. Path.* 1987; 11:343–350.

38. Drachman, D. B., and Sokoloff, L. The role of movement in embryonic joint development. *Develop. Biol.* 1966; 14:401–420.

39. Cheville, N. F. Inflammation and repair. In *Cell Pathology*, 2nd Ed., Iowa State University Press, Iowa City, 1983, pp. 236–297.

40. Keating, E. M., Marino, A. A., Albright, J. A., and Specian, R. D. Functional repair of rabbit gastrocnemius tendons using carbon fibers. *Clin. Orthop.* 1986; 209:292–297.

41. Alexander, H., Weiss, A. B., and Parsons, A. B. Absorbable polymer filamentous carbon composites: A new class of tissue scaffolding materials. In *Alloplastic Ligament Replacement*, C. Burri and L. Claes, Eds., Hans Huber, Bern, 1983, pp. 78–91.

42. Amis, A. A., Campbell, J. R., Kempson, S. A., and Miller, J. H. Comparison of the struction of neotendons induced by implantation of carbon or polyester fibers. *J. Bone Joint Surg.* 1984; 66B:131–139.

43. Forster, I. W., Ralis, Z. A., McKibbin, B., and Jenkins, D. H. R. Biological reaction to carbon fiber implants: The formation and structure of carbon induced "neotendon." *Clin. Orthop.* 1978; 131:299–307.

44. Jenkins, D. H. R. Ligament replacement in experiments on animals. In *Alloplastic Ligament Replacement*, C. Burri and L. Claes, Eds., Hans Huber, Bern, 1983, pp. 92–97.

45. Mendes, D. G., Soudry, M., Roffman, M., and Boss, J. H. Maturation of composite ligament. *Clin. Orthop.* 1988; 234:291–295.

46. Jenkins, D. H. R., and McKibbin, B. The role of flexible carbon-fibre implants as tendon and ligament substitutes in clinical practice: A preliminary report. *J. Bone Joint Surg.* 1980; 62B:497–499.

47. Aragona, J., Parsons, J. R., Alexander, H., and Weiss, A. B. Soft tissue attachment of a filamentous carbon absorbable polymer tendon and ligament replacement. *Clin. Orthop.* 1981; 160:268–278.

48. Claes, L., and Neugebauer, R. Mechanical properties of ligament replacement with carbon fibres. In *Alloplastic Ligament Replacement*, C. Burri and L. Claes, Eds., Hans Huber, Bern, 1983, pp. 28–36.

49. Wolter, D. Biocompatibility of carbon fibre and carbon fibre microparticles. In *Alloplastic Ligament Replacement*, C. Burri and L. Claes, Eds., Hans Huber, Bern, 1983, pp. 37–41.

50. Mendes, D. G., Iusim, M., Angel, D., Rotem, A., Mordochovich, D., Roffman, M., Lieberson, S., and Boss, J. H. Ligament and tendon substitution with composite carbon fiber strands. *J. Biomed. Mater. Res.* 1986; 20:699–708.

51. Hunt, M. S. An introduction to the use of carbon fibre reinforced composite material for surgical implants. *CSIR Report ME-1689*, Pretoria, South Africa, 1984.

52. Marino, A. A. Personal communication cited in Ref. 25.

53. King, J. B., and Bulstrode, C. J. K. Polyacetate-coated carbon fiber in extraarticular reconstruction of the unstable knee. *Clin. Orthop.* 1985; 196:139–142.

54. Parsons, J. R., Bhayani, S., Alexander, H., and Weiss, A. B. Carbon fiber debris within the synovial joint—A time dependent mechanical and histological study. *Clin. Orthop.* 1985; 196:69–76.

55. Demmer, P., Fowler, M., and Marino, A. A. Use of carbon fibers in the reconstruction of knee ligaments. *Clin. Orthop.* 1991; 271:225–232.

56. Goodship, A. E., Wilcock, S. A., and Shah, J. S. The development of tissue around various prosthetic implants used as replacement for ligaments and tendons. *Clin. Orthop.* 1985; 61:61–69.

57. Mendes, D. G., Soudry, M., Levine, E., Silbermann, M., Shoshan, S., Gross, U., Shajrawi, I., and Boss, J. H. The collagen composition of the carbon fiber composite ligament. An electron microscopical, biochemical, and immunohistological study. *J. Long-Term Eff. Med. Impl.* 1992; 1:305-319.

58. Boss, J. H., Shajrawi, I., Soudry, M., and Mendes, D. G. Histomorphological reaction patterns of the bone to diverse particulate implant materials in man and experimental animal. In *Particulate Debris from Medical Implants: Mechanisms of Formation and Biological Consequences*, ASTM STP 1144, K. R. St. John, Ed., American Society for Testing and Materials, Philadelphia, 1992, pp. 90-108.

59. King, J. B., and Bulstrode, C. J. K. Extra-articular carbon fibre at the knee. *J. Bone Joint Surg.* 1985; 67B:156-157.

60. Schiavone Panni, A., Fabbriciani, C., Delcogliano, C., and Franzese, S. Bone-ligament interaction in patellar tendon reconstruction of the ACL. *Knee Surg. Sports Traumatol. Arthroscopy.* 1993; 1:4-8.

61. Claes, L., and Neugebauer, R. *In vivo* and *in vitro* investigation of the long-term behavior and fatigue strength of carbon fiber ligament replacement. *Clin. Orthop.* 1985; 196:99-111.

62. Gleason, T. F., Barmada, R., and Ghosh, L. Can carbon fiber implants substitute for collateral ligament. *Clin. Orthop.* 1984; 191:274-280.

63. Boss, J. H., Shajrawi, I., and Mendes, D. G. The nature of the interface membrane of orthopaedic devices: A viewpoint of pathologists. *Orthopaedics Int. Ed.* 1993; 1:325-331.

64. Boss, J. H., Shajrawi, I., and Mendes, D. G. Intraosseous anchorage of the carbon fiber composite ligament by bony ingrowth. *J. Appl. Biomater.* 1991; 2:241-242.

65. Ling, R. S. M. Observations on the fixation of implants to the bony skeleton. *Clin. Orthop.* 1986; 210:80-96.

66. Jansen, J. A., van der Waerden, J. P. C. M., and DeGroot, K. Epithelial reaction to percutaneous implant materials: In vitro and in vivo experiments. *J. Invest. Surg.* 1989; 2:29-49.

67. Weiss, A. B., Blazina, M. E., Goldstein, A. R., and Alexander, H. Ligament replacement with an absorbable copolymer carbon fiber scaffold. Early clinical experience. *Clin. Orthop.* 1985; 160:268-278.

68. Maekisalo, S., Paavolainen, P., Holmstroem, T., and Skutnaab, K. Carbon fiber as a prosthetic anterior cruciate ligament. A biochemical and histological study. *Am. J. Sports. Med.* 1989; 17:459-462.

69. Neugebauer, R., and Claes, L. The biological reaction of the tissue to carbon fibre ligament prosthesis in sheep knee. In *Alloplastic Ligament Replacement*, C. Burri and L. Claes, Eds., Hans Huber, Bern, 1983, pp. 97-101.

70. Ricci, J. L., Gona, A. G., Alexander, H., and Parsons, J. R. Morphological characteristics of tendon cells cultured on synthetic fibers. *J. Biomed. Mater. Res.* 1984; 18:1073-1087.

71. Tayton, K., Phillips, G., and Ralis, Z. A. Long term effects of carbon fibers on soft tissue. *J. Bone Joint Surg.* 1982; 64B:112-114.

72. Shoshan, S., and Gross, J. Biosynthesis and metabolism of collagen and its role in tissue-repair processes. *Isr. J. Med. Sci.* 1974; 10:537-561.

73. Shoshan, S. Wound healing. *Intern. Rev. Connective Tis. Res.* 1981; 9:1-26.

74. Amiel, D., Akeson, W. H., Renzoni, S., Harwood, F., and Abel, M. Nutrition of cruciate ligament reconstruction by diffusion. Collagen synthesis studied in rabbits. *Acta. Orthop. Scand.* 1986; 57:201-203.

75. Wagner, B. M. Wound healing revisited: Fibronectin and company. *Human Path.* 1985; 16:1081.

76. Dunphy, J. E. *Wound Healing*, Medom Press, New York, 1974.

77. Cove, J. N., Cohen, K., and Diegelmann, R. F. Quantitation of collagen Types I and III during wound healing in rat skin. *Proc. Soc. Exp. Biol. Med.* 1979; 161:337-340.

78. Amiel, D., Kleiner, J. B., Roux, R. D., Harwood, F. L., and Akeson, W. H. The phenomenon of "ligamentization": Anterior cruciate ligament reconstruction with autogenous patellar tendon. *J. Orthop. Res.* 1986; 4:162–172.

79. Mendes, D. G. An overview of the use of carbon fibres in ligament reconstruction. *J. Orthop. Surg. Tech.* 1987; 3:53–65.

80. Bray, R. C., Flanagan, J. P., and Dandy, D. J. Reconstruction for chronic anterior cruciate instability: A comparison of two methods after six years. *J. Bone Joint Surg.* 1988; 70B:100–104.

81. Rushton, N., Dandy, D. J., and Naylor, C. P. E. The clinical, arthroscopic and histological findings after replacement of the anterior cruciate ligament with carbon-fibre. *J. Bone Joint Surg.* 1983; 65B:308–309.

82. Veth, R. P. H., den Heeten, G. J., Jansen, H. W. B., and Nielsoen, H. K. L. An experimental study of reconstructive procedures in lesions of the meniscus. Use of synovial flaps and carbon fiber implants for artificially made lesions in the meniscus of the rabbit. *Clin. Orthop.* 1983; 181:250–254.

83. Minns, R. J., Benton, M. J., Dunstone, G. H., and Sunter, J. F. An experimental study of the use of a carbon fibre patch as a hernia prosthesis material. *Biomaterials* 1982; 3:199–203.

84. Ward, R., and Minns, R. J. Woven carbon-fibre patch versus Dacron mesh in the repair of experimental defects in the lumbar fascia of rabbits. *Biomaterials* 1989; 10:425–428.

85. Thomas, N. P., Turner, I. G., and Jones, C. B. Prosthetic anterior cruciate ligaments in the rabbit. A comparison of four types of replacement. *J. Bone Joint Surg.* 1987; 69B:312–316.

86. Amis, A. A., Kempson, S. A., Campbell, J. R., and Miller, J. H. Anterior cruciate ligament in the dog: Biocompatibility and biomechanics of polyester and carbon fibre in rabbits. *J. Bone Joint Surg.* 1988; 70B:628–634.

87. Meyers, J. F., Grana, W. A., and Lesker, P. A. Reconstruction of the anterior cruciate ligament in the dog: Comparison of results obtained with three different porous synthetic materials. *Am. J. Sports Med.* 1979; 7:85–90.

88. Butler, H. C. Teflon as a prosthetic ligament in repair of ruptured anterior cruciate ligaments. *Am. J. Vet. Res.* 1964; 25:55–60.

89. Vaughan, L. C. A study of the replacement of the anterior cruciate ligament in the dog by fascia, skin and nylon. *Vet. Rec.* 1963; 75:537–541.

90. Sgaglione, N. A., Del Pizzo, W., Fox, J. M., Friedman, M. J., Snyder, S. J., and Ferkel, R. D. Arthroscopic-assisted anterior cruciate ligament reconstruction with the semitendinosus tendon: Comparison of results with and without braided propylene augmentation. *J. Arthroscop. Rel. Surg.* 1992; 8:65–77.

91. Claes, L., Burri, C., Neugebauer, R., Piehler, J., and Mohr, W. Animal experiments for comparison of various alloplastic materials in ligament replacements. In *Alloplastic Ligament Replacement*, C. Burri and L. Claes, Eds., Hans Huber, Bern, 1983, pp. 102–107.

92. Schiavone Panni, A., Denti, M., Franzese, S., and Monteleone, M. The bone-ligament junction: A comparison between biological and artificial ACL reconstruction. *Knee Surg. Sports Traumatol. Arthroscopy.* 1993; 1:9–12.

93. Davila, J. C., Lautsch, E. V., and Palmer, T. E. Some physical factors affecting the acceptance of synthetic materials as tissue implants. *Ann. N.Y. Acad. Sci.* 1968; 146:138–147.

94. Townley, C. O., Fumich, R. M., and Shall, L. M. The free synovial graft as a shield for collagen ingrowth in cruciate ligament repair. *Clin. Orthop.* 1985; 187:266–271.

95. Kurosaka, M., Yoshiva, S., and Andrish, J. T. Dacron-augmented anterior cruciate ligament reconstruction in dogs: A six-month follow-up study. *Am. J. Knee Surg.* 1993; 6:61–66.

96. Claes, L., Duerselen, L., Kiefer, H., and Mohr, W. The combined anterior cruciate and medial collateral ligament replacement by various materials: A comparative animal study. *J. Biomed. Mater. Res.* 1987; 21:319–334.

97. Contzen, M. Polyester ligament replacement in experiments on animals. In *Alloplastic Ligament Replacement*, C. Burri and L. Claes, Eds., Hans Huber, Bern, 1983, pp. 68–71.

98. Wirth, C. J. Temporary intraarticular knee stabilization with synthetic material (polyester-silicon) in the sheep. In *Alloplastic Ligament Replacement*, C. Burri and L. Claes, Eds., Hans Huber, Bern, 1983, pp. 58–63.

99. Lunkianov, A. V., Richmond, J. C., Barrett, G. R., and Gilquist, J. A multicenter study on the results of anterior cruciate ligament reconstruction using a Dacron ligament prosthesis in "salvage" cases. *Am. J. Sports Med.* 1989; 17:380–386.

100. Gilquist, J. Follow-up on 58 cases with Stryker–Meadox ligament prosthesis. *Advances in Cruciate Ligament Reconstruction of the Knee: Prosthetic Autogenous, Proc. 5th Intern. Symp.* 1988, pp. 155–164.

101. Lopez-Vazquez, E. Juan, J. A., and Debon, J. Reconstruction of the anterior cruciate ligament with a Dacron prosthesis. *J. Bone Joint Surg.* 1991; 73A:1294–1300.

102. Noble, C. A. The Stryker Dacon ligament in chronic anterior cruciate ligament tears. *Am. J. Sports Med.* 1989; 17:723.

103. Klein, W., and Jensen, K. U. Synovitis and artificial ligaments. *J. Arthroscopy Rel. Surg.* 1992; 8:116–124.

104. Desai, P., Steiner, G., Alexander, H., and Springer, S. Tissue response to prosthetic knee ligaments. *Proc. Impl. Retrieval Symp., Soc. Biomater,* 1992, 543.

105. Andrish, J. T., and Woods, L. D. Dacron augmentation in anterior cruciate ligament reconstruction in dogs. *Clin. Orthop.* 1984; 183:298–302.

106. Gupta, B. N., and Brinker, W. O. Anterior cruciate ligament prosthesis in the dog. *J. Am. Veter. Med. Assn.* 1989; 154:1057–1061.

107. Woods, G. W. Synthetics in anterior cruciate ligament reconstruction. A review. *Orthop. Clin. North Am.* 1985; 16:227–235.

108. Bolton, W., and Bruchman, B. Mechanical and biological properties of the Gore-Tex expanded polytetrafluoroethylene (PTFE) prosthetic ligament. In *Alloplastic Ligament Replacement*, C. Burri and L. Claes, Eds., Hans Huber, Bern, 1983, pp. 40–50.

109. Fujikawa, K., Iseki, F., Tomatsu, T., Takeda, T., and Seedhom, B. B. Microscopic and histological findings after reconstruction of the anterior cruciate ligament by the Leeds–Keio artificial ligament. *Knee* 1984; 10:35–40.

110. Markolf, K. L., Pattee, G. A., Strum, G. M., Gallick, G. S., Sherman, O. H., Nuys, V., and Dorey, F. J. Instrumented measurement of laxity in patients who have a Gore-Tex anterior cruciate-ligament substitute. *J. Bone Joint Surg.* 1989; 71A:887–893.

111. Glousman, R., Shields, C. Jr., Kerlean, R., Jobe, F., Lombardo, S., Yocum, L., Tibone, J., and Gambardella, R. Gore-Tex prosthetic ligament in anterior cruciate deficient knees. *Am. J. Sports. Med.* 1988; 16:321–326.

112. Alfield, S. K., Larson, B. L., and Collins, H. L. Anterior cruciate reconstruction in the chronically unstable knee using an expanded polytetrafluoroethylene (PTFE) prosthetic ligament. *Am. J. Sports Med.* 1987; 14:326–330.

113. Indelicato, P. A., Pascale, M. S., and Huegel, M. D. Early experience with the Gore-Tex polytetrafluorethylene anterior cruciate ligament prosthesis. *Am. J. Sports Med.* 1989; 17: 55–62.

114. Ferkel, R. D., Fox, J. M., Wood, D., Del Pizzo, W., Friedman, M. J., and Snyder, S. J. Arthroscopic "second look" at the Gore-Tex ligament. *Am. J. Sports Med.* 1989; 17:147–153.

115. Mueller-Mai, C. M., and Gross, U. M. Histological and ultrastructural observations at the interface of expanded polytetrafluoroethylene anterior cruciate ligament implants. *J. Appl. Biomater.* 1991; 2:29–35.

116. Bolton, C. W., and Bruchman, W. C. The Gore-Tex expanded polytetrafluoroethylene prosthetic ligament. An *in vitro* and *in vivo* evaluation. *Clin. Orthop.* 1985; 196:202–213.

117. Vireday, C., Settlage, R., and Bain, J. R. Tissue response to a porous ePTFE prosthetic ligament: Correlation of laboratory and clinical findings. *Abstr. Symp. on Retrieval and Analysis of Surg. Impl. Biomater., Soc. Biomater.,* 1988, 11.

118. Bruchman, W. C., Bain, J. R., and Bolton, C. W. Prosthetic replacement of the cruciate ligaments with expanded polytetrafluorethylene. In *The Cruciate Ligaments. Diagnosis and Treatment of Ligamentous Injuries of the Knee*, J. A. Feagan, Ed., Churchill Livingstone, New York, 1988, pp. 507–515.

119. Seedhom, B. B. The Leeds–Keio ligament: Biomechanics. In *Prosthetic Ligament Reconstruction of the Knee*, M. J. Friedman and P. M. Motta, Eds., W. B. Saunders, Philadelphia, 1988, pp. 118–127.

120. Seedhom, B. B., Fujikawa, K., and Atkinson, P. S. On fixation of Terylene to bone with special reference to the cruciate. *J. Bone Joint Surg.* 1987; 65B:660–665.

121. Marcacci, M., Gubellini, P., Buda, R., De Pasquale, V., Strocchi, R., Molgora, A. P., Zaffagnini, S., Guizzardi, S., and Ruggeri. Histologic and ultrastructural findings of tissue ingrowth. The Leeds–Keio prosthetic anterior cruciate ligament. *Clin. Orthop.* 1991; 267: 115–121.

122. Homsy, C. A., Prewitt, J. M. III, and Woods, G. W. Proplast ligament implants: Design and *in vitro* testing. In *Alloplastic Ligament Replacement*, C. Burri and L. Claes, Eds., Hans Huber, Bern, 1983, pp. 51–57.

123. James, S. L., Kellam, J. F., Slocum, D. B., and Larsen, R. L. The proplast prosthetic ligament stent as a replacement for the cruciate ligaments of the knee. In *Alloplastic Ligament Replacement*, C. Burri and L. Claes, Eds., Hans Huber, Bern, 1983, pp. 116–120.

124. Aichroth, P. M., Patel, D. V., Jones, C. B., and Wand, J. S. A combined intra- and extra-articular reconstruction using a carbon-Dacron composite prosthesis for chronic anterior instability. A two- to six-year follow-up study. *Intern. Orthop.* 1991; 15:219–227.

125. Aichroth, P. M., Jones, C. B., and Thomas, N. P. Carbon fibre and Dacron composites in the prosthetic reconstruction of the anterior cruciate ligament. *J. Bone Joint Surg.* 1986; 68B:841–847.

126. Kennedy, J. C., Roth, J. H., Mendenhall, H. V., and Sanford, J. B. Intraarticular replacement in the anterior cruciate ligament-deficient knee. *Am. J. Sports Med.* 1980; 8:1–8.

127. Barrett, G. R., and Savoies, F. H. Operative management of acute PCL injuries with associated pathology: Long-term results. *Orthopedics* 1991; 14:687–692.

128. Roth, J. H., Shkrum, M. J., and Bray, R. C. Synovial reaction associated with disruption of polypropylene braid-augmented intraarticular anterior cruciate ligament reconstruction. A case report. *Am. J. Sports Med.* 1988; 16:301–305.

129. Yamamoto, H., Ishibashi, T., Muneta, T., Furuya, K., and Mizuta, T. Effusions after anterior cruciate ligament reconstruction using the ligament augmentation device. *J. Arthroscop. Rel. Surg.* 1992; 8:305–310.

130. Daniel, D. M., Woodward, E. P., Losse, G. M., and Stone, M. L. The Marshall/Macintosh anterior cruciate ligament reconstruction with Kennedy ligament augmentation device: Report of the United States clinical trials. In *Prosthetic Ligament Reconstruction of the Knee*, M. J. Friedman and R. D. Ferkel, Eds., W. B. Saunders, Philadelphia, 1988, pp. 71–78.

131. Boss, J. H., Shajrawi, I., Soudry, M., Aunullah, J., Solomon, H., and Mendes, D. G. Studies on a novel anterior cruciate ligament polyethylene fiber prosthesis: The histomorphological pattern of organization and bony anchorage of a polyethylene fiber prosthesis in the stifle of the goat. *Clin. Mater.*, 1994; 15:61–67.

132. Shajrawi, I., Aunullah, J., Soudry, M., Solomon, H., Mendes, D. G., and Boss, J. H. Quantification of the tissue response to a polyethylene prosthesis of the ACL in the goat. A histomorphometric study. *Orthopaedics Intern. Edn.* 1993; 1:455–460.

133. Sennerby, L., Thomsen, P., and Ericson, L. E. Early tissue response to titanium implants inserted in rabbit cortical bone. Part I. Light microscopic observations. *J. Mater. Sci. Mater. Med.* 1993; 4:240–250.

134. Boss, J. H., Shajrawi, I., Aunullah, J., Solomon, H., Mendes, D. G., Schaefer, R., Soltesz, U., and Ulrich, D. Motion-induced inhibition of tissular organization and bony anchorage of a polyethylene anterior cruciate ligament prosthesis in the stifle of the goat. In *Biomedical*

Engineering, Recent Development, J. Vossoughi, Ed., University of the District of Columbia, Washington DC, 1994, pp. 1125–1128.

135. Boss, J. H., Shajrawi, I., and Mendes, D. G. Histological patterns of the tissue reaction to polymers in orthopaedic surgery. *Clin. Mater.* 1993; 13:11–17.

136. Boss, J. H., Shajrawi, I., and Mendes, D. G. The nature of bone-implant interface: The lessons learned from implant retrieval and analysis in man and experimental animal. *Med. Progr. Through Technology.* 1994; 20:119–142.

137. Ralis, Z. A., and Forster, T. W. Choice of the implantation site and other factors influencing the carbon fibre-tissue reaction. *J. Bone Joint Surg.* 1981; 63B:295–296.

138. Radford, W. J. R., and Amis, A. A. Biomechanical properties of a double prosthetic ligament in the anterior cruciate deficient knee. *J. Bone Joint Surg.* 1990; 72B:1038–1043.

139. Eriksson, E. Stalked patellar tendon graft in reconstruction of the anterior cruciate ligament. *Orthopedics* 1986; 9:205–211.

140. Macon, N. D., Lemons, J. E., and Niemann, K. M. W. Polymer particles *in vivo*: Distribution in the knee, migration to lymph nodes, and associated cellular response following anterior cruciate ligament replacement. In *Particulate Debris from Medical Implants: Mechanisms of Formation and Biological Consequences*, ASTM STP 1144, K. R. St. John, Ed., American Society for Testing and Materials, Philadelphia, 1992, pp. 189–199.

141. Davis, P. A., Huang, S. J., Ambrosio, L., Ronca, D., and Nicholais, L. A biodegradable composite artificial tendon. *J. Mater. Sci. Mater Med.* 1991; 3:359–364.

142. Strover, A. E. Carbon fibre. III. Operative techniques and instrumentation. In *Ligament Injuries and Their Treatment*, D. H. R. Jenkins, Ed., Chapman and Hall, London, 1985, pp. 269–297.

143. Jenkins, D. H. R. The repair of cruciate ligaments with flexible carbon fibre. *J. Bone Joint Surg.* 1978; 60B:520–522.

144. Allen, P. R., Amis, A. A., Jones, M. M., and Heatley, F. W. Evaluation of preserved bovine tendon xenograft: A histological, biomechanical and clinical study. *Biomaterials* 1987; 8:146–152.

145. Olson, E. J., Kang, J. D., Fu, F. H., Georgescu, H. I., Mason, G. C., and Evans, C. H. The biochemical and histological effects of artificial ligament wear particles: *In vitro* and *in vivo* studies. *Am. J. Sports Med.* 1988; 16:558–569.

146. Ratner, B. D. New ideas in biomaterials science—A path to engineered biomaterials. *J. Biomed. Mater. Res.* 1993; 27:837–850.

14

Yttria-Stabilized Zirconia for Improved Orthopedic Prostheses

Bernard Cales and Yves Stefani
Ceramiques Techniques Desmarquest
Evreux, France

I. INTRODUCTION

Orthopedic prosthesis implantation is becoming an increasingly common surgical procedure. Until recently, most orthopedic prostheses consisted of a combination of a polished metal bearing component, made of titanium alloy, Cr-Co alloy, or stainless steel, and an ultra-high molecular weight polyethylene (UHMWPE) counterbearing component. Although these combinations lead to a low-friction arthroplasty, metallic bearing components also induce a significant wear of UHMWPE and are subject to corrosion by the sinovial liquid. Resulting wear debris are almost always found in the surrounding tissue [1,2]. It has been shown that the UHMWPE debris are causing periprosthetic osteolysis [1,2]. These adverse tissue responses, which lead in extreme cases to prosthetic loosening, become the major problem with total hip arthroplasty 5 to 10 years after surgery [1,2]. Indeed, as pointed out by Jasty [1], because of prostheses loosening, between 10% and 30% of patients need reoperation after only 10 years. This situation, which is of particular concern for implantation in younger people, has led to the search for new friction combinations with reduced wear rates and reduced debris. Ceramic has been the most effective solution to date.

Ceramic components were in fact introduced in orthopedics in the 1970s, first by Boutin in France [3] and then by Griss and Heimke in Germany [4]. Several laboratory wear studies have clearly established that the wear rate of UHMWPE against alumina ceramic is significantly lower than against stainless steel [5] or Cr-Co alloy [6]. Semlitsch et al. reported an UHMWPE wear 20 times lower using alumina hip joint heads instead of Cr-Co alloy heads [7]. This behavior was confirmed by several clinical results [8–10].

However, alumina ceramics, even with fine microstructure and high chemical purity, remain brittle with low fracture strength and toughness when compared to metals. Alumina ceramics are therefore sensitive to microstructural flaws and have a low resistance to stress concentrations. As a consequence, in order to preserve a high reliability, only alumina femoral balls with a diameter higher than or equal to 28 millimeters (mm) [11] and with limited taper designs are currently manufactured. Small hip joint heads, with a diameter as low as 22.22 mm, which have been shown to give a lower UHMWPE wear rate [12,13], are not currently manufactured using alumina ceramics for reliability reasons.

To overcome these limitations, transformation-toughened ceramics were successfully introduced in orthopedics in 1985. The improved mechanical properties of zirconia ceramics, combined with excellent biocompatibility and wear properties, make this material the best choice for the new generation of orthopedic prostheses. Zirconia ceramics are already widely used in orthopedics in replacing alumina ceramics and, to a certain extent, metals. Today, over 150,000 zirconia ceramic hip joint heads have been implanted, mainly in Europe and in the United States.

The purpose of this chapter is to report on the physicochemical properties of zirconia ceramics used in surgical techniques and to describe current and possible future developments in the field of zirconia orthopedic prostheses.

II. PHYSICOCHEMICAL PROPERTIES AND BIOCOMPATIBILITY OF ZIRCONIA CERAMICS

A. Mechanical Properties of Zirconia Ceramics

1. Phase Transformation Toughening

Pure zirconia exhibits three polymorphic phases with increasing temperature: monoclinic, tetragonal, and cubic. The cubic phase is only thermodynamically stable at a high temperature ($> 2370°C$) and is brittle. The tetragonal phase transforms at low temperatures into the monoclinic phase, which is the stable phase at room temperature. Of greatest significance is the tetragonal-to-monoclinic (T-M) transformation, which is associated with a large volume change (3–5%) [14]. This transformation can be controlled by the addition of stabilizing oxides of bivalent metals M^{2+} (e.g., CaO, MgO) [15,16], trivalent metals M^{3+} (e.g., Y_2O_3) [17], or lanthanide oxides and some tetravalent metals M^{4+} like CeO_2 or TiO_2 [18]. Depending on the nature and content of the stabilizing oxide, a 100% tetragonal metastable solid solution (TZP) can be obtained at room temperature. It is essential here to distinguish between *metastable* transformation (that which can be controlled) and an *unstable* transformation, which is spontaneous.

In the field of orthopedic prostheses, a tetragonal yttria-stabilized zirconia polycrystal ceramic (Y-TZP), made of a ZrO_2-Y_2O_3 solid solution, is the most widely used. Some developments have also been made using magnesia-stabilized zirconia (Mg-PSZ) ceramics that offer similar mechanical properties to Y-TZP. However, due to the very high sintering temperature ($> 1700°C$) required for Mg-PSZ manufacturing, they are characterized by a coarse-grained microstructure containing a significant residual intragranular microporosity. In addition, the high sintering temperature can promote the diffusion of the impurities at grain boundaries to form a critical glassy phase that could affect the mechanical properties and wear behavior. For these reasons, the use of Mg-PSZ ceramics in surgery has remained limited.

The phase diagram of the ZrO_2-Y_2O_3 system (Fig. 1) displays a tetragonal single-phase field in which sintering should take place. Under the correct conditions of composition and temperature, a ceramic can be produced consisting of small tetragonal grains,

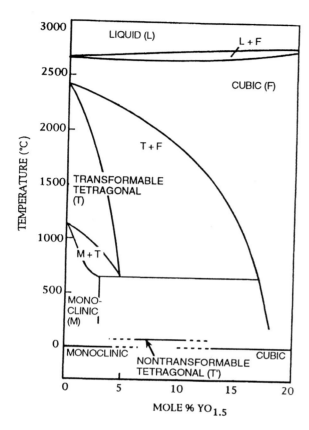

Figure 1   Phase diagram of the ZrO_2-Y_2O_3 system.

the metastability of which is directly related to several microstructural parameters (Fig. 2), (i.e., density, mean grain size, and Y_2O_3 content) [19]. Since these parameters are dependent on the manufacturing process, Y-TZP ceramics made by different sources can have very different properties. Generalizations need to be made with caution. Some papers have been quite misleading in this respect [20,21]. There has, for example, been much misunderstanding about the aging of Y-TZP ceramics.

The optimal metastable Y-TZP ceramics are achieved by the following:

- Density close to theoretical density (6.1 g·cm³)
- Mean grain size < <1 micrometer (μm)
- Y_2O_3 content close to 3 mole percent (mol%)

These conditions lead to outstanding mechanical properties. Indeed, in fully dense and fine-grained Y-TZP ceramics, the tetragonal-to-monoclinic (T-M) transformation of small grains, which would result in a volume increase, is resisted by the compressive stresses applied on these grains by their neighbors. The mechanism of toughening is considered to be a stress-induced T-M transformation of zirconia grains [22]. A propagating crack (Fig. 3), characterized by large tensile stresses at the crack tip, will produce a shear stress in the tetragonal particles that causes them to transform into monoclinic

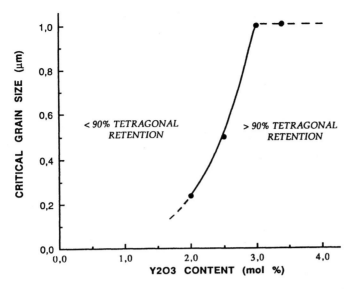

Figure 2   Influence of mean grain size and Y_2O_3 content on the stability of the tetragonal phase.

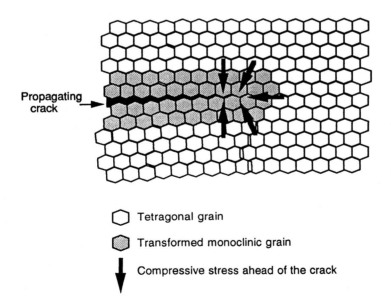

Figure 3   Scheme of the phase transformation toughening at the crack tip.

stable grains. The associated volume expansion ($>3\%$) of the transformed grains results in compressive stresses at the edge of the crack front. Extra energy is then required to move the crack through the ceramic, accounting for the increase in toughness and hence in strength. In the case of alumina ceramics, this mechanism does not exist. For this reason, Y-TZP ceramics with appropriate microstructure and chemical composition are currently characterized by flexural strength higher than 900 megapascal (MPa), which is two times higher than for alumina. As a direct consequence of these improved mechanical properties, the fracture strength of zirconia hip joint heads, press fit and loaded on metallic trunnions, is usually two times higher than the fracture strength of alumina heads having the same design [23].

The fracture strength of Y-TZP ceramics can further be improved by reducing toward zero the size of the intrinsic flaws, with the aid of an HIP (high isostatic pressure) treatment. The fracture strength of HIP treated Y-TZP ceramics can reach the outstanding value of 2000 MPa [24], while the toughness remains practically unchanged since the microstructure/chemical composition of the material is not modified.

2. Fracture Toughness and Slow Crack Growth

For crack resistance and lifetime prediction, the fracture toughness and the slow crack growth (SCG) behavior of Y-TZP materials are of prime importance. Fracture toughness can be measured by several techniques, leading to quite scattered results [25,26,71]. For this reason, it is necessary not only to report the fracture toughness value K_{IC} but also the measurement technique. The K_{IC} values measured by the indentation fracture technique vary greatly depending on the formula. Values between 4 and about 12 can be obtained depending on the toughness formula and the experimental error [27,71]. Though it strongly depends on the notch width [71], the single-edge notched beam (SENB) technique gives a more consistent result and a value of 10 ± 1 MPa$\sqrt{m}$ can be reached for Y-TZP ceramics with optimized microstructures [28]. This value must be regarded as a mean value because of the combined effect of both surface and bulk properties of Y-TZP.

Indeed, it has been recently shown by SCG analysis that the bulk and surface of Y-TZP ceramics could exhibit different SCG behaviors and fracture toughness [29]. Under given conditions of manufacturing (machining, grinding), tetragonal-to-monoclinic transformation could be induced in a thin surface layer [30,31], without extension inside the bulk (Fig. 4). Due to the volume expansion of the T-M transformation, a compressive layer at the surface of the Y-TZP samples could exist and modify the crack propagation characteristics and hence the toughness close to the surface. The thickness of this compressive layer depends on the severity of the surface treatment [65]. It could reach a few tens of micrometers for surfaces machined under "severe" conditions. On the other hand, the compressive layer can be eliminated by careful polishing of the surface.

A more recommended technique for toughness measurement in Y-TZP ceramics is that of the indentation strength [71]. The same bars prepared for flexural strength measurements can be used. The problem of residual stresses could be minimized by using the following technique [71]. A Vickers indentation under a load of 300 to 400 N is first applied in the middle of the bars. In order to have a large and stable crack after indentation, the indent is created through an oil drop (silicon oil) to avoid moisture penetrating the crack and the load is maintained for about 60 seconds (s). The bars are then fractured within 1 minute (min) with a 3- or 4-point flexural test. The fracture toughness is then obtained from the following formula:

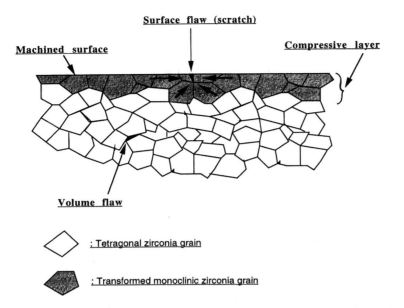

Machined surface

Surface flaw (scratch)

Compressive layer

Volume flaw

◇ : Tetragonal zirconia grain

⬠ : Transformed monoclinic zirconia grain

Figure 4 Scheme of a machined surface of a Y-TZP ceramic.

$$K_{IC} = 0.0186 \, (E/H)^{0.125} [\sigma(P)^{1/3}]^{0.75}$$

where
 E = the Young's modulus (GPa)
 H = hardness (GPa)
 P = the applied indentation load (N)
 σ = the measured residual flexural strength (MPa).

Fracture toughness values of 5.5 MPa$\sqrt{m}$, with a very low standard deviation (0.1 to 0.2 MPa$\sqrt{m}$) are typically obtained, using a 4-point flexural test. Such a toughness value is more representative of bulk properties of Y-TZP ceramics, as shown below.

The slow crack growth behavior of ceramic materials is currently described by the well-known relationship

$$V = A \, K_I^n$$

where
 V = the crack velocity
 K_I = the stress intensity factor
 A and n = constants (slow crack growth parameters).

In the case of Y-TZP ceramics, as explained above, due to the possible presence of a compressive layer at the surface of the material, bulk and surface SCG behaviors must be considered separately. Slow crack growth of volume flaws could be investigated using polished samples having 100% tetragonal phase at the surface. Thus, SCG of volume flaws in air exhibits a standard three-step diagram (Fig. 5), with

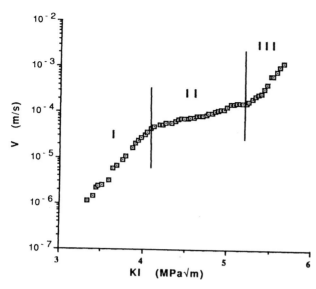

Figure 5   Typical three-step slow crack growth diagram for Y-TZP in air.

- Step I, at low crack velocity, corresponding to stress corrosion at the crack tip [32], the crack velocity being limited by the kinetics of the chemical reaction at the crack tip
- Step II, at higher crack velocity, in which SCG is controlled by the diffusion of the corrosive species up to the crack tip [32]
- Step III, at very high crack velocity, is not well known today

It may be noted that only Step I is representative of the normal fatigue situation in orthopedic components and of interest for lifetime prediction.

SCG behavior can be analyzed using various techniques, like double torsion, static fatigue, or dynamic fatigue [33]. The double-torsion technique is the most currently used, but must be optimized in the case of Y-TZP ceramics [29,34]. Indeed, the small groove machined in the double-torsion specimens generates a monoclinic compressive layer at the surface of the groove that hinders the study of volume flaws. A solution consists of making two Vickers indents close to the surface of the groove (Fig. 6) to generate a crack through the compressive layer. The bulk properties can then be studied. With such specimens, the scattering of the results is especially low, allowing for an accurate description of the slow crack growth parameters (Fig. 7) [29,34]. The fracture toughness obtained with the same double-torsion test and sample is 6.0 MPa√m for the bulk.

In Ringer's solution and water, only one stage of the SCG behavior is observed (Fig. 8). This has often been reported in water and suggests that the single mechanism responsible for the crack growth is the chemical reaction at the crack tip [32]. The scattering between different tests in Ringer's solution and in water is larger than that reported in air and is attributed to wetting [35]. The SCG behavior for bulk measured in air, Ringer's solution, and water are compared in Fig. 9 [29,34].

From this comparison, it may be concluded that, in Ringer's solution, like in air, the corrosive species appears to be water since experiments in pure water lead to the same

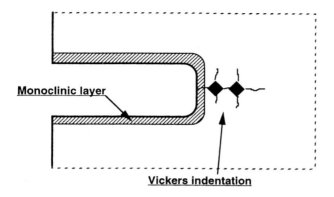

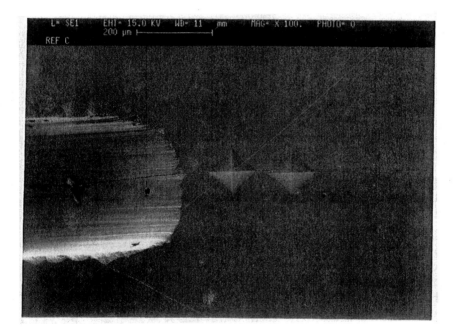

Figure 6   Scheme and micrograph of precracked double-torsion samples with the aid of two Vickers's indents.

single mechanism with identical crack growth parameter n (slope of the curve), which is also the same as in air experiments. The slow crack growth behavior is the same in Ringer's solution as in air. Therefore, aging of this material could be studied indifferently in air or in Ringer's solution.

A static fatigue experiment can also be used for very low fracture velocity measurements. For instance, SCG behavior for the bulk is depicted in Fig. 10 [29,34], down to 10^{-11} meter per second ($m \cdot s^{-1}$).

The "surface" fracture toughness measured by double torsion has been found to be

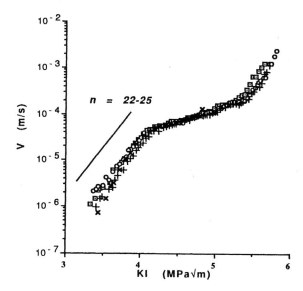

Figure 7   Slow crack growth in air of four samples of Y-TZP ceramic.

18 MPa√m̄ [29,34]. This is an apparent toughness that is the result of the superposition of the stress field by the crack and the compressive stress field induced by the transformation layer. This apparent toughness gives the significant strength of such a material when ground. The complete SCG diagram for Y-TZP ceramics, including bulk and surface contributions, is shown in Fig. 10. The high value of the stress exponent n (slope of the curve) reported for the surface flaws results from a compressive layer at the surface that leads to a threshold value of stress intensity factor K_I, below which no crack growth

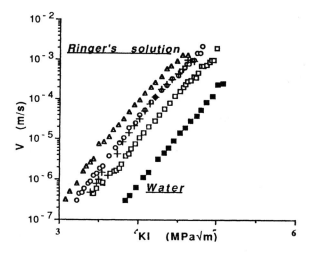

Figure 8   Slow crack growth in water and Ringer's solution of a Y-TZP ceramic.

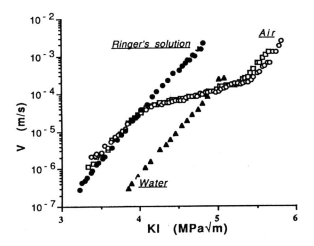

Figure 9 Comparison of the slow crack growth of a Y-TZP ceramic in air, water, and Ringer's solution.

occurs. This threshold value represents one of the best advantages of Y-TZP ceramics compared with other candidates such as alumina since it leads to a strong enhancement of lifetime. Indeed, this concerns the machining-induced surface flaws that could be responsible for the failure. Machining of the ceramics is critical in obtaining optimum fracture strength.

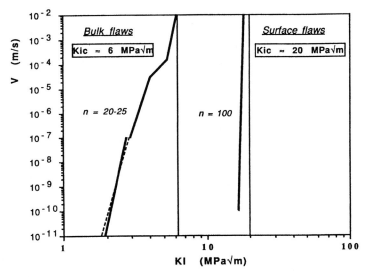

Figure 10 Complete slow crack growth diagram of a Y-TZP ceramic, including both bulk and surface contributions.

Table 1   Influence of the Sterilization Process on the Fracture Strength of Zirconia Ceramic (PROZYR®)

Sterilization process	Bending strength (MPa)	Standard deviation
Without	1039	107
Ethylene oxide	1186	76
Beta radiation	1069	100
Gamma radiation	1047	37
Autoclaving, 134°C, 2 bar	1106	110
Autoclaving, 121°C, 1 bar	1061	106

3.   Influence of Sterilization on Mechanical Properties

Before the implantation, zirconia ceramics are submitted to sterilization. Several sterilization techniques can be used and the sterilization may eventually be repeated several times in hospitals before use. However, no influence of sterilization on the fracture strength of Y-TZP ceramic has been detected. Table 1 summarizes the results for ethylene oxide, beta and gamma radiations (source of 50 kilo Gray), and autoclaving sterilizations. In order to evaluate the influence of repetitive sterilization operations, 20 autoclaving cycles were repeated on the same samples without any degradation in strength (Fig. 11). As mentioned above, this behavior is only representative of the material being studied, since it has been emphasized that low temperature degradation is strongly related to microstructure and chemical composition and to manufacturing process.

During sterilization by radiation (gamma or beta), the zirconia becomes colored. The

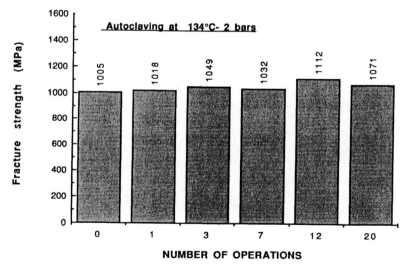

Figure 11   Influence of repetitive autoclaving on the flexural strength of PROZYR® Y-TZP ceramic.

change in color is induced by the ionizing radiation, which creates electrons and holes that can be trapped by traces of given elements [36] (a few parts per million [ppm]), such as rare earths. These color centers have no influence on the macroscopic properties of the material (strength, aging, etc.). A violet color has been often observed for sterilized Y-TZP ceramics; this could be attributed to traces of praseodymium. The same effect also has been reported previously for alumina [37] with different color changes (yellow to brownish).

B. Microstructure of TZP Ceramics and Other Properties

Y-TZP ceramics with outstanding mechanical properties require a fine-grained microstructure, with homogeneous grain size, such as that shown in Fig. 12. Mean grain size can be measured on flat polished and etched surfaces using the American Society for Testing and Materials (ASTM) 112-88 or the European EN/623 (Part 3) standards. The more recent EN/623 standard is preferred because it was written for advanced monolithic technical ceramics using the linear intercept technique. It should be noticed here that there is often a confusion between mean intercept length L (apparent grain size) and real average grain size G. Indeed, assuming the ceramic grains are near equiaxial, a polished surface will not cut through equatorial grain "diameters" and most of the grain will exhibit a lower cross section than reality (Fig. 13). The correction can be made by multiplying the mean intercept length measured on micrographs by a factor of 1.56 [38].

$$G = 1.56\, L$$

The standards only give recommendations for mean intercept length measurements.

In the case of Y-TZP ceramics, thermal etching is useful to reveal the microstructure. The thermal treatment needs to be previously optimized to avoid artificial grain growth. A temperature of 1350°C to 1400°C for 15 to 30 minutes is enough to etch the polished surface of Y-TZP ceramics.

Using these conditions, the mean grain size G of Y-TZP ceramics used in orthopedics

Figure 12   Typical microstructure of a Y-TZP ceramic.

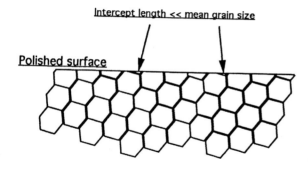

Intercept length << mean grain size

Polished surface

Figure 13   Scheme of a polished ceramic surface and apparent grain size.

is lower than 0.8 μm ($L < 0.5$ μm). However, it is not an objective to decrease the mean grain size to as small as possible. Indeed, it has been shown that, for mean grain size smaller than approximately 0.4 μm, the stress-induced phase transformation is no longer active [73], and lower fracture strength and toughness thus result. In addition, very small mean grain sizes are often observed on low density samples. A good objective for medical-grade Y-TZP ceramics is a mean grain size G of 0.5–0.7 μm ($L = 0.32$–0.45 μm). It will lead to both high mechanical properties and no aging effect in physiological conditions.

Other typical properties of a yttria-stabilized zirconia used in orthopedics (PRO-ZYR®) are summarized in Table 2. Among these properties, it may be noted that the

Table 2   Main Characteristics of a Zirconia Ceramic Used in Orthopedics and Related Standard Drafts

Properties	Units	ISO standard draft	ASTM standard draft	Zirconia ceramic[a]
Chemical composition				
ZrO_2	%	>94.2	>93.2	>93.5
Y_2O_3	%	5.1 ± 0.3	5.1 ± 0.2	5.1 ± 0.25
HfO_2	%	<5		<2
Al_2O_3	%	<0.5	<0.5	<0.5
Other	%	<0.5	<0.5[b]	<0.5
U, Th oxides	ppm	<20	<20	<5
Bulk density	g/cm³	>600	>6.00	>6.00
Open porosity	%			<0.1
Average linear intercept	μm	<0.6	<0.5	<0.5
Bending strength (4 points)	MPa	>900	>900	≥920
Biaxial strength	MPa	>550		>600
Fracture toughness[c]	MPa√m			5 ± 0.2

[a]PROZYR®
[b]Detail of chemical impurities to be confirmed
[c]Indentation strength technique (see text)

modulus of elasticity of zirconia is about two times lower than that of surgical-grade alumina. As a consequence, stress distribution generated in ceramics heads under loading on metallic trunnions are lower using Y-TZP zirconia instead of alumina, as shown by finite element analysis (FEA) [23]. Such a situation also contributes to higher fracture strength for zirconia hip joint heads.

The main physical properties recommended in the French standard on zirconia ceramic for surgical implant and those proposed for the ASTM and International Organization for Standardization (ISO) standard drafts are also summarized in Table 2.

C. Biocompatibility of Y-TZP Ceramics

Yttria-stabilized zirconias are very chemically stable ceramics that would exhibit a high biocompatibility in both *in vitro* and *in vivo* conditions. However, due to minor changes in composition from one Y-TZP to another (yttrium oxide content, impurities), it is not realistic to predict a general behavior for the *in vitro* and *in vivo* biocompatibility of these materials. Biocompatibility tests should be made by each manufacturer of Y-TZP.

As an indication, biocompatibility test results reported for the more extensively used surgical-grade Y-TZPs are summarized in Table 3. Most of these tests were conducted according to ASTM standards. The *in vitro* tests indicate no adverse reaction with cells or tissues. The short-term and long-term *in vivo* experiments also reveal an excellent biocompatibility. This is also supported by the numerous clinical results over a period of more than eight years, which confirm the absence of adverse tissue reaction.

Other *in vitro* and *in vivo* experiments on magnesia-doped zirconia (Mg-PSZ) [39] led to a similar conclusion for that material. Recent experiments on cell reactions with very fine zirconium oxide or hydroxide, resulting from metal hydrolysis, also show no inhibition of cell growth or proliferation [40].

D. Radioactivity of Zirconia Ceramics

The radioactivity of zirconia ceramics has been questioned because of the use, a few years ago, of rather impure zirconia powders as radio-contrast media in bone cement [41]. However, Y-TZP orthopedic implants are manufactured with very high purity zirconia

Table 3 Biocompatibility of a Surgical-Grade of Zirconia Ceramic

Biocompatibility test	Method used	Results
In vivo biocompatibility		
Short-term test	ASTM F 763/82	Very good
Long-term test	ASTM F 361	Very good
	ASTM F 469/78	
In vitro biocompatibility,		
general recommendations	ASTM F 748/82	
Cytotoxicity	NFS 90.702	Good cytocompatibility
Mutagenicity	Ames test/micronucleus	No mutagenic activity
Systemic toxicity	ASTM F 750/82	According to standard
Intracutaneous injection	ASTM F 749/82	No irritation
Sensitization	ASTM F 720/81	No sensitization
	Magnusson	

powders because a uniform chemical composition is required to achieve high mechanical properties. As a consequence, the resulting radioactivity is very low. Recently, several studies have been made of this issue [42–44].

Nevertheless, since zirconia implants remain in the body for a long period of time, it is essential to check that the radioactivity level of the zirconia powder used for Y-TZP manufacturing is as low as possible. In this objective, it may be considered that the mean radioactivity of the body or of human bones should not be exceeded by the implant. This is true for zirconia, but also for any other implanted materials (metals, alumina, ceramic coatings).

Concerning zirconia ceramics, traces of uranium and thorium oxides are generally detected. The level of these impurities depends on the zirconia raw material used and the purification route [42–44]. Uranium and thorium radionuclides are alpha, beta, and gamma emitters and the three types of radioactivity should normally be measured. In practice, however, due to the extremely low level of radioactivity to be measured, which is lower than the natural ambient radioactivity [42,43], only the gamma radioactivity could be measured quite easily. In addition, for given radionuclides, the gamma radioactivity level is related to the beta and alpha radioactivities. The beta and alpha radioactivities need to be measured by expert laboratories and the results are strongly dependent on the method used. This is not the case of gamma radioactivity, for which the value measured in human bones has been reported to be of the order of 80–100 $Bq \cdot kg^{-1}$ (Bequerel per kilogram) [44,64]. It is therefore recommended that the zirconia powder used for Y-TZP manufacturing be evaluated with gamma spectroscopy.

A comparison of various zirconia powders from different sources indicates large variations from one powder to another (Table 4) [42]. Only the powders prepared through an oxychloride route can have a gamma radioactivity lower than that for human bone. They can be accurately selected by gamma spectroscopy.

Another solution to control the final radioactivity of the product is to check the chemical composition, especially regarding the radionuclide contents (i.e., UO_2, ThO_2, eventually $^{40}K_2O$ for other materials, etc.). Indeed, uranium and thorium trace measurements could be achieved quite easily by inductively coupled plasma (ICP) or atomic absorption techniques currently used in many laboratories. In the case of yttria-stabilized zirconia for surgical implants, ISO and ASTM standard drafts recommend a total amount of uranium and thorium oxides lower than 20 ppm (Table 2). It is currently lower than 5 ppm for the best Y-TZP materials (Table 2).

III. IN VITRO AND IN VIVO BEHAVIOR OF ZIRCONIA CERAMICS

Of upmost significance for orthopedic applications is the long-term aging of zirconia ceramics. Indeed, long-term stability of physical properties is required to provide long implantation times.

Several papers have reported in the last few years [45] on the low temperature degradation (LTD) of zirconia ceramics at moderate temperature (150°C–400°C) in steam, and it was argued that LTD was a general behavior for Y-TZP ceramics. However, it must be recalled, as shown by the theoretical study of Lange [46], that the metastability and the resulting phase transformation toughening of Y-TZP ceramics are directly related to microstructural (grain size) and chemical (Y_2O_3 content) parameters. A review of low temperature degradation in Y-TZP ceramics has recently been made by E. Lilley [47].

Table 4   Gamma Massic Activity of Various Zirconia Powders

ZrO₂ source	Grade	Radionuclide	Massic activity (Bq/kg)	Manufacturing process (chemical route)
A		Ra-226	< 10	Oxychloride
		Ac-228	2.0	
		U-235	< 5	
B	1	Pb-212	7.0	Oxychloride
		Ac-228	3.3	
B	1	Ra-226	2.0	Oxychloride
		Ac-228	2.1	
B	2	Ra-226	< 11	Oxychloride
		Pb-212	8.2	
		Ac-228	4.5	
C	1	Ra-226	24.0	Other
		Pb-214	24.0	
		U-235	< 1.5	
C	2	Ra-226	248	Other
		Pb-214	243	
		U-235	< 5	
D		U-228	800	Other
		Th-232	39	
D		Ra-226	1221	Other
		U-235	27	
E				Other
F		Ra-226	2300	Other
		Ac-228	390	

Thus, two different Y-TZP ceramics, having different grain sizes and/or Y_2O_3 contents, will exhibit distinctly different LTD behaviors. This has been recently shown by Swab [48], who compared seven different commercial Y-TZP ceramics and found them to have significantly different LTD behaviors. For fine-grained ($\approx 0.5\ \mu m$), 3-mol% Y_2O_3-doped zirconia, there is essentially no low temperature degradation reaction under the severe conditions of more than 50 hours in steam at 200°C–400°C. Under physiological conditions (37°C, pH 7), LTD becomes nonexistent with such material. This behavior was confirmed by aging experiments in both *in vitro* and *in vivo* conditions on commercially available Y-TZP ceramics and in orthopedics [49,50].

The *in vitro* agings were performed by two laboratories, using Ringer's solution at 37°C at a pH of 7 [49]. Flexural test bars were machined directly from Y-TZP femoral heads (PROZYR®) and immersed in Ringer's solution for several months, up to two years. After aging, the fracture strength of Y-TZP, measured by either three-point or four-point bending, remained unchanged and equal to the value before aging (Fig. 14). This conclusion was emphasized by a statistical analysis of the fracture strength results using Weibull plots (Fig. 15). The Weibull modulus (slope of the curve), which is an estimate of the scatter in fracture strength, is not modified after aging more than one year. Similar results were reported by Shimizu et al. after aging another commercial Y-TZP ceramic for three years [51]. The fracture strength stability is due to the absence of T-M transformation under the physiological aging conditions. Indeed, measurement

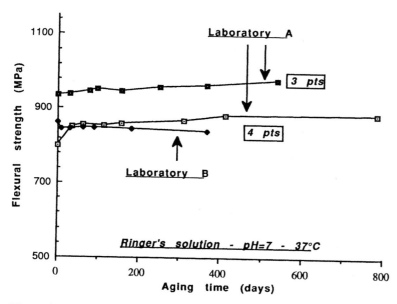

Figure 14   Influence of *in vitro* aging on the fracture strength of Y-TZP ceramic (PROZYR®).

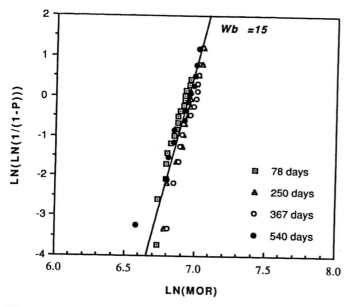

Figure 15   Weibull analysis of the fracture strength of a Y-TZP ceramic after various *in vitro* aging times.

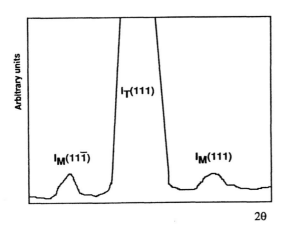

Figure 16 Scheme of the x-ray diffraction diagram with monoclinic and tetragonal [111] lines.

of monoclinic phase content by X-ray diffraction on polished and aged pellets clearly shows that no T-M transformation is induced by physiological aging [49]. The monoclinic fraction $M\%$ was calculated from the peak intensity [52]:

$$M\% = \frac{I_M(111) + I_M(11\bar{1})}{I_T(111) + I_M(111) + I_M(11\bar{1})}$$

where $I_{T,M}(111)$ is the intensity of the [111] tetragonal and monoclinic lines, as schematically shown in Fig. 16. After one year of aging, the monoclinic content remained extremely low, with the relative change before and after aging being close to zero (Fig. 17).

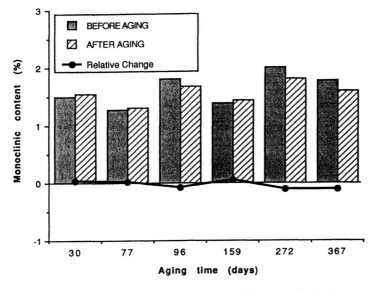

Figure 17 Influence of *in vitro* aging on the monoclinic phase content (absolute values before and after aging and relative change).

In vitro aging under stress was also performed on the same zirconia femoral heads. The heads were press fit on TA6V trunnions having a cylindrical hole along their axis to allow the Ringer's solution to wet the high-stressed zones at the top of the cone [53]. They were then axially loaded at 0, 10, 20, and 30 kN (kilo Newton) prior to immersion in Ringer's solution. After aging, the heads were loaded again until rupture according to a standardized burst test procedure. The fracture load of the heads before and after aging is plotted in Fig. 18. There is no significant change after one year aging in Ringer's solution. Indeed, a statistical analysis of the results, using a studentized test [54], leads to the conclusion that the fracture load is not degraded by static fatigue.

The same stability of mechanical properties was found after *in vivo* aging. Small, surgical-grade Y-TZP samples have been implanted up to 24–30 months in rats, rabbits, and sheep muscles or bones. The after-aging mechanical properties were measured by either the indentation fracture technique for the fracture toughness [49] or bending tests for the fracture strength [51]. The results of toughness measurements after various *in vivo* agings are shown in Fig. 19. Given the scattering of the toughness data (± 1 MPa√m), it was concluded that the zirconia ceramic studied was not sensitive to *in vivo* aging. The results reported after aging in sheep femurs are the most significant because of the stresses applied to the specimens within the sheep femurs. However, sheep implantation cannot be considered as fully representative of aging conditions in humans.

For this reason, analysis of retrieved implanted material should be considered as the best verification of aging behavior because it combines the influence of aging in physiological liquid to that of cyclic fatigue. Such an analysis has been done on retrieved zirconia hip joint heads after implantation times exceeding three years [55]. The machining of flexural test bars taken from retrieved heads allowed verification that the fracture strength of Y-TZP ceramic is unchanged after long-term aging in humans. Table 5 compares the flexural strength of the PROZYR® Y-TZP material before implantation and

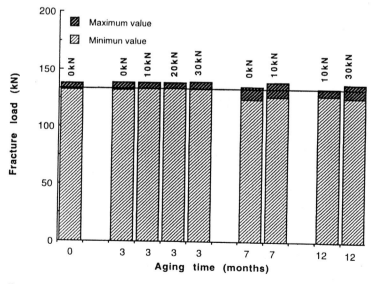

Figure 18 Influence of *in vitro* aging under stresses on the fracture strength of zirconia hip joint heads (PROZYR®).

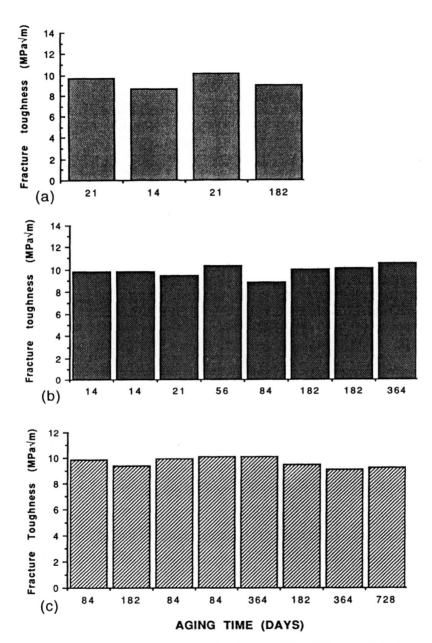

Figure 19 Influence of *in vivo* aging (a) rat; (b) rabbit; and (c) sheep implantation on the fracture toughness of Y-TZP ceramic (PROZYR®).

Table 5 Flexural Strength of PROZYR Zirconia Ceramic Before and After Two Years of Implantation

Flexural strength (MPa)	Before implantation	After two years of implantation
Mean value	1009	996
Standard deviation	85	57

after two years in humans, with test bars machined from femoral heads of the same batch and thus having exactly the same microstructure. In light of the standard deviation, it may be concluded that the modulus of rupture is very stable. The same conclusion was obtained after testing retrieved zirconia heads of the same origin, using a standard burst test, and comparing the fracture load to the current values measured by statistical process control (SPC) on several batches of heads with the same design (Fig. 20). After two to three years of implantation, the fracture load of the studied zirconia heads remained unchanged.

The *in vitro* and *in vivo* agings clearly show that Y-TZP ceramics, provided they have the appropriate microstructure and chemical composition, are sufficiently stable to resist aging and consequently constitute an outstanding class of material for orthopedic applications.

IV. SURFACE CHARACTERISTICS AND WEAR PROPERTIES OF ZIRCONIA CERAMICS AGAINST ULTRA-HIGH MOLECULAR WEIGHT POLYETHYLENE

The most important characteristic of materials used as bearing components for orthopedic applications is their capability to reduce wear debris and ion-release phenomena. The replacement of metallic bearing components by ceramic bearing components virtually eliminates the ion-release-related problem [56], while the quantity of UHMWPE debris is simultaneously decreased [10,57]. It is now well recognized that ceramics are superior materials for orthopedic uses in which wear debris is the critical issue [58].

Several studies have been done to compare the wear behavior of alumina and zirconia ceramics against UHMWPE [59–61]. However, most of these studies have been done on pin-on-disk laboratory tests and the results are somewhat contradictory. Kumar et al. obtained a lower year of polyethylene with zirconia than with alumina [60], while Streicher, Semlitsch, and Schön observed the opposite situation [59]. The disagreement results from differences in the experiments, but mainly from the origin of the various ceramic materials, which exhibit different surface characteristics, (microstructure, roughness, waviness, etc.). Furthermore, the experiments were often conducted on laboratory-made zirconia samples that cannot be regarded as representative of the commercially available zirconia implant materials.

In addition, it should also be noted that the wear properties of ceramic materials are dependent on the surface finish (roughness, waviness, roundness) and microstructure. These parameters are representative of the manufacturing and finishing route used by the zirconia ceramic producer and can vary from one source to another. For these reasons, it is not realistic to compare the wear behavior of ceramic materials of various origins

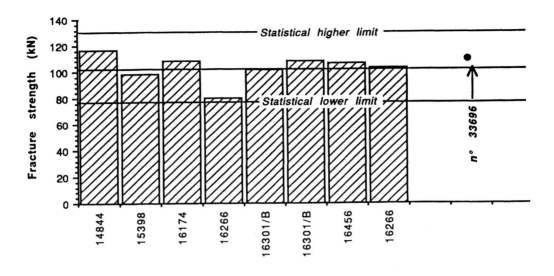

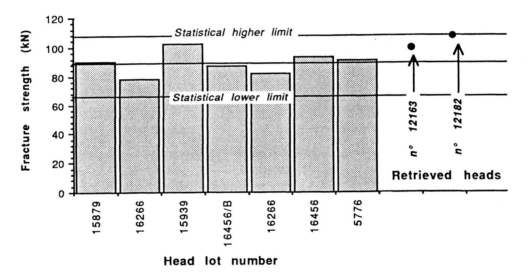

Figure 20 Fracture strength of retrieved heads compared with fracture strength of nonimplanted heads of the same design and of various lots (statistical process control).

or having a surface finish different from that of the real bearing components used in orthopedics.

Typical values of surface roughness and roundness for PROZYR® heads are summarized in Figs. 21 and 22 and compared with those of commercial alumina heads. The roughness R_a, R_z, and R_{max} (Fig. 21) were measured by three different laboratories on the same apparatus and the same heads and averaged for 25 samples. A good agreement was observed for R_a, R_z, and R_{max}. The roughness value R_a is of the order of 0.005 μm for a cutoff of 0.08 mm (ISO recommendations). The roundness was measured by a 3-D

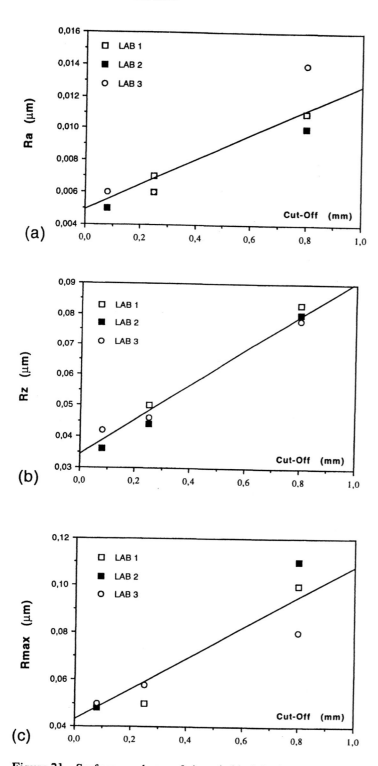

Figure 21 Surface roughness of zirconia hip joint heads (PROZYR®): (a) R_a; (b) R_z; (c) R_{max}.

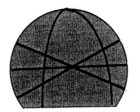

ROUNDNESS		ZIRCONIA HEAD (*)	ALUMINA HEAD
Mean Value (**)	(μm)	0.674	3.450
Maximum	(μm)	0.857	4.580
Minimum	(μm)	0.491	2.380
Range	(μm)	0.366	2.200
Standard Deviation	(μm)	0.146	0.790

Figure 22   Roundness of zirconia and alumina hip joint heads and scheme of measurement lines.

machine along five lines for each head (Fig. 22). The roundness deviation for the studied zirconia heads is extremely low. It is lower than 1 μm whatever the position of the measurement line (equatorial or meridian). Conversely, for the analyzed alumina heads, the roundness deviation is systematically higher and is close to the limit (5 μm) for the meridian position. The difference for the two types of heads lies in the manufacturing process (machining and polishing), which are basically different.

Investigation of wear properties of ceramic bearing components used in orthopedics requires performing these experiments using the same materials (heads and cups) and designs that reflect reality. In addition, as recently shown by Saikko et al. [74], it could be necessary, for the wear tests, to press fit the ceramic heads on the same trunnions used for implantation. Indeed, micromotion of the metallic trunnion inside the ceramic cone could generate abrasive metallic particles that can strongly affect the polyethylene wear [74].

Such an analysis was reported by McKellop et al. using a head-on-cup joint simulator with bovine serum as the lubricant [62]. The lubricant was complexed with ethylene diamine-tetraacetate (EDTA) to prevent calcium phosphate deposition onto the bearing surfaces. The wear of UHMWPE cups measured up to 5 million cycles is shown in Fig. 23 for the three studied heads (Cr-Co alloy, Howmedica; alumina: VITOX®, Morgan-Matroc; zirconia: PROZYR®, C. T. Desmarquest). The reproducible results indicate a lower wear rate with the zirconia heads than observed with the alumina and Cr-Co alloy heads.

Also surprising is the lower wear rate observed for the Cr-Co alloy heads compared with alumina heads. This situation could be due to the surface finish, which was slightly better on the studied Cr-Co heads than on the ceramic heads [62]. Indeed, it is well

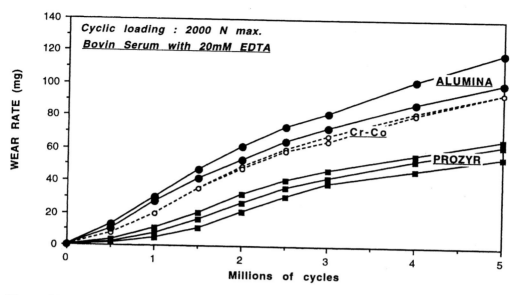

Figure 23   Results of head-on-cup wear experiment on zirconia, alumina, and Cr-Co heads. (After Ref. 62.)

known that abrasive wear, which has been reported to be the most significant mechanism of UHMWPE degradation, is directly dependent on head surface finish.

Finally, several studies have shown that wear of UHMWPE could be significantly reduced by using small 22.22-mm heads instead of 28- or 32-mm heads [12]. In this domain, because of their improved mechanical strength, Y-TZP ceramics offer a real advantage.

V. DEVELOPMENT OF ZIRCONIA HIP JOINT HEADS WITH CUSTOMIZED DESIGN

The use of yttria-stabilized zirconia for hip joint heads allows the manufacturing of numerous different heads, the design of which must be adapted and optimized to the metallic taper design. Because of the improved mechanical properties of Y-TZP ceramics, the geometrical parameters of the heads can be varied to a larger extent. It is, for instance, possible to manufacture small-diameter heads, down to 22.22 mm, with 8/10-mm or 10/12-mm cones, or heads with large cones, like 28-mm diameter heads with 14/16-mm cones. However, in order to guarantee the reliability of each design, it is necessary to know the stress distribution inside the head under loading. Indeed, the knowledge of the magnitude of the tensile stresses and their location is of prime importance because they affect the survival probability of the components.

This can be accurately achieved using finite element analysis (FEA) with appropriate contact elements to simulate the metallic taper/ceramic head interface. The finite element analysis of the real tensile stresses in a head under normal cyclic loading is extremely difficult because of the numerous loading situations (patient weight, motion rate, etc.). For this reason, it is essential to verify that the different geometries of heads fulfill

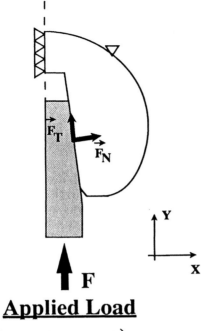

Applied Load

(▽ no displacement)

Figure 24   Scheme of the boundary conditions for finite element analysis.

the various requirements concerning fracture strength. For instance, the Food and Drug Administration (FDA) requires that ceramic hip joint heads have a mean rupture load, on a metallic taper, of 46 kN, with the minimum value higher than 20 kN, using a standardized uniaxial burst test.

Figure 24 shows the boundary conditions that can be used for such calculations. Since the ceramic head is fixed on the metallic taper by friction forces along the conical interface, sliding with friction is simulated at the interface by a Coulomb's law:

$$F_t = \mu F_n$$

where
μ = the friction coefficient
F_t = the tangential load
F_n = the normal load

The friction coefficient can be preliminarily estimated by press fitting and uniaxial loading of zirconia heads on metallic tapers. The measurement of the head/trunnion relative displacement using displacement transducers gives an estimate of μ. For zirconia heads on TA6V alloy trunnions, a value of μ of about 0.3 has thus been deduced. However, for precise FEA, the value of μ, or at least the relative displacement curve, would be determined in each case.

Under loading, tensile stresses are generated in the head in mainly two regions (Fig. 25), the first one located at the corner at the top of the taper, the second at the ceramic head/metallic trunnion interface. An FEA-optimized head/taper fitting should minimize the tensile stresses simultaneously in these two regions. This can be achieved by optimizing the contact area (location and extent) at the interface. Indeed, as shown by Seidelmann, Richter, and Soltész [63], the tensile stresses in the head depend strongly on the contact area at the interface.

The influence of the location and extent of contact area between a zirconia head and a TA6V trunnion on the maximum tensile stresses in the two critical regions mentioned above (Fig. 25) is shown in Fig. 26. It may be observed that, when increasing the surface of the contact or the distance d (Fig. 27) between the top of the taper and the top of the ceramic cone, the maximum tensile stresses decrease strongly in both regions (Figs. 26a and 26b). However, extending the surface contact to the bottom of the ceramic cone should be avoided. In such a case, the tensile stresses at the bottom of the head drastically increase (Fig. 26b).

A compromise design based on FEA should be defined for each type of head. In particular, ceramic/taper contact at the bottom of the cone could be avoided by an appropriate chamfer (Fig. 27). Another solution to increase the distance d without extending the contact to the bottom of the cone consists of reducing the thickness e at the top of the ceramic head (Fig. 27). Indeed, FEA clearly reveals that an increase of d by reduction of the thickness e, without modifying the geometry of the contact, leads to a significant decrease of the tensile stresses at the top of the cone (Fig. 28).

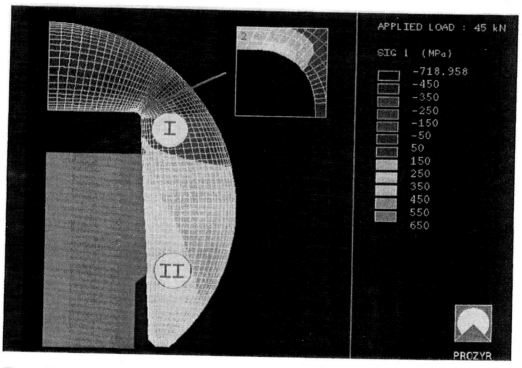

Figure 25   Typical stress concentration in hip joint heads under uniaxial loading.

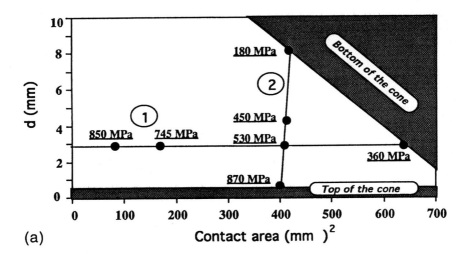

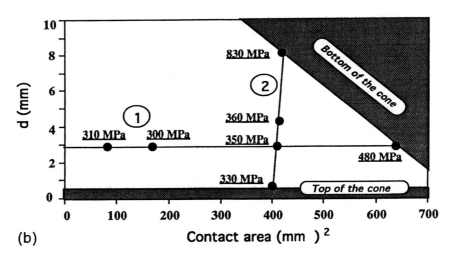

Figure 26 Diagram of the maximum tensile stresses versus contact area and distance d between the top of the metallic trunnion and the top of the ceramic cone: (a) at the top of the cone; (b) at the taper/head interface.

The introduction of a dome section at the top of the ceramic cone (Fig. 29) has been described as a favorable design modification that could lead to stress reduction when compared with other designs with a sharper angle at the top of the ceramic cone [70] (Fig. 29). In fact, a dome section at the top of the cone has no direct influence on the stress distribution, but can be associated with an increase of the distance d at the top of the ceramic cone. As shown above, only the increase of the distance d is responsible for a decease of the stress concentrations in the head. Indeed, two heads having the same design, one with a dome section and the other without, and characterized by the same

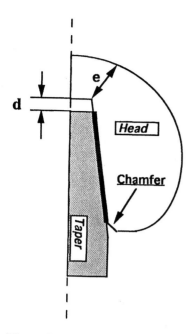

Figure 27   Scheme of a hip joint head press fit on a metallic trunnion.

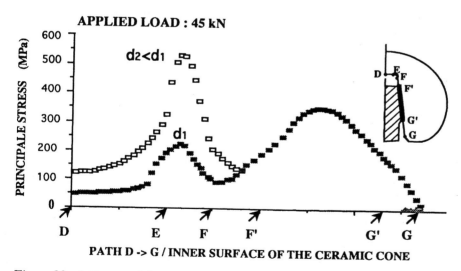

Figure 28   Influence of the distance *d* on the tensile stresses along the inner surface of the ceramic cone.

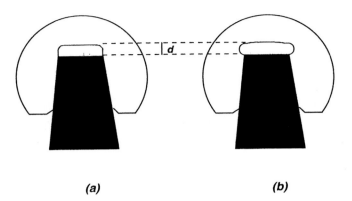

(a)   (b)

Figure 29   Comparison of two heads with the same design but (a) with or (b) without a dome section at the top of the cone.

distance d (Fig. 29) will exhibit the same stress concentrations and therefore the same rupture load. This is clearly shown in Fig. 30.

Tensile stresses inside the head can also be reduced by increasing the friction coefficient at the ceramic/taper interface, for instance, by modifying the surface characteristics of the metallic taper (roughness, thread) or the geometrical characteristics of the taper (angle). FEA using different friction coefficients μ clearly shows the reduction of tensile stresses when μ is increased (Fig. 31).

Thus, zirconia heads can be designed for various taper geometries after optimization of the head/taper contact parameters using FEA. Examples of such optimized zirconia hip joint heads are described below.

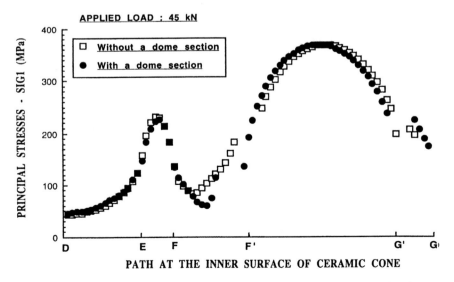

Figure 30   Comparison of the tensile stresses for the two heads shown in Fig. 29.

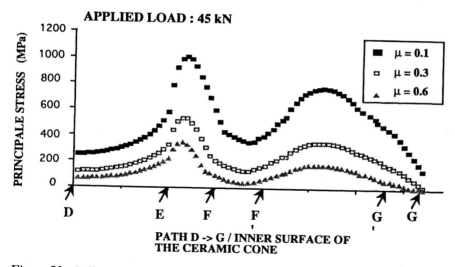

Figure 31   Influence of the friction coefficient on the tensile stresses along the inner surface of the cone.

VI.   CURRENT DEVELOPMENT IN ZIRCONIA HIP JOINT HEADS

The high fracture strength and toughness of yttria-stabilized zirconia ceramics (Y-TZP) allow the design of many reliable zirconia hip joint heads. The comparison of the stress maps obtained by finite element analysis to the values of rupture load effectively measured using a standardized burst test allows deduction of the value of the critical stress (stress leading to fast fracture) inside the zirconia heads. Such a comparison has been done on a large number of head geometries and clearly indicates that the critical stress is in the order of 800–850 MPa, close to the flexural strength value. It is therefore possible, using finite element analysis, to predict the fracture load of zirconia hip joint heads of a given design and to predict origin of the rupture. An iterative operation then allows optimization of the design of the heads and improvement of their fracture strength.

Table 6 summarizes the various possible designs for zirconia hip joint heads. The

Table 6   Design Possibilities for Y-TZP Zirconia Hip Joint Heads with Maximum Length Between Long and Short Neck

	Head diameter			
	32	28	26	22.22
Type of cone	Maximum length between long and short neck			
14/16	7 mm	7 mm	4 mm	
12/14	10 mm	8 mm	5 mm	0 mm
10/12	10 mm	10 mm	6 mm	3.5 mm
8/10	10 mm	10 mm	7 mm	5 mm

Shaded cases indicate current designs.

head diameter can vary from 32 to 22.22 mm, while different classes of cones, from 14/16 to 8/10, could be used. It should be noted that each class of cone covers a large number of slightly different real cone diameters corresponding to the geometries of the different commercially available metallic tapers. Table 6 also indicates for each ball/cone combination the maximum neck length that can be machined without reducing the performances of the head.

Of all combinations, the only one that cannot be achieved, for geometrical reasons, is the use of small, 22.22-mm zirconia femoral balls with large cones (i.e., 14/16 cones). All the other combinations are characterized, after design optimization, by a rupture load, under uniaxial loading, higher than 60 kN. However, the real rupture load depends not only on the zirconia head design, but also on the geometrical and physical properties of the metallic taper. A comparison of the measured rupture load for the same zirconia heads when uniaxially tested on TA6V or Cr-Co trunnions is shown in Fig. 32. This clearly shows that the use of a TA6V trunnion, having a lower Young's modulus than the Cr-Co trunnions, leads to a reduction in stress concentrations inside the heads and consequently to improved rupture loads. For this reason, the approval of a given zirconia hip joint head design should be submitted to a standardized burst test using metallic trunnions identical to the implanted prosthesis's stem trunnions and having the same specifications (metal composition, shapes, surface finish, etc.).

Examples of various geometries of manufactured zirconia hip joint heads, including different head diameters or classes of cone, are shown in Fig. 33. For instance, 28-mm zirconia femoral heads with a 12/14 cone of 5°43'30" are characterized, after design optimization, by a rupture load, when burst tested on TA6V trunnions, higher than 100 kN for three different neck lengths ($-3.5/0/+3.5$). Similarly, the rupture load of

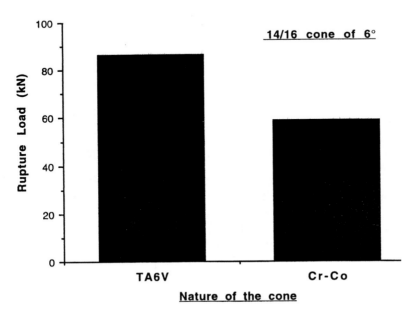

Figure 32 Comparison of the fracture strength of 28-mm zirconia heads on TA6V and Cr-Co trunnions with same design and same origin.

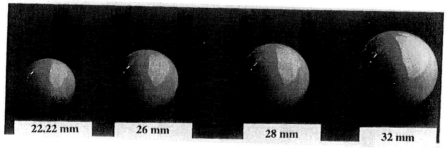

(a)

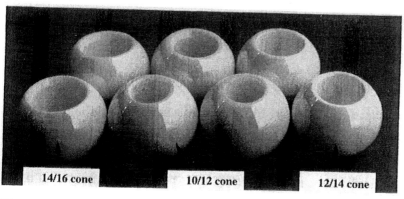

(b)

Figure 33 Examples of currently manufactured zirconia hip joint heads: (a) heads of different diameters, from 32 mm to 22.22 mm; (b) heads with different cone designs.

22.22-mm zirconia heads with an 8/10 cone of 6° can reach 95 kN in optimized conditions (head design, taper characteristics).

There are also limitations in the cone angles in order to obtain the best compromise between push-on and pull-off strength. Indeed, the relative displacement of the metallic taper inside the ceramic cone under loading directly depends on the cone angle (Fig. 34). Thus, for small cone angles (i.e., 3°), the metallic taper can more easily penetrate in the ceramic cone at relatively low loading. There is microscopic plastic deformation of the metallic taper at the interface that achieves some kind of "cold welding" and ensures high pull-off values. The real pull-off value is controlled by the taper characteristics. However, due to manufacturing tolerances in the ceramic and metallic cone diameters, small angles can lead to uncertainties in the final position of the taper inside the head. Large variations of the distance d between the top of the metallic taper and the top of the ceramic cone (Fig. 27) can consequently be introduced. As previously shown (see Section IV), such variations could have dramatic consequences on the stress concentration at the top of the ceramic cone (Fig. 28) and large scattering of the test rupture loads may be observed.

This problem is avoided in the case of larger angles (>10°). In this case, deviations from normal cone diameter size due to manufacturing tolerances do not generate such variation in the final position of the trunnion inside the head. But, in the case of such large angles, under a given loading, the penetration depth of the trunnion inside the head

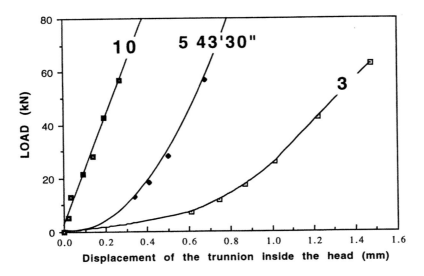

Figure 34   Displacement of the metallic trunnion inside zirconia heads for different cone angles.

is reduced when compared with small angles (Fig. 34). The plastic deformation of the trunnion at the trunnion/head interface could be reduced and lower pull-off values can result. This situation could be particularly sensitive when heads with large cone angle have to be fitted on trunnions with a smooth surface and/or a high elastic modulus (i.e., Cr-Co alloys or stainless steel). On the contrary, the pull-off load could be enhanced by increasing the trunnion surface roughness to promote local plastic deformation at the interface. Thin, machined grooves at the surface of the trunnions are frequently introduced for this reason.

In practice, intermediate cone angles in the range of 5° to 6° are the most widely used and give the best compromise between push-on and pull-off values.

The influence of other metallic taper parameters like straightness deviation and the like on the load-bearing capacity of ceramic femoral heads has been recently pointed out by Heimke [66] for alumina heads; the same conclusions apply for zirconia heads.

VII.   OTHER CURRENTLY USED ORTHOPEDIC COMPONENTS

Y-TZP ceramic is also currently used for new metatarsophalangeal implants. Indeed, severe metatarsophalangeal lesions could be treated mainly by two techniques [72]: the metatarsophalangeal pinning and the temporary interposition of a cup. However, these techniques are unsatisfactory for several reasons [72]. The removable button spacer cup was thus introduced by AMP Medical in metatarsophalangeal surgery to combine the advantage of the two previous techniques. They are made of a thickened cup with a hole in the center so that it could be used in association with metatarsophalangeal pinning (Fig. 35). Zirconia removable button spacer cups have been successfully used for two to three years in metatarsophalangeal surgery.

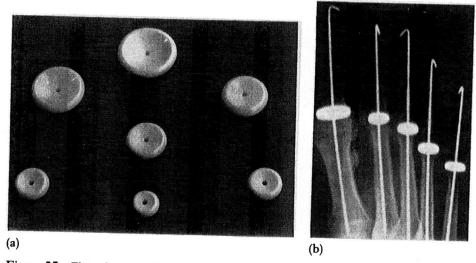

(a)   (b)

Figure 35   Zirconia removable button spacer cups: (a) from 18- to 8-mm diameter; (b) radiography of implanted removable button spacers with metatarsophalangeal pinning.

VIII.   FUTURE DEVELOPMENTS OF ZIRCONIA CERAMICS IN SURGERY AND OTHER APPLICATIONS

In the case of zirconia orthopedic components, several developments are expected in the future. First, improvements in the wear behavior of zirconia hip joint heads will still be made, with the development of new ceramic sockets as counterbearing components against zirconia heads. Indeed, ceramic against ceramic in total hip replacement has been shown to be an excellent tribological couple, as shown by clinical results of the alumina/alumina couple [67]. In the case of zirconia ceramics, a preliminary pin-on-disk test indicated an unfavorable behavior for zirconia/zirconia couple, compared with alumina/alumina (Table 7). However, as shown for the ceramic/polyethylene couple, the pin-on-disk tests are not representative enough of the real wear rate and contradictory results can be observed. For this reason, the zirconia/zirconia couple still needs to be investigated using head-on-cup-joint simulators. Furthermore, other ceramic/zirconia

Table 7   Wear Behavior of Some Ceramic/Ceramic Couples in Ringer's Solution Under 200 N

Roller	Plate	Weight loss		Friction coefficient
		Roller	Plate	
Alumina	Alumina	0.07	0.08	0.22
Y-TZP zirconia	Zirconia toughened alumina	0.3	0.58	0.72
Y-TZP zirconia	Silicon nitride	0.02	0.5	0.69
Y-TZP zirconia	Y-TZP zirconia	2.4	2.1	0.5
Y-TZP zirconia	Alumina	0.04	≈ 0	0.25

couples can exhibit wear rates equal to or lower than the alumina/alumina couple (Table 7). Here again, head-on-cup tests are required to verify the potential of such tribological couples. Progress is also expected with the use of zirconia heads with extremely high roundness, thus avoiding the costly issue of pairing.

Other potential applications are very promising in orthopedic surgery. For instance, Y-TZP zirconia ceramics can be employed to develop new shoulder prostheses, replacing conventional materials. The functional shapes of the shoulder heads are similar to those of hip joint heads and the experience obtained with hip joint heads can be easily transferred to shoulder prostheses.

Another very large field of application for toughened zirconia ceramics is knee prostheses. Serious UHMWPE wear and creep are reported with the use of metallic knee prostheses. Improvements are expected with ceramic components and clinical results have reported improved UHMWPE wear resistance using alumina knee prostheses [68]. However, because of the specific high stresses in knee prostheses, Y-TZP ceramics should be preferable to alumina ceramics for knee femoral components, the toughened mechanical properties of Y-TZPs leading to improved safety and reliability. Prototypes of Y-TZP knee femoral components have been studied [69], and preliminary wear tests are encouraging. However, a large research and development effort is still required to develop a reliable Y-TZP knee femoral component. Due to the complex shape of femoral components, a design optimization by finite element analysis is first needed and will require the experience of ceramists, prosthesis manufacturers, and surgeons. This will probably be the next challenge in orthopedic prosthesis development in the next 5–10 years.

Finally, it should be noted that zirconia ceramics have been successfully used as dental implants for more than 10 years. Hydroxyapatite-coated Y-TZP dental implants are now used without problem. Major developments are expected for Y-TZP ceramics in this field in the next years.

REFERENCES

1. Jasty, M., *J. Applied Biomat.*, 4:273–276 (1993).
2. Rose, R. M., et al., *J. Bone and Joint Surgery*, 62-A:537–549 (1980).
3. Boutin, P., *Rev. Chir. Ortop.*, 58:229–246 (1972).
4. Griss, P., and G. Heimke, *Arch. Orthop. Traumat. Surg.*, 98:157–164 (1981).
5. Dowson, D., *71st Meeting British Engineering Society*, Sept. 1978, Keele, United Kingdom.
6. Christel, P., et al., In *Bioceramics: Material Characteristics versus In Vivo Behaviour*, 523: 234–256, Ed. P. Ducheyne and J. E. Lemons, New York Academy of Sciences, New York (1988).
7. Semlitsch, M., M. Lehmann, H. Weber, E. Doerre, and H. Willert, *J. Biomed. Mater. Res.*, 11:537–552 (1977).
8. Zichner, L. P., and H.-G. Willert, *Clinical Orthop. Related Res.*, 292:86–94 (1992).
9. Clarke, I. C., *Clinical Orthop. Related Res.*, 282:19–30 (1992).
10. Schuller, H., and R. Marti, *Acta Orthop. Scand.*, 61:240–243 (1990).
11. Shimuzu, K., et al., *J. Biomed. Mater. Res.*, 27:729–734 (1993).
12. Clarke, I. C., A. Fujisawa, and H. Jung, *19th Annual Meeting Society for Biomaterials*, April–May 1993, Birmingham, AL.
13. Tateishi, T., and H. Yunoki, *Bull. Mechan. Engineer. Lab.*, 57 (1987).
14. Garvie, R. C., and J. R. Hellman, *J. Mat. Sci.*, 21:1253–1257 (1986).
15. Stubican, V. S., and M. F. Goss, In *Advances in Ceramics*, 3:25, Science and Technology of Zirconia, American Ceramic Society, Columbus, OH (1981).
16. Grain, C. F., *J. Am. Ceram. Soc.*, 50:288–290 (1967).

17. Miller, R. A., R. G. Smialek, and Garlick M. M., In *Advances in Ceramics*, 3:241, Science and Technology of Zirconia, American Ceramic Society, Columbus, OH (1981).
18. Tsukuma, K., and M. Shimada, *J. Mat. Sci.*, 20:1178–1184 (1985).
19. Lange, F. F., *J. Mat. Sci.*, 17:225–255 (1982).
20. Thompson, I., and R. D. Rawlings, *Biomaterials*, 11:505–508 (1990).
21. Drummond, J. L., *J. Am. Ceram. Soc.*, 72:675–676 (1989).
22. Evans, A. G., and A. H. Heuer, *J. Am. Ceram. Soc.*, 63:241–248 (1981).
23. Dingman, C. A., and G. Schwartz, *16th Annual Meeting Society for Biomaterials*, May 1990, Charleston, SC.
24. Masaki, T., and K. Shinjo, In *Advances in Ceramics*, 24:709–720. Science and Technology of Zirconia III, American Ceramic Society, Columbus, OH (1988).
25. Awaji, H., T. Yamada, and H. Okuda, *J. Ceram. Soc. Japan*, 99:403–410 (1991).
26. Quinn, G. D., et al., *J. Res. Natl. Inst. Stand. Technol.*, 97:579–583 (1992).
27. Liang, K., Study of cracking mechanisms of oxide ceramics, Thesis Institut National Sciences Appliquees, University of Lyon (1990).
28. Wang, J., W. M. Rainforth, I. Wadsworth, and R. Stevens, *J. Europ. Ceram. Soc.*, 10:21–31 (1992).
29. Chevalier, J., C. Olagnon, G. Fantozzi, B. Calès, and J. M. Drouin, *3rd European Ceramic Society Conference*, Madrid (1993).
30. Kondo, Y., Y. Kuroshima, Y. Hashizuka, A. Tsukuda, and S. Okada, *J. Ceram. Soc. Japan Inter. Ed.*, 95:1166–1168 (1987).
31. Masaki, T., M. Mizushina, Y. Kitano, Y. Mori, and G. Katagiri, *32nd Japan Congress on Mat. Research*, Soc. Mat. Sci., Kyoto, Japan (1989).
32. Wiederhorn, S. M., *J. Am. Ceram. Soc.*, 50:407–411 (1967).
33. Fett, T., and D. Munz, *J. Europ. Ceram. Soc.*, 6:67–72 (1990).
34. Chevalier, J., C. Olagnon, G. Fantozzi, and B. Calès, *J. Am. Ceram. Soc.* (in press).
35. Fuller, E. R., *Fracture Mechanics Applied to Brittle Materials*, ASTM STP 678, American Society for Testing and Materials, 3–18 (1979).
36. Kingery, W. D., H. K. Bowen, and D. R. Uhlmann, *Introduction to Ceramics—2nd Edition*, p. 678, Wiley-Interscience, New York (1976).
37. Willmann, G., In *Bioceramics and the Human Body*, pp. 250–255, Ed. A. Ravaglioli and A. Krajewski, Elsevier Applied Science, London (1992).
38. Wurst, J. C., and J. A. Nelson, *J. Am. Ceram. Soc.*, Feb:109 (1972).
39. Garvie, R. S., C. Urbani, D. R. Kennedy, and J. C. McNeuer, *J. Mat. Sci.*, 19:3224–3228 (1984).
40. Maurer, A. M., V. D. Le, S. G. Steinemann, H. Guenther, and J. Bille, *Proc. of 10th European Conference on Biomaterials*, Sept. 1993, Davos, Switzerland.
41. Hopf, Th., and B. Glöbel, *J. Applied Biomat.*, 1:315–316 (1990).
42. Heindl, R., and B. Calès, *Fourth World Biomaterials Congress*, April 1992, Berlin.
43. Calès, B., *Third Symp. Europ. Inst. Biomat. Microsurgery*, Oct. 1992, Nancy, France.
44. Burger, W., C. Piconi, A. F. Seda, A. Cittadini, and M. Boccalari, *Proc. of 10th European Conference on Biomaterials*, Sept. 1993, Davos, Switzerland.
45. Sato, T., S. Ohtaki, T. Endo, and M. Shimada, *High Tech Ceramics*, pp. 281–288, Ed. P. Vincenzini, Elsevier Science Publishers, Amsterdam (1987).
46. Lange, F. F., *J. Mat. Sci.*, 17:240–246 (1982).
47. Lilley, E., In Corrosion and Corrosive Degradation of Ceramics. *Ceramics Transactions*, 10:387–407, Ed. R. Tressler, M. McNallan (1990).
48. Swab, J. J., *J. Mat. Sci.*, 26:6706–6714 (1991).
49. Calès, B., and Y. Stéfani, *19th Annual Meeting Society for Biomaterials*, April–May 1993, Birmingham, AL. *J. Biomed. Mat. Res.*, 28:619–624 (1994).
50. Fantozzi, G., *Etude comparative et mise au point de matériaux pour prothèses osseuses*, Final Report, Ministry of Research, Contract No. 86-2-19-8-E, Ministry of Research, Paris, France (1988).

51. Shimizu, K., et al., *J. Biomed. Mat. Res.*, 27:729–734 (1993).
52. Mori, Y., Y. Kinato, and A. Ishitani, *J. Am. Ceram. Soc.*, 71:C322–C324 (1988).
53. Drouin, J. M., and B. Calès, *Proc. of 10th European Conference on Biomaterials*, Sept. 1993, Davos, Switzerland.
54. Lang-Michaut, C., *Practice of Statistical Tests—Analysis of Measurements*, Ed. Bordas, Paris (1990).
55. Calès, B., and Y. Stéfani, *Proc. of 10th European Conference on Biomaterials*, Sept. 1993, Davos, Switzerland. *J. Mat. Sci., Materials in Medicine*, 5:376–380 (1994).
56. Davidson, J. A., and P. Kovacs, *Proc. 8th So. Biomed. Engr. Conf.*, pp. 33–37, Richmond, VA (1989).
57. Oonishi, H., H. Igaki, and Y. Takayama, *Bioceramics*, 1:272–276 (1989).
58. Clarke, I. C., *Clin. Orthop. Relat. Res.*, 282:19–30 (1992).
59. Steicher, R. M., M. Semlitsch, and R. Schön, *Bioceramics*, 4:10–16, Ed. W. Bonfield, G. W. Hastings, and K. E. Tanner, Butterworth-Heinemann, London (1991).
60. Kumar, P., et al., *J. Biomed. Mater. Res.*, 25:813–828 (1991).
61. Tréheux, D., and A. Benabdallah, *Etude comparative et mise au point de matériaux pour prothèses osseuses*, Final Report, Ministry of Research, Contract No. 86-2-19-8-E, Ministry of Research, Paris, France (1988).
62. McKellop, H., B. Lu, P. Benya, and S. H. Park, *Orthopaedic Research Society Meeting*, Washington, DC, Feb. 1992.
63. Siedelmann, U., H. Richter, and U. Soltész, *Biomaterials 1980*, pp. 213–218, Ed. G. D. Winter, D. F. Gibbons, and H. Plenk, John Wiley & Sons, London (1982).
64. Capannesi, G., A. F. Sedda, C. Piconi, and F. Greco, In *Bioceramics and the Human Body*, pp. 211–216, Ed. A. Ravaglioli and A. Krajewski, Elsevier Applied Science, London (1992).
65. Kosmac, T., R. Wagner, and N. Claussen, *J. Am. Ceram. Soc.*, C72–C73 (1981).
66. Heimke, G., *Bioceramics*, 6:283–288, Ed. P. Ducheyne and D. Christiansen, Butterworth-Heinemann, Oxford (1993).
67. Sedel, J., R. Nizard, A. Meunier, J. M. Dorlot, and J. Witvoet, *Bioceramics*, 6:99–104, Ed. P. Ducheyne and D. Christiansen, Butterworth-Heinemann, Oxford (1993).
68. Oonishi, H., *Bioceramics*, 6:93–98, Ed. P. Ducheyne and D. Christiansen, Butterworth-Heinemann, Oxford (1993).
69. Cales, B., *Etude d'une prothèse de genou comportant un élément condylien en céramique de zircone*, Final Report, Ministry of Research, Contract No. 88-M-0268, Ministry of Research, Paris, France.
70. Middleton, J., G. N. Pande, H. G. Richter, and G. Willmann, *10th European Conference on Biomaterials*, Sept. 1993, Davos, Switzerland.
71. Smet, B. J., P. W. Bah, and P. P. A. C. Pex, *EURO-CERAMICS II*, 2:1155–1159, Ed. G. Ziegler and H. Hausner, Deutsche Keralische Gesellschaft, Köln (1993).
72. Barouk, L. S., The Metatarsophalangeal Removable Button Spacer, Brochure of AMP Medical.
73. Theunissen, G. S. A. M., J. S. Bouma, A. J. A. Winnbust, and A. J. Burggraaf, *J. Mater. Sci.*, 27:4429–4438 (1992).
74. Saikko, V., P. Paavolainen, M. Kleimola and P. Slätis, *Proc. Instn. Mech. Engrs.*, 206:195–200 (1992).

Enhanced Ultra-High Molecular Weight Polyethylene for Orthopedics Applications

A. R. Champion, K. Saum, W. Simmons, and E. Howard

E. I. duPont de Nemours, Incorporated
Wilmington, Delaware

I. INTRODUCTION

Orthopedic joint prostheses such as artificial hips, knees, and shoulders typically contain a highly polished metal or ceramic component articulating against a polymeric bearing surface. Ultra-high molecular weight polyethylene (UHMWPE) has been the bearing material of choice since the 1960s, when it was introduced in hip cups by Sir John Charnley [1]. Several other polymers, such as polytetrafluoroethylene (PTFE) [1,2], glass-filled PTFE [2], polyacetal [3], and carbon fiber reinforced UHMWPE [4,5], have been tested clinically, but none has equaled the long-term performance of UHMWPE.

Although UHMWPE has been the bearing material of choice for over two decades, it is recognized that damage can occur *in vivo*. Damage has been studied by analysis of retrieved orthopedic implants, for example. Wright et al. have characterized mechanical damage into several distinct types, such as creep deformation, scratching, abrasion, burnishing, pitting, delamination, and fracture [6,7]. Eyerer and Ke [8], Rose and Radin [9], Nagy and Li [10,11], Li, Nagy and Wood [12], and others, as well as Saum [13], have suggested that oxidation *in vivo* or from gamma sterilization may also contribute to damage of UHMWPE. Mechanical and oxidative damage can shorten implant lifetimes and can lead to the generation of wear debris *in vivo*. Wear debris has been linked to osteolytic activity and implant loosening [14–18]. Therefore, potential benefits could be gained if UHMWPE could be made with lower creep, greater abrasion resistance, higher strength, longer fatigue life, and greater oxidative stability. Such improvements should lead to longer implant lifetimes, offer increased benefit to patients, and provide more cost-effective joint reconstructions.

Until recently, commercially available UHMWPE was limited to the normal folded-chain structure with crystallinity of approximately 50%. Recent research has brought about advances in the processing of UHMWPE that led to materials with extended-chain

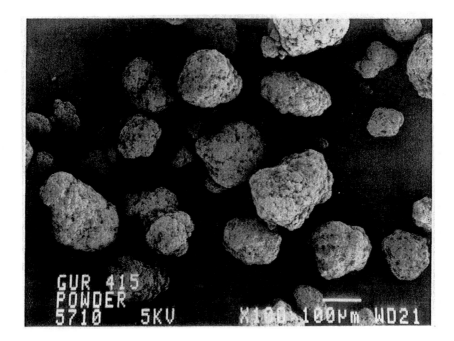

(a)

(b)

Figure 1   Scanning electron microscopy (SEM) photos of typical as-polymerized GUR 415 ultra-high molecular weight polyethylene (UHMWPE) powder: (a), ×100; (b), ×1000; (c), ×10,000.

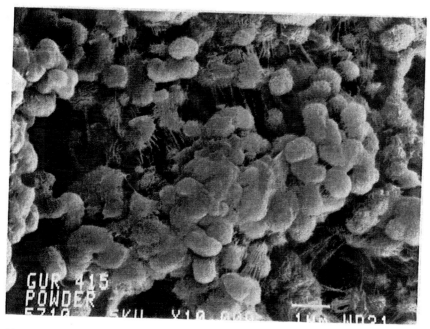

(c)

morphologies and higher crystallinity without sacrificing molecular weight [19,20]. The process involves subjecting conventional UHMWPE to a carefully controlled heating, pressure, and cooling cycle in an isostatic autoclave. The degree of crystallinity can be controlled by changing the process parameters. It has been found that altering the morphology and increasing the crystallinity of UHMWPE provides several changes in physical and mechanical properties that may be advantageous to total joint replacements. These changes address the mechanical and oxidative damage modes discussed above.

In this chapter, a brief review of conventional UHMWPE is presented. This is followed by a detailed discussion of the fabrication and properties of a new family of enhanced UHMWPEs that have recently become commercially available for use in total joint replacements.

II. CONVENTIONAL UHMWPE

A. UHMWPE Polymer

By definition, UHMWPE has a molecular weight greater than 1 million, and commercially available polymers are typically in the range of 2 to 6 million. The polymer is made in powder form by Ziegler–Natta polymerization [21–23]. The process, referred to as *suspension polymerization*, is carried out in a hydrocarbon liquid such as hexane. A highly active porous catalyst suspension is typically formed by reacting a transition metal compound such as $TiCl_4$ with a compound such as magnesium ethylate, $Mg(OC_2H_5)_2$. Catalyst particles have high surface area and are typically 7–30 microns in size. A cocatalyst such as triethyl aluminum is also used. A mixture of ethylene monomer ($CH_2=CH_2$) and hydrogen is introduced into the reaction vessel, and polymerization occurs on the catalyst particles. Reaction conditions are moderate, with temperatures less than 100°C and pressures up to a few atmospheres. Molecular weight tends to increase with decreasing reactor temperature and can also be influenced by catalyst composition, catalyst/cocatalyst ratio, ethylene/hydrogen ratio, pressure, and total reaction time.

Scanning electron microscopy (SEM) micrographs of a typical UHMWPE powder are shown in Fig. 1. Particles are about 50 to 250 microns in size (Fig. 1a). The bulk density of these particles is typically about 0.4 grams per cubic centimeter (g/cc). At higher magnifications (Figs. 1b and 1c), it can be seen that each particle is made up of many submicron particles and can contain filaments of polymer as well.

The most common UHMWPE materials available in the United States are GUR 412 and GUR 415 resins from Hoechst/Celanese and Himont's 1900 resins. GUR 412 and GUR 415 have viscosity average molecular weights of about 4 million and 6 million, respectively. Himont resins have molecular weights of about 3 to 6 million.

UHMWPE is a semicrystalline polymer (shown schematically in Fig. 2). Depending on the conditions of synthesis, part of the polymer crystallizes in the monoclinic, triclinic, or orthorhombic lattice [24]. The monoclinic or triclinic structure is obtained at relatively low synthesis temperatures (e.g., 30°C). At about 60°C or higher, the orthorhombic lattice is obtained. Also, the monoclinic form transforms irreversibly to the orthorhombic structure upon heating above 60°C. These crystalline regions are surrounded by a matrix of amorphous polymer in which the chains are more random and entangled. A DSC (differential scanning calorimetry) trace for GUR 415 UHMWPE powder is shown in Fig. 3. The crystalline melting endotherm has a peak at approximately 144°C. As-synthesized UHMWPE powders have relatively high crystallinity. Crystallinity can be estimated by comparing the enthalpy of fusion ΔH_m, obtained from the DSC trace, to the enthalpy of fusion for pure crystalline PE ($\Delta H_m^* = 290$ joules per gram [J/g]) [24]. The value of $\Delta H_m = 175.5$ J/g in Fig. 3 indicates a crystallinity of $\Delta H_m/\Delta H_m^* = 175.5/290$

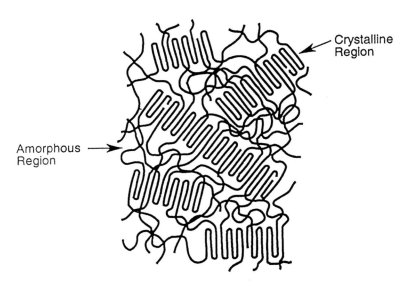

Figure 2 Schematic representation of the semicrystalline structure of ultra-high molecular weight polyethylene.

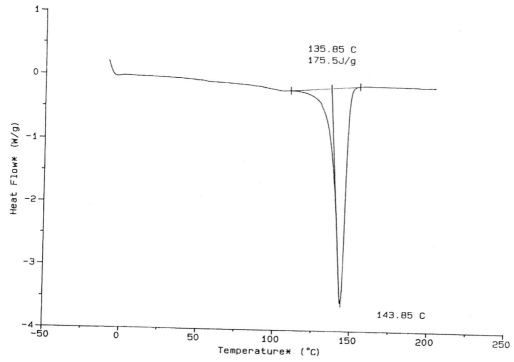

Figure 3 Differential scanning calorimetry (DSC) trace of GUR 415 powder (heating rate = 10°C/min in nitrogen).

= 61% for this particular sample. Crystallinities of 60–70% are typical for as-polymerized powders. The density of individual powder particles, measured by a density gradient column [25], is typically approximately 0.95 g/cc.

B. Consolidation

Because of the very high melt viscosity of UHMWPE, parts cannot be made by standard extrusion or injection molding processes used for ordinary thermoplastic polymers. Consolidation of UHMWPE is shown schematically in Fig. 4. UHMWPE powder is usually ram extruded into bars or compression molded into sheets, and orthopedic components are then machined from these raw stocks. Some manufacturers compression mold UHMWPE powder directly into bearing components. Consolidation is usually carried out well above the polymer melting point; temperatures are typically in the range of 180°C to 240°C. High pressures are also required to achieve good consolidation.

Consolidation conditions are very important for obtaining high quality UHMWPE material and components. If temperatures and pressures are not sufficiently high, the final product can contain unconsolidated regions in which neighboring powder particles are not well bonded. Examples of consolidation defects are shown in Fig. 5.

To see these defects, samples 50 microns thick were cut from UHMWPE raw stocks with a microtome, and optical micrographs were taken in transmitted light. It is our

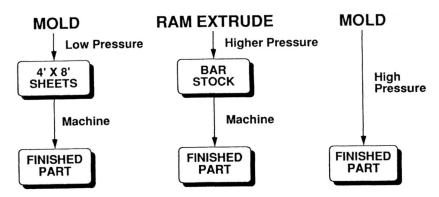

Figure 4 Methods of consolidating ultra-high molecular weight polyethylene polymer powder.

experience that the number of such defects is significantly greater in molded sheets than in extruded rods. This is believed to result from lower pressures and less uniform powder distribution being achieved in molding large sheets of material (typically 4 feet [ft] × 8 ft). The presence of such defects in orthopedic implants is believed to be undesirable because of the possibility that they can be a source of fatigue crack initiation. It is important for implant manufacturers to select high quality, well-consolidated raw materials for machining bearing components. Those who mold implants directly should inspect for consolidation defects and reject components with high defect levels.

When UHMWPE powders are consolidated above their melting points, the material recrystallizes in the orthorhombic lattice on cooling, but can have a different morphology from the original powder. The crystallization that occurs during synthesis produces morphologies in which the polymer chains are less entangled than melt recrystallized material, and the as-synthesized powder can contain extended-chain conformations [24,26]. Heating the powder above the melting point can increase entanglement density, which reduces chain mobility; this can hinder recrystallization and lamellar thickening. A DSC trace of a ram extruded GUR 415 UHMWPE sample is shown in Fig. 6. This differs from the DSC curve of the powder (Fig. 3) in two respects. First, the heat of fusion ΔHm is lower. The value of 155 J/g indicates a crystallinity of approximately 53% for this sample, compared with about 60–70% for starting powders. Crystallinities of extruded materials are typically 45–55%. Second, the peak of the melting endotherm occurs at a lower temperature, 135°C versus 144°C for nascent powder material. This difference is attributed to a folded-chain structure for the extruded material. Folded- and extended-chain morphologies are discussed in more detail below.

C. Mechanical Properties

Typical mechanical properties for conventional UHMWPE are shown in Table 1. GUR 412 and 415 and Himont 1900 are extruded bars, and RCH 1000 (Ruhr Chemie) is a molded sheet material made from GUR 412 resin. All properties were measured in our laboratory according to American Society for Testing and Materials (ASTM) standard test methods [27–30]. The GUR 412 and 415 extruded rods and the RCH 1000 molded sheet have comparable static properties. The Himont 1900 material has slightly higher density and yield strength and lower elongation and Izod impact strength due to its somewhat lower molecular weight. The properties shown in Table 1 are typical of UHMWPE materials currently used in orthopedic implants.

III. ENHANCED UHMWPE

A. Background

Several studies have reported that the morphology of polyethylene can be changed from the normal folded-chain form to extended-chain configurations by melting the polymer and recrystallizing under high pressure [31–34]. Pressure recrystallization also increases density and crystallinity and can lead to significant changes in mechanical properties such as yield and ultimate tensile strengths, elongation, elastic modulus, compressive behavior, creep, and impact strength.

The property changes that occur depend in part on the molecular weight of the starting polymer. For low molecular weight (MW) linear polyethylenes (e.g., MW less than about 200,000), pressure recrystallization can lead to materials with higher stiffness and creep resistance, but elongations are low and failure modes can be brittle. Early work by Lupton and Regester [31], however, showed that very tough materials with enhanced properties could be obtained for UHMWPE with molecular weights greater than about 2 million. Only small, laboratory-scale samples of enhanced UHMWPE were produced in their work, and these were not homogeneous due to temperature and pressure gradients during fabrication. We have extended this early work and report here developments that have led to commercial-scale processes for pressure recrystallized UHMWPE materials that are specifically tailored to the needs of orthopedic bearing surfaces.

For orthopedic applications, GUR 415 extruded rod stock has been selected as the starting material for the enhancement process. This material consistently has been found to have a very low level of consolidation defects, and GUR 415 resin is one of the highest molecular weight UHMWPEs commercially available. This UHMWPE material also meets ASTM specifications for mechanical and physical properties and trace element content for medical implants [30].

B. Pressure Recrystallization

Our processes, described in U.S. Patents [19,20,35], involve subjecting conventional UHMWPE to carefully controlled heating, pressure, and cooling cycles in an isostatic autoclave. The pressure-transmitting medium can be either gas or liquid. Pressures in the range of 20,000 to 60,000 pounds per square inch (psi) and temperatures from 160°C to 300°C have been investigated.

As discussed above, conventional folded-chain UHMWPE has a density of about 0.935 g/cc and is about 50% crystalline. With autoclave processing, a large family of extended-chain UHMWPE materials with densities of 0.94 to greater than 0.96 g/cc and crystallinities of 55% to greater than 80% have been produced. From this family of materials, two have been commercialized for orthopedic applications and are designated Hylamer® and Hylamer®-M (registered trademarks of E. I. duPont de Nemours, Inc.). Hylamer is designed for use in hip cups and as the glenoid component of shoulder prostheses, and Hylamer-M is designed for the tibial bearing surface in knee replacements. In the following sections, discussions focus on these two enhanced materials, and their morphology, microstructure, and properties are presented.

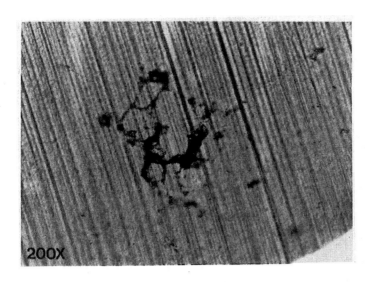

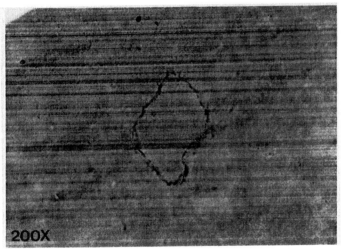

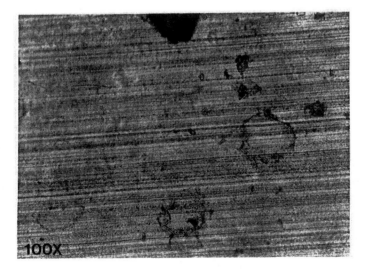

C. Polymer Morphology and Crystallinity

It was mentioned above that UHMWPE is a semicrystalline polymer (shown schematically in Fig. 2). In the crystalline regions of conventional UHMWPE, the linear polymer chains fold back on themselves to form the normal folded-chain (FC) conformation. Small angle x-ray scattering (SAXS) can be used to estimate the spacing between chain folds. Figure 7a is a typical SAXS plot of desmeared intensity I versus scattering angle 2Θ for conventional GUR 415 UHMWPE extruded rod. The spectrum shows a single broad peak corresponding to fold spacings in the range of about 450 angstroms ($\mathring{A}$) to 1000 $\mathring{A}$, with a maximum in the population at about 670 $\mathring{A}$.

Figure 7b shows an SAXS plot for Hylamer that has been enhanced by the high pressure autoclave process to a crystallinity of nearly 70%. This plot exhibits two distinct scattering peaks associated with fold spacings in the range of 4610 $\mathring{A}$ ($2\Theta = 0.0192°$) and 480 $\mathring{A}$ ($2\Theta = 0.184°$). The presence of the sharp peak at the lower angle indicates the presence of extended polymer chains, while the more diffuse, higher angle peak is characteristic of conventional folded-chain UHMWPE [36].

The presence of two different morphologies can also be seen by differential scanning calorimetry (DSC). Figure 6 showed a DSC trace for conventional ram extruded UHMWPE, which contains a single melting endotherm with a peak at 135°C. Figure 8 shows a DSC curve for Hylamer. The curve contains a peak at 148°C and a shoulder at a lower temperature. The 148°C peak is more like nascent polymer powder (Fig. 3). This large, high melting peak is indicative of the presence of a high percentage of extended chains. The lower temperature shoulder in Fig. 8 is associated with a small amount of residual folded-chain material. DSC is in agreement with the SAXS results above where both morphologies are present. The heat of fusion for this material indicates a crystallinity of about 67%.

Thus, it can be seen from SAXS and DSC measurements that the pressure enhancement process results in the conversion of folded-chain material to the extended-chain form and increases crystallinity. The amount of extended-chain material and the chain fold lengths depend on the operating conditions during pressure recrystallization. Figure 9 shows the DSC trace for a Hylamer-M sample. Here, two distinct peaks are seen, indicating significant amounts of both morphologies. Under very high pressure conditions, samples with crystallinities greater than 80% have been obtained, and chain fold lengths of the order of 10,000 $\mathring{A}$ have been reported [32].

Infrared (IR) spectroscopy can also be used to follow the effects of pressure recrystallization. For UHMWPE, the IR band at 1894 cm^{-1} is associated with CH_2 rocking in the crystalline regions, and the band at 1303 cm^{-1} is associated with CH_2 twisting in the amorphous regions [37]. A *crystallinity index* has been defined as the ratio of the heights of these two peaks [12]. For GUR 415 UHMWPE extruded rods, this ratio is typically about 0.25. As crystallinity is increased by pressure enhancement, the crystallinity index increases approximately linearly. Hylamer-M has a crystallinity index of approximately 0.35, and Hylamer has a value of about 0.47. The relationship between crystallinity obtained from DSC measurements and the infrared crystallinity index is shown in Fig.

Figure 5 Consolidation defects in ultra-high molecular weight polyethylene (UHMWPE). Unconsolidated regions such as these can occur if proper temperatures and pressures are not used during fabrication of solid materials from UHMWPE powder.

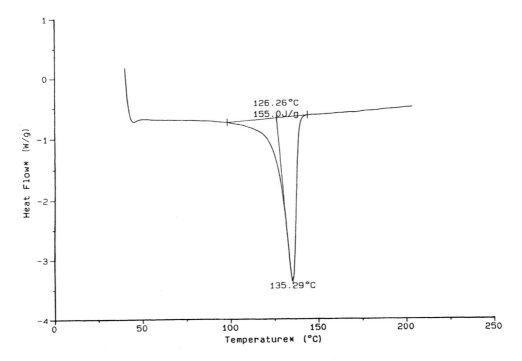

Figure 6 Differential scanning calorimetry (DSC) trace of a typical extruded rod of GUR 415 UHMWPE (heating rate = 10°C/min in nitrogen).

10. The infrared technique provides a rapid quality control method for estimating crystallinity of enhanced UHMWPE materials.

D. Crystalline Lamellar Structure

The crystalline lamellar structure of conventional and enhanced UHMWPE has been investigated by transmission electron microscopy (TEM) [38]. TEM specimens were prepared by the method of Kanig [39] to enhance contrast at the crystal/amorphous

Table 1 Typical Properties of UHMWPE Materials

Property	Extruded rods			Molded sheet
	GUR 415	GUR 412	Himont 1900	RCH 1000
Density (g/cc)	0.935	0.935	0.937	0.935
Tensile modulus (kpsi)	201	206	220	198
Tensile strength (kpsi)	6.0	5.9	5.3	5.2
Yield strength (kpsi)	3.38	3.41	3.58	3.42
Elongation (%)	340	320	180	320
Izod (ft-lb/in)	18	18	12	20

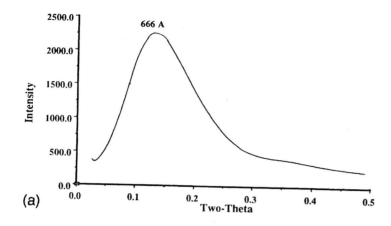

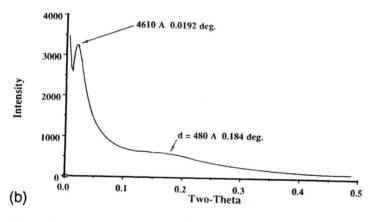

Figure 7   Small angle x-ray scattering (SAXS) plots of ultra-high molecular weight polyethylene (UHMWPE): (a), conventional UHMWPE; (b), pressure recrystallized UHMWPE.

interfaces. The technique involves chlorosulfonation of the polymer, sectioning with diamond knives, and staining with phosphotungstic acid. Images were obtained on a JOEL 2000FX TEM operated at 120-kV (kilovolt) accelerating voltage.

TEM images of conventional GUR 415, Hylamer-M and Hylamer are shown in Fig. 11. The crystalline lamellae can be clearly seen. Table 2 shows the lamellar thicknesses and lengths measured from the micrographs.

For each material there is a range of lamellar dimensions, but definite differences can be seen between conventional and enhanced samples, and qualitative comparisons can be made. Conventional UHMWPE, with its folded-chain structure, generally has lamellae that are less than about 35 nm (nanometers) thick and about 1 micron or less in length. For Hylamer-M, there is a mixture of large and small lamellae. The large lamellae, corresponding to extended-chain regions, have thicknesses of about 75 to 100 nm and lengths in the order of 3 to 4 microns. The smaller lamellae are characteristic of folded-

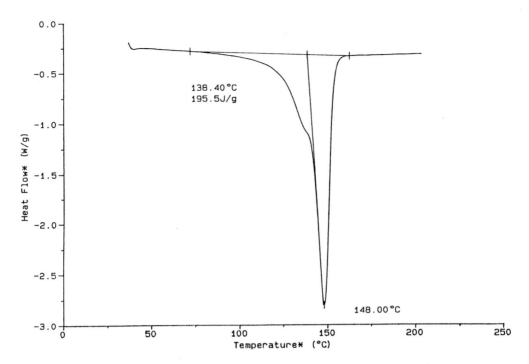

Figure 8 Differential scanning calorimetry (DSC) trace of a Hylamer sample pressure recrystallized to approximately 67% crystallinity. The material is converted predominantly to the extended-chain form. Only a small amount of folded-chain structure remains.

chain material (20–35 nm). In Hylamer, there is also a mixture of large and small lamellae. The larger generally are greater than about 120 nm in thickness and are also about 3 to 4 microns long, and the smaller are again characteristic of folded-chain material (20–35 microns). The volume fraction of extended-chain lamellae is qualitatively larger in Hylamer than in Hylamer-M. More quantitative analyses are in progress.

TEM thus provides additional evidence that pressure enhancement of UHMWPE increases the degree of crystallinity and the dimensions of the crystalline regions.

E.   Physical and Mechanical Properties

The above changes in morphology and crystallinity produced by pressure recrystallization led to significant changes in the physical and mechanical properties of UHMWPE. Several important properties are summarized in Table 3, in which Hylamer and Hylamer-M are compared with conventional GUR 415 UHMWPE. All values were determined by ASTM standard test methods [25,27–29].

Table 3 shows that Hylamer-M and Hylamer have melting points (determined from peaks in DSC curves) that are 12°C to 14°C higher than conventional UHMWPE as a result of pressure recrystallization. Because crystalline regions of UHMWPE have higher density than amorphous regions, increasing the crystallinity also raises the density of the final material significantly, as shown in Table 3.

An important benefit of pressure recrystallized UHMWPE is significantly reduced

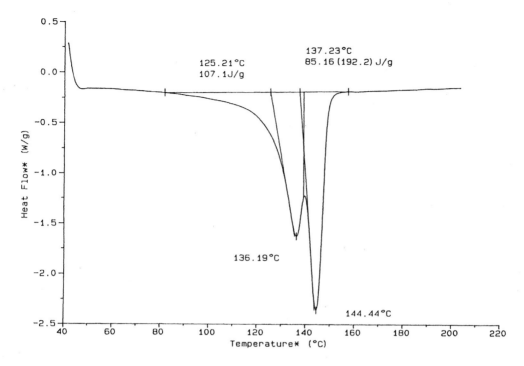

Figure 9   Differential scanning calorimetry (DSC) trace of a Hylamer-M sample. The two peaks indicate the presence of extended-chain and folded-chain morphologies.

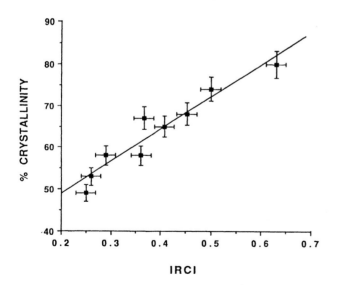

Figure 10   Crystallinity determined by differential scanning calorimetry (DSC) measurements (obtained from ΔH_m) versus infrared crystallinity index.

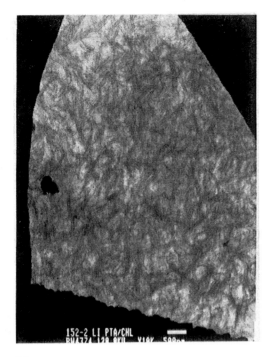

(a)

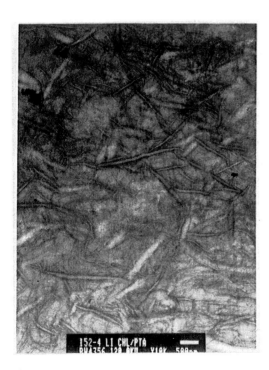

(b)

Figure 11 Transmission electron microscopy (TEM) images of lamellar structures: (a), GUR 415 UHMWPE; (b), Hylamer-M; (c), Hylamer.

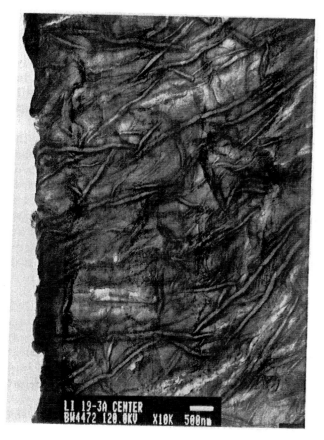

(c)

creep. Creep deformation has been identified as one of the damage modes in retrieved implants [6,7]. The data in Table 3 show that Hylamer-M and Hylamer have 25–44% lower creep than conventional UHMWPE. Measurements were made on 0.5 × 0.5 × 0.5 inch (in) samples at 1000 psi for 24 hours (h) at 23°C and 50% relative humidity (RH) [29].

Table 2 Lamellar Dimensions of Conventional and Enhanced UHMWPE

Material	Lamellar thickness (nm)	Lamellar length (μm)
Conventional GUR 415	≤35	≤1
Hylamer-M	75–100	3–4
	20–35	
Hylamer	≥120	3–4
	20–35	

nm, nanometers; μm, micrometers

Tensile properties are also enhanced by the autoclave process. Stress-versus-strain curves for Hylamer, Hylamer-M, and conventional material are shown in Fig. 12a. Data were obtained according to ASTM D-638 [27], using Type 1 tensile specimens and a crosshead speed of 2 in/min. Table 3 shows that yield strengths of Hylamer and Hylamer-M are 23% and 14% greater, respectively, than conventional UHMWPE. Increased yield strength allows the materials to be loaded to higher stresses before plastic deformation occurs. The data of Table 3 also show that ultimate tensile strengths are increased somewhat.

It is particularly important to note that elongation to break is not decreased by the Hylamer process. It was mentioned above that pressure recrystallization of *low* molecular weight polyethylenes can result in brittle materials with no yield point and elongations of only a few percent [31]. This is not the case for UHMWPE recrystallized under proper conditions. Elongations to break of Hylamer and Hylamer-M are greater than 300% and are comparable to conventional UHMWPE specimens measured in identical tests. Thus, the excellent toughness of UHMWPE, as indicated by the area under the stress-strain curve, is maintained. The high toughness can also be seen from the Izod impact strengths reported in Table 3. Izod values for Hylamer and Hylamer-M are equal to or greater than conventional UHMWPE and show that increasing crystallinity to the levels achieved in these materials results in no loss of impact performance.

Tensile modulus, measured as the initial slope of the stress-strain curves, is also increased by pressure recrystallization. Figure 12b shows expanded initial portions of the stress-strain curves of Hylamer, Hylamer-M, and conventional UHMWPE. Strains were measured with a linear variable differential transformer (LVDT) for increased accuracy. Crosshead speed was 0.2 in/min as specified in the ASTM test method. Moduli were obtained by fitting a straight line to the steepest portion of the curves. While increased modulus can lead to increased contact stress, this tends to be offset by the higher yield strength of the materials. Finite element models of hip and knee joints have shown that stress/yield strength ratios are less than or equal to those for conventional UHMWPE. In addition, the increased modulus can be taken into account by proper joint design.

Table 3   Mechanical and Physical Properties

Property	Hylamer	Hylamer-M	UHMWPE
Crystallinity (from DSC) (%)	68 ± 3	57 ± 3	50 ± 3
ΔH_m (J/g)	198 ± 9	166 ± 8	145 ± 9
Melting point (°C)	148.7 ± 0.5	147.0 ± 1.3	135 ± 1.5
Density (g/cc)	0.955 ± 0.001	0.946 ± 0.001	0.934 ± 0.001
Creep (24 hrs at 1000 psi) (%)	0.9 ± 0.1	1.2 ± 0.2	1.6 ± 0.3
Tensile yield strength (kpsi)	4.15 ± 0.10	3.85 ± 0.10	3.38 ± 0.07
Ultimate tensile strength (kpsi)	5.9 ± 0.6	5.5 ± 0.7	4.9 ± 0.5
Elongation (%)	334 ± 22	369 ± 28	339 ± 25
Modulus (kpsi)	365 ± 35	291 ± 34	201 ± 19
Izod (ft-lb/in)	22.4 ± 1.1	21.9 ± 0.9	17.8 ± 0.5

±values = 1 standard deviation

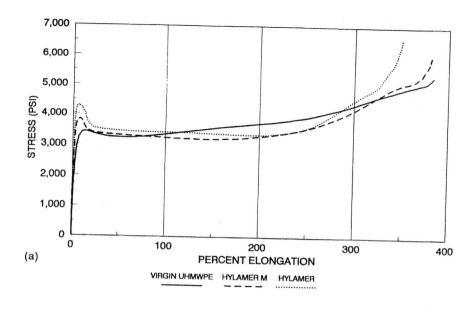

(a)

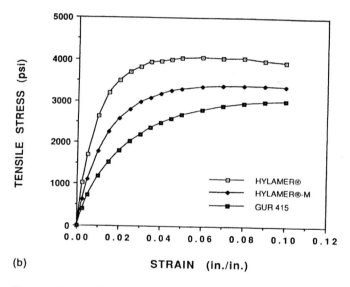

(b)

Figure 12 Typical tensile stress-versus-strain curves for Hylamer, Hylamer-M, and GUR 415 UHMWPE: (a), complete curves to failure (cross-head speed = 2 in/min); (b), initial portion measured at 0.2 in/min crosshead speed.

The data in Table 3 represent the averages and standard deviations of measurements from 2000 bars of Hylamer and 750 bars of Hylamer-M produced commercially in the autoclave process. Each bar is 5 ft long and 3–4 inches in diameter. The low standard deviations in Table 3 indicate that the process is well controlled and reproducible.

Compressive data have also been obtained using the ASTM method [40]. Figure 13a shows compression stress-versus-strain curves obtained with cylindrical specimens 0.50 inches in diameter by 1 inch long. Strain was obtained from crosshead motion to 50% compression. As with the tensile experiments, the curves show a higher yield strength for Hylamer and Hylamer-M compared with conventional UHMWPE. Figure 13b shows the initial portion of the curves in greater detail. Samples were 0.50-in diameter by 2-in long in order to allow attachment of a strain transducer.

Initial compressive moduli were obtained by fitting a straight line to the steepest portion of the curves. Values are shown in Table 4. In compression, the yield point is not as clearly defined as in the tensile tests, for which there is an unambiguous peak. Therefore, a 2% offset yield stress was calculated for each material; values are also given in Table 4. Compressive yield strengths of Hylamer and Hylamer-M are 76% and 37% higher, respectively, than conventional UHMWPE. Finally, the initial portions of the tensile and compressive stress-strain curves are superimposed in Figure 13c, and it can be seen that the initial portions of the curves are nearly identical to about 3% strain.

F. Fatigue Crack Growth Behavior

Fatigue crack propagation has been implicated as a mechanism for the pitting, delamination, and fracture of UHMWPE observed in retrieved orthopedic implants [6,7,41]. Therefore, it is important to determine the effects of the pressure recrystallization process on crack growth behavior.

Center-notched tension specimens 30 mm (millimeters) wide by 10 mm thick by 100 mm long were tested in accordance with ASTM E-647 [42]. A 15-mm crack was introduced by drilling a 5-mm diameter hole at the center, making cuts with a jeweler's saw, and cutting the final 1 mm of each tip with a razor blade. The specimen is shown in Fig.

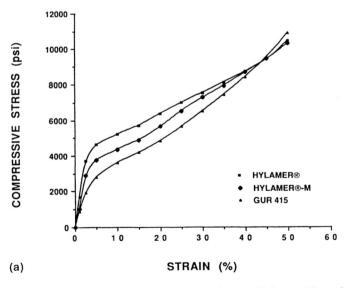

(a)

Figure 13 Compressive curves for Hylamer, Hylamer-M, and GUR 415: (a), to 50% compression, with strain measured by crosshead motion; (b), initial portion measured with a dual sensor strain transducer (DSST); (c), initial portions of tensile and compressive curves superimposed.

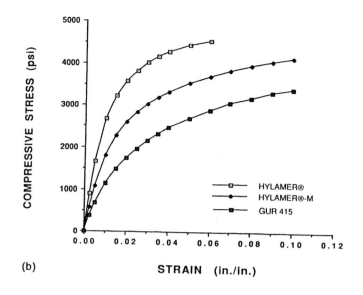

(b)

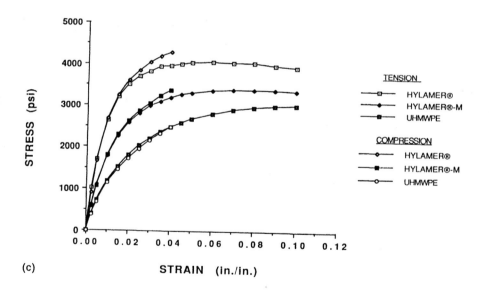

(c)

14. Samples were loaded in cyclic tension using a square waveform at a frequency of 2 Hertz (Hz) and a minimum/maximum stress ratio of $R = 0.15$. Initial maximum stresses were 18.9 megapascal (MPa) for Hylamer and Hylamer-M and 15.6 MPa for conventional GUR 415 UHMWPE. Tests were stopped periodically, and crack length was measured with a traveling optical microscope.

A series of fatigue crack growth tests was conducted at room temperature in air as an initial screening experiment to determine if there were any differences in behavior among Hylamer, Hylamer-M, and GUR 415 [43]. Results for unsterilized materials are shown in

Table 4   Compressive Properties

	Initial modulus (kpsi)	2% Offset yield stress (kpsi)
Hylamer	359 ± 13	4.07 ± 0.09
Hylamer-M	235 ± 19	3.15 ± 0.18
GUR 415	157 ± 14	2.30 ± 0.20

Fig. 15. Crack growth rates (da/dN) in meters/cycle are plotted against the stress intensity factor range ΔK (MPa√m). Results indicate that changing the crystallinity and morphology of UHMWPE by pressure recrystallization can lead to slower fatigue crack growth. Figure 15 shows that, for a given value of stress intensity range ΔK, crack growth rates in Hylamer-M and Hylamer are approximately one and two orders of magnitude lower, respectively, than for conventional GUR 415 UHMWPE.

Pressure recrystallized samples with higher crystallinity than Hylamer were also evaluated at room temperature. Fatigue crack growth tests were carried out on two materials with 74% and 83% crystallinity (versus ~68% for Hylamer). At 74% crystallinity, the da/dN curve was identical to that for Hylamer. The material with 83% crystallinity, however, exhibited unstable crack growth even when initial stress levels were reduced 20% below the level used for the other materials. Thus, while properties such as density, yield strength, modulus, and creep resistance continue to increase with increasing crystallinity, it is possible to have decreased fatigue performance when crystallinity is higher than about 80%. Izod impact strength has also been observed to decrease to less than 10 ft-lb/in (foot-pounds per inch of notch) for materials with greater than 80% crystallinity. Figure 16 shows fatigue crack growth rates (da/dN) versus crystallinity for a constant stress intensity value of $\Delta K = 1.7$ MPa√m. The data indicate that there is a minimum in crack growth rate when crystallinity is about 65–75%. Hylamer appears to be at this optimum condition.

Samples were then tested in distilled water at 37°C as a closer approximation to *in*

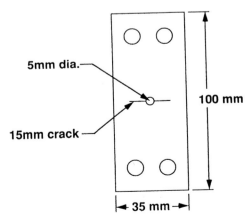

Figure 14   Center-cracked tensile specimen geometry for fatigue crack growth tests.

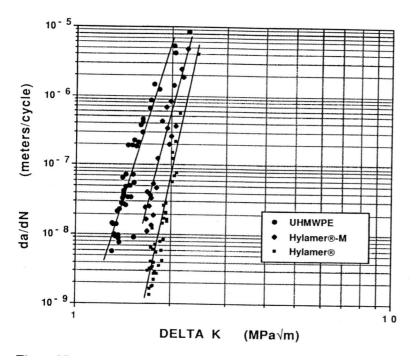

Figure 15 Fatigue crack growth results for Hylamer, Hylamer-M, and conventional UHMWPE at room temperature in air (unsterilized).

vivo conditions [44]. Figure 17 shows the results for unsterilized samples at 37°C. All samples were allowed to soak at temperature for at least two weeks prior to fatigue testing and were immersed at 37°C during cycling. Unsterilized samples were evaluated in order to determine the effects of crystallinity uncomplicated by the effects of gamma irradiation. As with the room temperature results above, the data at 37°C show that the enhanced materials exhibit slower crack growth. For a given stress intensity range ΔK, crack growth rates da/dN in Hylamer-M and Hylamer are approximately 1/10 and 1/50, respectively, of conventional UHMWPE.

Figure 18 compares results for sterilized and unsterilized samples in 37°C water. In this figure, the data points are for gamma-sterilized materials, and the solid lines are least-squares fits to the unsterilized 37°C data of Fig. 17. The figure shows that, for conventional UHMWPE, crack growth rates in the sterilized samples are about five times the rates in unsterilized material. This increase is believed to result from oxidation damage caused by gamma irradiation [45]. For Hylamer-M and Hylamer, there is no significant difference between sterilized and unsterilized samples. This is shown by the fact that the data points for the sterilized samples fall on top of the lines for the unsterilized samples. This result is consistent with the greater oxidation resistance observed for the more crystalline materials [46]. Eyerer et al. also reported that pressure recrystallized UHMWPE is significantly more stable against oxidation [47]. Further discussion about oxidation of these enhanced materials during gamma irradiation is given below.

These fatigue crack growth results show another significant benefit of pressure recrystallization of UHMWPE when proper conditions are chosen. Decreases of 1 to 2 orders

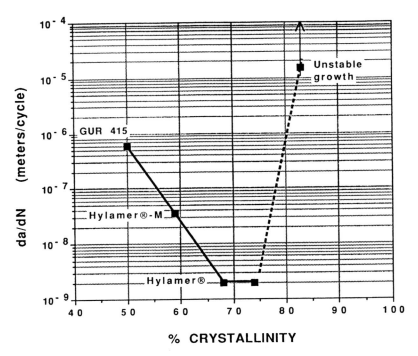

Figure 16 Fatigue crack growth rates of enhanced UHMWPE versus crystallinity. A value of ΔK = 1.7 MPa$\sqrt{m}$ was used for this comparison.

of magnitude in fatigue crack propagation rates should lead to longer implant lifetimes *in vivo*.

G. Wear Behavior

Wear of UHMWPE bearing surfaces, by mechanisms such as scratching, burnishing, and abrasion, is another important damage mode seen in retrieved implants [6,7]. Therefore, it is important to investigate the wear behavior of pressure recrystallized UHMWPE materials and to determine if the changes in polymer morphology and crystallinity provide an improvement. Wear behavior has been evaluated by pin-on-disk tests and with a hip simulator.

1. Pin-on-Disk Tests

One station of a custom-built laboratory tri-pin-on-disk apparatus is shown schematically in Fig. 19. Three pins of enhanced or conventional UHMWPE were mounted 120° apart in the bottom of a cup as shown. Pins were 0.300-in diameter by 0.06-in thick. A polished Co-Cr counterface was loaded against the three pins. The constant counterface load was adjusted to give a bearing stress of 1460 psi for all tests.

Tests were carried out with the counterface/pin system submerged in bovine calf serum at 37°C. The counterface was driven in an oscillatory motion at 1 Hz, resulting in an average interface speed of 0.056 meters per second (m/s) (11 ft/min). The test appara-

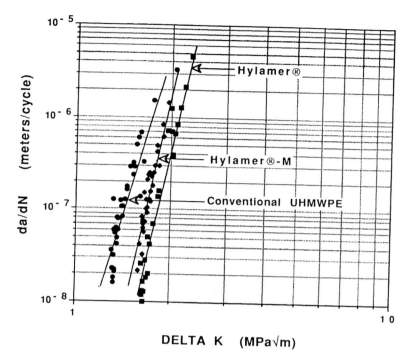

Figure 17   Fatigue crack growth rates *da/dN* versus stress intensity ΔK at 37°C in distilled water (unsterilized).

tus contains 6 of these dynamic stations and an additional six stations for static measurements to generate creep and fluid absorption data used to correct the dynamic results to give true wear rates.

All static and dynamic stations were interrupted at four-day intervals (330,000 cycles) for independent measurements of wear by changes in both weight and thickness. Wear factors obtained from weight and thickness changes were generally in close agreement. The serum was replaced at each interval. Testing was continued for a total of 3.3 million cycles, corresponding to a sliding distance of 185 kilometers (km).

The quality of polishing on the Co-Cr counterface was found to be a significant variable in these tests. Figure 20 shows wear factors for enhanced UHMWPE as a function of the Co-Cr counterface roughness in microinches (μin). The results show that a surface roughness of 7 μin can give wear factors that are five to six times greater than wear rates produced by high quality surfaces with roughness less than 1 μin. Therefore, when reporting wear data, it is important for investigators to characterize counterface surfaces thoroughly to insure self-consistent data and to avoid reaching incorrect conclusions when comparing results from different investigators.

A series of pin-on-disk tests was carried out to compare Hylamer with conventional GUR 415 UHMWPE using the above protocol. All counterfaces were polished to less than 1 microinch. A total of 18 Hylamer samples and 12 GUR 415 control samples were tested to 3.3 million cycles. Results are shown in Figure 21a. Wear factors for conven-

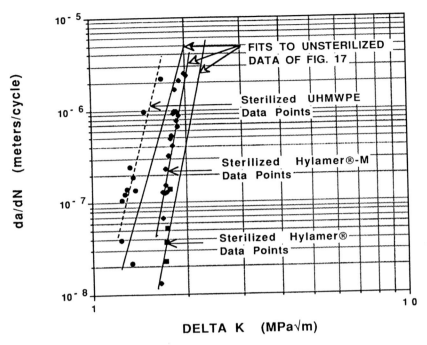

Figure 18 Comparison of fatigue crack growth rates for sterilized versus unsterilized materials at 37°C in distilled water.

tional UHMWPE and Hylamer were -3.56×10^{-8} and -2.43×10^{-8} cubic millimeters per Newton-meter (mm^3/N-m) respectively. This represents a 32% lower wear rate for Hylamer than for conventional UHMWPE ($p \leq 0.05$).

The results of a test of six Hylamer-M versus six conventional UHMWPE samples are shown in Fig. 21b. Counterfaces were again polished to a roughness of less than 1 microinch, and testing was continued to 3.3 million cycles. The average wear factor for conventional UHMWPE was -3.41×10^{-8} mm^3/N-m compared to -2.23×10^{-8} mm^3/N-m for Hylamer-M. This corresponds to a 35% lower wear rate for Hylamer-M than for GUR 415 UHMWPE ($p \leq 0.05$).

In a second test of Hylamer-M versus conventional UHMWPE, in which the Co-Cr counterface roughnesses were 2 to 3 μin (Fig. 21c), the conventional material had a wear factor of -7.61×10^{-8} mm^3/N-m ($N = 6$), while the value for Hylamer-M was -4.28×10^{-8} mm^3/N-m ($N = 12$). This represents a 44% reduction in wear rate for Hylamer-M versus GUR 415 ($p < 0.05$). The higher wear factors for this test compared with the previous tests again illustrate the important effect of surface finish on wear behavior. Additional tests of Hylamer-M versus GUR 415 are in progress.

2. Hip Simulator Studies

The wear behavior of Hylamer was also investigated on a hip simulator [48]. Acetabular cups having inside diameters of 32 mm were machined from bars of Hylamer and conventional GUR 415 UHMWPE and were sterilized with 2.5 megarad (Mrad) of gamma radiation. Three cups of each material were wear tested against Co-Cr alloy hip balls that

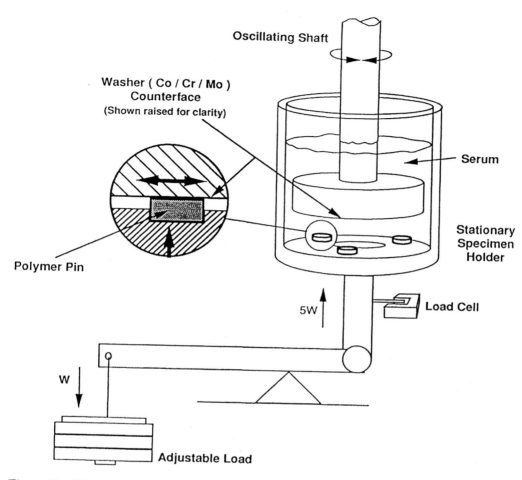

Figure 19 Schematic of dynamic tri-pin-on-disk test station.

had been polished to surface roughnesses of 2 to 3 μin. Cups were immersed in bovine blood serum and oscillated at approximately 1 Hz under a physiological hip cycle with a maximum load of 2000 Newtons (N). Tests were continued to 5 million cycles. At intervals of 500,000 cycles, cups were removed from the tester, cleaned, dried, and weighed along with 3 cups of each material that was soaked in serum. The static soak controls were used to correct the dynamic tests for fluid absorption.

An initial break-in period was observed in which wear rates increased slightly during the first 1.5 million cycles. Between 1.5 and 4 million cycles, wear rates were relatively stable. Hylamer exhibited an approximately 3.8% lower wear rate (30.4 vs. 31.6 mm^3/10^6 cycles for conventional UHMWPE), but this was not felt to be a statistically significant difference ($p > 0.4$) [48]. Between 2.5 and 5 million cycles, the wear rate of Hylamer was about 9% lower than conventional UHMWPE (27.3 vs. 29.9 mm^3/10^6 cycles, $p > 0.2$) [49]. This suggests that the difference in wear rate between Hylamer and conventional UHMWPE is becoming more apparent with increased testing time on the simula-

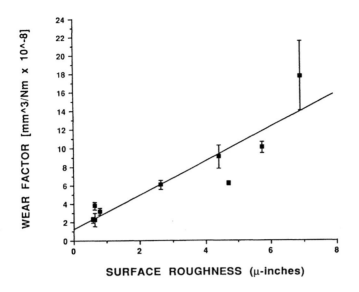

Figure 20   The effect of Co-Cr counterface roughness on wear rate observed in pin-on-disk tests.

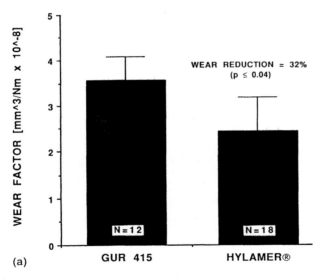

(a)

Figure 21   Wear rates from pin-on-disk tests in bovine serum at 37°C versus conventional ultra-high molecular weight polyethylene (UHMWPE): (a) Hylamer (counterface roughness <1 μin); (b) Hylamer-M (counterface roughness <1 μin; (c), Hylamer-M versus conventional UHMWPE with counterface roughness equal to 2 to 3 μin.

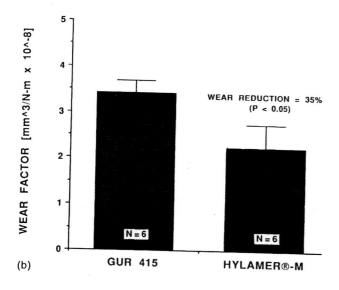

(b)

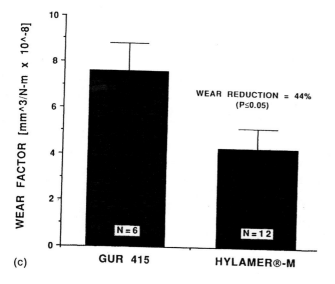

(c)

tor. With only three samples of each material, however, it is difficult to obtain high levels of statistical significance. Additional hip simulator data will be obtained.

Both pin-on-disk and hip simulator studies indicate that the pressure recrystallized materials have lower wear rates than conventional UHMWPE. This provides additional evidence that these materials have the potential for longer implant lifetimes and less debris generation.

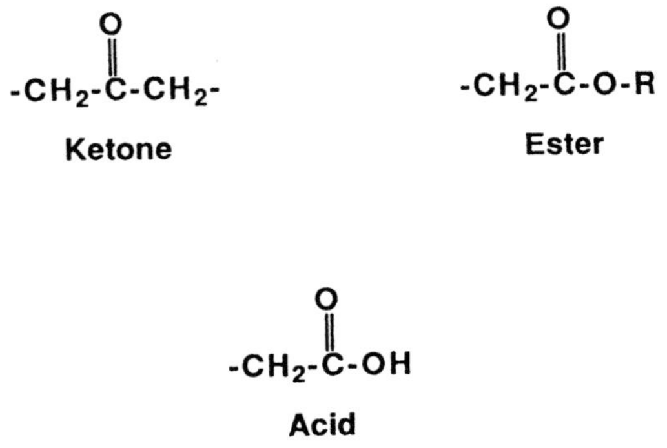

$$\text{-CH}_2\text{-}\overset{\overset{\displaystyle O}{\|}}{\text{C}}\text{-CH}_2\text{-}$$

Ketone

$$\text{-CH}_2\text{-}\overset{\overset{\displaystyle O}{\|}}{\text{C}}\text{-O-R}$$

Ester

$$\text{-CH}_2\text{-}\overset{\overset{\displaystyle O}{\|}}{\text{C}}\text{-OH}$$

Acid

Figure 22 Oxygen-containing species formed after gamma sterilization of UHMWPE in air. Infrared analysis shows that ketones are the predominant species, but ester and acid groups are also present.

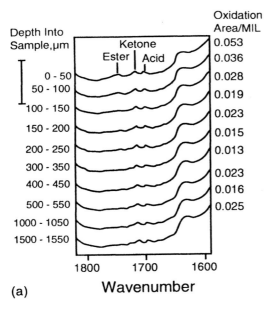

(a)

Figure 23 Carbonyl bands of Fourier transform infrared (FTIR) spectra: (a), unsterilized ultrahigh molecular weight polyethylene (UHMWPE) showing little oxidation at any depth; (b), UHMWPE one month after gamma sterilization at 2.5 megarads (Mrad) in air with significant oxidation present and ketones the predominant species produced; (c), UHMWPE three years after gamma sterilization in air with oxidation levels greater at all depths. The bar at the left of each set indicates an absorbance of 0.1.

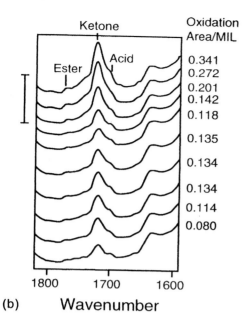

(b) Wavenumber

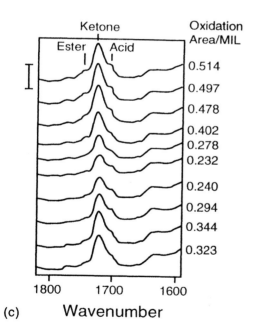

(c) Wavenumber

H. Oxidation

Oxidation has been observed in UHMWPE after sterilization by gamma radiation in air, during storage of components on the shelf, and in retrieved implants [8–13]. Oxidative degradation has a detrimental effect on material performance such as fatigue lifetimes and crack growth rates. High levels of oxidation are frequently associated with high levels of damage in retrieved implants [50].

We have studied oxidation of conventional UHMWPE, Hylamer, and Hylamer-M by sterilizing samples in air with 2.5 Mrad of gamma radiation and determining the amount of oxidation by Fourier transform infrared (FTIR) spectroscopy. When UHM-WPE is gamma sterilized, free radicals are formed and, if oxygen is present, it can combine with these radicals to form carbonyl groups such as ketones, esters, and carboxylic acids. These species are shown in Fig. 22. The formation of acid groups results in chain scission and a lowering of molecular weight. Formation of ketones and esters does not lower molecular weight, but these can be sites of further degradation *in vivo*.

A microspectrometric FTIR technique for analyzing oxidation in UHMWPE was developed by Nagy and Li [10]. A vertical slice, 250-μm thick, was taken through an UHMWPE sample with a microtome. IR spectra were obtained with a UMA 300 infrared microscope, a Digilab 60A FTIR spectrometer, and a narrow-range MCT detector. The microscope was equipped with a motorized stage capable of moving in 10-μm steps. The adjustable aperture window was set to 50 × 200 μm, and spectra were obtained at 50-μm intervals between the surface and a depth of 2000–6000 μm into the specimens. At each step, 100 scans were made, with a resolution of 4 cm^{-1}. The ester, ketone, and carboxylic acid species produced by oxidation have peaks in the infrared region at 1738, 1720, and 1696 cm^{-1}, respectively. The degree of oxidation can be estimated by integrating the total area of this carbonyl band between 1660 and 1800 cm^{-1} and normalizing by the sample thickness. The carbonyl area/mil (0.001 inch) is taken as a measure of oxidation.

Figure 23 shows this carbonyl region of the IR spectrum for three conventional GUR 415 UHMWPE tibial components. A 250-μm thick vertical slice was taken through each component, and FTIR spectra were obtained in 50-μm steps from just below the articulating surface to a depth of 2 mm. Figure 23a is the spectrum for an unsterilized component one month after manufacture. Only very small peaks are present, indicating very little oxidation in a new unsterilized specimen at any depth. Figure 23b is the carbonyl region for a component one month after gamma sterilization in air at 2.5 Mrad. Oxidation is present at the surface and decreases with depth into the sample. Ketones are the predominant oxidative species, but traces of ester and acid groups are also present. Figure 23c is the spectrum for a gamma-sterilized component after three years on the shelf in commercial packaging. The level of oxidation is measurably higher than for the recently sterilized specimen of Fig. 23b and indicates that oxidation of UHMWPE continues as components are exposed to air before implantation.

Intuitively, one might expect that increasing the crystallinity of UHMWPE will increase oxidation resistance because oxygen can diffuse less rapidly into the more tightly packed crystalline regions than into the amorphous regions of the polymer. Eyerer et al. exposed thin films of UHMWPE to 3% hydrogen peroxide solutions and determined the effects of oxidation by measuring changes in density and modulus and by IR measurements of the formation of ester groups [47]. They report that pressure recrystallized materials, fabricated under conditions similar to Hylamer, were significantly more stable

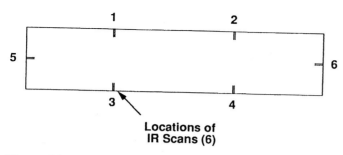

Figure 24 Diagram showing locations of Fourier transform infrared (FTIR) measurements on microtome slices through Hylamer, Hylamer-M, and conventional UHMWPE specimens. Oxidation to a depth of 750 μm was determined at each location, and the six values were averaged to obtain a value for the level of oxidation of each material after gamma sterilization in air.

against oxidation than normally processed UHMWPE. The oxidation behavior of Hylamer and Hylamer-M has, therefore, been investigated by the FTIR technique.

Disks of Hylamer, Hylamer-M, and UHMWPE 0.25-in thick were sterilized with 2.5 Mrad of gamma radiation. A microtomed slice was taken through each disk, and oxidation as a function of depth was measured at six locations around the perimeter (see Fig. 24). The total oxidation down to a depth of 750 μm was determined for each location, and a grand average was calculated for the amount of oxidation on each sample. The results are shown below.

	Oxidation (peak area/mil)
Hylamer	1100
Hylamer-M	1150
Conventional UHMWPE	1460

These results show that the Hylamer samples have about 25% less oxidation than the conventional GUR 415 UHMWPE. Additional studies of oxidation in Hylamer and Hylamer-M are ongoing. Analysis of retrieved components will be reported as they become available.

IV. CONCLUSIONS

Ultra-high molecular weight polyethylene can be enhanced significantly by pressure recrystallization. The changes in physical and mechanical properties that result from the changes in polymer morphology and crystallinity offer potential benefits in orthopedic applications. The improvements in creep resistance, yield strength, crack growth behavior, wear, and oxidative stability all address the need for improved orthopedic bearing surfaces. These improvements are accomplished without sacrificing molecular weight or toughness and without the use of any additives to the polymer.

Well-controlled commercial-scale processes have been developed at duPont to produce Hylamer enhanced UHMWPE. Orthopedic components are available through De Puy/duPont Orthopaedics, Incorporated, a joint venture between De Puy and duPont formed in 1989. To date, over 55,000 hip cups, tibial trays, and shoulder glenoids have been implanted and appear to be performing well. Research and development programs are continuing in an ongoing effort to provide better orthopedic bearing materials. As retrievals become available, thorough analyses will be made in order to gain an ever-improving understanding of these materials.

ACKNOWLEDGMENTS

The authors gratefully acknowledge J. Trentacosta, W. Lilly, and B. Moran, duPont Central Science and Engineering, for their pin-on-disk wear studies; B. Wood, duPont Corporate Center for Analytical Sciences, for the transmission electron microscopy work; D. Kasprzak and R. Martin for infra-red analysis; and L. Berger, duPont Central Research and Development, for the SAXS studies. The technical assistance of J. Reid and M. Coates is also gratefully acknowledged.

REFERENCES

1. Charnley, J., *Low Friction Arthroplasty of the Hip*, Springer-Verlag, New York (1979).
2. Charnley, J., Tissue Reactions to Polytetrafluorethylene, *Lancet*, 2:1379 (1963).
3. Hastings, G. W., Load Bearing Polymers Used in Orthopaedic Surgery, *Brit. Polymer J.*, 10: 251–255 (1978).
4. Poly Two™ Carbon Polyethylene Composite: A Carbon Fiber Reinforced Molded Ultra-High Molecular Weight Polyethylene, Zimmer U.S.A. Research and Development Division Report, Warsaw, Indiana (Jan. 1977).
5. Ainsworth, R., Farling, G., and Bardos, D., An Improved Bearing Material for Joint Replacement Prostheses: Carbon Fiber Reinforced UHMW Polyethylene, *Trans. Orthop. Res. Soc.*, 2:120 (1977).
6. Wright, T. M., Hood, R. W., and Burstein, A. H., Analysis of Material Failures, *Orthop. Clin. North Am.*, 13:33–44 (1982).
7. Wright, T. M., and Bartel, D. L., The Problem of Surface Damage in Polyethylene Total Knee Components, *Clin. Orthop.*, 205:67–74 (1986).
8. Eyerer, P., and Ke, Y. C., Property Changes of UHMW Polyethylene Hip Cup Endoprostheses During Implantation, *J. Biomed. Mater. Res.*, 18:1137–1151 (1984).
9. Rose, R. M., and Radin, E. L., A Prognosis for Ultra High Molecular Weight Polyethylene, *Biomaterials*, 11:63–67 (1990).
10. Nagy, E. V., and Li, S., A Fourier Transform Infrared Technique for the Evaluation of Polyethylene Orthopaedic Bearing Materials, *Soc. for Biomaterials Transactions*, 109 (1990).
11. Nagy, E. V., and Li, S., Analysis of Retrieved Knee Components via Fourier Transform Infrared Spectroscopy, *Soc. for Biomaterials Transactions*, 274 (1990).
12. Li, S., Nagy, E. V., and Wood, B. A., Chemical Degradation of Polyethylene in Hip and Knee Replacements, *Trans. Orthop. Res. Soc.*, 17:41 (1992).
13. Saum, K. A., Oxidation versus Depth and Time for Polyethylene Gamma Sterilized in Air, *Trans. Orthop. Res. Soc.*, 19:174 (1994).
14. Howie, D. W., Vernon-Roberts, B., Oakeshott, R., and Manthey, B., A Rat Model of Resorption of Bone at the Cement-Bone Interface in the Presence of Polyethylene Wear Particles, *J. Bone and Joint Surg.*, 70A:257–263 (1988).
15. Mirra, J. M., Marder, R. A., and Amstutz, H. C., The Pathology of Failed Total Joint Arthroplasty, *Clin. Orthop.*, 170:175–183 (1982).
16. Dannenmaier, W. C., Haynes, D. W., and Nelson, C. L., Granulomatous Reaction and Cystic Bony Destruction Associated with High Wear Rate in a Total Knee Prosthesis, *Clin. Orthop.*, 198:224–230 (1985).
17. Willert, H. G., and Semlitsch, M., Reactions of the Articular Capsule to Wear Products of Artificial Joint Prostheses, *J. Biomed. Mater. Res.*, 11:157–164 (1977).

18. Wroblewski, B. M., Wear of High Density Polyethylene on Bone and Cartilage, *J. Bone and Joint Surg.*, 61B:498–500 (1979).
19. Li, S., and Howard, E. G., U.S. Patent 5,037,928 (1991).
20. Howard, E. G., and Champion, A. R., patent pending.
21. Bohm, L. L., Reaction Model for Ziegler–Natta Polymerization Processes, *Polymer*, 19:545–552 (1978).
22. Bohm, L. L., Ethylene Polymerization Process With a Highly Active Ziegler–Natta Catalyst: 1. Kinetics, *Polymer*, 19:553–561 (1978).
23. Bohm, L. L., Ethylene Polymerization Process With a Highly Active Ziegler–Natta Catalyst: 2. Molecular Weight Regulation, *Polymer*, 19:562–566 (1978).
24. Ottani, S., and Porter, R. S., A Calorimetric Investigation on High Molecular Weight Polyethylene Reactor Powders, *J. Polymer. Sci., B*, 29:1179–1188 (1991).
25. American Society for Testing and Materials, ASTM D-1505, Standard Test Method for Density of Plastics by the Density-Gradient Technique (1985).
26. Chanzy, H., Day, A., and Marchessault, R. H., Polymerization on Glass-Supported Vanadium Trichloride: Morphology of Nascent Polyethylene, *Polymer*, 8:567–588 (1967).
27. American Society for Testing and Materials, ASTM D-638, Standard Test Method for Tensile Properties of Plastics (1989).
28. American Society for Testing and Materials, ASTM D-256, Standard Test Methods for Impact Resistance of Plastics and Electrical Insulating Materials (1984).
29. American Society for Testing and Materials, ASTM D-621, Standard Test Methods for Deformation of Plastics Under Load. (1976).
30. American Society for Testing and Materials, ASTM F-648, Standard Specification for Ultra-High-Molecular Weight Polyethylene Powder and Fabricated Form for Surgical Implants (1984).
31. Lupton, J. M., and Regester, J. W., Physical Properties of Extended-Chain High-Density Polyethylene, *J. Appl. Polymer Sci.*, 18:2407–2425 (1974).
32. Lupton, J. M., and Regester, J. W., Exceptionally Rigid and Tough Ultrahigh Molecular Weight Linear Polyethylene, U.S. Patent 3,944,536 (1976).
33. Basset, D. C., and Turner, B., On the Phenomenology of Chain-Extended Crystallization in Polyethylene, *Phil. Mag.*, 29:925–955 (1974).
34. Eyerer, P., Kurth, M., Ellwanger, R., Madler, H., Federolf, H.-A., and Siegmann, A., Ultrahigh Molecular Weight Polyethylene for Replacement Joints, *Kuntstoff*, 77:617–622 (1987).
35. Simmons, W., and Howard, E., Pressure Vessel, U.S. Patent 5,236,669 (1993).
36. Berger, L. L., and Wilson, F., internal communication, E.I. duPont de Nemours (1988).
37. Raff, R. A. V., and Doak, K. W., eds., *Crystalline Olefin Polymers*, Part 1, pg 719, Interscience Publishers, New York (1965).
38. Wood, B. A., Crystalline Lamellae in UHMWPE Measured by TEM, Analytical and Physical Measurements Section, E. I. DuPont de Nemours, internal communication (1991).
39. Kanig, G., New Electronmicroscopic Investigations of the Morphology of Polyethylene, *Progr. Colloid & Polymer Sci.*, 57:176–191 (1975).
40. American Society for Testing and Materials, ASTM D-695, Standard Test Method for Compressive Properties of Rigid Plastics (1989).
41. Connelly, G. M., Rimnac, C. M., Wright, T. M., Hertzberg, R. W., and Manson, J. A., Fatigue Crack Propagation Behavior of UHMWPE, *J. Ortho. Res.*, 2:119–125 (1984).
42. American Society for Testing and Materials, ASTM E-647, Standard Test Method for Measurement of Fatigue Crack Growth Rates (1988).
43. Bunzey, G., Warner, R., and Andrews, W. R., Fatigue Crack Growth in UHMW Polyethylene, Materials Characterization Laboratory Report No. MCL92013-1 to E. I. DuPont (April 1992).
44. Bunzey, G., Warner, R., and Andrews, W. R., Fatigue Crack Growth in Sterilized UHMW Polyethylene, Materials Characterization Laboratory Report No. MCL92013-3 to E. I. DuPont (July 1992).

45. Roe, et al., *J. Biomed. Mater. Res.*, 15:209 (1981).

46. Li, et al., Chemical Degradation of Polyethylene in Hip and Knee Replacements, *Trans. ORS*, 17:41 (1992).

47. Eyerer, P., Ellwanger, R., Federolf, H.-A., Kurth, M., and Madler, H., Polyethylene. In *Concise Encyclopedia of Medical and Dental Materials*, D. Williams, Editor, MIT Press, Cambridge (1990).

48. McKellop, H., Lu, B., and Li, S., Wear of Acetabular Cups of Conventional and Modified UHMW Polyethylenes Compared on a Hip Joint Simulator, *Transactions of the 38th Annual Meeting, Orth. Res. Soc.*, 356 (1992).

49. McKellop, H., private communication, University of Southern California (1992).

50. Rimnac, C. M., Klein, R. W., Khanna, N., and Weintraub, J. T., Post-Irradiation Aging of UHMWPE, *Soc. for Biomaterials Transactions*, (1993).

III
METALS IN ORTHOPEDICS

16
Bone-Metal Interaction

Uri Oron
Tel Aviv University
Tel-Aviv, Israel

I. INTRODUCTION

The use of biomaterials in reconstructive surgery has grown exponentially each decade since World War II. This tremendous progress has taken place due to the need for strengthening or replacing of body components that transplantation cannot accommodate, and through technological advances throughout the years. It is now well understood that the successful employment of artificial material for the replacement of structural components in the body has to be a result of interdisciplinary research by physicists, chemical engineers, biologists, and clinicians. Currently, biomaterials of a wide range of mechanical strength and chemical and physical properties are used in medicine. These include polymers as vascular and cardiovascular materials, tricalcium phosphate (TCP) and hydroxyapatite (HA) bioceramics as bone graft substitutes, biosensors, and electrical devices, and various metal alloys as prosthetic devices in orthopedics and dentistry [Hanker and Giammara 1988]. This chapter focuses primarily on metal prosthetic devices and their interaction with bone.

II. FIXATION OF METAL PROSTHETIC COMPONENTS TO BONES IN HUMANS

The functional restoration of joints damaged by trauma or disease is obtained by prosthetic surgery. In particular, the implementation of a hip prosthesis is regarded as routine in orthopedic surgery [McKee 1982] and thorough research has been developed in the field. The prosthetic replacement of the knee, and even more so the ankle or elbow, occurs less frequently in clinical practice, and has been studied less intensively.

Artificial replacement of joints relies on good anchorage between the prosthetic components and the host bone in order to obtain a good functional performance of the

489

joint for long periods of time. The loosening of these components with time is the most frequent complication in total hip replacement. One method that has been used for many years to bond these components to bone is the use of acrylic bone cement. The other methods rely on biological fixation (cementless joints) by the growth of bone to porous or other shaped types of implants. Dental implants are always implanted without the use of cement.

Reviewing the orthopedic literature on the subject of joint prosthesis loosening in the case of a cemented prosthesis is a demanding task because of the different interpretations given to the term *failure* and, consequently, to the term *loosening*. From various reports of long-term follow-up of loosening after hip replacement, it appears that the numbers vary from 1.5% to 32.7% of the patients for whom the loosening was reported [Pizzoferrato et al. 1991]. The above variability indeed reflects the complexity of the definition and the phenomenon of the implant loosening. Furthermore, it was difficult to find a direct relationship between the loosening and a specific factor like the kind of prosthesis or other factors. However, it was generally agreed from reviewing and follow-up of hip replacement in young patients (under the age of 40) that the incidence of loosening occurs in this group to a much higher degree. Despite the constant trials to improve the cementation technique [Mulroy and Harris 1990] in order to prevent this loosening, or impregnation of the polymethylmethacrylate cement with growth hormone to promote bone growth next to the implants [Downes et al. 1990], there is a widespread trend to insert cementless prostheses in young patients to avoid the failures related to the use of cement.

In summary, while replacement of cemented artificial joints has already been performed for many years with rather good results, it is agreed that the bone/cement interface is the point of failure in these implants. Thus, biological fixation may prove to be a viable alternative to the acrylic cement and is already a preferable alternative in joint replacement in young patients.

III. BIOLOGICAL FIXATION OF METAL IMPLANTS

The basic principles of the process of bone growth to porous metal implants have been previously reviewed [Pilliar 1987; Albrektsson and Lekholm 1989; Albrektsson and Zarba 1993]. The surface as well as the shape of the implants has been altered in order to achieve a proper functional performance and good bonding between the bone and the implants. Thus, the surface may be porous, contain grooves, be plasma sprayed, or contain fiber mesh to improve bonding between the growing bone and the implant. This direct bonding was defined as *osseointegration* to indicate direct apposition of the bone on the metal implant without the interface of connective tissue. Indeed, in past years, many studies have reported progressive bony ingrowth to metal implants in experimental animals and in retrieved, cementless implants in humans. These studies demonstrated, mainly by histological methods, the basic phenomenon of bone growth to metal implants that are inserted to long bones in experimental animals either intramedullary or transcortically.

Sumner et al. (1986) and Turner et al. (1986) compared the effect of surface macroscopic alternation of the implants on their bonding strength. They found that fiber mesh on the implants gave a better bonding strength to host bone over implants with a porous surface up to six months after surgery. Jasty et al. (1986) have shown in hip joints in dogs that contained porous titanium mesh surfaces that, as soon as three weeks after insertion, woven bone is formed in between the titanium fibers. Recently, Stulberg et al.

(1991) observed that, after cementless titanium porous-coated knee joints were implanted to dogs, connective tissue was formed between the implants and the newly formed bone.

It has been shown that micromotion between the implants and the host bone inhibits bone growth to them [Cameron, Pilliar, and McNab, 1973; Heck et al. 1986]. Aspenberg et al. (1992) recently used a unique model to show this effect on bony ingrowth in general. They studied bone growth to a 1-mm (millimeter) canal through a titanium chamber implanted in the proximal tibia of rabbits. The central part of the canal could be moved in relation to its end. During a 30-second period once a day, 20 cycles of 0.5-mm movements caused the canal to be filled mainly by connective tissue as opposed to cancellous bone in a "nonmovement" situation.

IV. BONE GROWTH TO VARIOUS ALLOYS

Bone growth to metal implants is also dependent on the metal alloy itself. The normal process of primary bone formation during bone healing after ablation of bone as a regular process for preparation of the bone for implant insertion may be affected by the presence of the implant in the site of mineralization. It was recently shown by Kohavi et al. (1992) that the maturation of extracellular matrix vesicles around titanium implants inserted into the tibia of rats was delayed when compared with normal primary bone formation during bone healing. The delay in mineralization is compensated by an increase in vesicle production, resulting in an enhancement of primary mineralization by the titanium. We have shown in our experimental model in the rat (see Section VI) that the enzymatic activity of alkaline phosphatase (a marker for osteoblasts) in the newly formed tissue after reaming of the medullary canal of the femur in rats (procedure of preparation for implant insertion) was higher than that of the tissue formed around the control Ti6A1-4V implants and similar to the activity around the heat-treated (prior to implantation) implant. This is another example that the implant itself and its chemical surface characteristics can affect the adjacent milieu of cells and normal repair response of ablated bone marrow.

In another study by Johansson, Sennerby, and Albrektsson (1991), it was shown that bone apposition to commercially pure titanium (cp-Ti) and Ti-6A1-4V alloy is different using transmission electron microscopy on thin sections of these metals that were sputtered on polycarbonate plastic implants; the interface zone of cp-Ti demonstrates more organized bone than the Ti-6A1-4V implants and the collagen-free proteoglycan layer was narrower (200–400 angstroms [Å]) in the cp-Ti than in the Ti-6A1-4V alloy (500–1000 Å). Orr, de Bruijn, and Davies (1992) studied the bone interface between cp-Ti and titanium alloy implants inserted transfemorally in rats using scanning electron microscopy of specimens that were freeze fractured in liquid nitrogen. In this study, too, a greater adherence was demonstrated to titanium implants as compared with no adherence to titanium alloy implants.

In another study, Johansson, Hansson, and Albrektsson (1990) investigated tissue response to tantalum, niobium, and cp-Ti implanted in the tibial metaphysis of rabbits. The ground substance layer had a thickness in the range of 40 to 60 nanometers (nm) for niobium implants and 20–40 nm of collagen filaments close to the cp-Ti implants. Histomorphometric analysis of bony contact around niobium and titanium screws inserted in the rabbit bone showed almost no differences between the two metals [Johansson and Albrektsson 1991].

Torque strength of screw-shaped implants of cp-Ti and Co-Cr alloy (Vitallium) implants were analyzed three months after implantation to the tibial metaphysis [Johansson, Sennerby, and Albrektsson 1991]. The torque strength of the cp-Ti was higher (24.9 n/cm) than the Vitallium (11.7 n/cm). Moreover, the histomorphometric study revealed more bone-to-metal contact for the cp-Ti implants. Several other studies compared the bone apposition to various metals and also between metal alloy used in orthopedics and ceramic or polymers. Comparison of the removal torque between screw-shaped implants of cp-Ti and polymerized methyl methacrylate in the rabbit tibia showed the greatest value for the titanium implants [Moreberg and Albrektsson 1991]. In another study comparing the reparative process in femurs of cats around cp-Ti and glass-ceramic-coated implants, only the titanium implants became osseointegrated [Barth, Johannson, and Albrektsson 1990].

In our experimental model we have also shown that the shear strengths of Ti-6A1-4V implants are two- to three-fold significantly higher than the identical stainless steel 316L implants inserted to the medullary canal of rats up to 35 days after implantation (Hazan and Oron 1990a).

In summary, it can be concluded that the metal alloys, ceramics, or polymers currently used in orthopedics cannot be considered to have identical biocompatibility to the body tissue or fluids. Moreover, different alloys can elicit different responses of an identical biological milieu in which they are inserted. Currently, based on recent studies, cp-Ti appears to be the metal of choice when only osseointegration is under consideration. The precise mechanisms by which the osteogenic cells respond so differently to various metals are not clearly understood, but again stress the significance of the host-implant interface, discussed below.

V. THE BONE-METAL INTERFACE

The investigation of bone-metal interface involves a multidisciplinary research that can attract biologists, chemists, physicists, material scientists, and clinicians. The tissue reaction to metal implants is different from chemically reactive glass. The bone-metal interface has been studied previously by several authors [Kasemo and Lausmaa 1986; Pilliar 1987; Williams 1987; Albrektsson and Jakobsson 1986, 1987; Albrektsson and Lekholm 1989; Galante et al. 1991; Albrektsson and Zarba 1993]. Kasemo and Lausmaa (1986) also defined in their review the interface zone between the implant and the tissue as the whole region in which the implant may induce changes in the biological system that may in turn, via surface reactions, induce changes in the implant material. Williams (1987) and Parsegian (1983), based on theoretical calculations, claimed that the initial bonding between the biological tissue and the implant is hydrophilic. Later, these bonds are exchanged by electrostatic bonds that better interconnect the molecules adjacent to the implant.

Kasemo (1983) also claimed that hydrophilic chemical bonds are relatively weak and temporary bonds with energy of 10 kilojoules per mole (kj/mol), while covalent electrostatic chemical bonds are stronger and have a much higher energy (50–500 kj/mol), and therefore are probably the constant and stable bonds between the molecules and the implants. Later, Kasemo and Lausmaa (1986) claimed that, considering the variation of chemical composition occurring at an implant surface and the very large spectrum of molecules present in the biological system, it is likely that all types of bonding occur at the interface between molecules and the metal, from weak van der Waal's interaction through H bonding, to strong ionic and covalent bonding. This assumption also suggests that there is a dynamic rather than a static state at the interface since there is a strong relationship between bonding strength and the time that a molecule stays adsorbed to the surface.

A novel approach that was first introduced by Albrektsson and his colleagues [Albrektsson and Hansson 1986] gave a better insight on the interface phase between metals and the bone. In this system, metal was sputtered on polycarbonate plugs in order to obtain a section of approximately 50 nm that could be viewed by transmission electron microscope. According to this work, the morphologically distinguishable bone tissue (an extracellular matrix comprised of mineralized collagen) was separated from the implant surface by a layer of extracellular matrix ground substance said to contain proteoglycans and glycosaminoglycans. The width of this layer varied in the case of pure titanium from 200 Å to 1000 nm but was never less than 400–600 Å on gold and several thousand angstrom on stainless steel. Recently, Orr, de Bruijn, and Davies (1992) took a different approach, examining the interface zone by scanning electron microscopy after fixation and freeze fracturing the specimens to enable examination of the tissue immediately adjacent to the implant without decalcification. Using the above technique, they were able to show that the tissue abutting the implant was a cement-line-like layer that separated the implant from the surrounding bone proper. In the case of hydroxyapatite rods, this cement-line-like layer was composed of globular accretions that were clearly visible on the smooth-grained surfaces of the hydroxyapatite.

Kasemo and Lausmaa (1986), in an excellent review paper, have addressed all aspects of the surface properties (chemical and physical properties to the atomic scale, such as chemical composition, cleanliness, texture, surface energy, corrosion resistance, and tendency to denaturate proteins) of metal implants and their possible significance to the integration of the implant in host tissue. It is evident from this review and many other studies that biomolecules interact quite differently with different solid surfaces. The formation of the oxide layer of metals upon exposure to air is very rapid. According to Kasemo and Lausmaa (1986), the first step is adsorption of O_2 molecules, which immediately dissociate to oxygen atoms at the surface. Within a few milliseconds (ms), the first monolayer of oxygen may be formed. Within about 1 ms, an oxide layer of 1-mm thickness may have grown, and within a few seconds the oxide growth is virtually completed on the metal surface.

It should be noted that oxidation proceeds by oxygen ion diffusion into the metal and/or by metal ion diffusion in the reverse direction. The surface oxide stops growing for kinetic reasons (i.e., due to slow transport of oxygen and metal atoms), and not because of thermodynamics. Therefore, the oxide growth will increase in rate if the oxygen and/or metal atom transport is accelerated (e.g., by an increase in temperature or by the presence of certain impurities that enhance the ion transport and/or O_2 dissociation). Certain strong oxidants (ozone, peroxides, singlet O, etc.) may also accelerate oxidation. This means, in the context of metal, that a direct contact is never established between the implant metal and the host tissue but, rather between the tissue and the surface oxide of the implant.

Various methods are currently being used in industry to control the chemical properties of the oxide layer. Anodic oxidation (electrochemical oxidation) and plasma oxidation (O plasma is used instead of liquid electrolytes) are the most common. Ion implantation, in which the desired ions are formed in a vapor accelerator and directed toward the sample, is another more sophisticated method to affect the chemical characteristics of the surface layer of the metals. In the case of corrosion-resistant implants that do not induce violent tissue reactions, however, the interface zone probably only penetrates about 1 micrometers or less into the implant and less than about 1 mm into the tissue.

Valuable information about the influence of different preparation procedures (cleaning and passivation process, sterilization, etc.) on the nature of the surface oxide and the contamination level can be gained by surface analysis of implants before implantation. Important information about changes in the surface oxide layer and its possible significance after implantation can be gained by analysis of retrieved implants. McQueen et al. (1982) used the Auger electron spectroscopic (AES) technique in combination with argon ion sputtering to study the surface oxides on titanium dental implants removed after 0.5 and 8 years of clinical function. Their results show that the thickness of the surface oxide increases considerably throughout the entire implantation period. According to this work, the oxide thickness in these implants after six years was 200 nm, as opposed to about 5 nm in an unimplanted sample. Varying amounts of calcium, phosphorus, and sulfur were found to be incorporated into the surface oxides.

Sundgren, Boda and Lundstrom (1986), using AES in combination with ion sputtering, measured the thickness and chemical composition of the surface oxides on samples implanted in various tissues of humans. Implants located in bone contained calcium and phosphorus in the oxide layer. The oxide thickness of implants in cancellous bone remained unaffected, while for implants in bone marrow it increased by a factor of 3 or 4. Implants located in soft tissue had an oxide thickness of about 1.5 times that of the original implant, and in some cases it also contained sulfur. Thus, the thickness and nature of the oxide layer was found to depend on both calcium and phosphorus. We [Hazan 1991] have also studied possible alternation of the surface chemical composition of control and heat-treated (280°C) stainless steel 316L and Ti-6A1-4V plates (1 cm × 1 cm) that were incubated *in vitro* (DMEM medium at 37°C, 95% O_2 + CO_2, with multiple changes of the medium) up to 30 days using the AES technique. No significant changes were observed in these plates with time by the incubation *in vitro*.

According to Kasemo and Lausmaa (1986) the continued growth of the oxygen layer must take place via metal ion diffusion from the metal-oxide interface to the oxide-liquid interface and/or by oxygen ion diffusion in the reverse direction. The source of oxygen can be strongly oxidizing agents such as the peroxide species (H_2O_2) and singlet O ($^1O_2$), which are known to be produced by the immune system and in inflammatory responses.

There is no simple explanation for the phenomenon of oxide growth and ion incorporation to it. The results, however, provide evidence that the interaction between the implant surface and the host tissue is a dynamic process that takes place over long periods of time and may be dependent on the biological nature of the host tissue.

VI.   ATTEMPTS TO IMPROVE THE BONDING OF METAL IMPLANTS TO BONE

Several attempts have been made in the past to enhance bony ingrowth to metal implants. Impregnation of porous implants with calcium phosphate did not affect the rate of bone growth to them [Berry et al. 1986], whereas carbon coating of implants prior to their insertion had minimal enhancement effect on bone growth to them [Anderson et al. 1984]. It was already shown by Halstead, Jones, and Rawlings (1979) that, in carbon-coated implants retrieved from humans, the tissue that apposed the carbon coating was scar and connective tissue rather than newly formed bone. Other studies made use of electric currents [Berry et al. 1986] and electromagnetic fields [Schutzer et al. 1990] in order to augment bony ingrowth to metal implants. None of the above methods yielded a higher interface bond strength than control, nontreated implants. The most common approach was coating or impregnating the implants with various matrices similar to those in natural bone to achieve a better growth and attraction of the presumptive osteoblasts or osteoblasts to the metal implants.

The most extensively studied among these matrices were hydroxyapatite (HA) [Lemons 1988; Oonishi 1991] and tricalcium phosphate (TCP). Many studies have investigated the effect of precoating of the metal implants with HA prior to their insertion on the bonding strength of the implants to bones using mechanical (pull-out force) and histological methods in experimental animals. Thomas et al. (1987) studied the effect on the bonding strength of the implant to bone up to 32 weeks postinsertion in experimental animals and found no significant effect over the control implants. In general, however, other studies have shown that the initial bonding strength of the coated implants to the bone was higher than the control, uncoated specimens, but there was no difference in long-term experiments.

It was shown [Oonishi et al. 1990] that, in rabbits and goats, porous Ti-6A1-4V implants coated with HA gave approximately four times greater bonding strength than uncoated implants at two weeks postinsertion, twice as much at four weeks, and a similar strength at 12 weeks. In another study [Gottlander and Albrektsson 1991], threaded HA-coated and uncoated pure titanium screws were inserted to the rabbit tibial metaphysis. It was found that, after six weeks, there was more (not significant) direct bony contact around the HA-coated implants than around the control. At a one-year time interval, there was more direct bone-to-implant contact with the uncoated pure titanium controls. A histomorphometric study on unthreaded HA-coated and titanium-coated implants in rabbit bone revealed significantly more direct bone contact after six months in the HA-coated implants [Gottlander, Albrektsson, and Carlsson 1992]. Hydroxyapatite-coated implants are also used clinically in cementless hip and knee joints, as well as in dental implants. Long-term studies of the clinical success of the coated implants are not yet available.

Oonishi et al. (1990) have reported improved results with HA-coated porous metal implants and also the use of HA granules between the bone and bone cement in order to obtain a bioactive interfacial bone concentration. Nevertheless, it is known that HA peels off with time after insertion to humans as evident from retrieved implants. Indeed, in a study by Muller-Mai, Voist, and Gross (1990) in which dense HA implants were investigated after implantation to the distal femur in rabbits by scanning and transmission electron microscopy, it was shown that changes in surface morphology of the HA are caused by leaching (increasing pore diameter), corrosion (particulate disintegration), and active resorption by osteoclasts.

We have recently investigated the possibility that the nature of chemical surface characteristics of the outer layer of the metal implants may determine the tissue response to it [Hazan and Oron 1990b; Hazan, Brener, and Oron 1993; Hazan and Oron 1993]. We have hypothesized that a simple process such as heat treatment, which alters the surface oxide layer of metals in general, may affect the process of bony ingrowth to them. To test the hypothesis, we have developed a simple experimental model in rats in which metal screwlike implants are inserted to the medullary canal of the femur through the knee joint [Hazan and Oron 1991]. In this model, the implant is in a practically unloaded situation so that we are able to obtain simultaneously mechanical (pull-out force), biochemical, and histological results with rather low variability within a short period of time and with a large number of animals.

The screw implants were driven (not screwed) axially by impaction to the medullary canal of the femur so that they could be withdrawn with minimal force immediately postinsertion. New bone was deposited between the ridges of the screw, as evident by histological examination [Hazan and Oron 1991]. Thus, after measurement of shear strengths of the screw implants, the newly formed bone that remained between the ridges of the screw implant, which was pulled out from the bone (Fig. 1), could be extracted and calcium content and alkaline phosphatase activity (a marker for bone-forming cells, osteoblasts) could be determined. Furthermore, the newly formed bone could also be collected and used for further *in vitro* incubation to measure ^{45}Ca incorporation (see below).

The above model was used to test the effect of heat treatment of the implants on their shear strength in the medullary canal at various time intervals after insertion. A progressive and significant ($p < 0.01$) increase in bony ingrowth into the grooves between the ridges of the screw implant as reflected by shear strength was observed with time after implantation for both control (not heated) and heat-treated (under dry airflow) Ti-6A1-4V implants (Fig. 2). The values were negligible at the time of insertion, and reached values of 1.04 ± 0.16 (mean $\pm$ SEM [standard errors of the mean]) and 2.13 ± 0.16 MPa at 10 and 35 days after surgery, respectively, in control Ti-6A1-4V implants (Fig. 2). The values of the heat-treated implants were significantly higher ($p < 0.05$) than

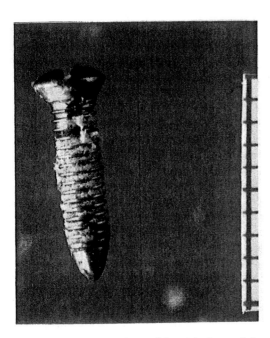

Figure 1   Screw implant with newly formed tissue around it. Note the newly formed tissue between the ridges of the screw after it was pulled out of the femur and the shear strength was measured ($\times 10$, length of scale on right side is 1 cm).

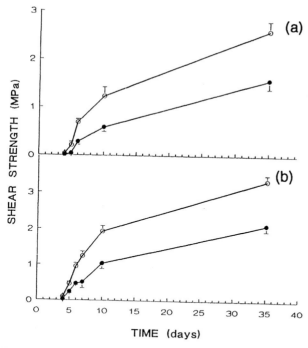

Figure 2 Shear strengths of control (● — ●) and heat-treated (○ — ○) implants as a function of time after insertion to the medullary canal in the femur: (a) stainless steel 316L; (b), Ti-6Al-4V (each point is mean ± SEM of 7–9 rats).

those of the controls at all time intervals after surgery, comprised of values of 3.7-, 1.9-, 2.0-, 2.4-, and 1.9-fold over controls at 4, 5, 6, 7, and 10 days postsurgery, respectively, and a 60% increase at 35 days after implantation. A similar augmentation phenomenon to that obtained for the Ti-6Al-4V implants was noticed also when the implants made of stainless steel 316L were heat treated in an identical procedure to the Ti-6Al-4V implants prior to insertion into the rats (Fig. 2). In this case, too, the shear strength of the heat-treated implants was significantly higher ($p < 0.05$) at all time intervals, reaching values of 3.0-, 5.3-, 2.5-, 2.1-, and 1.7-fold over the control at 4, 5, 6, 10, and 35 days postsurgery, respectively.

Using the above model, it was also possible to determine the enzymatic activity of alkaline phosphatase, which is a good marker of active osteoblasts in the newly formed tissue around the implant. In Table 1, the results of this activity around control, heat-treated, and in sham-operated femurs (reaming of the femur as for implant insertion, but without insertion of the implant) are presented. The peak activity of alkaline phosphatase in newly formed tissue around the heat-treated implants, which coincides with the activity around the control implants but shows a 1.6-fold higher activity, lends credence to the possibility that there are more osteoblasts next to the heat-treated implants at this stage of bone formation. The similar specific activity of alkaline phosphatase activity in the sham-operated and heat-treated implants may indicate that these implants are indeed more biocompatible than the controls, and that the amount of osteoblasts next to them is

Table 1 Shear Strength of Control and Heat-Treated Porous Ti-6Al-4V and Co-Cr Cylinders Inserted Transcondyllarly to the Femur in Dogs

Alloy	Time (weeks)	Shear strength (MPa) (M ± SEM)	
		Control	Heat treated
Ti-6Al-4V (Tivanium)	0	0.24 ± 0.1 (9)	0.53 ± 0.15 (10)
	4	1.85 ± 0.3 (11)	2.66[a] ± 0.32 (12)
Co-Cr (Vitalium)	0	0.33 ± 0.05 (8)	0.31 ± 0.07 (9)
	4	1.60 ± 0.27 (12)	2.49[a] ± 0.22 (12)

Heat-treated implants (2 to 3 implants per leg) were inserted transcondyllarly to the femur, while the control implants were inserted to the contralateral leg of 4 dogs. Pull-out forces were measured immediately and 4 weeks after insertion. Results are expressed in MPa and number of implants in parentheses.
[a]Statistically ($p < 0.05$) different from control.

similar to that of repair tissue in an intact bone (without the presence of an implant) in response to injury.

We have also performed a study to follow the rate of calcification in the newly formed tissue around the control and heat-treated screw implants by incubating the tissue collected from retrieved implants inserted as above to rats as an organ culture in a synthetic medium containing ^{45}Ca *in vitro*. The rate of calcification in the tissues collected at various time intervals following insertion is presented in Fig. 3. It can be seen that the rate of calcification increases from Day 5, reaching a peak at Day 7 postinsertion, and then declines to Day 10. These results corroborate with the maturation of bone around these implants from woven to primary mature bone, which takes place during the second week postinsertion of the implants.

The effect of heat treatment of implants prior to their insertion on bony ingrowth to them was also investigated in porous coated (three layers of beads on a core cylinder) implants inserted transcondyllarly to the femur of dogs (Table 1). The result indicated that the pull-out forces did not differ statistically between the heat-treated and control implants when they were analyzed immediately following insertion. These results indicate that the heat treatments do not cause any physical changes or distortion in the outermost layers of the beads, as was also shown previously [Hazan 1991] by using scanning electron microscopy. However, four weeks after insertion the shear strength of the heat-treated implants was significantly ($p < 0.05$) higher than the control nonheated implants, both in the Ti-6A1-4V and the Vitallium alloy implants.

In order to obtain information on the alterations in the surface chemical characteristics of the metal alloys by the heat treatment, Auger electron spectroscopic (AES) analyses were made on control and heat-treated implants (Figs. 4–6). It can be seen that the most significant change caused by the heat treatment in general was the increase in thickness of the oxide layer. This increase does not occur when implants are heated during

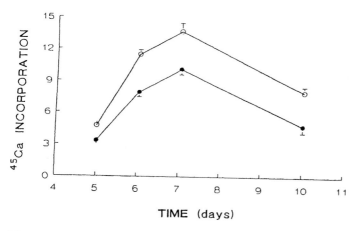

Figure 3 Rate of calcification in an *in vitro* system of the tissue collected around control and heat-treated Ti-6Al-4V implants. Newly formed tissue around the implants that were inserted to the medullary canal of rats (Hazan and Oron 1993) were collected at 5, 6, 7, and 10 days postinsertion. The tissue from three implants (rats) was pooled together and three such samples were used at each time interval for the control of heat-treated implants. The tissue was transferred to 2-ml artificial medium (DMEM) containing 4.5 milligrams per liter (mg/l) synthetic medium (saturated by 95% O_2 and 5% CO_2) and were incubated for 3 h at 37°C in the presence of 1.5 microcurie (μCi/ml) ^{45}Ca in the medium. The amount of ^{45}Ca that incorporated to calcified tissue was determined at the end of incubation by the homogenizing, centrifuging, and extensive wash of the sediment as described by Reddi and Sullivan (1980). The rate of calcification in each sample is expressed in cpm per mg wet weight tissue incubated tissue. Results are mean ± SEM of three pooled samples (as described above) from three rats at each time interval.

sterilization by autoclaving (to about 130°C), as seen in Fig. 5, but heating to 280°C caused an increase of approximately two-, four-, and three-fold in the oxide layer in Ti-6Al-4V stainless steel 316L and Co-Cr alloys, respectively. Further heating of the stainless steel alloy to 550°C markedly increased the thickness of the oxide layer (Fig. 4c) as was also the case with Ti-6Al-4V alloy (Hazan, Brener, and Oron 1993). In the case of the stainless steel alloy, chemical alterations in the outermost layer of the oxide also took place. While in the control samples the surface oxide consisted predominantly of chromium oxide (Fig. 4a), in the heat-treated implants ferum oxide was the dominant oxide (Fig. 4c). In general, it can be seen that there are differences in the oxide layers among the alloys in control nonheated samples with the highest oxide layer in the Ti-6Al-4V alloy (~60Å), followed by the Co-Cr and stainless steel alloys with thicknesses of about 15Å (Figs. 4–6).

The correlation between the Auger electron spectroscopic analysis of the surface chemical characteristics of the metals and the mechanical, biochemical, and histological results is complex. A further investigation of the surface chemical characteristics of the metal by more sophisticated methods like energy dispersive analysis of x-ray (EDAX), secondary ion mass spectrometry (SIMS), and the like may shed light on the molecular levels of the surface chemical changes by the heat treatment of the implants. The mechanism(s) by which the heat treatment of the implant induces the enhancement of bony ingrowth into it is not yet clearly understood. The course of tissue reaction, namely,

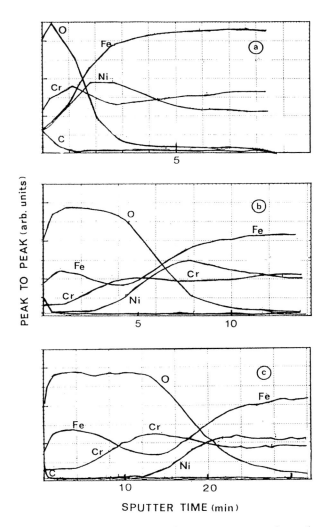

Figure 4 Scanning Auger electron spectroscopic peak-to-peak height/depth profiles of control and heat-treated stainless steel 316L implants: (a), control (autoclave) sample; (b), heat-treated (280°C, 20 min) implant; (c), heat-treated (550°C, 20 min) implant. Note a progressive increase in the thickness of the oxide layer in Fig. 4b and a further increase in Fig. 4c relative to the control sample. The oxide layer in autoclaved implants consists predominantly of chromium oxide, while in the heat-treated implants ferum oxide is the outermost oxide layer. The sputtering rate was approximately 5 Å /min.

osteoprogenitor cells, to the implants is a complex sequence of events that may be mediated by a variety of biochemical substances. These substances are, in turn, affected by the physicochemical interaction of the outermost layer of the metal with the molecules and cells in the adjacent milieu.

Indeed, it has been suggested previously that molecules of the extracellular matrix (proteoglycans) are the molecules in immediate contact with the metal oxide of the

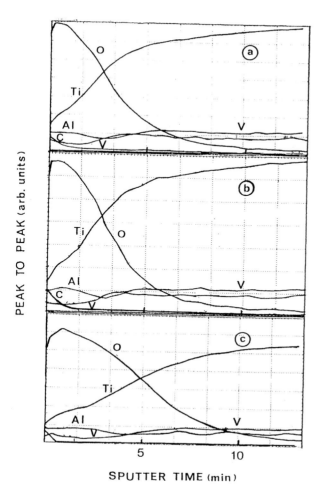

Figure 5 Scanning Auger electron spectroscopic peak-to-peak height/depth profiles of control and heat-treated Ti-6Al-4V implants: (a), control (as-it-is) sample; (b), autoclaved sample; (c), heat-treated (280°C, 180 min) implant. Note that there is no change in the oxide layer thickness when the control ("virgin") sample is heated by autoclaving. The sputtering rate was approximately 10 Å/min relative to the control sample.

implants and also associated with the collagen bundles next to the formed bone [Albrekts-son and Jacobsson 1987]. However, since it was found that the heat treatment does not change the morphologic (roughness) properties of the surface of the implants [Hazan 1991; also see above], it is postulated that this treatment alters the oxide layer characteris-tics (thickness, chemical nature, electric properties, etc.).

Thus, the alteration of the oxide layer characteristics (Figs. 4–6) may indeed be a significant factor that determines the final rate of bone apposition next to the implants. The fact that bony ingrowth to control, nonheated implants is significantly higher next to Ti-6Al-4V implants than to the stainless steel (Fig. 2) may also support the above con-

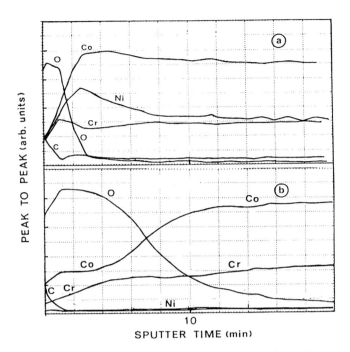

SPUTTER TIME (min)

Figure 6 Scanning Auger electron spectroscopic peak-to-peak height/depth profiles of control and heat-treated Co-Cr (Vitallium) implants: (a), control (autoclaved) sample; (b), heat-treated (280°C, 180 min) implant. Note increase in the oxide layer in the heat-treated sample as compared with the control sample. Note also the marked reduction of nickel oxide in the outer oxide layers in the heat-treated implants as compared with the control.

cept. Indeed, the thickness of the oxide layer of the nonheated Ti-6A1-4V alloy is higher than stainless steel; this may suggest that the thickness of the oxide layer in conjunction with other chemical properties of the outer layer of each alloy may play a significant role in determining the rate of bony ingrowth to a certain alloy. The general correlation between enhancement of bone growth and increase of the oxide layer in all three alloys tested (Figs, 2, 4–6; Table 2) corroborates the above hypothesis. However, the thickness of the oxide layer and its chemical characteristics have, most probably, some "optimality" in terms of enhancement of bone growth since a further increase in the oxide layer by heating to 550°C in stainless steel and Ti-6A1-4V alloy [Hazan, Brener, and Oron 1993] resulted in a decrease in bone growth to them.

The significance of the oxide layer in bone apposition next to metal implants has also been previously addressed by several authors. Sundgren, Bodg and Lundstrom (1986) found that calcium and phosphate were embedded in the oxide layer of the implants and that the oxidation process of the implants occurred for up to several years in titanium implants embedded in bone marrow in humans. Recent preliminary observations by Hanawa (1991) suggest that both cp-Ti and Ti-6A1-4V surface oxides can selectively adsorb phosphate and calcium ions from mixed ionic solutions, and that the crystallographic structures of the resultant calcium phosphate phases are different on the two oxides. Thus, chemical reactions at the surface of titanium-based metals may predispose to the accumulation of calcium-phosphate-enriched surfaces, but the structure of these

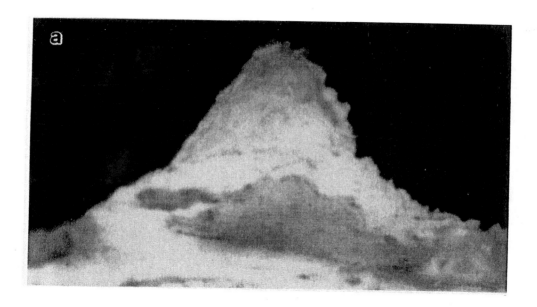

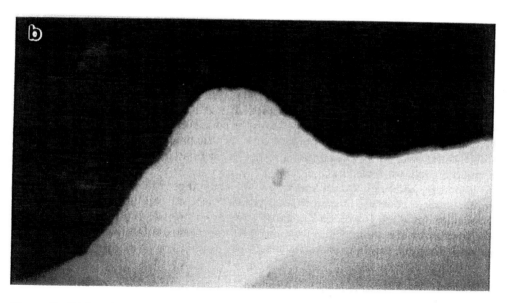

Figure 7 Light micrographs of longitudinal sections of control (a) and heat-treated (b, c) implants and the newly formed bone opposed to it at 35 days postinsertion to the femur. The sections were prepared from rats in which the heat-treated implants were inserted into one leg (femur) and the control implants were inserted to the contralateral leg. Rats were injected (intraperitoneally) with tetracycline (Ledramycine 25 mg/kg body weight) as a marker for calcification zone [Speer et al. 1991] one and four days before sacrifice. The tibias with the implants were fixed in Millonig's fixative for 24 h, embedded in Historesin, sectioned in the longitudinal midline, and viewed with a microscope with epilumination fluorescence [Bab et al. 1984]. Note the immature bone next to the nontreated implant (P) in Fig. 7a. In Figs. 7b and 7c, note the osseointegration with the heat-treated implants at 35 days postsurgery. In Fig. 7c, an osteocyte is located less than 10 μm from the metal zone (arrow) (C, compact bone; a, b, $\times$150; c $\times$350).

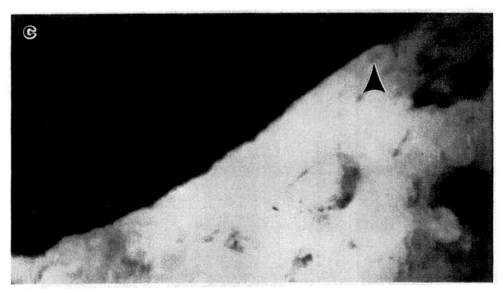

Figure 7   Continued.

phases may, in view of a calcium-phosphate-rich, cementlike interfacial tissue, provide subtle differences in the bony interface formed. It was recently shown by Wisbey et al. (1991) that heat treatment ($\sim 400\,^{\circ}C$) increases the corrosion resistance of titanium alloy. The possibility that this phenomenon may also affect the processes associated with osteoblast differentiation from osteoprogenitor cells and/or bone growth and maturation next to the implant cannot be ruled out.

In summary, although the enhancement of bony ingrowth to metal implants by altering the surface chemical characteristics may be a new concept in bone-metal interactions, considerable work is needed to characterize more precisely both the modification of metal oxides by the biological milieu and also the chemical interaction between the organic and inorganic components of the interfacial cement line of modified oxide layers.

Table 2   Specific Enzymatic (Unit/mg Protein) Activity of Alkaline Phosphatase in Tissue Extracts

Days past insertion or marrow ablation	Control implants	Specific activity (mean ± SEM)	
		Heat-treated implants	Sham-operated femur
5	4.1 ± 1.2	7.1[a] ± 0.6	9.2[a] ± 1.4
6	9.8 ± 2.1	16.5[a] ± 3.8	15.7[a] ± 4.1
7	4.2 ± 2.3	7.9[a] ± 1.3	5.0 ± 1.7

Each point is the mean ± SEM of 5–7 femurs.
[a]The level of statistical significance is $P < 0.05$ from control femurs.

VII. CONCLUDING REMARKS AND FUTURE RESEARCH

The primary interaction at the implant-tissue interface occurs within a distance of atomic dimensions from the implant surface. As time proceeds, the healing process commences and the nature of the biosystems surrounding the implant changes accordingly. New biological molecules appear and replace those originally adsorbed on the surface, and a new secondary reaction can be induced in the biological system that, in turn, may influence the structure of the tissue that is developing around the implant. Some tissue will eventually approach and may connect to the surface of the implant. The primary interaction at the interface itself, via a secondary reaction, thus influences the tissue development on the macroscopic scale.

Many questions may be asked in light of the results presented in this chapter (from the reviewed literature and our own studies). What makes the tissue respond differently to different materials? How do the chemical characteristics of the outermost layer of the implant at the molecular and atomic levels affect the sequence of events as detailed above and the final type of tissue next to the implant? These questions may currently require more theoretical answers, but the results of other studies as well as our own show a dramatic change in rate of bone growth to metal implants when surface chemical characteristics are changed. Thus, it may be postulated that the short time interval after implantation and the implant surface status (contamination, composition, etc.) prior to implantation may be of crucial importance for the long-term development of the implant-tissue interface.

It can be stated that, in the field of biomaterial-tissue interfaces, the molecular approach is still in its infancy. New, sophisticated methods of analyzing surface chemical characteristics should be used in the future in conjunction with molecular biological methods (*in vitro* and *in vivo*) to analyze the first few layers of molecules that adsorb on an implant surface and to ascertain their importance in the final bonding strength of the implant in the host tissue. Such studies could make a significant contribution to a better understanding of the bone-metal implant interaction.

REFERENCES

Albrektsson, T., and H. A. Hansson. 1986. An ultra-structural characterization of the interface between bone and sputtered titanium or stainless steel surface. *Biomaterials* 7:201–205.

Albrektsson, T., and M. Jakobsson. 1986. An ultra-structural characterization of the interface between bone and sputtered titanium or stainless steel surface. *Biomaterials* 7:201–205.

Albrektsson, T., and M. Jakobsson. 1987. Bone-metal interface in osseointegration. *J. Prosthet. Dent.* 57:597–607.

Albrektsson, T., and U. Lekholm. 1989. Osseointegration: Current state of art. *Dent. Clin. North Amer.* 33:537–554.

Albrektsson, T., and G. A. Zarba. 1993. Current interpretations of the osseointegrated response: Clinical significance. *Int. J. Prosthodont.* 6:95–105.

Anderson, R. C., C. D. Cook, A. M. Weinstein, and R. J. Haddad, Jr. 1984. An evaluation of skeletal attachment of LTI pyrolytic carbon, porous titanium, and carbon-coated porous titanium implants. *Clin. Orthop. Rel. Res.* 182:242–257.

Aspenberg, P., S. Goodman, S. Toksuig-Larsen, L. Ryd, and T. Albrektsson. 1992. Intermittent micromotion inhibits bone ingrowth. Titanium implants in rabbits. *Acta Orthop. Scand.* 63: 141–145.

Bab, I., B. A. Ashton, M. E. Owen, and A. Boyde. 1984. Incident light microscopy of surfaces of plastic embedded hard tissues. *J. Microscopy* 134:49–53.

Barth, E., C. Johannson, and T. Albrektsson. 1990. Histologic comparison of ceramic and titanium implants in cats. *Int. J. Oral Maxillofac. Implants* 5:227–231.

Berry, J. L., J. M. Geiger, J. M. Moran, J. S. Skraba, and A. S. Greenwald. 1986. Use of phosphate or electrical stimulation to enhance the bone-porous implant interface. *J. Biomed. Mater. Res.* 20:65–77.

Cameron, H. U., R. M. Pilliar, and I. McNab. 1973. The effect of movement on the bonding of porous metal to bone. *J. Biomed. Mater. Res.* 7:301–311.

Downes, S., D. J. Wood, A. J. Malcolm, and S. Y. Ali. 1990. Growth hormone in polymethylmethacrylate cement. *Clin. Orthop.* 252:294–298.

Galante, J. O., J. E. Lemons, M. Spector, P. D. Wilson, Jr., and T. M. Wright. 1991. The biological effects of implant materials. *J. Orthop. Res.* 9:760–775.

Gottlander, M., and T. Albrektsson. 1991. Histomorphometric studies of hydroxylapetite-coated and uncoated CP titanium threaded implants in bone. *Int. J. Oral. Maxillofac. Implants* 6: 399–404.

Gottlander, M., T. Albrektsson, and L. V. Carlsson. 1992. A histomorphometric study of unthreaded hydroxylapetite-coated and titanium-coated implants in rabbit bone. *Int. J. Oral. Maxillofac. Implants* 7:485–490.

Halstead, A., C. W. Jones, and R. D. Rawlings. 1979. A study of the reaction of human tissue to proplast. *J. Biomed. Mater. Res.* 13:121–134.

Hanawa, T. 1991. Titanium and its oxide film: Substrate for formation of apatite. In *The Bone-Biomaterial Interface*. J. E. Davis (ed.), University of Toronto Press, Toronto, pp. 49–61.

Hanker, J. S., and B. L. Giammara. 1988. Biomaterials and biomedical devices. *Science* 242:885–892.

Hazan, R. 1991. Regulatory mechanisms of bone growth to metal implant. Ph.D. thesis, Tel Aviv University.

Hazan, R., and U. Oron. 1990a. Differential rate of bone growth to titanium alloy and stainless steel implants. In *Interface in Medicine and Mechanics,-2*, K. R. Williams, A. Toni, J. Middleton, and G. Pallott, eds., Elsevier Applied Science, London, pp. 29–34.

Hazan, R., and U. Oron. 1990b. Enhancement of bony ingrowth to titanium and titanium alloy orthopaedic implants in experimental model in the rat. In *Interface in Medicine and Mechanics-2*, K. R. Williams, A. Toni, J. Middleton, and G. Pallott, eds., Elsevier Applied Science, London, pp. 35–42.

Hazan, R., and U. Oron. 1991. Bone growth around a metal implant inserted to the medullary canal: A new experimental model in the rat. *Clin. Mater.* 7:45–49.

Hazan, R., R. Brener, and U. Oron. 1993. Bone growth to metal implants is regulated by their surface chemical characteristics. *Biomaterials* 14:570–574.

Hazan, R., and U. Oron. 1993. Enhancement of bone growth to metal implants inserted to the medullary canal of the femur in rats. *J. Orthop. Res.* 11:655–663.

Heck, D. A., I. Nakajima, P. J. Kelly, and E. Y. Chao. 1986. The effect of load alteration on the biological and biomechanical performance of a titanium fiber-metal segmental prosthesis. *J. Bone Joint Surg.* 68-A:118–126.

Jasty, M., H. E. Rubash, G. Paiement, C. Bragdon, T. P. Harrigan, and W. H. Harris. 1986. Distribution of bone ingrowth into proximally coated, femoral porous canine total hip replacements. In *32nd Annual ORS*, New Orleans, Louisiana, 17–20.

Johansson, C. B., H. A. Hansson, and T. Albrektsson. 1990. Qualitative interfacial study between bone and titanium, niobium or commercially pure titanium. *Biomaterials* 11:277–280.

Johansson, C. B., and T. Albrektsson. 1991. A removal torque and histomorphometric study of commercially pure titanium and titanium implants in rabbit bone. *Clin. Oral Implants Res.* 2:24–29.

Johansson, C. B., L. Sennerby, and T. Albrektsson. 1991. A removal torque and histomorphometric study of bone tissue reactions to commercially pure titanium and Vitallium implants. *Int. J. Oral. Maxillofac. Implants* 6:437–441.

Kasemo, B. 1983. Biocompatability of titanium implants: Surface science aspects. *J. Prosthet. Dent.* 49:832–837.

Kasemo, B., and L. Lausmaa. 1986. Surface science aspects on inorganic biomaterials. *CRC Crit. Rev. Biocompa.* 2:335–380.

Kohavi, D., Z. Schwartz, D. Amir, C. M. Mai, U. Gross, and J. Sela. 1992. Effect of titanium implants on primary mineralization following 6 and 14 days of rat tibial healing. *Biomaterials* 13:255–260.

Lemons, J. E. 1988. Hydroxyapatite coatings. *Clin. Orthop. Rel. Res.* 235:220–223.

McKee, G. K. 1982. Total hip replacement — Past, present and future. *Biomaterials* 3:130–135.

McQueen, D., J. E. Sundgren, B. Ivarsson, I. Lundstrom, B. af-Ekenstam, A. Svensson, P. I. Branemark, and T. Albrektsson. 1982. Auger electron spectroscopic studies of titanium implants. In *Advances in Biomaterials*, Vol. 4, A. J. Lee, T. Albrektsson, and P. I. Branemark, eds., John Wiley and Sons, New York, p. 179.

Moreberg, P., and T. Albrektsson. 1991. Removal torque for bone-cement and titanium screws implanted in rabbits. *Acta Orthop. Scand.* 62:554–556.

Muller-Mai, C. M., C. Voigt, and U. Gross. 1990. Incorporation and degradation of hydroxyapatite implants of different surface roughness and surface structure in bone. *Scanning-Microsc.* 4:613–622.

Mulroy, R. D., and W. H. Harris. 1990. The effect of improved cementing techniques on component loosening in total hip replacement. An 11 year radiographic review. *J. Bone Joint Surg.* 72B:757–760.

Oonishi, H., M. Yamamoto, H. Ishimaru, E. Tsuji, S. Kushitani, M. Aono, and Y. Ukon. 1990. The effect of hydroxyapatite coating on bone growth into porous titanium alloy implants. *J. Bone Joint Surg.* 71-B:213–216.

Oonishi, H. 1991. Orthopaedic application of hydroxyapatite. *Biomaterials* 12:171–178.

Orr, R. D., J. D. de Bruijn, and J. R. Davies. 1992. Scanning electron microscopy of the bone interface with titanium, titanium alloy and hydroxyapatite. *Cell. Mater.* 2:241–251.

Parsegian, V. A. 1983. Molecular forces governing tight contact between cellular surfaces and substrates. *J. Prosthet. Dent.* 49:838–842.

Pilliar, R. M. 1987. Pourous-surface metallic implants for orthopedic applications. *J. Biomed. Mater. Res.* 21:1–33.

Pizzoferrato, A., G. Ciapetti, S. Stea, and A. Toni. 1991. Cellular events in the mechanism of prosthetic loosening. *Clin. Mater.* 7:51–81.

Reddi, A. H., and N. E. Sullivan. 1980. Matrix-induced endochondral bone differentiation: Influence of hypophysectomy, growth hormone and thyroid-stimulating hormone. *Endocrinology* 107:1291–1299.

Schutzer, S. F., M. Jasty, C. R. Bragdon, T. P. Harrigan, and W. H. Harris. 1990. A double-blind study on the effects of a capacitively coupled electrical field on bone ingrowth into porous-surfaced canine total hip prosthesis. *Clin. Orthop. Rel. Res.* 260:297–304.

Speer, K. P., L. D. Quarles, J.M. Harrelson, and J. A. Nunley. 1991. Tetracycline labelling of the femoral head following active intracapsular fracture of the femoral neck. *Clin. Orthop. Rel. Res.* 267:224–228.

Stulberg, B. N., J. T. Watson, S. D. Stulberg, T. W. Bauer, and M. T. Manley. 1991. A new model to assess tibial fixation. II. Concurrent histologic and biomechanical observations. *Clin. Orthop. Rel. Res.* 263:303–309.

Sumner, D. R., T. M. Turner, R. M. Urban, and J. O. Galante. 1986. Bone ingrowth into titanium fiber metal and bead surfaces in a total hip arthroplasty model. *32nd Annual ORS*, New Orleans, Louisiana, p. 342.

Sundgren, J. E., P. Bodo, and I. Lundstrom. 1986. Auger electron spectroscopic studies of the interface between human tissue and implants of titanium and stainless steel. *J. Coll. Inter. Sci.* 110:9–20.

Thomas, K. A., J. F. Kay, T. Cook, and S. D. Jarcho. 1987. The effect of surface macrotexture and hydroxyapatite coating on the mechanical strengths and histologic profiles of titanium implant materials. *J. Biomed. Mater. Res.* 21:1395–1414.

Turner, T. M., D. R. Sumner, R. M. Urban, D. P. Rivero, and J. O. Galante. 1986. A comparative study of porous coated in a weight-bearing total hip-arthroplasty model. *J. Bone Joint Surg.* 68A:1396–1409.

Williams, D. F. 1987. Review, tissue-biomaterial interactions. *J. Mater. Sci.* 22:3421–3445.

Wisbey, A., P. J. Gregson, L. M. Peter, and M. Tuke. 1991. Effect of surface treatment on the dissolution of titanium-based implant materials. *Biomaterials* 12:470–473.

17
Metals in Orthopedic Surgery

Ravi H. Shetty and Walter H. Ottersberg
Zimmer, Inc.
Warsaw, Indiana

I. INTRODUCTION

Implanted biomedical prosthetic devices are intended to perform safely, reliably, and effectively in the human body for prolonged periods of time. Stability under the imposition of repetitive loading in a hostile environment places unique demands on the materials, designs, and manufacturing methods used to create the implant. Materials used for orthopedic devices should possess good biocompatibility, adequate mechanical properties, and sufficient corrosion resistance, and be manufacturable at a reasonable cost. Metals, because of their unique properties, have found successful application in the field of orthopedics as prosthetic and fracture fixation devices.

In the text following, after a brief historical summary of the development of metals in the orthopedic field, the three major contemporary groups of metals used in the majority of orthopedic products—titanium and its alloys, cobalt-based alloys, and stainless steels are discussed. Additional information on specific materials may be obtained from the references cited in this article.

II. HISTORICAL BACKGROUND

The earliest written record of an application of metal in surgical procedures is from the year 1565 when Petronius recommended the use of gold plates for the repair of cleft palates. In 1666 Fabricius described the use of gold, bronze, and iron wires in surgical procedures. A variety of materials and designs were tried by Bell in 1804. In 1829 Levert made the first study of tissue tolerance to metals and concluded that platinum was the best-tolerated metal. In 1849 Malgaigne unsuccessfully attempted to overcome the problem of infection.

The last two decades of the 19th century heralded two developments in medical

509

science that significantly accelerated the progress of orthopedic surgery. Around 1883 Lister developed his antiseptic surgical techniques, sharply reducing the incidence of infection in open fracture reduction procedures. Closely following, around 1895, Roentgen's x-ray techniques allowed the surgeon to visualize fractured bones.

Visualization and antiseptic surgery—enabling the surgeon to perform safe, precise reductions of fractures—spurred the development of metal implants. Research into the tolerance of tissue to various materials began to make headway. In his investigations of plates, screws, bands, and wires in a variety of metals, Lambotte recommended the use of soft steel with nickel and gold plating. In 1908 Von Baeyer reported on cellular reaction to metals implanted in the environment of the human body. Many materials were tried, such as ivory plates, brass plates, and steel bands and screws. While such appliances frequently failed, their use met with a success sufficient for that era. It was ca. 1912 that Sherman, head of United States Steel's Medical Department, performed his landmark work. Following a series of procedures in which the bone plates fractured intraoperatively, it became obvious to Dr. Sherman that a better bone plate was needed. He enlisted the aid of U.S. Steel's metallurgical staff in the development of an improved material for bone plates. For the first time, surgeons and engineers joined forces in attacking the implant problem. This biomechanical partnership has continued to the present day, with spectacular benefit to the patient.

From this joint endeavor came the well-known Sherman, vanadium steel, bone plates, and screws. These appliances were such a dramatic improvement over what had been available that their use became widespread. They became a standard purchase item of the federal government and the Department of Commerce published commercial specification number CS-37-31 covering vanadium steel bone plates. Publication of a specification was another landmark in orthopedic surgery. It was the beginning of what has developed into a substantial number of government specifications covering a variety of implants and internal fixation devices.

While the mechanical problems appeared to have been solved, the problem of body compatibility continued. In 1913 Hey-Groves published a study on tissue tolerance to metals, recommending that implants be made of nickel-plated steel.

In 1914 Lane published his work on the "no-touch" technique, which became the foundation for subsequent orthopedic procedures. He demonstrated the need for exceptionally sterile practices when inserting metal into the human body. This marked a major milestone on the road to successful orthopedic surgery. In 1921 Stanley and Gatellier demonstrated the migration of metal ions from metal implants into the adjacent tissue.

In 1926, 18-8 stainless steel was brought to America from Germany. It generated immediate interest as an implant material since it was stronger than vanadium steel and had better biocompatibility. While this stainless steel's compatibility was far superior to vanadium steel, it still had some limitations when exposed to saline environments. In 1927 Strauss received a patent on 18-8 SMO stainless steel, which was essentially the 18-8 stainless with molybdenum. The symbol *SMO* on a device became the hallmark of the finest surgical implants.

In 1929 dental laboratories in the United States developed the cobalt-based alloys for dental appliances. Good performance of these alloys for this application resulted in their first use in orthopedic implants in 1936. Today the cobalt-based alloys are widely used in orthopedic surgery.

As work was carried on stainless steels, it became apparent that a further modification of 18-8 SMO stainless was desirable. In 1941 the National Research Council assigned a research project to C. R. Murray and C. G. Fink at Columbia University to determine the most desirable metal or alloy for the internal fixation of fractures. This study resulted in recommendation of type 302 and 316 stainless steels in 1943. Further research at several medical centers across the nation prompted the American College of Surgeons at its 1946 meeting to endorse 316 stainless steel for use in surgical implants.

In 1954 Jergesen reported on his investigation of titanium as an implant material. This is probably the latest development in the history of orthopedic materials. Today, titanium and its alloys are the most versatile metals available for use as surgical implants. They have superior biocompatibility, can be fabricated by a variety of methods, and have excellent mechanical properties.

In the 1960s the F-4 committee of the American Society for Testing of Materials (ASTM) was formed to standardize materials used in surgical implants. The ASTM F-4 committee is comprised of surgeons, manufacturers, and research personnel working together to develop and standardize the best possible surgical implants and materials. It was their efforts that resulted in the present availability of the wide variety of surgical implant materials.

III. METALS AND ALLOYS IN ORTHOPEDICS

A. Titanium and Titanium-Based Alloys

Titanium and titanium alloys are relatively new materials compared to stainless steels and cobalt-based alloys. Titanium metal was discovered in 1791 by Gregor and was named in 1795 by Kloproth. Titanium exhibited attractive physical, mechanical, and chemical properties that prompted interest in the extraction of the metal from its ores. The first successful extraction attempt was made in 1887 by Nilson and Patterson. Their product, however, was not very pure. In 1910 Hunter was able to produce 99.9% pure titanium on a laboratory scale. Titanium metal remained a laboratory curiosity for a considerable time until Kroll developed the technique of reducing titanium tetrachloride ($TiCl_4$) with metallic magnesium (Mg). The Kroll process has revolutionized titanium extraction technology and has become the major method of extracting sponge titanium from its ore.

As a result of large-scale production of titanium metal by the Kroll process, extensive efforts were made to develop new and improved alloys of this metal. Many alloys were developed, particularly for use in aerospace applications. Among these, the Ti–6Al–4V alloy was found to be the most versatile and has become the most widely used titanium alloy to date in both aerospace and other industries. The interest in this alloy as a potential orthopedic material began as early as 1957 when Zimmer initiated a project at the Armour Research Foundation of the Illinois Institute of Technology to evaluate the properties of several alloys for implant applications.

1. Types and Compositions of Titanium and Titanium-Based Alloys

Four grades of unalloyed titanium are used for implant applications, as shown in Table 1 [1]. These are classified according to their interstitial contents. The interstitial elements used in this classification are oxygen, nitrogen, and iron. Among these interstitials, oxygen has the greatest influence on strength and ductility of the metal.

Among titanium alloys, Ti–6Al–4V alloy has been widely used in the manufacture of orthopaedic implants. Its chemical composition is given in Table 2 [2]. Three other alloys used to a lesser extent in orthopaedic implant applications are Ti–3Al–2.5V, Ti–5Al–2.5Fe, and Ti–6Al–7Nb alloys.

Table 1   Chemical Compositions of Commercially Pure Titanium

	Composition, wt%			
Element	Grade 1	Grade 2	Grade 3	Grade 4
Nitrogen, max	0.03	0.03	0.05	0.05
Carbon, max	0.10	0.10	0.10	0.10
Hydrogen, max	0.015	0.015	0.015	0.015
Iron, max	0.20	0.30	0.30	0.50
Oxygen, max	0.18	0.25	0.35	0.40
Titanium	Balance	Balance	Balance	Balance

2.   Structure and Properties of Titanium and Titanium-Based Alloys

At room temperature, titanium exists as a hexagonal close-packed (HCP) crystal structure. When heated above 883°C, it transforms to a body-centered cubic (BCC) crystal. The HCP structure is called *alpha* (α) titanium and the BCC structure is called the *beta* (β) phase.

The addition of aluminum to titanium stabilizes the α-phase and addition of vanadium stabilizes the β-phase. The relative amounts of these two phases and their phase morphology in the alloy are usually governed by alloy chemistry and thermomechanical treatments.

The effect of temperature and the percentage of alloying elements on α- and, β-phase stabilization is illustrated by the schematic phase diagram in Fig. 1 indicating the wide range of alloys possible with different physical and mechanical properties. These alloys are classified primarily on the basis of the phases present, such as α-alloys, β-alloys, and ($\alpha + \beta$)-alloys. Ti–6Al–4V alloy is an ($\alpha + \beta$)-alloy.

Ti–6Al–4V alloy is generally used in one of three conditions: wrought, forged, or cast.

Wrought Alloy.   Wrought alloy is available in standard shapes and sizes from the metal producer or fabricator and mill annealed at 730°C for 1 to 4 h, furnace cooled to 600°C, and then air cooled to room temperature. Mill annealing generally produces a fine-grained equiaxed ($\alpha + \beta$) microstructure (Fig. 2). The volume fraction of the β-

Table 2   Chemical Composition of ELI-Grade Ti–6Al–4V Alloy

Element	Composition, wt%
Nitrogen, max	0.05
Carbon, max	0.08
Hydrogen, max	0.012
Iron, max	0.25
Oxygen, max	0.13
Aluminum	5.50–6.50
Vanadium	3.50–4.50
Titanium	Balance

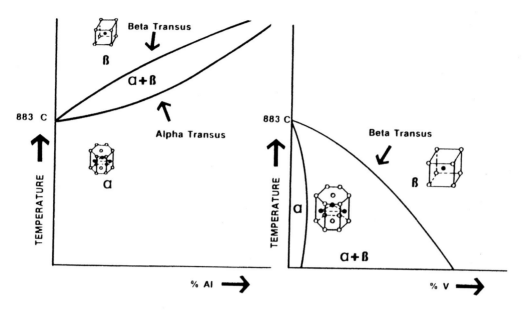

Figure 1 Typical phase diagrams for α-stabilized (with Al) and β-stabilized (with V) titanium systems.

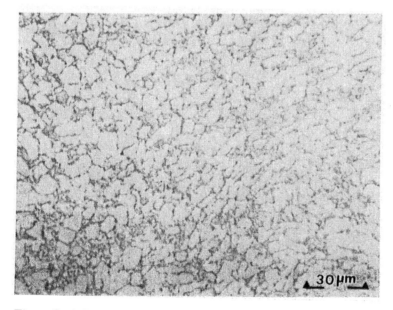

Figure 2 Mill-annealed Ti–6Al–4V alloy microstructure.

phase depends on the composition of the alloy and the annealing temperature. In alloys containing a high percentage of Al, furnace cooling causes the precipitation of Ti$_3$Al (α_2) in the α-phase. The α_2-phase is generally not resolvable by optical microscopy.

Forged Alloy.   Ti–6Al–4V alloy is usually hot-forged at temperatures where both α- and β-phases are stable. The typical hot-forging temperature is between 900° and 980°C. Hot forging produces a fine-grained α-structure with a dispersion of very fine β-phase, as shown in the accompanying photomicrograph (Fig. 3). A final annealing treatment is often given to the alloy to obtain a stable microstructure without significantly altering the properties of the alloy.

Cast Alloy.   The investment-casting method has been widely used to produce complex titanium shapes [3]. Difficulties arise when casting this alloy since titanium readily reacts with its environment, including the container used for holding the liquid metal. Once these difficulties are overcome and castings are produced, a somewhat different microstructure from that described in the previous section is formed upon cooling. Because the β-phase is the stable solid phase immediately after the metal solidifies, the ($\alpha + \beta$) structure observed at room temperature is the result of a transformation of β-phase to the duplex ($\alpha + \beta$) structure. As the solid material cools below the β-transformation temperature, transformation occurs by nucleation and growth process. Alpha particles are nucleated at the β-grain boundaries and along certain nucleation-preferred crystallographic orientations. As cooling continues, these α-particles grow into a needle-like, or "acicular," shape.

To provide a metallurgically stable, homogeneous structure, castings are annealed at approximately 840°C. This treatment also provides a means whereby stresses introduced during solidification of the castings are relieved. The typical cast and annealed Ti–6Al–

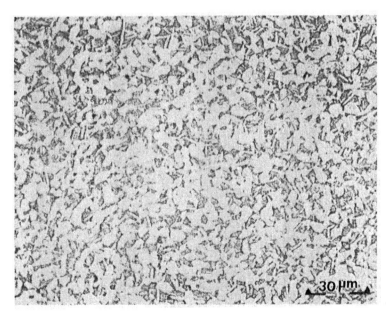

Figure 3   Forged and annealed Ti–6Al–4V alloy showing a fine-grained α-matrix with a fine dispersion of intergranular β-phase.

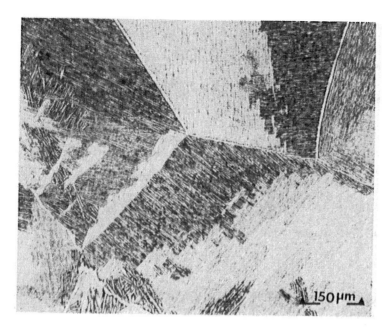

Figure 4 Typical cast and annealed Ti--6Al-4V alloy microstructure.

4V alloy microstructure is shown in Fig. 4. Cast Ti-6Al-4V alloy has slightly lower values for mechanical properties than the wrought alloy. This may be attributed to the nature of the $\alpha + \beta$ duplex structure in cast Ti-6Al-4V. All Ti-6Al-4V castings are hot isostatic pressed (HIPed) to ensure structural integrity.

3. Properties of Titanium and Titanium Alloys

Tensile Properties.   The tensile properties of commercially pure (CP) titanium and Ti-6Al-4V alloy are given in Tables 3 and 4. The modulus of elasticity of these materials is around 16×10^6 psi, which is one half the value of cobalt-based alloys and stainless steels. From Table 3 it is clear that higher impurity content in CP titanium leads to higher strength and lower ductility. The yield and ultimate tensile strengths of Ti-6Al-4V alloy are substantially higher than that of commercially pure titanium.

Table 3   Tensile Properties of CP Titanium[a]

Grade	Hardness	Tensile properties[b]		
		YS (ksi)	UTS (ksi)	Percent elongation
Grade 1	R_B70-87	25.0	35.0	24.0
Grade 2	R_B88-92	40.0	50.0	20.0
Grade 3	R_B95-99	55.0	65.0	18.0
Grade 4	R_C23-29	70.0	80.0	15.0

[a]Minimum properties
[b]YS, yield strength; UTS, ultimate tensile strength

Table 4 Tensile Properties of Ti–6Al–4V Alloy[a]

| Alloy condition | Tensile properties[b] | | |
	YS (ksi)	UTS (ksi)	Percent elongation
Wrought			
Mill anneal (MA)	120.0	130.0	15.0
Solution treating			
and aging (STA)	140.0	150.0	10.0
Cast[c]			
Mill anneal	110.0	120.0	10.0
HIPing and mill anneal	115.0	125.0	12.0

[a]Typical properties
[b]YS, yield strength; UTS, ultimate tensile strength
[c]Approximate values

Fatigue Properties. Fatigue properties are of critical importance in implant applications, particularly those applications in which the implant will be subjected to cyclic loading. Fatigue fracture is defined as progressive fracture of a part under repeated cyclical or fluctuating loads. Cyclic stress can cause failure at a significantly lower level of stress than required to cause failure in static loading as measured by tensile testing. The actual microscopic process by which fatigue fracture occurs is primarily of theoretical interest. However, the fatigue strength of a material is definitely an important characteristic of the material. Table 5 summarizes the fatigue properties of CP- titanium and Ti–6Al–4V alloy under the most severe test condition with fully reversed stress ($R = -1$).

Corrosion Properties. Titanium is one of the most corrosion resistant engineering materials available today. Very low levels of corrosion are observed in near-neutral pH solutions,

Table 5 Fatigue Properties of CP Titanium and ELI-Grade Ti–6Al–4V Alloy[a]

Metal or alloy type	Condition	Fatigue limit at 10^7 cycles and $R = -1$ (ksi)
CP titanium	Grade 1	18.0[b]
	Grade 2	28.0[b]
	Grade 3	39.0[b]
	Grade 4	49.0[b]
Ti–6Al–4V alloy	Wrought	
	Mill anneal (MA)	80
	Solution treating and aging (STA)	90[b]
	Cast[b]	
	Mill anneal	70.0
	HIPing and mill anneal	75.0

[a]Typical properties
[b]Approximate values

especially those containing chloride ions. Titanium derives its resistance to corrosion from the formation of a thin, adherent, solid oxide film that passivates the material [4].

Wear Properties.   The wear properties of titanium are important to the long-term success of titanium implants. The significance of titanium wear resistance was recognized early by researchers in this field [5]. Malkin [6] reported that the higher coefficient of friction resulting from fretting fatigue at moderate levels of contact stresses could lead to increased wear and loosening of total joint prostheses.

Initial research into the wear behavior of Ti–6Al–4V/polyethylene wear couples raised questions concerning this material combination when used in total joint replacements [7–9]. More recent experiments have, however, demonstrated the efficacy of Ti–6Al–4V/polyethylene wear couples. Miller et al. [10] first reported that properly polished and passivated Ti–6Al–4V produced slightly lower wear rates when coupled with ultrahigh molecular weight polyethylene (UHMWPE) than either stainless steel or cobalt–chromium–molybdenum alloy. These findings were substantiated by McKellop et al. [11]. McKellop's pin-on-disk experiments showed that the wear rates of UHMWPE against Ti–6Al–4V were slightly lower than those of stainless steel.

Clarke et al. [12] examined the abrasive wear characteristics of the Ti–6Al–4V/UHMWPE wear couple. These tests were performed on a hip simulator using bovine serum as a lubricant. Tests were run with and without acrylic bone cement particles present in the serum. There was no abnormal wear of the metallic component under either condition. Acrylic bone cement particles were found embedded in the UHMWPE cup. These results indicated that Ti–6Al–4V alloy performed satisfactorily under laboratory conditions when compared with 316L stainless steel or cobalt–chromium–molybdenum alloy.

Rostoker and Galante [13] found that with proper surface treatment (i.e., surface passivation), titanium alloy may be successfully used for prosthetic joints with wear rates as low as 316L stainless steel or cobalt–chromium–molybdenum alloy. In recent years, several surface-hardening processes have been developed to improve wear properties of titanium alloys. Among them, nitrogen ion implantation [14,15] and the Ti-Nidium™ [16,17] surface hardening processes have been successfully used on titanium alloy implants with significant benefits.

Biocompatibility.   The biocompatibility of titanium and titanium alloys has been documented for over 40 years [18]. In 1940 Bothe, Beaton, and Davenport [19] reported that unalloyed titanium samples implanted in cat femora were equally as well tolerated as Co–Cr alloy and stainless steel implants.

Leventhal [20] implanted titanium bars subcutaneously in rabbits and titanium screws in rat femora, and left the bars and screws for various periods of time up to 16 weeks. No infection of the tissue surrounding the implant was seen. From this study, he concluded that titanium is an ideal metal for fracture fixation devices.

In animal studies, porous as well as nonporous titanium implants in bone tissue showed excellent biocompatibility in all cases [21–25]. All investigators reported that undesirable fibrous encapsulation of the implants was minimal to nonexistent.

In 1967 Laing, Ferguson, and Hodge [26] performed biocompatibility studies using accepted and unaccepted implant materials. Biocompatibility was ascertained by a histological measurement of membrane thickness around each implanted material. Tissue reaction to titanium and titanium alloy implants was remarkable for the consistently thin pseudomembrane and minimal fibrosis around the implants.

Niles [27] implanted porous Ti–6Al–4V void metal composites (VMC) in goat femora to investigate the possible use of this material in knee prosthesis fixation. Evaluations were made biomechanically and histologically at 6 weeks and 5 months. Implant acceptance was indicated by the lack of inflammatory response, fibrous encapsulation sheath, and bone resorption. He concluded that readily identifiable new bone structure, strong fixation, and excellent biocompatibility were typical. Some subarticular implants in joints appeared to induce normal hyaline cartilage overgrowth.

Autian [28] evaluated acute toxicity of Ti–6Al–4V alloy in rabbits and compared results with standard control substances. His study concluded that Ti–6Al–4V alloy is noncytotoxic and can be used safely as an implant material.

Raab et al. [29] made a comparative study of the surface degradation of different orthopaedic alloys at bone cement–implant interfaces and concluded that Ti–6Al–4V alloy is least sensitive to surface degradation when compared to either 316L stainless steel or Co–Cr–Mo alloy. This may be a critical factor in establishing the superiority of Ti–6Al–4V alloy over other orthopaedic alloys.

4. Manufacturability

The availability of Ti–6Al–4V is an important consideration in its widespread use as a surgical implant material. This titanium alloy is a common one utilized by numerous other industries that require its outstanding properties for their applications. The aerospace industry, the largest user of the alloy, has created a large enough demand for the material that titanium alloy manufacturers can justify producing substantial quantities of Ti–6Al–4V to supply sufficient alloy for orthopedic applications as well.

Titanium alloy producers commonly provide required mill shapes in the annealed condition. The alloy in the stable, annealed condition is machineable and requires no additional thermal treatment after fabrication of finished products from the raw material. The alloy may also be forged. This type of treatment imparts optimum values to all mechanical and physical properties of the alloy. The alloy may be fabricated by many other commonly practiced manufacturing techniques into finished products. It may be polished to a high luster or may be finished to a satin sheen. Regardless of its surface condition, Ti–6Al–4V alloy maintains its outstanding corrosion resistance.

Ti–6Al–4V alloy may also be cast. Although there are technical difficulties concerning the casting technology of the alloy, the significant point to be considered here is that even if the alloy is cast, it is identical in composition to the so-called wrought, annealed, or forged Ti–6Al–4V alloy.

There are slight differences in some of the mechanical properties of each, depending on manufacturing methods. Machining operations on the alloy must be performed with proper and specific manufacturing tools and equipment. The alloy requires a very sharp cutting implement and the appropriate feed rate for the removal of stock. When the alloy is shaped with the use of an abrasive grinding disk, precautions must be taken that sparks generated do not create a fire hazard. Frequently, in the titanium industry, sparks or other small debris from manufacturing operations are collected in a wet container. Very finely dispersed alloy particles, such as grinding particles, may ignite and burn with an intense flame. However, there is no danger whatsoever of the bulk material igniting.

Porous Coatings for Implant Fixation by Bony Ingrowth. Orthopedic devices have traditionally been implanted using bone cement (polymethylmethacrylate—PMMA). The fixation afforded by bone cement is primarily mechanical in nature. The cement locks into small surface irregularities on the implant and in the interstices of cancellous bone.

In many cases there is little adhesive bond between an implant and bone cement. The failure of the implant–bone cement interface has continued to be a problem.

Porous coated implants [30] offer promise for alleviating bone–cement interface problems. The porous coatings without bone cement can provide implant fixation via bony ingrowth [22].

Sintered metal beads, plasma flame sprayed metal powders, and diffusion bonded fiber metal pads are examples of porous surfaces being applied to orthopedic implants.

Sintered-Bead Surfaces. Porous surfaces composed of uniform, spherical beads generally have a consistently organized arrangement of pores due to the orderly manner in which the beads tend to pack together. Pore size is a function of, and approximately one third of, the bead diameter. The shape of the pores is dictated by how the beads pack together and the necking that occurs between the beads as a result of the sintering process.

Porous beaded surfaces can be manufactured by attaching two to three layers of beads to a metallic substrate using a suitable binder and then subjecting this composite structure to temperatures that are 90–95% of the melting point of the substrate. At these temperatures, the binder is vaporized and the beads become sintered to each other and the substrate. Ti–6Al–4V alloy and CP titanium are generally used for beaded titanium surfaces (Fig. 5).

Plasma Flame Spraying. Plasma flame sprayed surfaces are typically irregular and rough in appearance. The size and distribution of pores in a plasma-sprayed surface are more random than in sintered bead surfaces. The fused metal powder particles that compose this surface create interconnected peaks and valleys on the substrate surface. Plasma-sprayed porous surfaces have an inherent advantage over beaded surfaces because plasma flame spraying is a highly versatile manufacturing process, capable of applying a porous coating to substrates of complex geometry.

Plasma flame spraying uses an electric arc to ionize gas, turning it into a high-temperature plasma. Metal powder is introduced to this plasma and ejected at high speed in a molten state onto the substrate. The plasma-sprayed coating initially bonds to the substrate by mechanical interlocking. A subsequent sintering operation ensures a metallurgical bond between particles and substrate. The porosity and pore size of such coatings varies with the thickness of the coating. For a typical coating thickness of 500 to 800 μm, the peak-to-valley distances of the surface are in the range of 200 to 400 μm, while the

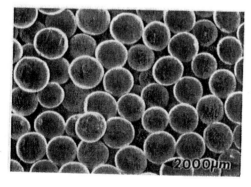

Figure 5 Titanium-beaded surface.

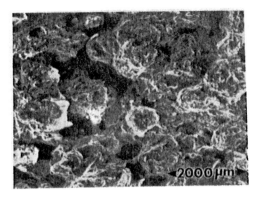

Figure 6   Plasma flame sprayed titanium surface.

pore size ranges from 20 to 200 μm. Variation in the surface porosity from 25% to 50% is to be expected from the nature of the process (Fig. 6).

Titanium Fiber Metal Pads.   The complex appearance of porous titanium fiber metal pads makes them distinctly different from other types of porous surfaces (Fig. 7). The surface pores are highly convoluted and interconnected within the pad, and are randomly arranged. A certain degree of linearity is lent to this porous structure because of its fibrous nature.

Porous titanium fiber metal pads are created by the compaction and diffusion bonding of randomly oriented titanium wires. The diffusion bonding is done much below the melting temperature of the substrate material. The porosity of the pad can be tailored by controlling parameters during the compaction process. A typical pad provides 50% porosity and the pore size is variable, with a typical average value of 400 μm.

5. Product Applications

Titanium and titanium alloys are used in the manufacture of a variety of orthopedic implants, as described in Table 6. Photographs of Ti–6Al–4V alloy hip and knee implants are presented in Figs. 8 and 9, respectively.

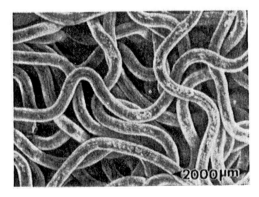

Figure 7   Fiber metal bonded titanium surface.

Table 6 Titanium Implants

Titanium and titanium alloys	Typical applications
CP titanium	Porous coated devices; suture wire
Ti–6Al–4V alloy	Hip stems, knees, shoulder joint, elbow joint, and fracture fixation devices such as I/M nail, hip screws, bone plates, bone screws
Ti–3Al–2.5V alloy	Fracture fixation devices
Ti–6Al–7Nb alloy	Hip and knee joints

B. Cobalt-Based Alloys

The initial medical use of cobalt-based alloys was in the manufacture of dental castings. An excellent resistance of this material to degradation in the oral environment attracted the attention of orthopedic surgeons. Consequently, the material was evaluated for use in the body and found to have good compatibility. It was, however, an extremely difficult material to fabricate and for this reason its use was limited. Continuing work led to the development of specialized casting methods. Today cobalt-based alloys are in general orthopedic use.

1. Types and Composition of Cobalt-Based Alloys

The Co–Cr–Mo alloys are widely used in the manufacture of orthopedic implants. Two basic compositions of Co–Cr–Mo alloy fall within ASTM F-75 [31] and ASTM F-799 [32] specifications. These are: (1) Co–Cr–Mo alloy strengthened by carbides and (2) Co–Cr–Mo alloy strengthened by the addition of nitrogen. Typical compositions of these alloys are given in Tables 7 and 8. In addition to these alloys, wrought Co–Cr–W–Ni [33] and Co–Ni–Cr–Mo [34] alloys are used in orthopaedic surgery to a lesser extent. The chemical compositions of these alloys are given in Tables 9 and 10, respectively.

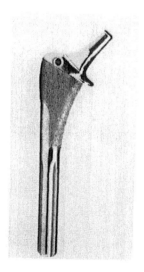

Figure 8 A porous coated Ti–6Al–4V alloy hip stem.

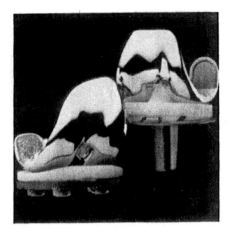

Figure 9 Porous coated Ti–6Al–4V alloy femoral and tibial components of a total knee system. Also seen in the picture are UHMWPE tibial inserts for articulation.

2. Structure of Cobalt-Based Alloys

Cobalt forms solid solutions with chromium and molybdenum. The cobalt-based alloys generally contain about 30 wt% of chromium and around 7 wt% of molybdenum. These alloys are used in one of three conditions: cast, wrought, or forged.

Cast Alloy. All Co–Cr alloy castings used in orthopedic implants are fabricated by investment casting [35,36]. In the investment-casting process, a wax model of the implant is made and a ceramic shell is built around the wax model. When wax is melted away, the ceramic mold has the shape of the implant. The ceramic shell is hot fired to obtain the required mold strength. Molten metal is then poured into the shell, the shell and metal are allowed to cool, and the shell is removed to reveal a solid metal implant. Because the metal part can be cast very close to the final shape, relatively little machining or polishing is required to complete the fabrication.

Table 7 Chemical Composition of Cast Co–Cr–Mo Alloy

Element	Composition, wt%	
	min	max
Chromium	27.0	30.00
Molybdenum	5.0	7.00
Nickel	—	1.00
Iron	—	0.75
Carbon	—	0.35
Silicon	—	1.00
Manganese	—	1.00
Cobalt	Balance	Balance

Table 8   Chemical Composition of Wrought
Co–Cr–Mo Alloy

Element	Composition, wt%	
	min	max
Chromium	26.0	30.00
Molybdenum	5	7
Nickel	—	1.0
Iron	—	0.75
Carbon	—	0.35
Silicon	—	1.0
Manganese	—	1.0
Nitrogen	—	0.25
Cobalt	Balance	Balance

The casting process produces large grains and metallurgical imperfections in the castings. Due to the presence of these metallurgical imperfections and large grains, castings exhibit lower mechanical properties than wrought alloys and forgings.

In the as-cast condition, Co–Cr–Mo alloy exhibits a microstructure consisting of $M_{23}C_6$ interdendritic primary carbides in a matrix of Co–Cr–Mo face-centered cubic (FCC) solid solution (Fig. 10). The size and distribution of these primary carbides are a function of alloy carbon content, metal pouring temperature, section thickness, and mold preheat temperature. Castings produced by this method exhibit adequate strength, good corrosion properties, and excellent wear resistance for implant applications. The mechanical properties of cast Co–Cr can be improved by hot isostatic pressing (HIPing). HIPing, in general, does produce some improvement in the mechanical properties of castings. Cast Co–Cr alloy can also be heat treated to improve its chemical homogeneity and mechanical properties. Heat treatment provides only limited benefit to the casting.

Table 9   Chemical Composition of Wrought
Co–Cr–W–Ni (L-605) Alloy

Element	Composition, wt%	
	min	max
Carbon	0.05	0.15
Manganese	1.00	2.00
Silicon	—	0.40
Phosphorus	—	0.040
Sulfur	—	0.030
Chromium	19.00	21.00
Nickel	9.00	11.00
Tungsten	14.00	16.00
Iron	—	3.00
Cobalt	Balance	Balance

Table 10   Chemical Composition of Wrought
Co–Ni–Cr–Mo (MP-35N) Alloy

	Composition, wt%	
Element	min	max
Carbon	–	0.025
Manganese	–	0.15
Silicon	–	0.15
Phosphorus	–	0.015
Sulfur	–	0.010
Chromium	19.0	21.0
Nickel	33.0	37.0
Molybdenum	9.0	10.5
Iron	–	1.0
Titanium	–	1.0
Cobalt	Balance	Balance

Wrought Alloy.   The wrought alloy possesses a uniform single-phase microstructure with fine grains. Wrought Co–Cr–Mo alloy (HS21) can be further strengthened by cold work. The other two wrought Co–Cr alloys, namely L-605 (HS25) and MP-35N, can also be strengthened by cold work as well as precipitation hardening heat treatment.

Forging.   The Co–Cr forging is produced from a hot forging process. In the mid-1970s, it was discovered that it was possible to hot forge Co–Cr–Mo alloy with almost the exact

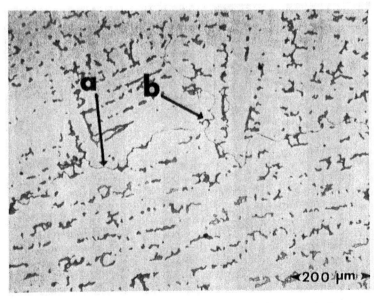

Figure 10   Microstructure of cast Co–Cr–Mo alloy. Grain boundary and carbide are shown by arrows (a) and (b), respectively.

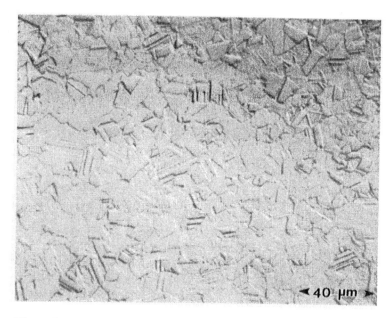

Figure 11 Forged Co–Cr–Mo alloy microstructure.

chemical composition as the cast alloy [37] A low-carbon version of ASTM F-75 is used in forging. In addition to lower carbon content in the alloy (usually 0.05 wt% or lower), the alloy contains chromium content of 26.0 to 30.0 wt% as compared to 27.0 to 30.0 wt% for ASTM F-75 alloy. Furthermore, a small quantity of nitrogen (0.25 wt% maximum) is added to the alloy to improve its strength and corrosion resistance. This new alloy in a thermomechanically processed condition (Fig. 11), is designated as ASTM F-799. The forging of Co–Cr–Mo alloy requires a sophisticated press and complicated tooling. These factors make it more expensive to fabricate a device from a Co–Cr–Mo forging than from a casting.

3. Properties of Cobalt-Based Alloys

Tensile Properties. The tensile properties of Co–Cr alloys are evaluated using a standard tensile test method. Material properties such as yield strength, ultimate tensile strength, Young's modulus, and percentage elongation are calculated using these test data. The mechanical properties of cobalt-based alloys are summarized in Tables 11 through 14.

Table 11 Tensile Properties of Cast Co–Cr–Mo Alloy

Alloy condition	Tensile properties[a,b]		
	YS (ksi)	UTS (ksi)	Percent elongation
As-cast	75.0	105.0	10.0

[a]Typical properties
[b]YS, yield strength; UTS, ultimate tensile strength

Table 12   Tensile Properties of High-Strength Co–Cr–Mo Alloy

| Alloy condition | Tensile properties[a,b] | | |
	YS (ksi)	UTS (ksi)	Percent elongation
Hot-forged	130.0	180.0	14.0

[a]Typical properties
[b]YS, yield strength; UTS, ultimate tensile strength

Fatigue Properties.   The fatigue strength of the alloy is evaluated using a standard fatigue test. The most common form of data generated in fatigue testing is the so-called S–N curve. In most materials, the S–N curve does not become truly constant at a stress value. In these cases, a certain number of cycles, usually 10 million, is arbitrarily selected as the test limit. The maximum stress a material will endure without fracture for this given number of cycles is known as the *endurance limit, fatigue limit*, or *fatigue strength* of the material. The typical fatigue strengths of Co-based alloys are given in Table 15.

Corrosion Properties.   The corrosion resistance of Co-based alloys is evaluated using *in vitro* and *in vivo* test methods [4]. *In vitro* tests include short-term electrochemical, and long-term immersion testing. *In vivo* corrosion testing is conducted in laboratory animals. Laboratory corrosion test data and clinical information indicate that Co-based alloys possess adequate corrosion resistance in the body environment.

Wear Properties.   Wear is a deterioration of an implant surface due to removal of material caused by relative motion between the implant surface and a contacting surface. Therefore, wear properties of an implant alloy are very important to the success of total hip and knee joint replacements.

   The wear properties of cobalt-based alloys are evaluated using a pin-on-disk wear tester and hip and knee simulators [38]. Laboratory test data and clinical experience indicate that cobalt-based alloys possess adequate wear resistance for orthopaedic applications.

Biocompatibility.   Biocompatibility is the first important test the material must successfully undergo before it can become an implant material. Various *in vitro* and *in vivo* tests

Table 13   Tensile Properties of L-605

| Alloy condition | Tensile properties[a,b] | | |
	YS (ksi)	UTS (ksi)	Percent elongation
Annealed or solution treated[a]	66.0	139.0	60.0
Solution-treated + 10% CW[c]	103.0	147.0	44.0
Solution-treated + 15% CW[c]	122.0	158.0	28.0
Solution-treated + 20% CW[c]	138.0	174.0	18.0

[a]Typical properties
[b]YS, yield strength; UTS, ultimate tensile strength
[c]Approximate value

Table 14 Tensile Properties of MP-35N

Alloy condition	Hardness	Tensile properties [a,b]		
		YS (ksi)	UTS (ksi)	Percent elongation
Annealed	R_B90–100	60.0	135.0	70.0
40% CW + aged	R_c40–45	240.0	270.0	10.0

[a]Typical properties
[b]YS, yield strength; UTS, ultimate tensile strength

have indicated that Co–Cr–Mo, Co–Cr–Ni–W, Co–Ni–Cr–Mo are biocompatible and are suitable for use as surgical implants [4,39]. The long-term effects of metal ions on the body are not known and more studies are required to shed light on this subject.

4. Manufacturability

The high-carbon version of Co–Cr–Mo alloy (ASTM F-75) can be investment cast. This manufacturing method allows considerable freedom in implant design and its flexibility has been an important factor in the widespread application of the alloy for orthopedic implants.

The low-carbon version of Co–Cr–Mo alloy (ASTM F-799) can be machined or forged from wrought Co–Cr–Mo alloy. The devices manufactured from wrought alloy possess much higher strength properties than cast alloy. Therefore, forged Co–Cr–Mo alloy implants are extensively used in orthopedics for high-strength applications. Similarly, wrought Co–Cr–Ni–W and Co–Ni–Cr–Mo alloys can also be machined or forged similar to wrought Co–Cr–Mo alloy.

Porous Coatings for Implant Fixation by Bony Ingrowth. Like titanium implants, porous coated Co–Cr implants have been extensively used for bony ingrowth application [30]. The techniques used to apply porous coatings to orthopedic implants can have a dramatic effect on the microstructure and properties of the implants.

Table 15 Fatigue Properties of Cast Co–Cr–Mo Alloy, High-Strength Forged Co–Cr–Mo Alloy, L-605 and MP-35N

Material	Fatigue limit [a] at 10^7 cycles and $R = -1$ (ksi)
1. Cast Co–Cr–Mo Alloy	40.0
2. High-strength forged Co–Cr–Mo alloy	110.0
3. L-605	
Annealed or solution treated	30.0
Solution treated + 10% CW	46.0
Solution treated + 15% CW	55.0
Solution treated + 20% CW	62.0
4. MP-35N	
Annealed	27.0
40% CW + aged	108.0

[a]Approximate values

Sintered beads, plasma flame sprayed metal powders, and diffusion bonded fiber metal pads are different types of coatings used on Co–Cr orthopedic implants.

Sintered Beaded Surfaces.   Spherical beads of Co–Cr are gravity sintered onto Co–Cr implants to obtain porous coated implants. Gravity sintering is carried out at temperatures that approach the melting point of the implant, typically at 90–95% of the implant melting point.

Exposing fine-grained forged or wrought Co–Cr–Mo alloy to temperatures reaching 90–95% of its melting point, as required in gravity sintering, results in grain growth and microstructural modifications. Since exposure to gravity-sintering conditions transforms fine-grained structures into structures having the grain size of cast material, forged implants are generally not used as substrates for porous coating. Most gravity-sintered Co–Cr–Mo implants are investment-cast devices. The effect of high sintering temperatures on cast Co–Cr–Mo is rather different. Cast Co–Cr–Mo already exhibits a coarse grain structure, so grain growth during sintering is not a major problem for this material. Cast Co–Cr–Mo contains chromium carbide second-phase particles, however, which have a different chemical composition than the bulk material. This chemical inhomogeneity is important in sintering because local inhomogeneities exhibit lower melting points than the bulk material. It is not unusual, therefore, to observe melted areas in cast Co–Cr–Mo implants with sintered bead coatings (Fig. 12). This effect is known as *incipient melting*. The extent of incipient melting in such implants depends on variables such as casting quality and sintering temperature control. Incipient melting can occur anywhere on the implant. The presence of incipient melting on Co–Cr coatings will lower the fatigue strength of the implants.

Plasma Spray Coating.   Co–Cr–Mo alloy can be plasma sprayed similar to CP titanium and Ti–6Al–4V alloy. The porosity of the coating varies with the thickness of the coating, and pore sizes in the range 20–200 μm can be obtained from the process.

Co–Cr Fiber Metal Pads.   The Co–Cr–Mo fiber metal pad (Fig. 13) is bonded to its substrate using a diffusion-bonding process. This process is similar to the process used to produce titanium fiber metal bonded to Ti–6Al–4V alloy. Pressure and temperature are used to metallurgically bond the fiber metal to itself and to the substrate. Because of the application of pressure, it is possible to keep the temperature relatively low (65–75% of the melting point), which avoids the significant microstructural changes that occur during gravity sintering of beads.

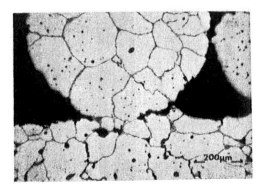

Figure 12   Gravity-sintered Co–Cr–Mo alloy beads on Co–Cr–Mo alloy substrate.

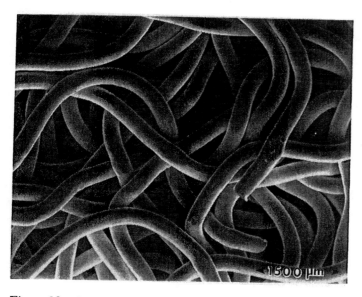

Figure 13   Co–Cr–Mo alloy fiber metal pad.

5.   Product Applications

Co–Cr alloys are used in the manufacture of various orthopedic implants. Some of the implants manufactured from Co-based alloys are given in Table 16. Figures 14 and 15 are pictures of Co–Cr–Mo alloy hip and knee implants, respectively.

C.   Stainless Steels

Stainless steel was discovered in 1904 by Leon Guillet. His early work was concentrated on iron–chromium alloys containing carbon. These alloys were classified into *ferritic* and *martensitic* stainless steels. In 1906 Guillet developed iron–chromium–nickel alloy, more commonly known today as *austenitic* stainless steel. The use of stainless steel in surgical applications began in 1926 when Strauss patented the 18-8 Mo stainless steel containing

Table 16   Cobalt-Based Alloy Implants

Co-based alloys	Typical applications
Co–Cr–Mo Alloy (ASTM F-75)	Hip stems, knees, shoulder joints, elbow joints, porous coated devices, and fracture fixation devices such as bone plates, hip screws, and bone screws
Low-carbon Co–Cr–Mo alloy (ASTM F-799)	Hip stems, shoulder joints, elbow joints, fiber metal porous coated devices, and fracture fixation devices
Co–Ni–Cr–Mo alloy	Hip stems and fracture fixation devices
Co–Cr–Ni–W alloy	Fracture fixation devices

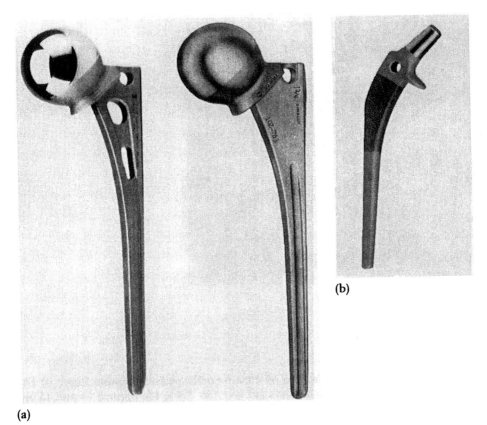

(b)

(a)

Figure 14   Co–Cr–Mo alloy hip stems. (a) Cast Co–Cr–Mo alloy hip stems. (b) High-strength forged Co–Cr–Mo alloy, precoat hip stem.

2% to 4% molybdenum and a very low percentage of carbon. The use of stainless steel revolutionized orthopedic surgery.

1.   Types and Compositions of Stainless Steels

Two types of stainless steels are used in orthopedics. These are 316L and 22-13-5 stainless steels. The chemical compositions of these steels are given in Tables 17 and 18 [40,41].

2.   Structure of Stainless Steels

At room temperature, iron exists in a BCC crystal structure. When heated above 910°C, it transforms to a γ-FCC crystal and the FCC crystal transforms again to the δ-BCC crystal structure at higher temperature.

Chromium is added to iron to improve the corrosion resistance of iron. Nickel is added to iron–chromium alloy to stabilize the austenitic phase. Molybdenum is also added to the alloy to improve corrosion resistance in saline and acidic environments. 316L stainless steel alloy used for surgical implants contains 17–19% chromium, 12–14% nickel, and 2–3% molybdenum. The carbon content in 316L stainless steel should not exceed 0.03 wt% to maintain good corrosion resistance. Maximum corrosion resistance is

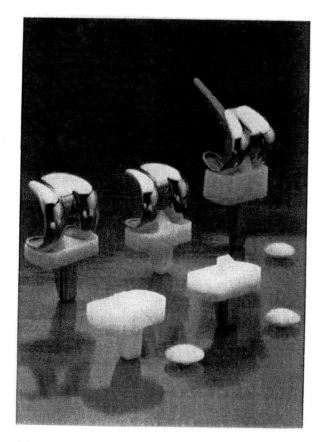

(a)

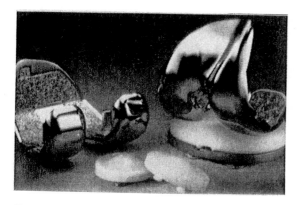

(b)

Figure 15   Co–Cr–Mo alloy knees. (a) Cast Co–Cr–Mo alloy femoral and tibial components of a knee system. Also seen in the picture are UHMWPE tibial inserts, all-poly tibial components and patellar domes. (b) Fiber metal porous coated Co–Cr–Mo alloy femoral components. Also seen in the picture are a Ti–6Al–4V alloy tibial component, an UHMWPE tibial insert, and metal-backed UHMWPE patellar domes.

Table 17   Chemical Composition of 316L Stainless
Steel

Element	Composition, wt%
Carbon	0.030 max
Manganese	2.00 max
Phosphorus	0.025 max
Sulfur	0.010 max
Silicon	0.75 max
Chromium	17.00–19.00
Nickel	13.00–15.50
Molybdenum	2.00–3.00
Nitrogen	0.10 max
Copper	0.50 max
Iron	Balance

obtained when the carbon is in solid solution and when there is a homogeneous single-phase microstructure. A homogeneous single-phase austenitic microstructure is obtained by annealing 316L stainless steel in the temperature range of 1038–1093 °C and quenching in water. A rapid cooling is essential to keep the carbon in solution. Slower cooling will result in chromium carbide precipitation along grain boundaries in the temperature range of 450° to 900°C, resulting in poor alloy corrosion resistance. The formation of these grain boundary carbides in stainless steels is known as *sensitization*. The low-carbon stainless steels have a lesser tendency for sensitization than high-carbon stainless steels.

A number of high-strength stainless steels have been developed for many commercial applications in recent years. Among them, 22Cr–13Ni–5Mn (22-13-5) stainless steel [41,42] possesses attractive properties for implant applications. The 22-13-5 stainless steel contains more chromium, manganese, and nitrogen, and less nickel, than does 316L. It

Table 18   Chemical Composition of 22-13-5
Stainless Steel

Element	Composition, wt%
Carbon	0.030 max
Manganese	4.00 to 6.00
Phosphorus	0.025 max
Sulfur	0.010 max
Silicon	0.75 max
Chromium	20.50–23.50
Nickel	11.50–13.50
Molybdenum	2.00–3.00
Nitrogen	0.20–0.40
Niobium	0.10–0.30
Vanadium	0.10–0.30
Copper	0.50 max
Iron	Balance

also contains niobium (columbium) and vanadium, which are not present in the latter. Nitrogen is added to this alloy to stabilize the austenitic microstructure and to improve strength and corrosion resistance.

The stainless steels are generally used in two conditions: wrought or forged.

Wrought Alloy.   Wrought alloy possesses a uniform microstructure with fine grains [43] (Figs. 16 and 17). In the annealed condition it possesses low mechanical strength properties. The alloy can be strengthened by cold working. Stainless steels work harden rapidly and increase in strength properties with cold work. A typical cold-worked microstructure of 316L stainless steel is given in Fig. 18.

Forged Alloy.   Stainless steels can be hot forged to shape rather easily because of their high ductility. They can also be cold forged to shape to obtain required strength properties. Forging processes similar to those used with cobalt-based alloys may be applied to stainless steels.

3. Properties of Stainless Steels

Tensile Properties.   The tensile properties of annealed 316L and 22-13-5 stainless steel are given in Tables 19 and 20. The measured yield strength of 22-13-5 stainless steel is about 2 times greater and the measured ultimate tensile strength is about 70% higher than that of annealed 316L stainless steel. The reduction in cross-sectional area of 22-13-5 stainless steel is comparable to, but the percentage elongation is lower than, that of 316L stainless steel.

The cold-worked 316L and 22-13-5 stainless steels have a broader range of tensile strength depending upon the fabrication history of the product. Highly cold-worked wire products, for example, will exhibit higher strength than bar stock that is used in the fabrication of larger items. Figure 19 shows the effects of varying degrees of cold working on the static mechanical properties of both 316L and 22-13-5 stainless steels. It is clear

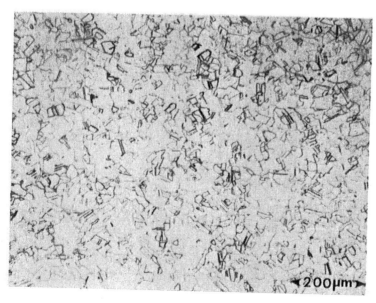

Figure 16   Annealed or hot-forged 316L stainless steel microstructure.

Figure 17   Annealed or hot-forged 22-13-5 stainless steel microstructure.

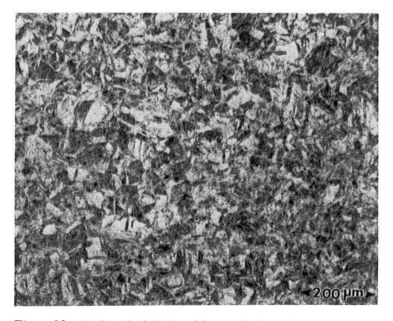

Figure 18   Cold-worked 316L stainless steel microstructure.

Table 19   Tensile Properties of 316L Stainless Steel

Percent cold work	Hardness	Tensile properties [a,b]		
		YS (ksi)	UTS (ksi)	Percent elongation
0	R_B75–100	35.0	80.0	55.0
30	R_C25–30	120.0	130.0	20.0
60	R_C30–35	145.0	180.0	12.0
80	R_C40–45	155.0	195.0	10.0

[a]Typical properties
[b]YS, yield strength; UTS, ultimate tensile strength

Table 20   Tensile Properties of 22-13-5 Stainless Steel

Percent cold work	Hardness	Tensile properties [a,b]		
		YS (ksi)	UTS (ksi)	Percent elongation
0	R_C25–30	110.0	140.0	35.0
30	R_C30–35[c]	170.0	180.0	15.0
60	R_C35–40[c]	215.0	230.0	9.0

[a]Typical properties
[b]YS, yield strength; UTS, ultimate tensile strength
[c]Approximate values

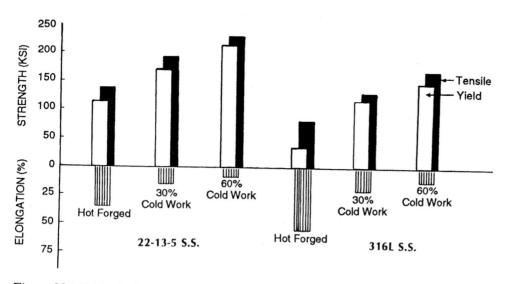

Figure 19   Mechanical properties of 22-13-5 and 316L stainless steels at different levels of cold work.

from the data that increased strengthening of the 22-13-5 alloy is seen at all cold-work levels. The increased strength, however, makes it much more difficult to achieve the higher cold-work levels in usable materials forms.

Fatigue Properties.   The fatigue properties of 316L and 22-13-5 stainless steels are presented in Table 21. The fatigue strength of hot-forged 22-13-5 stainless steel is twice the fatigue strength of hot-forged 316L stainless steel. The fatigue strengths of these steels can be further increased through cold work (Table 21).

Corrosion Properties.   The corrosion properties of stainless steels are usually evaluated by electrochemical tests [4]. Typical potentiodynamic anodic polarization plots for annealed 316L and 22-13-5 stainless steels in Ringer's solution are given in Fig. 20.

The 22-13-5 stainless steel exhibited a wide stable passive region with a breakdown potential of about 900 mV. When the potential sweep was reversed, the protection potential observed was essentially at the breakdown potential. The protection potential theory suggests that for potential values below the protection potential, pits will be neither initiated nor propagated. Potential values between the protection potential and breakdown potential will result in propagation of existing pits but not in initiation of new pits. Potential values above the breakdown potential will result in initiation and propagation of new pits. If pits form on a corroding specimen, a hysteresis loop will result upon potential sweep reversal. The area of hysteresis and, hence, the observed value of the protection potential will depend in part on the extent of pitting on the specimen. Therefore, the observation of the protection potential at the breakdown potential and a very small hysteresis loop indicates that pits did not form on the sample surface at the breakdown potential. This is a good indication of the relatively high resistance of 22-13-5 stainless steel to pitting corrosion.

The results of polarization tests on 316L stainless steel are quite different. While the equilibrium potential was about the same as that for 22-13-5 stainless steel, this alloy exhibited a small passive region with a breakdown potential of 400 mV. When the potential sweep was reversed, the protection potential observed was lower than the equilibrium corrosion potential. This alloy also exhibited a large hysteresis loop. The observation of the protection potential below the equilibrium corrosion potential and a large hysteresis loop for 316L stainless steel indicates that pitting did occur on the specimen surface.

The results of the electrochemical polarization tests on 22-13-5 stainless steel are reinforced by immersion test results. An immersion test based on the crevice test method

Table 21   Fatigue Properties of 316L and 22-13-5 Stainless Steels

Stainless steel alloy	Percent cold work	Hardness	Fatigue limit[a] at 10^7 cycles and $R = -1$ (ksi)
316L	0	$R_B75-100$	26.0
	30	R_C25-30	55.0
	60	R_C30-35	65.0
	80	R_C40-45	70.0
22-13-5	0	R_C25-30	55.0
	30	R_C30-35	77.0
	60	R_C35-40	97.0

[a]Approximate values

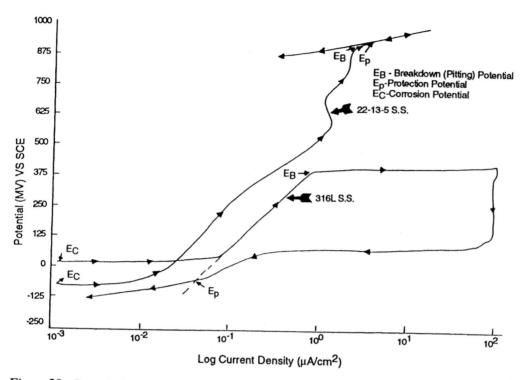

Figure 20 Potentiodynamic anodic polarization curves for 22-13-5 and 316L stainless steels.

developed by the International Nickel Company (INCO) [44] was used to evaluate the crevice corrosion resistance of the alloy in Ringer's solution. The test results after 14 weeks of immersion indicated that the 22-13-5 stainless steel was superior in performance compared to 316L stainless steel.

Wear Properties. 316L and 22-13-5 stainless steels exhibit adequate wear resistance against an ultrahigh molecular weight polyethylene (UHMWPE). The wear properties of stainless steels are comparable to Co–Cr–Mo alloy [39].

Biocompatibility. Various *in vitro* and *in vivo* tests have indicated that 316L and 22-13-5 stainless steels are biocompatible and suitable for use as surgical implants [4,45]. The long-term effects of metal ions on the body are, however, less clear.

Table 22 Stainless Steel Implants

Stainless steel	Typical applications
316L (ASTM F-138)	Hip stems and fracture fixation devices such as IM rods, spinal rods, hip screws, bone plates, bone screws
22-13-5 (ASTM F-1314)	Hip stems and fracture fixation devices such as hip screws, bone plates, spinal rods, IM nails

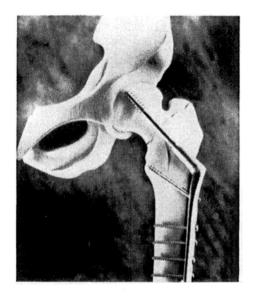

(a)

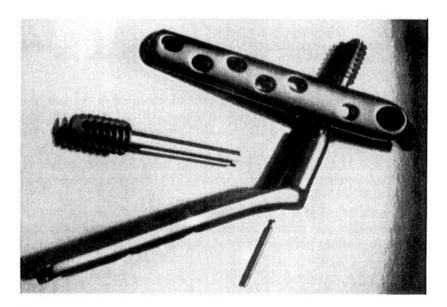

(b)

Figure 21   Stainless steel compression hip screws. (a) Compression hip screw implanted in a femur. (b) Compression tube and plates, lag screws, and a locking pin.

4. Manufacturability

Stainless steel implants can be easily manufactured by forging or machining from wrought mill products. Forging requires forging presses and dies, while machining requires conventional metal-working processes. Modern machining techniques such as computer numerical control (CNC) combined with computer-aided design/computer-aided manufacturing (CAD/CAM) allow parts to be rapidly produced directly from drawings without requiring many intermediate handling steps. Essentially, no metallurgical changes occur during conventional machining, so the mechanical properties of a machined part are identical to the properties of the bar from which it was machined. Forgings, however, can be produced by hot- or cold-forging methods.

5. Product Applications

316L and 22-13-5 stainless steels are used in the fabrication of different types of implants. Some of the implants manufactured from these two alloys are given in Table 22. Pictures of stainless steel implants are presented in Fig. 21.

REFERENCES

1. ASTM F67: Standard specification for unalloyed titanium for surgical implant applications, *Annual Book of ASTM Standards*, 13.01: 3–5 (1993).
2. ASTM F136: Standard specification for wrought titanium 6Al–4V ELI alloy for surgical implant applications, *Annual Book of ASTM Standards*, 13.01: 19–21 (1993).
3. Newman, J. R., D. Eylon, and J. K. Thorne, Titanium and titanium alloys, *Metals Handbook*, 15: 824–835 (1988).
4. Fraker, A. C., Corrosion of metallic implants and prosthetic devices, *Metals Handbook*, 13: 1324–1335 (1987).
5. Duff-Barclay, I., and D. Spillman, Total human joint prostheses — A laboratory study of friction and wear, *Proc. Instn. Mech. Engrs.*, 181: 90–103 (1966-1967).
6. Malkin, S., D. P. Majors, and T. H. Courtney, Surface effects during fretting fatigue of Ti-6Al–4V, *Wear, 22*: 235–243 (1972).
7. Laing, P. G., Compatibility of biomaterials, *Orthop. Clin. N. Am.*, 4: 249–273 (1973).
8. Swanson, S. A. V., M. A. R. Freeman, and J. C. Heath, Laboratory tests on total joint replacement prostheses, *Journal of Bone and Joint Surgery*, 53B: 759–773 (1973).
9. Galante, J. O., and W. Restoker, *Acta Orthop. Scand., Suppl.*: 145 (1973).
10. Miller, E., et al., A comparative evaluation of the wear of ultrahigh molecular weight polyethylene abraded by Ti-6Al–4V, *Wear, 28*: 207–216 (1974).
11. McKellop, H. A., et al., Wear screening tests with potentially superior prosthetic bearing materials, *Trans. 23rd Orthopaedic Res. Soc.*,, 1977. p. 163.
12. Clarke, I. C., et al., Wear of Ti-6Al–4V implant alloy, written communication (1981).
13. Restoker, W., and J. O. Galante, The influence of titanium surface treatments on the wear of medical grade polyethylene, *Biomaterials, 2*: 221–224 (1981).
14. Sioshansi, P., Improving the properties of titanium alloys by ion implantation, *Journal of Metals, 42*: 30–31 (1990).
15. Crowninshield, R., et al., Simulating total knee replacement wear *in vitro*: Comparison of Ti-6Al–4V and nitrogen ion implanted Ti-6Al–4V, *Orthop. Trans., 14*: 470–471 (1990).
16. Shetty, R. H., et al., Method of surface hardening orthopaedic implant devices, U.S. Patent 5,192,323 (1993).
17. Improved abrasion resistance of nitrogen-hardened titanium alloy surfaces, *Current Topics in Orthopaedics Technology* (Zimmer, Inc., Warsaw, IN), 3: 5 (1990).
18. Williams, D. F., Titanium and titanium alloys, *Biocompatibility Clin. Implant Mater., 1*: 9–44 (1981).
19. Bothe, R. T., L. E. Beaton, and H. A. Davenport, Reaction of bone to multiple metallic implants, *Surg. Gyn. Obstet., 71*: 598–602 (1940).

20. Leventhal, G. S., Titanium a metal for surgery, *JBJS, 33A*: 473–474 (1951).
21. Hahn, H., and W. Palich, Preliminary evaluation of porous metal surfaced titanium for orthopaedic implants, *J. Biomed. Mater. Res., 4*: 571–577 (1970).
22. Galante, J., et al., Sintered fiber composites as a basis for attachment of implants to bone, *JBJS, 53A*: 101–114 (1971).
23. Rhinelander, F. W., N. Ronweyha, and R. C. Milner, Microvascular and histogenic responses to implantation of a porous ceramic into bone, *J. Biomed. Mater. Res., 5*: 81–112 (1971).
24. Predecki, P., B. A. Auslaender, and J. E. Stephan, Attachment of bone to threaded implants by ingrowth and mechanical interlocking, *J. Biomed. Mater. Res., 6*: 401–412 (1972).
25. Niles, J. L., and M. Lapitsky, Biomechanical investigations of bone porous carbon and porous metal interfaces, *J. Biomed. Mater. Res. Symp., 4*: 66–84 (1973).
26. Laing, P. G., A. B. Ferguson, and E. S. Hodge, Tissue reaction in rabbit muscle exposed to metallic implants, *J. Biomed. Mater. Res., 1*: 135–149 (1967).
27. Niles, J. L., *Porous titanium alloy as a sub-articular support in the knee*, Presented at the Fifth Annual Biomaterials Symposium, Clemson University, April 14–18, 1973.
28. Autian, J., Private communication, University of Tennessee, Memphis, TN (1972).
29. Raab, S., A. M. Ahmed, and J. W. Provan, The quasistatic and fatigue performance of the implant/bone cement interface, *J. Biomed. Mater. Res., 16*: 159–182 (1981).
30. Andersen, P. J., Medical and dental applications, *Metals Handbook, 7*: 657–663 (1984).
31. ASTM F75: Standard specification for cast cobalt–chromium–molybdenum alloy for surgical implant applications, *Annual Book of ASTM Standards*, 13.01: 6–7 (1993).
32. ASTM F799: Standard specification for thermomechanically processed cobalt–chromium–molybdenum alloy for surgical implants, *Annual Book of ASTM Standards*, 13.01 :236–238 (1993).
33. ASTM F90: Standard specification for wrought cobalt–chromium–tungsten–nickel alloy for surgical implant applications, *Annual Book of ASTM Standards*, 13.01: 11–13 (1993).
34. ASTM F562: Standard specification for wrought cobalt–nickel–chromium–molybdenum alloy for surgical implant applications, *Annual Book of ASTM Standards*, 13.01: 99–101 (1993).
35. Pruitt, T. J., and M. J. Hanslits, Cobalt based alloys, *Metals Handbook*, 15: 811–814 (1988).
36. Pilliar, R. M., Manufacturing processes of metals: the processing and properties of metal implants, *Met. Ceram. Biomater., 1*: 79–105 (1984).
37. Hollander, R., and J. Wulf, New technology for mechanical property improvement of cast Co–Cr–Mo–C surgical implants, *J. Biomed. Mater. Res., 9*: 367–369 (1975).
38. McKellop, H. A., and I. C. Clarke, Evolution and evaluation of materials-screening machines and joint simulators in predicting *in vivo* wear phenomena, *Functional Behav. Orthopaed. Biomater., 2*: 51–85 (1984).
39. Williams, D. F., The properties and clinical uses of cobalt-based alloys, *Biocompatibility Clin. Implant Mater., 1*: 99–127 (1981).
40. ASTM F138: Standard specification for stainless steel bar and wire surgical implants, *Annual Book of ASTM Standards*, 13.01: 22–24 (1993).
41. ASTM F1314: Standard specification for wrought nitrogen strengthened, high manganese, high chromium stainless steel bar and wire for surgical implants, *Annual Book of ASTM Standards*, 13.01: 694–696 (1993).
42. Carpenter 22Cr–13Ni–5Mn stainless steel, *Carpenter Technology Handbook*, 1991, pp.107–109.
43. Bardos, D. I., Stainless steels in medical devices, *Handbook of Stainless Steels*, 42: 1–10 (1977).
44. Anderson, D. B., Statistical aspects of crevice corrosion in seawater: Galvanic and pitting corrosion-field and laboratory studies, *STP 576, American Society for Testing and Materials*, 1976, pp. 231–242.
45. Sutow, E. J., and S. R. Pollack, The biocompatibility of certain stainless steels, *Biocompatibility Clin. Implant Mater., 1*: 45–98 (1981).

18

Titanium and Zirconium Alloys in Orthopedic Applications

Denes I. Bardos
Smith & Nephew Richards
Memphis, Tennessee

I. INTRODUCTION

The development of aseptic surgical procedures and antibiotics during the 1940s gave significant impetus for accelerated development of surgical procedures of the musculo-skeletal system. Surgical techniques for the repair and reconstruction of bone and joints advanced rapidly during the past five decades. Materials development was manifested in the introduction of various metals and metal alloys with the attributes necessary to support the exacting specifications and the myriad demands placed on orthopedic implant devices. A correlation can be seen between the clinical success of orthopedic procedures and the material properties of currently used alloys. A brief chronological summary of the formerly and currently used alloys is presented in Table 1.

The prominent performance characteristics that appear to have driven the introduction of new materials were improved corrosion resistance and biocompatibility, and increasing the strength of load-bearing devices. The clinical performance of metallic biomaterials can only be evaluated on a device-specific basis, including such important parameters as the location of the device in the skeletal system, surgical technique, fixation methodology, and long-term biological manifestations. In this chapter the orthopedic applications of titanium and zirconium alloys are presented in light of our current understanding of these complex issues.

II. UNALLOYED TITANIUM

Unalloyed or commercially pure titanium (cp Ti) is available in four grades. These were selected based on oxygen content, which determines the mechanical properties of the material. ASTM standard F76 sets forth the chemical composition and minimum mechanical properties of this material. A brief summary of the relevant properties is presented in Table 2.

Table 1   Chronology of Metal Alloys in Orthopedic Applications

Alloy	Year	Application	Performance Issues
Vanadium steel	1912	Bone plates	Corrosion problems
Cast Co–Cr–Mo	1937	Dental devices	Well accepted
Cast Co–Cr–Mo	1938	Orthopedic implants	Well tolerated, adequate strength
302 stainless steel	1938	Bone plates/screws	Corrosion resistance
316 stainless steel	1946	Trauma implants	Better corrosion resistance and strength
Titanium	1965	Hip implants (England)	Corrosion resistance, tissue acceptance
316LVM stainless steel	1968	Trauma implants	Further improvements in corrosion resistance, strength
MP35N	1972	European hip prostheses	High strength
Ti–6Al–4V	1974	Trauma implants	High strength, biocompatibility
Ti–6Al–4V	1976	Hip prostheses	High strength, low modulus
Forged Co–Cr–Mo	1978	Hip prostheses	Highest fatigue strength
22-13-5 stainless steel	1981	Hip implants, trauma	High strength, forgeability
Ti–6Al–7Nb	1982	Hip implants	High strength, biocompatibility
Cold-forged 316LVM	1983	Compression hip screw	High strength
Zirconium 2.5Nb (zirconia coated)	1994	Joint prostheses	Improved wear resistance, biocompatibility

The ductility of cp titanium enables the fabrication of a variety of wire and cable products from this material. Corrosion resistance and relatively high strength were among the reasons for selecting titanium wire and cable in surgical procedures requiring the approximation of bony fragments, osteotomies, or other procedures that require stabilization of bone while fusion or healing takes place. Successful patient outcomes have been reported with cp titanium wire in a variety of surgical procedures. Long-bone fractures, pelvic repair, and spinal fusion present the need for high strength and the stable fixation of several month's duration that can be provided by these devices.

The most common material selected for wire and cable applications is Grade 2 because of the trade-off between higher strength and decreasing ductility. During orthopedic surgery, frequently it is required to tie a knot or otherwise fasten the wire and cable after it has been applied to the surgical site. Titanium is difficult to form into knots or to

Table 2   Unalloyed Titanium

	Grade 1	Grade 2	Grade 3	Grade 4
% oxygen, max	0.18	0.25	0.35	0.40
Tensile strength, MPa (ksi)	240 (35)	345 (50)	450 (65)	550 (80)
Yield strength, MPa (ksi)	170 (25)	275 (40)	380 (55)	485 (70)
Ductility, % elongation	24	20	18	15

twist together for the purpose of fastening the ends. Frequently, a sleeve-type device is provided into which the ends are threaded and subsequently crimped. Figure 1 illustrates a typical cp titanium cable and fastening device that can be utilized in a variety of orthopedic applications.

Hip prostheses were fabricated from unalloyed titanium soon after it became commercially available in the 1950s. The outstanding corrosion resistance, light weight, and biocompatibility were the motivating factors in selecting this material. Clinical experience was limited to relatively few centers. Similarly, fracture fixation devices in the form of bone plates and bone screws were evaluated in this time period. Minimal tissue response and the absence of any adverse systemic reaction encouraged further developments.

For the surgical correction of scoliosis, titanium cables and screws have been used with significant clinical success. The titanium devices known as the *Dwyer system* utilize screws and staples that are inserted into the vertebrae of the area of curvature of the spine. After the mechanical straightening of the segments of the spine, the eyes of the screw heads are crimped to secure the cable in the correct position. The ductility of

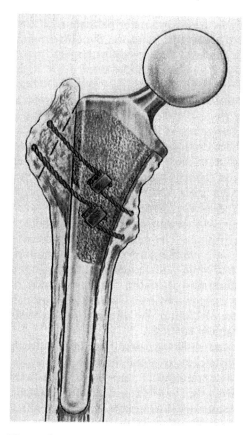

Figure 1 Unalloyed titanium, Grade 2, cable for the reattachment of the greater trochanter. After the cable is tightened the sleeves are crimped, providing secure fixation of the bone segments.

unalloyed titanium enables this crimping to take place without cracking of the screw heads. This procedure was performed with an anterior approach to the spinal column. More recently, procedures with a posterior approach have become widespread, diminishing the use of unalloyed titanium in this application. Contemporary procedures utilize stainless steel hooks, rods, and screws that can be combined for stable constructs of the various segments of the spinal column.

III. TITANIUM ALLOY

Adding alloying additions to titanium accomplishes a significant increase in the mechanical strength characteristic of the material. A variety of alloys have been utilized with great success in commercial applications, especially in the highly technologically demanding aerospace and military fields. The most widely used alloy in the fabrication of jet aircraft is the titanium–6 aluminum–4 vanadium grade (Ti–6Al–4V). This alloy was selected for orthopedic prosthetic implant applications and was readily available commercially in a variety of mill products such as bars and plates. The standard specification (ASTM F136 and ISO5832-III) set forth exacting compositional limits in order to ensure reproducibility in mechanical properties.

Total hip prostheses are made from titanium 64 alloy in order to achieve high resistance to metal fatigue breakage of implants in highly active, younger patients who may subject a device to very high, repeated physiological loads. Furthermore, the biomechanical compatibility between the low modulus of bone and the high-modulus implant material can be improved by the selection of this alloy. The elastic modulus of other high-strength implant metals such as cobalt and stainless steel is twice that of titanium alloy. Therefore, a better approximation of the elastic modulus is accomplished in an attempt to transmit more physiologically normal forces to the surrounding cortical bone. This is necessary to ensure bone viability and to reduce disuse atrophy in long-term applications.

The high-strength characteristics of these devices proved adequate; however, clinical complications such as loosening and fragmentation of the bone cement surrounding the prosthesis prompted the development of porous coated devices. Commercially pure titanium beads are attached to the high-strength alloy stem, utilizing a high-temperature sintering process. The resultant metallurgical bond ensures a high-strength attachment of 51 MPa (7500 psi). Hip prostheses of such design can be implanted in the medullary cavity of the femur in a firm press-fitting manner (Fig. 2). This provides an opportunity for bone to grow into the pores of the beaded surface, enabling a permanent fixation of the device through this biologic bonding of metal and bone. This is due, in large measure, to the electrochemical surface properties of titanium and its alloys. The propensity of titanium to form highly stable oxides [1,2] ensures a chemically stable surface of ceramic-like composition that does not provoke any adverse reaction in the adjacent tissue. Bone cells have been observed growing into and onto titanium surfaces.

Some patients may be allergic to metals in contact with their skin. Similarly, allergic reactions of various severity are known to occur subsequent to metal implantation. Cases of eczematous dermatitis related to the long-term implantation of some metal prostheses have been known to occur. There is some evidence that even the corrosion-resistant materials used in orthopedic implants, such as stainless steel and cobalt–chromium alloy, may produce some minute quantities of corrosion products and release metal ions in the process, which may be responsible for these allergic reactions. The exact immunologic mechanism triggering hypersensitivity is not clearly understood. Surgical removal of the

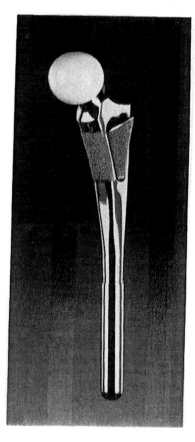

Figure 2   Total hip prosthesis comprised of Ti–6Al–4V alloy stem for strength and cp titanium sintered bead surface for biologic fixation, and zirconia ceramic head for optimum friction and wear performance.

implant frequently eliminates the symptoms, thus establishing a clear causative relationship. The alloying elements such as cobalt, nickel, and perhaps chromium have been suspected as sensitizing agents. Titanium and titanium alloys do not contain known sensitizing elements. Titanium alloy is the most widely recommended choice for patients suspected of being sensitive to metals. Outstanding clinical success in this regard prompted the utilization of titanium in numerous medical applications in addition to orthopedics.

Titanium alloys have been utilized in the fabrication of total-knee prostheses. In this application, highly polished titanium femoral components articulate against an ultrahigh molecular weight polyethylene tibial part. Due to the high stresses and the continuous rubbing motion, the inert oxide layer from titanium can be rubbed off. In this process, the exposed titanium repassivates; that is, it forms a new oxide layer, and the cycle is repeated. Large quantities of oxide debris can accumulate in the adjacent tissues and the joint capsule. This can also act as a third-body abrasion, further aggravating the problem. Therefore, in articulating joint configurations, cobalt alloy is recommended (Fig. 3). A

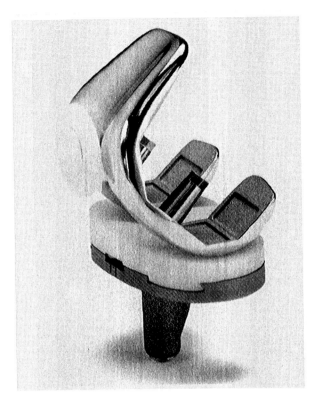

Figure 3   Total knee prosthesis made of cobalt alloy femoral component and Ti–6Al–4V alloy tibial reinforcing tray for high-strength support of the construct.

variety of attempts have been made to strengthen the surface characteristics; however, long-term solutions have not been found.

In orthopedic fracture fixation devices, stainless steel has been the predominant choice of material. Recently, titanium has been introduced in some limited applications. Titanium (cp) with slight cold working to improve mechanical strength is offered in bone plate and bone screw applications. Ti–6Al–4V alloy is utilized in intramedullary rods and for the internal fracture reduction of the proximal femur. Unlike prosthetic applications, the strong attachment of the device to bone in temporary implants is not desirable, and if it does occur, removal of the fracture fixation appliance is complicated and difficult. Clinical advantages of titanium trauma devices await long-term observations.

IV. NEW ALLOY DEVELOPMENT

The utilization of the most biocompatible alloying elements prompted the development and introduction of a new titanium alloy containing 13% niobium and 13% zirconium [1]. The three elements comprising this alloy promise the most biocompatible alloy developed for orthopedic applications. The elastic modulus of this material is lower than any other metal alloy for implant applications. The mechanical properties are compared in

Table 3 Typical Mechanical Properties of Various Titanium and Zirconium Alloys

Alloy	Strength,[a] MPa		Ductility, % elongation	Elastic modulus, GPa	Fatigue strength, MPa
	UTS	YS			
Ti–6Al–4V	980	850	12	115	515
Ti–13Nb–13Zr	1030	900	15	79	530
Ti–5Al–2.5Fe	860	780	10	115	500
Ti–6Al–7Nb	1050	900	12	105	500
Zr–2.5Nb (zirconia coated)	600	400	42	97	520

[a]UTS, ultimate tensile strength; YS, yield strength

Table 3 to other titanium alloys intended for orthopedic applications. Clinical utilization of the material includes bone plates and bone screws, as well as proximal femoral fracture reduction devices.

Two additional alloy development efforts have been reported by orthopedic implant manufacturing companies aimed at substituting niobium or iron for vanadium in the Ti 64 alloy.

V. ZIRCONIUM ALLOY

The unsurpassed clinical success of metal oxide ceramics such as aluminum oxide and zirconium oxide [3,4] prompted the development of zirconium alloy for orthopedic applications. Highly polished ceramic-bearing surface articulating against ultrahigh molecular weight polyethylene reduces not only the frictional forces, but the rate of wear of the polyethylene component as well. The applications of high-ceramic monolithic components are limited due to current manufacturing technology. The fabrication of ceramic femoral knee prostheses, for example, is not practical. The desirable attributes of metal alloys combined with those of ceramics can be achieved utilizing the unique property of zirconium in its ability to be oxidized to form a dense, hard, biocompatible, low-friction, low-wear, well-bonded, ceramic-bearing surface of ZrO_2.

During oxidation of the zirconium alloy, a blue–black microcrystalline monoclinic ZrO_2 oxide film forms. Depending on the manufacturing technology, a dense oxide thickness of about 2 to 6 μm can be obtained. The ceramic-like properties are transitioned gradually to the ductile metal substrate [5], as the transition from the surface zirconia oxide to the base metal is through a diffusion layer characterized by high strength and outstanding bonding.

REFERENCES

1. Kovacs, P., and Davidson, J.A., The electrochemical behavior of a new titanium alloy with superior biocompatibility, *Titanium '92, Science and Technology*, The Minerals, Metals & Materials Society, 1993.
2. Solar, R.J., Corrosion resistance of titanium surgical implant alloys: a review, *ASTM STP 684*, 1979, pp. 259–273.
3. Christel, P., Meunier, A., Heller, M., Torre, J.P., and Peille, C.N., Mechanical properties and

short-term in-vitro evaluation of yttrium-oxide-partially stabilized zirconia, *JBMR*, Vol. 23, No. 1, Jan. 1989, pp. 45–62.

4. Mittelmeier, H., Total hip replacement with the autophor cement-free ceramic prosthesis, in *The Cementless Fixation of Hip Endoprostheses*, E. Morscher, ed., Springer-Verlag, Berlin, Heidelburg, 1984, pp. 225–240.

5. Davidson, J.A., Asgian, C.M., Mishra, A.K., and Kovacs, P., Zirconia (ZrO_2)-coated zirconium-2.5Nb alloy for prosthetic knee bearing applications, Proc., 5th International Symposium on Ceramics in Medicine, Kyoto, Japan, Nov. 28–30, 1992, *Bioceramics, 5*, 1993.

19
Bone-Anchored Biomaterials in Experimental and Applied Research

Tomas Albrektsson, Bjorn Albrektsson, Lars V. Carlsson,
Magnus Jacobsson, and Tord Rostlund
University of Gothenburg
Gothenburg, Sweden

I. INTRODUCTION

Biomaterials research is often performed by basic scientists working in isolation from clinicians. Questions of interest to basic researchers may be very different from those of the clinical specialist. But clinicians, while alert to patient needs, often lack sufficient biomaterials knowledge to conceive of new biomaterials and treatment principles. Thus, most basic researchers currently investigate physical or biological principles far removed from practical medicine. Conversely, clinicians have frequently been unable to participate in the development of new biomaterials, a stagnant situation exemplified by the soft tissue anchored blade-vent implants in clinical dentistry and by some types of uncemented implants in orthopedic surgery. In contrast, with more than 20 years of close collaboration between theoretical and clinical researchers, we have been able to introduce the concept of osseointegration, currently utilized in craniofacial implantology with excellent long-term clinical results.

The isolated basic research laboratory is rarely the source of initiatives in the development of new biomaterials. We believe that the development of new clinical biomaterials requires the special spirit of close co-operation between basic scientists and clinical researchers. New biomaterials will require testing in the biological environment, including perhaps the cell culture, and in the engineering laboratory. However, a new biomaterial, will have to pass further scrutiny in carefully monitored animal experiments. But these are not the last hurdles to pass. With substantial experimental support for new biomaterials, clinical trials may be initiated, which must be extensive and rigorously controlled. Despite meticulous cell culture and animal experiments, the clinical trials are liable to reveal new and unexpected behaviour often in contradiction of the best-controlled cell culture or animal studies. After 5 years or more of clinical work (the most important part of the scientific investigation), we may finally have proved our new biomaterial.

The present chapter outlines our approach to the development of new biomaterials. This overview includes developments in basic and clinical science. The common theme of our experimental and clinical implants is direct bone anchorage—*osseointegration*. In oral implantology and ear, nose, and throat (ENT) surgery, osseointegration is a well-known concept, whereas it is insufficiently investigated in orthopedic surgery. We conclude this chapter with comments on our first clinical experience with osseointegrated implants in arthroplasty operations.

II. EXPERIMENTAL MODELS FOR VITAL MICROSCOPY OF BONE

During the 1970s a vital microscopic implant for *in vivo* and *in situ* investigations of bone tissue—the optical bone chamber (Fig. 1)—was developed at our laboratories [1]. The implant consists of a hollow titanium screw of a diameter of 4 mm. Inside this screw one long and one short glass rod are glued so as to leave a space of 150 μm in between. Using very gentle surgical technique, the implant is inserted into the long bone of an experimental animal, allowing bone to incorporate the foreign material—*osseointegration*. At the same time some of this newly formed bone will grow through the space between the glass rods. This ingrown bone tissue is thin enough to be transilluminated in a light microscope. Thereafter, the animal is examined weekly. In this manner Eriksson [4] was able to investigate acute and long-term effects of a defined heat stimulus. This new experimental model made it possible, in principle, to investigate living bone at the resolution level of the light microscope over unlimited follow-up periods. Bone remodeling after osteotomies was studied [2] and, for the first time, it was possible to document creeping substitution in living cortical bone. Cutting cones were seen to invade the bone at a rate of some 30 μm a day, whereas regenerating vessels in cancellous bone grew at an approximate rate of

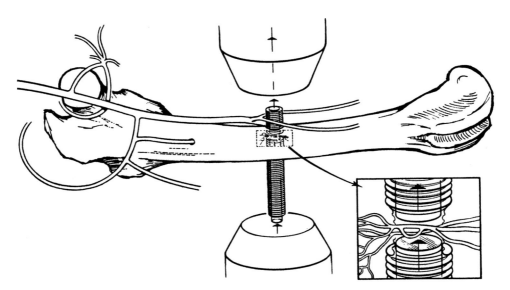

Figure 1   The optical bone chamber enables the study of bone microcirculation and bone remodeling *in situ* at the light microscopical resolution level.

0.2–0.4 mm/day [3]. This vital microscopic bone chamber model has since been used by us in a number of versions for investigations of bone remodeling under various conditions. Eriksson also studied the effect of temperature on heat injury and the bone tissue response. This utilized a modification of the originally described bone chamber, where a thermistor was placed parallel to the top glass rod and in contact with the ingrown bone tissue. Eriksson also developed an electric heat-stimulating device that could be attached to the chamber. By having one investigator observing through the vital microscope during heating up to temperatures varying between 45° and 55°C, it was possible to study the tissue reactions during the application of the heat stimulus and show that the critical temperature–time relationship for bone injury is 47°C applied for 1 min [5].

Jacobsson [6] investigated the bone tissue response to irradiation. He utilized one advantage with the optical bone chamber: repeated observation of precisely the same bone sample before and after irradiation over a long follow-up. Jacobsson [6] reported that immature bone was much more sensitive to an irradiative trauma than was ordered lamellar bone. He found a delayed lamellarization pattern in bone irradiated at therapeutic dose levels compared to control bone [7]. Buch [8] used the vital microscopic chamber with two platinum electrodes on each side of the chamber, connected to a DC stimulator placed under the dorsal skin of the rabbit. Stimulating with a direct current of 50 μA, Buch [8] could demonstrate a negative tissue reaction resulting in bone resorption. However, he demonstrated that DC currents of 5 and 20 μA magnitude were capable of stimulating bone growth inside the chambers [9], and that the same type of electrical stimulation resulted in a vascular leakage [10].

The test chamber [11] was further developed to function as an *in situ* model for the study of the influence of different drugs on bone tissue (Fig. 2). This chamber model had a titanium microplug inserted parallel to the top glass rod. The tissues were first inspected in the vital microscope. Thereafter, the microplug was withdrawn from the chamber, and curing bone cement was gently injected down to contact the ingrown tissues. In this manner, curing bone cement was found to cause emboli that were actually seen forming inside veins and then being transported out of the field of observation [12]. In fact, it has since been verified that central venous emboli may be routinely detected after clinical use of bone cement in major arthroplasties [13]. Bone resorption and fat-cell degeneration were observed in the first few months after cement insertion. Morberg [14] reported such adverse tissue reactions to bone cement and followed the same tissue compartment for up to 2 years after cementation with repeated vital microscopy [15].

The great advantage with the vital microscopic chamber is the possibility of performing simultaneous studies of bone remodeling and vascular reactions. Bone blood flow velocity may be measured in individual capillaries utilizing, for instance, a superimposed video frame technique. Or the investigator may prefer to register an overall average blood flow with the laser Doppler technique [12]. The laser Doppler unit may be directly coupled to the bone chamber, thereby avoiding two potential errors of this method, namely the exact orientation and the potential tissue pressure of the laser Doppler probe.

III. THE HARVEST CHAMBER FOR QUANTIFIED EVALUATIONS OF BONE INGROWTH

During the 1980s we developed other types of experimental implants, the so-called Bone Growth Chambers [16] and the Harvest Chambers [17]. The Bone Growth Chamber is original in the sense that it was first constructed for clinical tests by one of our clinical

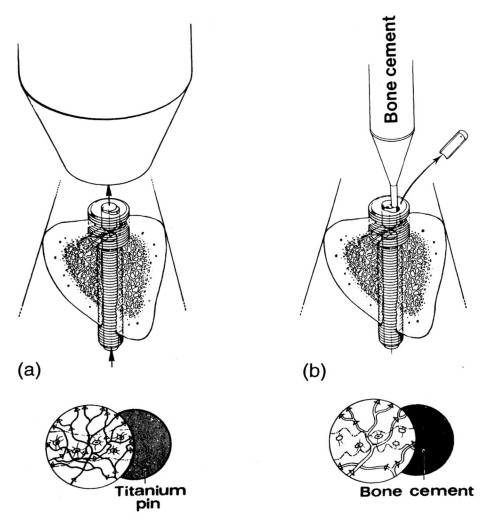

Figure 2 The test chamber is a modification of the original optical bone chamber. The chamber is inserted in a long bone of the animal and allowed to incorporate during a time of some months (a). At onset of the experiments, a titanium pin is withdrawn from its position immediately adjacent to the top glass rod of the chamber. Curing bone cement is then injected down to contact the tissue that has grown into the chamber. This enables repeated observations of the acute and long-term effects of curing bone cement (b).

team members [18]. Divisable titanium chambers were implanted in the tibia and in the temporal bone of volunteering patients suffering from certain types of hearing disorders with missing ossicular bone. Inside the chambers we formed open cavities shaped like the missing ossicular bones. After implantation, bone invaded these canals so that, on removal of the chamber, it was possible to harvest these "man-molded" ossicles with minimal surgical trauma and transplant them to the middle ear [19, 20]. Some 10 patients were treated in this manner and when evaluated in the 5-year follow-up were found to have splendid hearing [21]. This clinical work inspired the experimental part of our laboratory to develop Bone Growth chambers for the study of the influence of the fibrin adhesive system (FAS) on bone healing [16]. We mixed FAS according to the instructions from the manufacturer and used one bone growth chamber in one leg as a control and another chamber in the contralateral extremity for FAS injection. Four weeks after commencement the chambers were removed with a trephine and split open, and the tissue that had invaded the canals was collected. Each chamber produced two specimens, one canal in the cortical and one in the marrow space. The collected bone specimens were microradiographed and then evaluated with the help of an IBAS computer. In the 4-week period, it was evident that this drug tended to retard bone growth rather than acting in a stimulating manner as suggested previously [22]. Bone growth chambers were utilized in other studies that established a dose–response relationship for bone regeneration after irradiative trauma [23].

However, the bone growth chamber had one drawback: the construction of the implant necessitated implant removal and animal sacrifice when collecting bone samples. To encompass more dynamic bone studies, we therefore developed the harvest chamber [17]. The harvest chamber is equipped with a lid and a penetrating canal. The lid may be removed, without animal sacrifice, thereby giving access to the implant canal, from which the ingrown bone may be harvested (Fig. 3). The lid is then replaced and new bone will invade the canal for another harvest 3–4 weeks later. In this way, animals have yielded repeated harvests over a whole year. Test and control harvest chambers have been inserted in experimental animals and the ingrown bone has been quantified with microradiograms [24] as well as histomorphometrical data. We used this method to analyze bone formation after single-dose irradiation to 15 Gy, using an experimental design similar to that of the bone growth chambers. One chamber was inserted in one leg and acted as control, whereas an identical chamber inserted by the same surgeon in the contralateral extremity was subjected to a controlled cobalt-60 irradiation dose. With this method we demonstrated that bone formation impairment was greater immediately after the irradiation trauma than 1 year later [25]. This inspired our clinical work with the insertion of craniofacial implants in irradiated bone beds, today a routine procedure at our university in treatment with extraoral implants to restore the craniofacial skeleton after tumour surgery. Another experimental–clinical connection originally tested in harvest chambers relates to divers' chambers. Animals were placed in the hyperbaric environment during a couple of hours daily and every animal served intermittently as test or control. A typical schedule was that an animal was placed in the divers' chamber during two periods of 3 weeks and thereafter served as control during two other periods of 3 weeks. In the experimental setup we could see a clearly enhanced bone formation in chamber-treated animals compared to controls, a finding that was attributed to the artificially enhanced P_{O_2} levels [26]. This has motivated a diver's chamber project with irradiated patients to be treated with implants [27].

The harvest chamber has been used in modified forms to test the effects of bone growth factors (Fig. 4) and micromotion. Experiments with local, repeated applications of IGF-1 did not increase the amount of mineral in the harvest chamber model [28,29]. In the micromotion experiment the implant canal, when subjected to 20 cycles of 0.5 mm movement applied during a 30-sec period once daily, showed ingrowth of vascularized fibrous tissue and only small amounts of bone in comparison to control chambers [30]. Figure 5 represents an overview of different implant models developed at our laboratories for *in situ* bone studies.

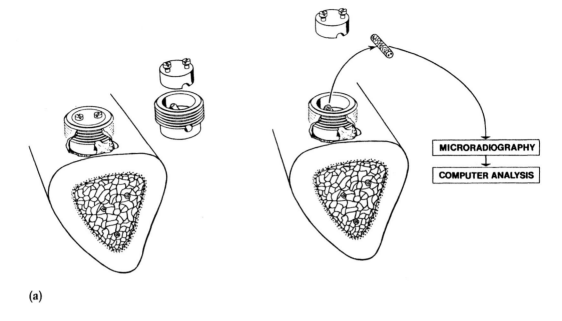

(a)

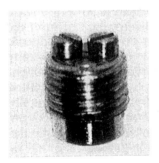

(b)

Figure 3 The harvest chamber has a penetrating canal that goes straight through the implant body. The implant is inserted in the long bone of the rabbit and, for example, 3 weeks later, the lid is lifted off the chamber and soft tissues that have penetrated the canal are harvested for microradiographical and histomorphometrical analyses. The lid is replaced and another harvest may be collected 3 weeks later. Studies are usually performed with two harvest chambers inserted in two long bones of the animal in a test-and-control fashion. Animals may give repeated harvests over yearlong observation periods (a). The assembled harvest titanium chamber has an outer diameter of 6 mm (b). Histological representation of tissue collected from a harvest chamber. The amount of bone is determined with a microradiographical or a histomorphometrical technique (c).

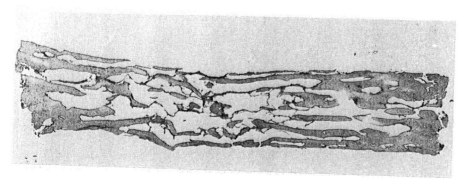

(c)

IV. CURRENT CLINICAL APPLICATIONS OF OSSEOINTEGRATED IMPLANTS

Results from vital microscopic studies of bone at the Laboratory of Experimental Biology, where the senior authors worked in the 1960s, led to the introduction of a new oral implant system, today referred to as the *Nobelpharma implant*. Until the 1980s treatment with oral implants was not regarded as *lege artis* at most university clinics. The implant developed at our university was anchored in bone, in contrast to other oral implant devices that were tried at the time. Excellent documented clinical results [31–3] enabled the Nobelpharma implant to be the first accepted by the American Dental Association, and to date, more than 1 million of these implants (Fig. 6) have been inserted in patients all over the world. We continue to work in close co-operation with clinical colleagues to expand current indications for oral implants, for example, in severely resorbed or irradiated bone beds.

Based on combined laboratory–clinical investigations at our university, our first permanent skin-penetrating implants were inserted clinically in 1977. Clinical indications for treatment with implant-based facial epistheses include congenital disorders and trauma or cancer surgery. An additional indication for skin-penetrating implants is certain types of hearing disorders, where a bone conduction hearing aid is coupled to the bone-anchored titanium implant. Clinical reports verify the aesthetic and functional advantages [34–37] of bone-anchored, skin-penetrating epistheses (Fig. 7). The incidence of soft-tissue disorders is low despite the permanent skin penetration [38]. In the case of directly coupled-bone anchored hearing aids, there has been significant increase in patient hearing threshold level, as well as cosmetic advantages [38]. This clinical material represents the first controlled study ever of permanently skin-penetrating implants. Our longest follow-up to date is 17 years, and the Gothenburg technique of inserting skin-penetrating, osseointegrated implants is now applied all over the world [39].

From observations with various types of vital microscopic and harvest-type chambers we have gained knowledge on bone reactions to various stimuli that we subsequently have applied clinically. Albrektsson et al. [40] and Albrektsson and Albrektsson [1] have, used these studies to present data on six different factors that govern the incorporation of experimental implants in bone. These factors relate to the biocompatibility, design and surface conditions of the implant, the state of the host bed, the surgical technique at

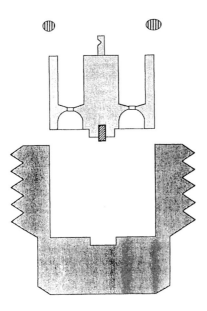

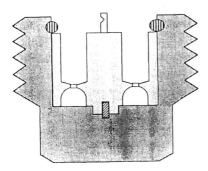

Figure 4 A modification of the harvest chamber allows repeated injection of bone growth factors into the canals in the bottom of the chamber lid.

installation, and the loading conditions applied afterward. To check the individual importance of these various parameters for implant security, we have developed various types of torque gauge manometers (Fig. 8).

V. OSSEOINTEGRATED IMPLANTS IN ORTHOPEDIC SURGERY

Building on the experience gained from experimental laboratory work and clinical practice with dental and craniofacial implants, we have developed a hip joint arthroplasty system. Technology transfer is well known to be a complicated and cumbersome task.

The results with current hip arthroplasties, show that there is a great need for reliable,

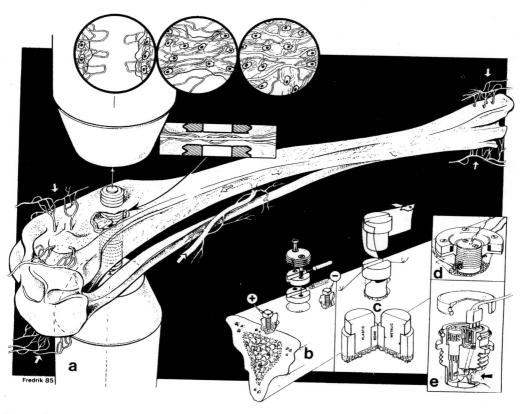

Figure 5 One great advantage of the optical chamber is the ability to repeatedly study the same bone segment during, for instance, the phase of bone accretion. (a). Bone growth chambers have been used in studies of the effects of electrical stimuli (b). The polycarbonate plug method allows for analysis of the bone–metal interface at the electron microscopic resolution level (c). A modified harvest chamber used to study the effects of heat on bone regeneration (d). A specially constructed titanium implant with enclosed electronics utilized in a study of bone marrow pressure (e).

long-term fixation methods based, not only on engineering principles, but to a greater degree on biological principles than has hitherto been the case (Fig. 9). Although in elderly patients [41] cemented Charnley-type arthroplasties may provide excellent function, even up to 10 years after implantation, the results for younger patients are discouraging. In a national study conducted in Sweden of 92,675 hip arthroplasties performed in the period 1978–1990, Malchau and co-workers [41] found that the revision rate for males with osteoarthrosis in the age group 55–64 years (8098 hips) was over 20% after 10 years. This takes no account of malfunctioning arthroplasties deemed ineligible for revision surgery. For women over 75 years of age with osteoarthrosis (7810 hips) the revision rate was only 7% after 10 years. This can be compared to women with rheumatoid arthrosis younger than 55 years (1118 hips) where the revision rate was close to 20% after 10 years.

The concept for our hip arthroplasty system is based on the principles postulated

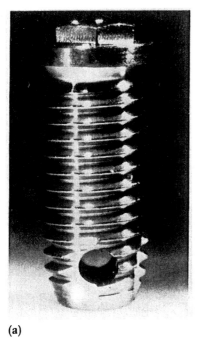

(a)

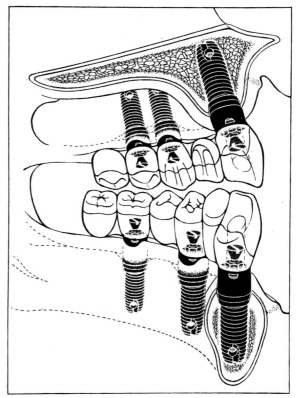

(b)

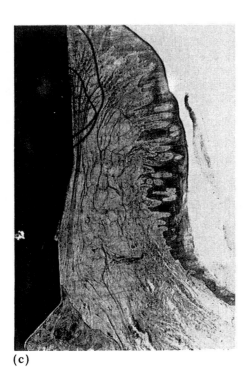

(c)

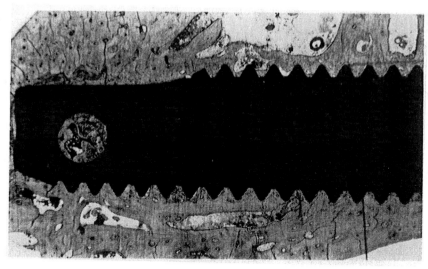

(d)

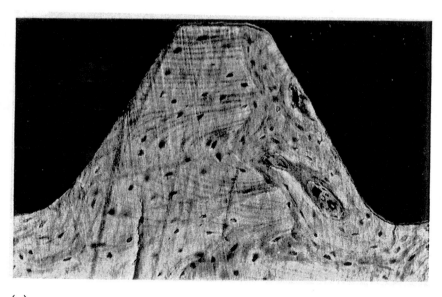

(e)

Figure 6   The Nobelpharma oral implant originally developed at our university (a). The implant is used in partly or fully edentulous cases and has demonstrated 98% success rate for 5 and 10 years of follow-up in the mandible (b). The implant penetration of the mucosal membranes is generally without clinical problem, presumably due to the stable anchorage of the device (c). Retrieved oral implants have demonstrated a very high degree of bone-to-implant contact, in different cases varying between 60% and 99% of the implant surface (d). Higher-power ground section with osteocytes in close proximity to the implant surface (e).

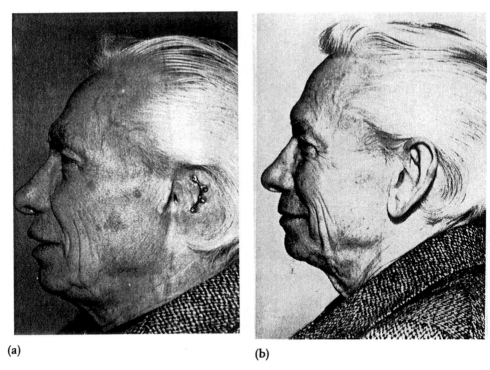

(a)   (b)

Figure 7 An example of first routine usage of skin-penetrating implants known to the present authors. After surgical removal of this patient's pinna for tumor, four implants were inserted in the temporal bone (a) and later a silicone ear prosthesis was attached to these. Five- and 10-year survivals of such skin-penetrating implants have been in the order of 95% (b).

[40,42,43] to facilitate osseointegration. Albrektsson et al. [40] in 1981 reviewed clinical retrieved implants from humans placed in such different sites as the mandible, maxilla, tibia, temporal bone, and iliac bone. A total of 38 stable and integrated implants were investigated using radiography, scanning electron microscopy (SEM), transmission electron microscopy (TEM), and histology. It was concluded that to guarantee osseointegration, threaded, unalloyed titanium implants should be used. In addition the authors suggested a delicate surgical technique be used. Carlsson [42] could demonstrate in animals that screw-shaped commercially pure (cp) titanium implants developed more contact with the bone than did T-plates and cylinders. It was also concluded that a close initial fit between bone and implant is necessary to achieve direct bone contact, and also that smooth-surfaced implants have less resistance to unscrewing than rough-surfaced ones. Another important conclusion was that titanium screw-shaped implants may develop direct bone contact although they are immediately dynamically loaded. Rostlund [43] pointed out the importance of using biocompatible materials, of which cp titanium is one, in order to achieve osseointegration. Other factors of importance are macroscopic implant design (a threaded form being preferable) and the status of the host bed; long-term prospects are reduced by osteoporosis, previous radiation treatment, or diabetes, although these conditions are not absolute contraindications.

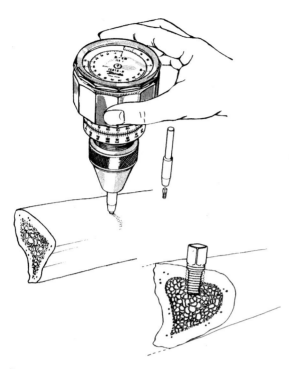

Figure 8 The original torque gauge manometer utilized to test the anchorage strength of implants. An electrically controlled torque device has been developed.

In the present project we have chosen to use cp titanium, a metal that is considered to be among the most biocompatible and with vast documentation in both experimental and clinical practice but is softer and weaker than most orthopedic materials. Because of this, modelling and stress analysis using finite element methods were essential in the early construction phases. On this basis, given the theoretical and practical limitations of finite element analysis, the design was developed to ensure that it would fulfill loading, healing, and functional demands.

The implant orientation follows the natural loading pattern in the normal proximal femur, thus avoiding fractures and stress shielding. This was also confirmed by finite element studies. The results of the finite element analysis were validated in bench tests with a cyclical load of 4 kN over 10 million cycles, with no untoward effects on the implants.

The macroscopic design of the implant was known to be important. It has rotational symmetry and is externally threaded, allowing it to be screwed into position in the femur. We know from the literature [44,45] that a threaded implant will provide greater initial stability than a smooth cylinder. In a review of different dental implant systems, Albrektsson [44] concluded that unthreaded implants of a cylindrical shape may not establish a steady state with peri-implant bone. Using photoelastic stress analysis, Deines et al. [45] concluded that a screw-shaped implant will distribute the stresses evenly along the entire length of the implant interface, in contrast to a cylindrical, nonthreaded design where

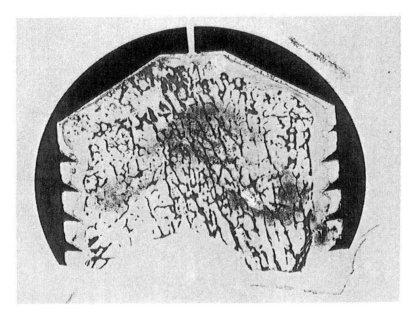

(a)

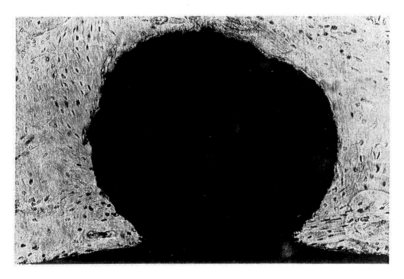

(b)

Figure 9   Cement-free hip constructions have generally failed to demonstrate direct bone-to-implant contact (a). This does not mean that all of the interface exhibits soft tissue contact, as demonstrated by an illustration of a porous coated implant hip retrieved from a patient (b). However, as is demonstrated on a retrieved specimen of a tibial component, the bone ingrowth is generally restricted to specific regions of the implant (c).

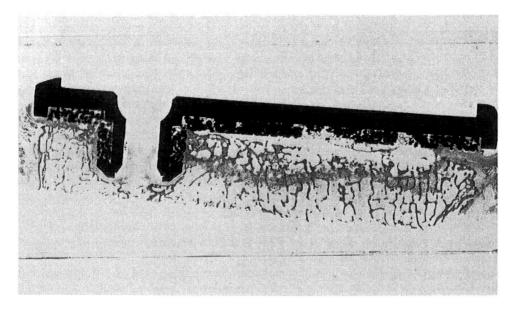

(c)

stress concentrations occurred in the apical area alone. In a study of the interface zone between implants and bone tissue *in vivo*, Albrektsson et al. [46] found that initial stability is of utmost importance if direct anchorage of an implant (without intervening soft tissue) is to be achieved in hard tissue.

In the present project the structure of the implant surface is somewhat roughened by blasting. Carlsson et al. [47], using an animal model, measured the removal torques for two different surface textures (as-machined and electropolished) and examined the histological appearance of CP titanium implants 6 weeks after implantation in rabbit femora. Significantly higher removal torques were shown for the rough implants, with no difference in the amount of bone apposition.

The correct loading conditions are essential for any implant to become fully integrated into hard tissue. To satisfy this condition the implant is threaded, as mentioned above, and we allow extra time postoperatively for healing before full weight bearing is allowed.

One of the most neglected factors in implant applications today is the surgical technique. Even minor manipulation of bone tissue will cause heat formation, let alone reaming, sawing, and curing of polymethylmethacrylate (PMMA). In a combined clinical and experimental study, Eriksson and co-workers [48] investigated heat caused by drilling in cortical bone. With a drill speed of 20,000 rpm and saline cooling, average temperatures of 40°C in rabbits, 56°C in dogs, and 89°C (with a maximum registration of 96°C) in humans were recorded at a distance of 0.5 mm from the periphery of the drill hole. It is not unusual to heat the bone tissue to 90°–100°C during these procedures. On the other hand, that ample cooling with agents such as saline can reduce or prevent any temperature rise was demonstrated in a clinical study [49]. Placing a thermocouple 0.5 mm from the drill surface, the temperature rise in the mandible of patients was measured. The mean temperature rise during drilling, using adequate cooling technique with saline solution, was only 1.1°C (from 29.2° to 30.3°C). In order to reduce the surgical trauma we are extremely careful to use only very sharp instruments and generous cooling. The rotational symmetry of the implant simplifies the surgical procedure and eases control of surgical trauma. With the improved visibility enabled by our design, the rotational speed and pressure applied during bone cutting can be controlled much more readily than with the blind reaming of the femoral shaft, as in conventional femoral replacement.

When introducing a new hip arthroplasty, showing the viability of the concept over long periods of time is always a problem. It is now 30 years since Charnley introduced his revolutionary methods of hip surgery, and a vast body of knowledge and information has been accumulated over the time on surgical techniques, implant materials, cementing techniques, and follow-up and evaluation procedures, to name but a few areas.

Roentgenstereophotogrammetric analysis (RSA), a method developed by Selvik and co-workers [50], can be used to overcome the lack of detail inherent in many other methods of evaluation of implant performance. Both conventional radiography and clinical evaluation of stability are crude in the sense that impairment of implant function will not become evident until long after its onset.

Measurements of conventional radiographs can have a resolution of 1–5 mm and 1–6 degrees, depending on the technique employed, the anatomic region investigated, and the number of examinations. RSA of metallic markers implanted in the skeleton and prosthesis permits analysis of very small movements to much greater accuracy.

RSA can be separated into four stages:

1. *Implantation of tantalum markers*: Special tantalum balls with a diameter of 0.8 or 1 mm, are inserted in bone and prosthesis using a special spring-loaded piston. At least 3 noncolinear markers must be implanted in both skeleton and prosthesis; usually 5 or more markers are used.

2. *Radiographic examination*: Simultaneous exposures are taken by two roentgen tubes while the patient is inside a Plexiglas calibration cage fitted with tantalum markers at exactly known positions. The radiation doses at RSA examinations have proved to be low compared with equivalent conventional radiographic examinations.

3. *Measurements on radiographs*: The images of markers are numbered according to a standardized pattern. The two-dimensional position of each point is measured and stored in a computer. A digitizing tablet is used.

4. *Mathematical calculations*: The mathematical computations are performed with the aid of a personal computer. One computer program (X-ray) calculates the three-dimensional positions of the markers from the measured film coordinates. Another computer program (Kinerr®), detects and corrects erroneous identification of tantalum markers. This program also identifies and ignores loose tantalum balls. A further program (Kinlab), differentiates between three-dimensional point motion and rigid body motion. The film coordinates are transformed to a three-dimensional coordinate system using a projector of similarity transformation. Calculated movements of the rigid body can then be analyzed by the computer program Kinlab, which can represent them as rotation about and translations along three coordinate axes or a single axis called the *screw axis*. Relative movement between an optionally chosen, fixed reference segment (usually the skeleton) and movements of one or several rigid bodies or single tantalum balls can be calculated. Segment motion and translation of the rigid body can also be measured and analyzed.

The accuracy depends on the quality of the calibration equipment, image quality, film flatness, the position of the measuring instruments, and the number and configuration of the tantalum markers. The accuracy can be as high as 10 to 150 μm or 0.03° to 0.6°. The accuracy for examinations of hip joint prostheses is usually 0.3 to 0.4 mm and 0.4° to 0.6°.

Employing the RSA technique on conventional hip arthroplasties in prospective studies [51], it has been shown that implant function and survival can be predicted early to a high degree of accuracy. In other words, if the implant is initially stable, it will remain so over time, whereas an implant that demonstrates early movements in relation to the bone tissue of the implant site, will become increasingly loose with time and often eventually fail.

In a continuing pilot study using our newly designed hip arthroplasty, follow-up for over a year shows that implant stability and osseointegration can be achieved using our method of direct bone anchorage outlined above.

VI. THE GOTHENBURG OSSEOINTEGRATED HIP: CASE HISTORY

The follow-up is currently limited to less than 2 years; the Gothenburg osseointegrated hip system is still in the phase of clinical development and trial. One typical case is presented here. The patient is a male who was 66 years old at the time of operation. Preoperatively he had a Harris hip score (HHS) of 47, with severe pain at rest and during activity. He was using a crutch as support during outdoor walking. Maximal walking distance was less than 500 m. He was operated with a Gothenburg osseointegrated femoral component utilizing a modified Hardinge incision. The hip was dislocated and, using a specially constructed guide instrument, an osteotomy of the femoral neck was performed. A unique centralizing system and drill guide were used to drill a 10-mm hole starting in the cut femoral neck and extending through the lateral cortex. Using a guide rod placed in this 10-mm hole, the proximal 30 mm was reamed to a final diameter with optimal calcar contact. The acetabulum in this case was replaced with an Optifix (Smith and Nephew) acetabular component. All surgery was performed with a minimally traumatizing technique in accordance with the osseointegration protocol [40]. With trial reduction, leg length was controlled and stability was checked. Thereafter the hip was marked with 0.8 mm tantalum markers for the postoperative roentgenstereophotogrammetric (RSA) analysis. Gothenburg guide and cylindrical fixtures of appropriate length and diameter were connected and firmly fixed into each other to obviate fretting corrosion between the two fixtures. The assembled component was then inserted and screwed home until the collar rested firmly on the calcar. A ceramic acetabular head was added, the hip was reduced, and the wound was closed.

The postoperative progress was uneventful. The patient was allowed partial weight bearing using crutches for 3 months. Postoperatively at 3, 6, and 12 months RSA analyses were performed and, in addition, clinical evaluations were completed. The patient was totally pain-free at 3, 6, and 12 months of follow-up. The HHS increased to 93 at 12 months. He was not using any walking aids, had a range of movement of more than 90° of flexion, and walked without a limp. Radiographically there was some rounding off of the most proximal part of the calcar, but otherwise there were no changes in the bone or implant position during the first year. There were no radiolucent lines. RSA analyses demonstrated no migration in any direction. With such excellent clinical, radiographical, and RSA results, we conclude that it is possible to achieve good initial stability and

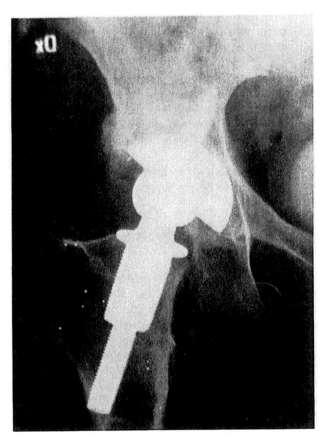

Figure 10   An osseointegrated hip model developed at our laboratories. Also visible are the small tantalum markers inserted for RSA measurements.

adequate clinical function without an intramedullary stem in the femoral diaphysis (Fig. 10). When clinical trials have been successfully completed, the system will be released for wider availability.

REFERENCES

1. Albrektsson, T., and Albrektsson, B., Osseointegration of bone implants. A review of an alternative mode of fixation, *Acta Orthop. Scand.,* *58,* 567–577, 1987.
2. Albrektsson, T., Repair of bone grafts. A vital microscopic and histological investigation, *Scand. J. Plast. Reconstr. Surg., 14,* 1–12, 1980.
3. Albrektsson, T., *In vivo* studies of bone grafts., *Acta Orthop. Scand., 51,* 9–17, 1980.
4. Eriksson, R. A., Heat-induced bone tissue injury. An in vivo investigation of heat tolerance of bone tissue and temperature rise in the drilling of cortical bone, Ph.D. thesis, University of Gothenburg, Sweden, 1984.
5. Eriksson, R. A., and Albrektsson, T., Temperature threshold levels for heat-induced bone tissue injury, *J Prosth. Dent., 50,* 101–107, 1983.

6. Jacobsson, M., On bone behaviour after irradiation, Ph.D. thesis, University of Gothenburg, Sweden, 1985.

7. Albrektsson, T., Jacobsson, M., and Turesson, I., Irradiation injury in bone tissue, *Acta Radiol. Oncol., 19,* 235–240, 1980.

8. Buch, F., On electrical stimulation of bone tissue, Ph.D. thesis, University of Gothenburg, Sweden, 1985.

9. Buch, F., Nannmark, U., and Albrektsson, T., A vital microscopic description of the effects of electrical stimulation of bone tissue, *J. Bioelectr., 5,* 105–128, 1986.

10. Nannmark, U., Buch, F., and Albrektsson, T., Vascular reactions during electrical stimulation. Vital microscopy of the hamster cheek pouch and the rabbit tibia, *Acta Orthop. Scand., 56,* 52–56, 1985.

11. Albrektsson, T., and Linder, L., A method for short- and long-term *in vivo* study of the bone–implant interface., *Clin. Orthop., 159,* 269–273, 1981.

12. Albrektsson, T., Implantable devices for long-term intravital microscopy of bone tissue, *CRC Crit. Rev. Biocompatibility, 3,* 25–51, 1987.

13. Ulrich, C., and Heinrich, H., Intrafemoral pressure in total hip replacement, in *Implant–Bone Interface* (J Older, ed.), Springer-Verlag, London, 1990, pp. 95–100.

14. Morberg, P., On bone tissue reactions to acrylic cement, Ph.D. thesis, University of Gothenburg, 1991.

15. Morberg, P., and Albrektsson, T., Bone reactions to intramedullary insertion of methylmethacrylate cement. A vital microscopic long-term *in vivo* study, *Eur. J. Exp. Musculoskel. Res., 1,* 11–17, 1992.

16. Albrektsson, T., Bach, A., Edshage, S., and Jonsson, A., Fibrin adhesive system (FAS) influence on the bone healing rate. A microradiographical evaluation using the bone growth chamber, *Acta Orthop. Scand., 53,* 747–753, 1982.

17. Albrektsson, T., Jacobsson, M., and Kalebo, P., The harvest chamber—A newly developed implant for analysis of bone remodelling *in situ,* in *Biomaterials and Biomechanics 83* (P. Ducheyne, G. van der Perre, and A. E. Aubert, eds.) Advances in Biomaterials 5, 1984, pp. 283–288.

18. Tjellstrom, A., Tympanoplasty with preformed autologous ossicles, Ph.D. thesis, University of Gothenburg, 1977.

19. Tjellstrom, A., Lindstrom, J., Albrektsson, T., Branemark, P.-I., and Hallen, O., A clinical pilot study on preformed, autologous ossicles I, *Acta Otolaryngol. (Stockholm), 85,* 33–39, 1978.

20. Tjellstrom, A., Lindstrom, J., Albrektsson, T., Branemark, P.-I., and Hallen, O., A clinical pilot study on preformed, autologous ossicles II, *Acta Otolaryngol. (Stockhohm), 85,* 232–242, 1978.

21. Tjellstrom, A., and Albrektsson, T., Five-year follow-up of preformed, autologous ossicles in tympanoplasty, *J. Laryngol. Otol., 99,* 729–733, 1985.

22. Albrektsson, T., Bach, A., Edshage, S., and Jonsson, A., Letter to the editor, *Acta Orthop. Scand., 54,* 656–658, 1983.

23. Jacobsson, M., Jonsson, A., Albrektsson, T., and Turesson, I., Dose–response for bone regeneration after single doses of ^{60}cobalt irradiation, *Int. J. Radiol., Oncol., Biol. Phys., 11,* 1963–1969, 1985.

24. Kalebo, P., On experimental bone regeneration in titanium implants. A quantitative, microradiographic and histologic investigation using the bone harvest chamber, Ph.D. thesis, University of Gothenburg, Sweden.

25. Jacobsson, M., Jonsson, A., Albrektsson, T., and Turesson, I., Short- and long-term effects of irradiation on bone regeneration, *Plast. Reconstr. Surg., 76,* 841–848, 1985.

26. Nilsson, L. P., Granstrom, G., and Albrektsson, T., The effect of hyperbaric oxygen treatment of bone regeneration, *Int. J. Oral Max. Fac. Implants, 3,* 43–48, 1987.

27. Granstrom, G., and Jacobsson, M., Titanium implants in the irradiated tissue. Benefits from

hyperbaric oxygen., in *First International Winter Seminar on Implants in Craniofacial Rehabilitation and Audiology* (T. Albrektsson, ed.), Lech, Austria, 1991, pp. 42–47.

28. Aspenberg, P., Albrektsson, T., and Thorngren, K.-G., Local applications of growth-factor IGF-1 to healing bone, *Acta Orthop. Scand., 60,* 607–610, 1989.

29. Roos, J., Sennerby, L., and Albrektsson, T., A modified harvest chamber for the study of the influence of local administration of growth factors on bone regeneration, submitted for publication, 1994.

30. Aspenberg, P., Goodman, S., Toksvig-Larsen, S., Ryd, L., and Albrektsson, T., Intermittent micromotion inhibits bone ingrowth, *Acta Orthop. Scand., 63,* 141–145, 1992.

31. Zarb, G. (ed.), Proceedings of the Toronto conference on osseointegration in clinical dentistry., *J. Prosth. Dent., 50,* 1983.

32. Branemark, P.-I., Zarb, G., and Albrektsson, T. (eds.), *Osseointegration in Clinical Dentistry,* Quintessence Publ., Chicago, 1985.

33. Albrektsson, T., Dahl, E., Enbom, I., Engevall, S., Engquist, B., Eriksson, R. A., Feldmann, G., Freiberg, N., Glantz, P.-O., Kjellman, P., Kristersson, L., Kvint, S., Kondell, P.-A., Palmquist, J., Werndahl, L., and Astrand, P., Osseointegrated oral implants. A Swedish multicenter study of 8139 consecutively inserted Nobelpharma implants, *J. Periodontol., 59,* 287–296, 1988.

34. Tjellstrom, A., Osseointegrated implants for the placement of absent or defective ears, *Clin. Plast. Surg., 17,* 355–366, 1990.

35. Tjellstrom, A., and Portmann, D., Application des implants osteointegres dans les epitheses et la prothese auditive, *Rev. Laryngol., 113,* 439–445, 1992.

36. Albrektsson, T., Branemark, P.-I., Jacobsson, M., and Tjellstrom, A., Present clinical applications of osseointegrated percutaneous implants, *Plast. Reconstr. Surg., 79,* 721–730, 1987.

37. Tjellstrom, A., and Jacobsson, M., Clinical applications of percutaneous implants, in *High Performance Biomaterials* (M. Szycher, ed.), Technomic Publ., Basel, 1991, pp. 207–230.

38. Tjellstrom, A., and Granstrom, G., Long-term follow-up with the bone anchored hearing aid: A review of the first 100 patients between 1977 and 1985, *ENT J., 73,* 21–23, 1994.

39. Granstrom, G., Bergstrom, K., and Tjellstrom, A., The BAHA and BAE in the rehabilitation of congenital ear malformations in *Third International Winter Seminar Implants in Craniofacial Rehabilitation and Audiology* (T. Albrektsson, M. Jacobsson, and A. Tjellstrom ,eds.), Selva, Val Gardena, Italy, 1993, p. 50.

40. Albrektsson, T., Branemark, P.-I., Hansson, H.-A., and Lindstrom, J., Osseointegrated implants. Requirements for ensuring a long-lasting, direct bone anchorage in man, *Acta Orthop. Scand., 52,* 155–170, 1981.

41. Malchau, H., Herberts, P., and Ahnfelt, L., Prognosis of total hip replacement in Sweden. Follow-up of 92,675 operations performed 1978–1990, *Acta Orthop. Scand., 64,* 497–506, 1993.

42. Carlsson, L., On the development of a new concept for orthopaedic implant fixation, Ph.D. thesis, University of Gothenburg, Sweden, 1989.

43. Rostlund, T., On the development of a new arthroplasty, Ph.D. thesis, University of Gothenburg, Sweden, 1990.

44. Albrektsson, T., On long-term maintenance of the osseointegrated response, *Aust. Prosthodon. J. 7*(suppl.), 1524, 1993.

45. Deines, D. N., Eick, J. D., Cobb, C. M., Bowles, C. Q., and Johnson, C. M., Photoelastic stress analysis of natural teeth and three osseointegrated implant designs, *Int. J. Periodont. Rest. Dent., 13,* 541–549, 1993.

46. Albrektsson, T., Branemark, P.-I., Hansson, H.-A., Kasemo, B., Larsson, K., Lundstrom, I., McQueen, D., and Skalak, R., The interface zone of inorganic implants *in vivo*: Titanium implants in bone, *Ann. Biomed. Eng. 11,* 1–27 (1983).

47. Carlsson, L., Rostlund, T., Albrektsson, B., and Albrektsson, T., Removal torques for polished and rough titanium implants, *Int. J. Oral Max. Fac. Implants, 3,* 21–24, 1988.

48. Eriksson, R. A., Albrektsson, T. and Albrektsson, B., Heat caused by drilling cortical bone. Temperature measured *in vivo* in patients and animals, *Acta Orthop. Scand.*, *55*, 629–631, 1984.

49. Eriksson, R. A., and Adell, R., Temperatures during drilling for the placement of implants using the osseointegration technique, *J. Oral Maxillofac. Surg.*, *44*, 4–7, 1986.

50. Selvik, G., A roentgen stereophotogrammetric method for the study of the kinematics of the skeletal system, Thesis, University of Lund, Sweden 1974; reprinted *Acta Orthop. Scand.*, *60*, suppl. 232 (1989).

51. Snorrason, F., Fixation of total hip arthroplasties. A clinical, radiographic and roentgen stereophotogrammetric analysis. Thesis, Umea University, Sweden, 1990.

IV
BONE REPAIR AND JOINT REPLACEMENT

20

Design Considerations for Cementless Total Hip Arthroplasty

Timothy McTighe
Joint Implant Surgery and Research Foundation, Chagrin Falls, Ohio

Lorence W. Trick
University of Texas Health Science Center, San Antonio, Texas

James B. Koeneman
Orthologic, Phoenix, Arizona

I. INTRODUCTION

"Technique, technique, technique" is a quote from David Hungerford, M.D. Technique is more important than design or material. In order for a surgical procedure to be considered a success, it must provide reproducible, satisfactory clinical results, reproducibility being the key word. The best implant put in poorly is not as good as the worst implant put in well.

Many varieties of designs for cementless total hip replacement are currently available and provide good to excellent results in the hands of their developers (Fig. 1). However, the challenge comes when these individual designs and techniques expand into the general marketplace. Too often general orthopedists do not appreciate the required technique for a given design. In addition, they often have less experience, and tend to overextend indications. Certainly clinical results have been less satisfactory in the young, active patient population [16,15,29].

There is no question that bone cement has made and continues to make a significant contribution to the success of total hip replacements. However, it is important to recognize its inherent biological and mechanical limitations (low modulus, low fatigue strength, potential toxicity, and propensity for late hematogenous infection). At this time, there continues to be a significant controversy about cement versus cementless fixation. This chapter reviews only cementless considerations.

This review covers anatomy, materials, testing, history, surgical technique, and a look into the immediate future for cementless total hip implants. It is our hope that this text will offer guidelines to students, residents, implant developers, and surgeons, as well as the orthopedic hip specialist.

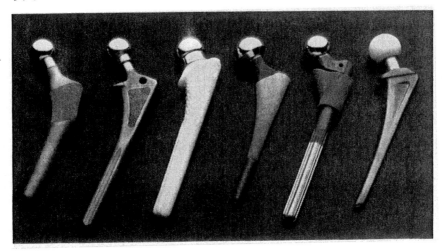

Figure 1 Varieties of cementless stems.

II. ACETABULAR CONSIDERATION

The hip joint is not a perfect ball-and-socket joint; the femoral head is oval in shape and the articular surface of the acetabulum is horseshoe shaped. The dome of the acetabulum, which has been considered a weight-bearing area, is in fact flexible (Fig. 2). The horns of the acetabulum can thus close up and contact the femoral head when the

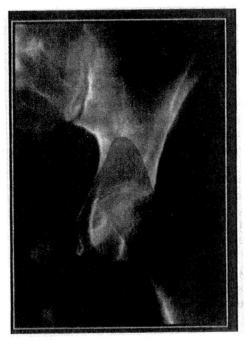

Figure 2 Radiolucent triangle.

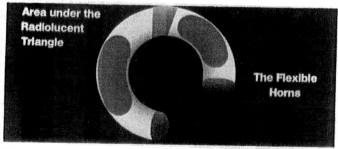

Figure 3 Principal weight bearing areas of the acetabulum.

joint is loaded [33,70]. The degree of this movement is dependent upon age, load, and femoral anteversion. This mobility of the acetabular horns could explain biomechanically the development of aseptic loosening that occurs around acetabular components.

Pauwels describes a radiolucent triangular space above the dome of the acetabulum [59] (Fig. 3). The shape of this triangle is subject to modifications that are dependent upon femoral loading orientation. In advanced osteoarthritis of the hip the surface area of this triangle decreases and vanishes. It is interesting to note that with age, the hip becomes more congruent and the radiolucent triangle disappears while a trabecular pattern becomes apparent.

Apart from the initial stability at the acetabular implant bone interface, some time after initial implantation is needed for the acetabular horns to become mobile again. This corresponds to radiographic evidence of radiolucent lines in zones 1 and 3 [8,27] (Fig. 4). In fact, clinical analysis of cemented devices demonstrates considerable progression of acetabular component loosening beyond the 12th year and even earlier in young, active patients [12,17,15,20,26]. This mobility might further explain finding little or no bone ingrowth on retrieved cementless implants [19,61,21,22,23]. Mobility of the acetabular horns must be considered in design parameters if long-term fixation is to be

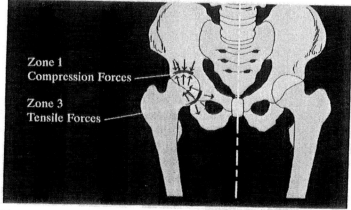

Figure 4 Compressive and tensile forces acting on acetabular components.

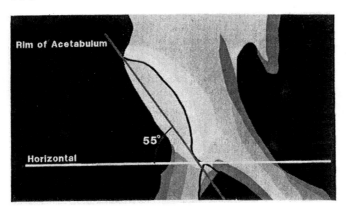

Figure 5 Orientation of acetabulum.

achieved. Fixation is enhanced if the prosthesis is set in a position of less than 45° abduction to promote compression and eliminate tension at the interfaces.

The acetabulum is generally spherical in shape (Fig. 5) and its opening is oriented closer to 55° than 45°, downward in the coronal and sagittal plane, and anteverted approximately 15° to 20° in the midsagittal plane.

Initial acetabular component stability is affected by the cup's ability to engage with the host bone. This is a function of cup design, size, and surgical technique. Cups of a true hemispherical design are more stable than low-profile designs [1]. Adjunct screw fixation can enhance initial stability but may contribute to osteolysis in the long term. Care should be taken to not penetrate intrapelvic structures by screws or drill bits. A study by Perona et al. demonstrated that the ilium provides the least amount of intrinsic support to cup fixation, while the anterior and posterior columns provide more stability [60]. Current technique attempts to press fit 1-2 mm of a hemispherical design and only use adjunct screw fixation when necessary. If a modular design is used with dome screw fixation, the anterior superior quadrant of the acetabulum should be avoided because it is the highest-risk area due to the medial intrapelvic vascular structures [73,40] (Fig. 6). When possible, peripheral screws should be used over dome screws due to their greater ability to restrict micromotion of the anterior and posterior columns in addition to being placed in a more appropriate safe zone away from intrapelvic vascular structures.

A. Acetabular Components

Cementless acetabular components are gaining popularity in the United States and in the rest of the world. These implants are indicated for both primary and revision surgery. It appears the bony matrix of the acetabulum is well suited for cementless fixation. Cementless fixation is best accomplished in the well-formed acetabulum where the shape is hemispheric and the implant can be placed in close apposition with the trabecular bone.

Historically, Phillipe Wiles is credited with implanting the first total hip replacement in 1938 [74]. The surgery was performed in London, England, and the implant consisted of two steel components. It was McKee, however, who began to popularize this procedure, beginning his development work in 1940 [49,50]. By 1951 only a limited clinical experience existed. His design consisted of a metal acetabular component that was secured by screw fixation. During this time, McKee helped to identify one of the key prob-

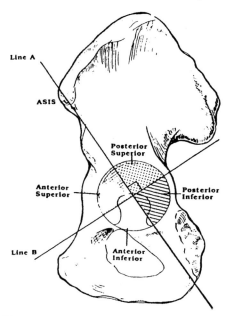

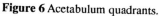

Figure 6 Acetabulum quadrants.

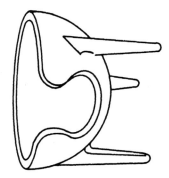

Figure 7 Urist cup.

lems in total joint fixation, namely, the distribution of forces at the interface between prosthesis and bone.

In 1957 Urist [72] evolved an acetabular cup endoprosthesis similar to the earlier Smith-Peterson cup (Fig. 7). His clinical results, however, were not encouraging since most patients required revision after 2-3 years.

In 1956 Sivash [38], of the Soviet Union, began work on an all-metal total hip design. By 1957 his acetabular model provided a helical thread on its outer surface with a 7 mm pitch and a 110 mm depth. This design proved to be difficult to insert and evolved into a 1962 modification. The 1962 design included four rows of circumferential blades (Fig. 8). Surgical technique required reaming the acetabular rim 3 mm smaller than the diameter of the prosthesis, which allowed the sharp edges to be impacted and rotated into the bony rim. Additional fixation was achieved by the use of screws placed through the rim of the prosthesis [68].

In 1969 Boutin, of France, introduced the use of porous ceramics as a means of attachment [10,11]. At about the same time, the Judet brothers began an acetabular design that achieved fixation through a series of bone screws but rapidly failed because of the acrylic head [39].

These developments created the initial interest in the search to find a satisfactory and enduring method of skeletal attachment for acetabular components. However, the introduction of acrylic bone cement for fixation by Charnley soon led to its widespread use and the abandonment of attempts to develop cementless designs [18]. As clinical reports of long-term cemented hip replacements began to emerge, concerns were raised about the mechanical longevity and the osteolytic potential of fragmented bone cement [75,36]. In an attempt to overcome some of these problems, Harris began a clinical series in the early 1970s utilizing a metal-backed component to be used with acrylic bone cement (Fig. 9). The metal-backed design sought to reduce peak stresses at the bone-cement

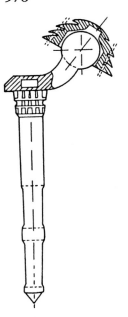

Figure 8 Sivash 1962 design.

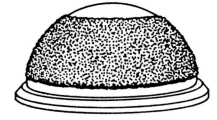

Figure 9 Harris cup.

interface, to contain and support the poly insert, and to reduce cold flow with the option of insert replacement due to wear [34].

In 1982 Noiles introduced the S-ROM™ threaded design that was evolved from the earlier Sivash design (Fig. 10). The design featured a low-profile, self-cutting cup that was inserted through impaction and torque. This was the first acetabular component that offered optional angled poly inserts to enhance joint stability.

Mallory, McTighe, and Noiles [51] further collaborated on the S-ROM by adding regionally placed porous coatings (Fig. 11). This design, called the Super Cup™, offers immediate mechanical skeletal fixation by the feature of threads and also allows for the potential of long-term bone ingrowth into the porous beads. This design continues to be used in the United States.

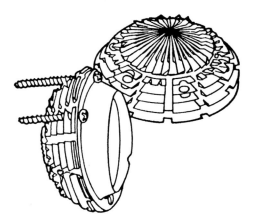

Figure 10 1982 S-ROM design.

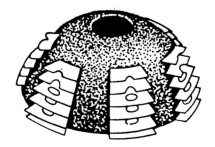

Figure 11 Super Cup design.

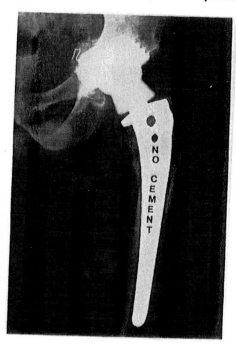

Figure 12 Mittelmeier ceramic cup and press fit stem.

Threaded acetabular components, as compared to porous press-fit designs, have had the longer history of cementless application in total hip arthroplasty. The Europeans have pioneered and championed this concept in both primary and revision surgery.

Lord [46] and Mittelmeier [56,57,58] have both reported comparable results, with approximately 90% good to excellent results for primaries and 75% good to excellent results for revisions. Mittelmeier continues to use his ceramic threaded device today (Fig. 12). The success of the Europeans spurred enthusiasm in usage in the United States and by 1986 threaded designs were being promoted by most implant companies.

Bierbaum, Capello, Engh, Mallory, Miller, and Murray are a few of the pioneers of clinical usage of threaded devices in the United States [51]. Each has encountered different degrees of success with various designs. As of this writing, none of these surgeons are currently using threaded devices for primary or revision surgery.

The lack of a full understanding of the design features and the required surgical technique, along with proper indications and contraindications, predisposed some of these devices to failure. First and foremost in the successful implantation of a cementless device, and particularly a threaded device, are exposure and surgical technique. Acetabular exposure must be greater for these devices than for conventional cemented cups. Threaded components have a major, or outside, diameter larger than that of the prepared dimensions of the acetabulum. It is therefore necessary to directly face the acetabulum for insertion of these threaded devices.

There are four basic classifications of threaded cup designs. It is crucial to understand the differences in these designs and most of all to understand the particular design chosen for implantation. A complete understanding of the design will enable the surgeon to maximize surgical techniques to achieve a good result.

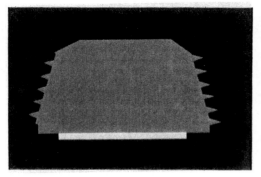

Figure 13 Truncated cone.

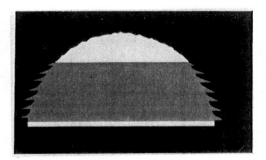

Figure 14 Hemispherical ring.

B. Threaded Cups

Classification of Threaded Cups

This section discusses four classifications of threaded cups:
- Truncated cone (Fig. 13)
- Hemispherical ring (Fig. 14)
- Hemispherical shell with conical threads (Fig. 15)
- Hemispherical shell with spherical threads (Fig. 16)

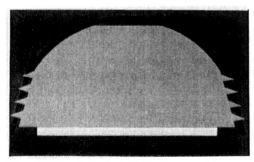

Figure 15 Hemispherical shell with conical threads.

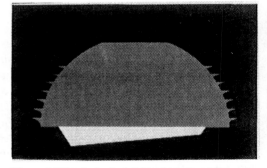

Figure 16 Hemispherical shell with spherical threads.

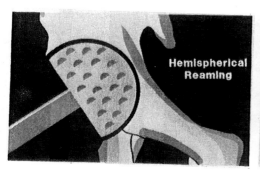

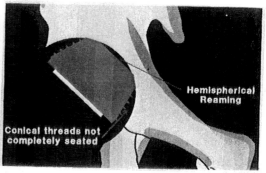

Figure 17 Hemispherical reaming.

Figure 18 Hemispherical reaming with truncated cup.

1. Truncated Cone

The truncated cone is the design of most European systems, including both Lord and Mittelmeier devices. Whether the truncated cone design is a cup or a ring, the geometry of a truncated cone makes the design inherently very stable. However, it does require more bone removal than a hemispherical design (Fig. 17).

Although very successful in Europe, these designs have not met with great acceptance in North America. The surgical technique required to ensure proper seating for a truncated cone is quite demanding. If reamed spherically, the threads engage very little bone (Fig. 18). If deepened with the reamer, contact between implant and bone is increased. However, bone stock is sacrificed. It appears the device must penetrate subchondral bone in the medial wall to ensure maximum purchase (Fig. 19).

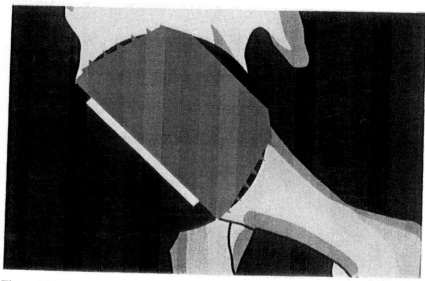

Figure 19 Proper position for truncated cone cup.

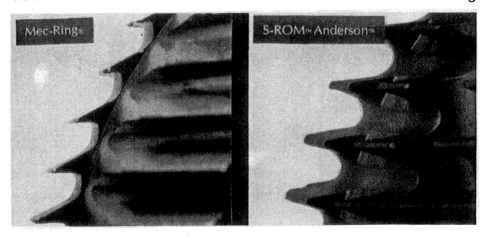

Figure 20 Thread profiles.

2. Hemispherical Ring

The Mec-ring™ from Germany appears to be the most popular ring design. It is a threaded ring, spherical in shape, with a large apical hole. This apical hole allows the poly insert to protrude through the ring, thus interfacing with the prepared acetabular bony bed.

A close look at this design raises some questions and concerns. The thread buttress angle provides for maximum pull-out resistance. However, this is not the mode of loading for threaded cups. Since the majority of the loads placed on the acetabular component are in compression, a horizontal thread profile would be more appropriate for proper load transfer (Fig. 20). An extremely large apical hole allows for more load transfer to the thin fossa as compared to designs that have either a small hole or an enclosed dome (Fig. 21).

The designs with a smaller hole do not allow the poly inserts to protrude through the hole. These are classified as cups, not rings.

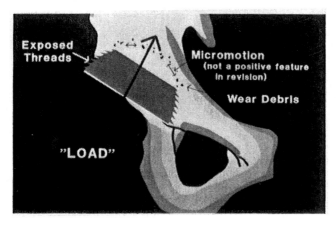

Figure 21 Threaded ring.

In revision situations where the subchondral bone is diminished or lost, loading should be transferred to the periphery to protect or shield this area.

Earlier designs had only neutral-angle poly inserts requiring a more horizontal orientation of the cup to ensure joint stability. This type of positioning can compromise bony coverage of the implant, resulting in less implant fixation. In addition, if any micromotion occurs between poly insert and bone, the possibility of wear debris exists [71,43].

3. Hemispherical Shell with Conical Threads

This is the design of most U.S. manufacturers. The hemispherical shell has an advantage over a truncated cone because it allows preservation of the subchondral bone by reaming hemispherically. The conical threads are much easier to design and manufacture as compared to spherical threads. However, the conical thread does compromise maximum potential for seating the entire thread into a hemispherically reamed acetabulum.

4. Hemispherical Shell with Spherical Threads

The S-ROM Anderson™ Cup was the first hemispherically domed shell with spherical threads. Note that the thread buttress angle provides maximum resistance to the compression loads going into the acetabulum. The apical hole is small enough to reduce

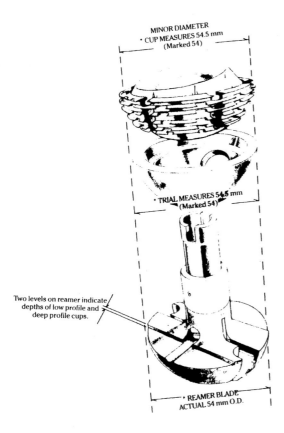

Figure 22 Reamer versus threaded cup diameter.

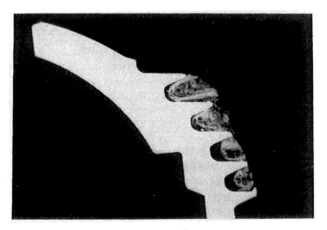

Figure 23 Cross section of retrieved threaded cup.

loads that are transferred through the apex; however, the hole is still large enough for visualization and access for bone graft material.

The major diameter of the thread is 5 mm greater than the diameter of the trial. Therefore, the penetration of each thread is 2.5 mm relative to the dome and flute spherical surface. The actual thread minor diameter, or root diameter, is such that the root of each thread lies 0.5 mm below the dome and cutting flute's spherical surface, thus allowing 0.5 mm space for bone chips from thread cutting to accumulate (Fig. 22).

By 1990 most threaded devices, with the exception of the S-ROM Super Cup, had been discontinued from routine use in both primary and revision surgery (Fig. 23).

It is important to note that threaded acetabular components are not all the same, just as porous and cemented designs are not all the same. Only full understanding of the chosen design and the required technique for that design will ensure a good, long-lasting result.

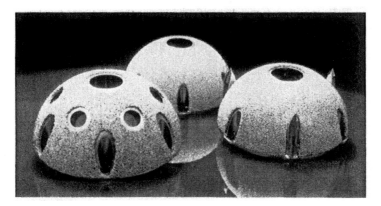

Figure 24 Porous cups.

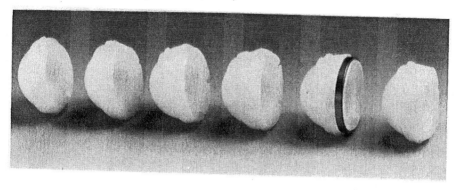

Figure 25 Polyethylene lines available in different angles.

C. Modular Acetabular Components

Two-piece, modular porous acetabular components have gained major market acceptance in total hip arthroplasty (Fig. 24). The main advantage over threaded devices is ease of insertion. Adjunct fixation can be enhanced by bone screw fixation. Polyethylene liners come in a variety of head diameters as well as offering different offset angles to enhance head coverage (Fig. 25). However, as pointed out by Krushell et al., elevated polyethylene liners are not without problems [42]. Elevated rim liners increase range of motion in some directions and decrease range of motion in other directions. They do not in any global sense provide greater range of motion than a neutral liner. Therefore, routine use of an elevated rim liner is not recommended. If a cup is malpositioned, a liner might offer some immediate implant stability; however, polyethylene is not a good material for structural support, and cold flow, deformation, disassociation, and late joint dislocation are real probabilities. It is preferable to reposition the metal cup rather than relying on polyethylene to function under high loads.

However, these modular designs are not without problems. Since their introduction, osteolysis due to particulate debris has increased in cementless total hip arthroplasty.

The most common cause of proximal, femoral bone loss is due to osteolysis [52,9] (Fig. 26). Although the specific cause of lysis is not known, it has been attributed to a variety of factors such as motion of the implant. Foreign-body reaction to particulate debris, in particular to polymeric debris, probably plays the greatest role. It has been almost two decades since Willert et al. first described the problem of polyethylene wear

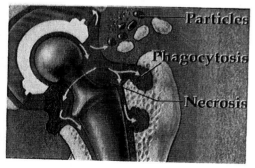

Figure 26 Osteolysis.

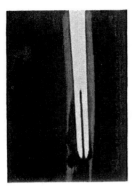

Figure 27 Bone loss due to particulate debris generated osteolysis.

leading to periprosthetic inflammation, granuloma, bone resorption, and implant loosening [75]. Since then, many studies have documented the finding of particulate bone cement and polyethylene in periprosthetic tissue [36,66].

In normal-wearing artificial joints, linear wear rates of 0.05-0.2 mm per year result in the generation of about 25-100 mm (25-100 mg) of polyethylene debris annually. On a basis of known dimensions of polyethylene particles found in tissue around the hip prosthesis, this equates to the annual production of tens to hundreds of billions of particles [9].

Variations of polyethylene wear rates probably relate to acetabular implant design, femoral head size, femoral head material, and at least in part to the quality of the polyethylene used [44,2]. Wide variations are known to exist between batches of polyethylene and between different polyethylene suppliers [76].

Metal particulate debris generated from the stem or cup in sufficient quantities could activate macrophage-mediated osteolysis. More likely the cause is the migration of metallic debris into the articulation, resulting in increased third-body wear of polyethylene (Fig. 27). Additional poly debris can be generated by poor modular designs, incomplete conformity of the liner within the metal cup, thin polyethylene resulting in cold flow, and wear through and abrasion of screw heads against the convex polyethylene surface (Fig. 28).

Problems with excessive wear due to titanium bearing surfaces have been reported (Fig. 29). In addition, clinical evidence indicates higher volumetric wear with 32 mm heads.

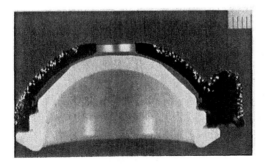

Figure 28 Incomplete conformity of cup and poly insert.

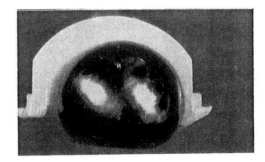

Figure 29 Excess wear due to titanium head.

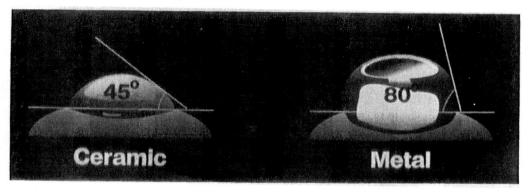

Figure 30 Wettability of ceramic versus metal.

Ideally, the bearing surface for most sliding (Fig. 30), rotating, or articulating bearing surfaces will be made from material having relatively high strength, high wear, and corrosion resistance; a high resistance to creep; and low frictional movements. In reality no one material presently exhibits all of these characteristics. Therefore, with present bearing systems compromises are typically made between these various characteristics. There are, however, some immediate steps that can be taken to reduce the generation of particulate debris.

1. Use ultra-high molecular weight polyethylene with high ratings in key mechanical and physical properties.
2. Use non-modular, molded acetabular components.
3. Use modular components with:
    *   High conformity and support.
    *   Secure locking mechanism.
    *   Minimum polyethylene thickness 6-8 mm.
4. Use a 28 mm or smaller head diameter.
5. Do not use titanium alloy as a bearing surface.
6. Minimize modular sites on femoral side to reduce chances of third-particle wear debris.

III. FEMORAL CONSIDERATION

The femoral head is slightly larger than one half of a sphere, and the shape is more oval than spherical. The stresses on the femoral head usually act on the anterior superior quadrant, and surface motion can be considered as sliding on the acetabulum. Two important angles need to be considered: the neck shaft angle and the angle of anteversion. In addition to these two angles, the joint reaction force is affected by femoral head offset [28,65,37]. It is also important to remember that while static force is considerably greater than body weight, even greater force is generated posteriorly in dynamic situations such as acceleration and deceleration: manifest in negotiating stairs or inclines, in changing from a sitting to a standing position or vice versa, and in other routine activities of daily living that load the hip in flexion.

The biological response of bone to stress greatly affects the outcome of cementless total hip arthroplasty. The adaptive bone remodeling process, "Wolff's law", must be taken into consideration in deciding on material, geometry, and size selection for cementless femoral components. Many clinical and radiological studies have demonstrated the sensitivity of this adaptive remodeling process [31] (Fig. 31).

It has been shown that trabecular microfracture and remodeling is a major mode of accelerated remodeling in response to changes in mechanical demands on the bone [32]. Trabeculae that fail, either by fatigue mode or by overloading, will disappear if the ends do not contact each other and if the resulting trabecula bears no load (disuse atrophy). However, if the fractured trabecula realigns itself and the fracture site still maintains control such that the structure is able to transmit load, the trabecula will remodel in the new direction much more quickly than through the mechanism of ordered resorption and apposition. Interfaces created surgically within the structure and subsequently loaded by mechanical means result in severe overloading of the remaining cancellous structure.

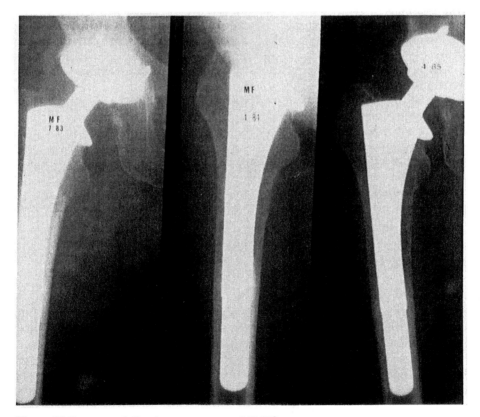

Figure 31 Bone remodeling in a porous coated AML® stem.

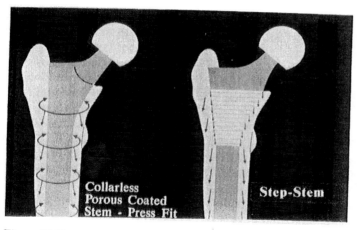

Figure 32 Hoop stresses versus compressive stresses.

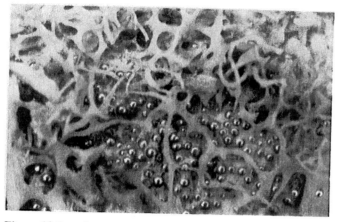

Figure 33 Bone ingrowth into a porous surface.

Cancellous bone is a poor material for structural support of a prosthesis. Cancellous bone is a biological engineered material, and its strength depends on its having the entire bulk of the structure intact. The creation of an interface with areas of cancellous bone disproportionately weakens the structure. In addition, interfacing an implant with cancellous bone merely serves to increase the stress at the interface to a level that causes fatigue failure of the bone [62].

Through proper design and surgical technique, one can achieve significant enhancement of the mechanical properties of the procedure consistent with basic biomechanical principles. It is recommended that most, if not all, of the cancellous bone be removed. Structuring the surface of an implant will minimize the surface shear stresses. In addition, structuring will transfer hoop stresses into compression stresses within the femur (Fig. 32). For an uncemented femoral component to be successful it is universally agreed that initial stability is essential. In addition, there must be a mechanism to ensure long-term bony fixation (Fig. 33).

During the past three decades, techniques, materials, and prosthetic designs for cementless total hip arthroplasty have been improved significantly. During the last 15 years in particular, there has been a growing movement into more complex cementless designs, particularly in the area of modularity. (Fig. 34). Not all cementless designs are equal, and it is important to understand certain design features that segregate individual implants into specific categories within the cementless group. Some appear to be successful whereas others have failed rapidly. To date, all current cementless designs have one feature in common — a modular head. So the simplest of designs features a unibody stem with a modular head that takes either a metal or ceramic articulation (Fig. 35). However, there is a fast-growing trend to add additional modular features to aid in achieving initial implant-to-bone stability by better fit and fill criteria, that is, maximization of endosteal contact.

Replacement of the normal position of the femoral head is essential for correction of mechanical balance between abductor forces. This is addressed by vertical height, version angle, and medial offset of the head relative to the axis of the stem (Fig. 36). If vertical height is too short, joint stability is a problem. If too long, patient complaints result and nerve palsy is possible. Incorrect version angle can result in reduced range of

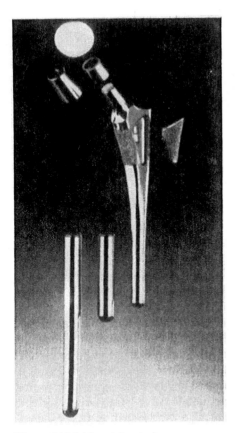

Figure 34 Multimodular design.

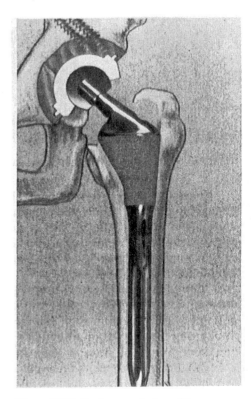

Figure 35 Unibody stem design with modular head.

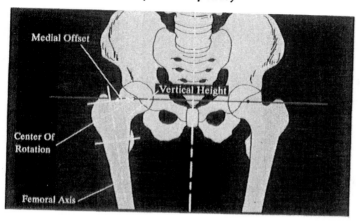

Figure 36 Biomechanical function.

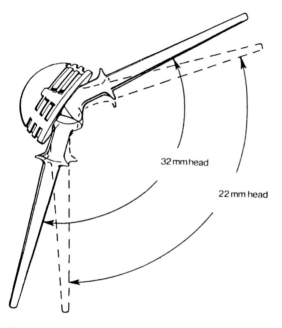

32 mm head

22 mm head

Figure 37 Range of motion.

motion and possible hip dislocations. Medial offset that is too short will cause shortening of the abductor moments, and there will be greater resultant force across the hip joint. If offset is too great, increased torsional forces will be placed on the femoral implant. For a femoral component to be successful it must have initial torsional stability with or without cement.

Modular head diameters are available from 22 to 32 mm. Charnley strongly advocated a 22 mm head due to its lower frictional properties [17]. However, joint stability is not as good as in a larger-diameter head (Fig. 37). Most designers and surgeons now compromise on a 26 or 28 mm diameter, which provides adequate polyethylene thick-

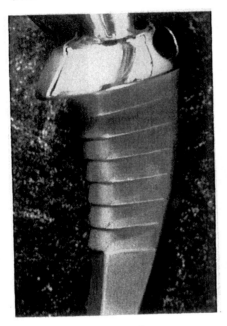

Figure 38 Betchel stepped stem.

ness on the acetabular bearing side, as well as improved range of motion and stability compared with a 22 mm diameter [44].

Normally the femur is loaded from the outside cortex, and stresses are transferred internally. However, in a stemmed reconstruction the biomechanical loading has been changed to an internal loading mechanism. Intramedullary stems place an unnatural hoop stress on the bone. This hoop stress must be transferred into compressive loads to the

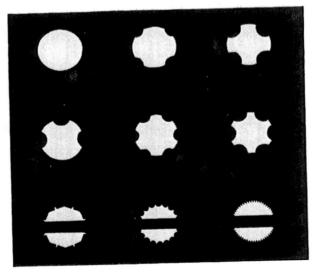

Figure 39 Distal Cross-Sectional Geometry.

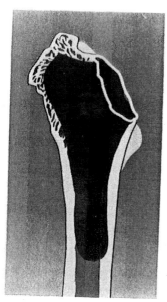

Figure 40 Femoral cavitary and segmental defect.

proximal femur. One way to help accomplish this is to design proximal steps into the femoral component. Early endoprosthetic stems were developed by Bechtol in 1954, the "Stepped Prosthesis"™, and a later one by Townley also featured this stepped-design concept (Fig. 38). However, the idea was not revisited until Pughs' work in 1981 led to the OmniFit™ design and his additional work that led to the 1984 S-ROM proximal sleeve design [62,63].

A. Femoral Components

The objective for cementless total hip stems of long-term pain-free stability is dependent on both primary and secondary fixation of the implant to the bone. An effective cementless stem should resist subsidence, tilting and torsional forces.

Primary mechanical stability is, therefore, a prerequisite for long-term success. Torsional fixation of the femoral component is considered the most important criteria for long-term success [48]. It is only logical that design features that improve fixation are likely to improve clinical results.

Although there may be advantages in bone remodeling by initial stability by proximal fixation, irregularity in shape and structure of the bone in the metaphyseal area can compromise stability. It has been previously reported that a constant proportional relationship is not present between the shape and size of the metaphysis and diaphysis. In addition the revision situation results in alterations in the normal bony architecture, making fit and fill more difficult to achieve [47,67]. Distal stem stability enhances overall initial stability of the implant in both primary and revision total hip arthroplasty. (Fig. 39).

With cavitary and segmental bone damage it is difficult to achieve stability of the implant (Fig. 40). In this situation some authors have previously recommended distal fixation. It is our opinion that distal stability is preferable over distal fixation. This can be achieved by fluting the distal end of the stem. Whiteside [48] and Koeneman [45] have shown that fluting offers more initial stability in torsion as compared to a fully porous coated stem.

It is generally agreed that the better the fit and fill ratio of the femoral component, the better the initial stability and potential for long-term fixation. Over the past 10 years fit and fill has taken several approaches: (1) a large quantity of sizes (unibody); (2) modularity; and (3) custom (intraoperative or preoperative).

B. Unibody Stems

Due to concerns that modular sites generate particulate debris along with social-economical pressures, there is a strong movement back to one-piece stem designs, especially for routine primary hip reconstruction. The challenge for unibody designs as with all designs is to optimize fit and fill, to ensure optimal loading of stress to the proximal femur, to avoid the problems of torsional and axial instability while providing for reproducible surgical technique.

Currently there is considerable controversy as to straight (Fig. 41) vs. anatomical (Fig. 42) and collar vs. collarless stem designs. In an attempt to appeal to both mentalities, newer geometric designs (Fig. 43) are emerging. These designs feature straight stems with anterior flares and anteverted necks.

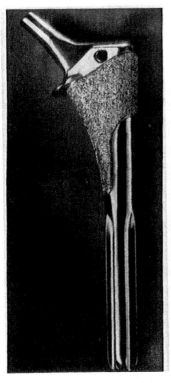 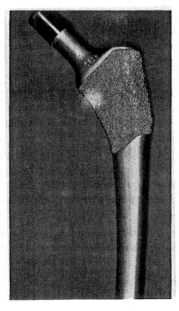 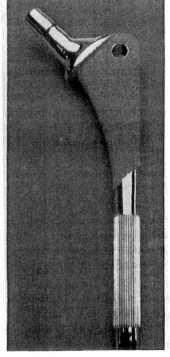

Figure 41 Multilock™ straight stem. **Figure 42** PCA™ Anatomic stem. **Figure 43** Replica™ geometric stem.

C. Modular Stems

The concept of modularity is to provide for intraoperative customization of fit and fill with each individual femur. There are a variety of modular designs available, from modular necks (Fig. 44), proximal (Fig. 45) and distal sleeves (Fig. 46), and mid-stem tapers (Fig. 47). Each design has specific features and benefits and requires complete knowledge of each individual design and surgical technique.

While modular designs represent an advance in the ability to precisely fit the implant to the bone, the mechanical integrity of the assembled component must be fully tested prior to clinical usage. Machining methods, tolerances, surface characteristics, materials, electrochemical environment and mechanical environment are all critical factors that

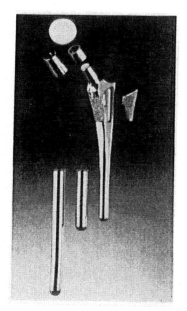

Figure 44 Modular neck.

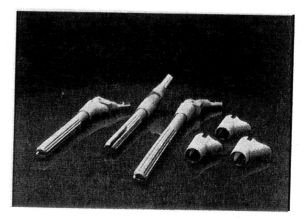

Figure 45 S-ROM stem.

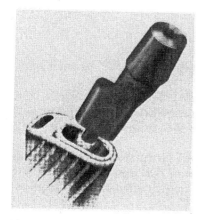

Figure 46 Example modular distal sleeves.

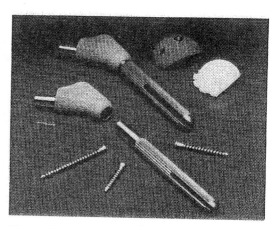

Figure 47 Mid-stem taper design.

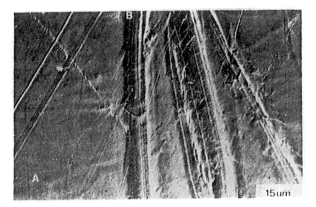

Figure 48 Example of increased wear of bearing surface.

need careful consideration in evaluating the long-term performance of modular inter-faces [69].

In evaluating the mechanical performance of cementless femoral stems, there is no single test that can adequately represent the various bony conditions that a hip stem may be subjected to invivo. This in part explains the wide variance in testing methods found today.

Recently, concern about particulate debris generated by modular interfaces has been raised. In fact, we are now beginning to see published reports concerning in-vitro testing of modular designs [41,24]. One major concern of metal particulate debris, is the possibility of increasing the rate bearing surfaces wear (Fig. 48).

Modularity has been shown to be cost-effective and offers many intraoperative custom capabilities [47,67]. Short-term results are very encouraging and have high appeal

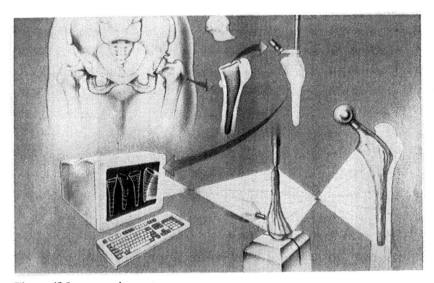

Figure 49 Intraoperative custom.

for revisions and difficult primaries such as congential dysplasia [14]. However, modularity has made surgical technique more demanding.

D. Custom Stems

Customs offer great versatility; however, intraoperative customs reduce surface treatments such as hydroxyapatite (HA) or porous surfaces (Fig. 49). In addition, there is the concern of increased operating room time and the difficulty in achieving reproducible, clinical and surgical results [30]. As for preoperative customs, again, in routine cases there are no outcome data to support this approach over standard off-the-shelf designs, which generally speaking are less costly. It will take another 10 years of clinical comparison to judge whether customs have an advantage over standard off-the-shelf cementless devices. This is one problem in total joint surgery that does not seem to exist in other medical disciplines. In the meantime, it follows that advances must be made based mainly on theoretical grounds, good solid, basic science, and animal experimentation rather than on short-term clinical evaluations by the implant-developing surgeon in a small number of patients.

Obviously there is a need for all three types of implant modalities: unibody, modular, and customs (although these are not necessary with adequate modularity).

However, the surgeon must be aware of all the design features and pick and choose the appropriate design indicated for individual patients. No one design is going to fill all the needs that are found in total hip replacement surgery today. The future challenge will be to address growing indications in a restricted health care financial market.

IV. MATERIAL CONSIDERATION

Biomedical materials are synthetic polymers, biopolymers, natural macromolecules, metals, ceramics, and inorganics such as hydroxyapatite. For materials to be used successfully in the body, they must have minimal degradation in the body, they must be compatible with the biological environment, and they must be strong enough to perform their intended purpose.

Stainless steel, especially 316L, has been used for many years as an implant material [3,5]. Early total joint replacements and current internal fracture fixation devices utilize stainless steel. In some designs this material has shown crevice corrosion. Cobalt-chrome alloys have been popular as implant materials because of their corrosion resistance and good wear properties. CoCrMo alloy is typically used in devices that are cast.

Forged parts are made from CoNiCrMo alloy. These alloys have relatively high elastic moduli. A desire for a lower modulus material led to the use of titanium and its alloys. Commercially pure titanium is used because of its corrosion resistance, but it is not used in applications that require high structural strength. The titanium alloy that has been most widely used in orthopedic applications is the Ti6Al4V alloy. This material has good fatigue properties but is softer and has lower resistance to wear, especially when extraneous materials are introduced [2,6]. Surface treatments of these alloys have shown improved wear resistance. Titanium alloys with moduli even lower than the Ti6Al4V alloy are beginning to be used. Specialty applications that utilize a change in part shape after implantation use an alloy that is approximately one half nickel and one half titanium, which returns to an original shape under body temperature. These materials are tolerated well by body tissues. Tantalum has excellent biocompatibility and is used for markers

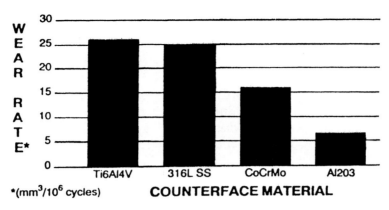

Figure 50 Wear rates.

because of its high radiodensity. With all metals there has been a concern for long-term protein-metal interactions and hypersensitivity of individuals to some of the metal ions that diffuse into body tissues.

Aluminum oxide ceramics have been used extensively as bearing surfaces in artificial joints because of its excellent wear properties [25,57,64] (Fig. 50). It has not been used extensively for other structural applications because of its high elastic modulus and brittleness. Zirconia has been introduced recently as an alternative to aluminum oxide.

Polymeric composite materials have been investigated as implant materials. Carbon, glass, quartz, and polymeric fibers have been used for the reinforcing phase, and carbon (carbon-carbon composites), epoxy, polyetheretherketone (PEEK), polybutadiene, and polysulfone have been used as matrices.

Initial testing of artificial implants was prompted by a fatigue fracture rate of about 3% in early (1970s) femoral stems of artificial hip implants [6] (Fig. 51). The test methods that were developed simulated the failure mode of these early implants. Both the American Society for Testing and Materials (ASTM) and the International Standardiza-

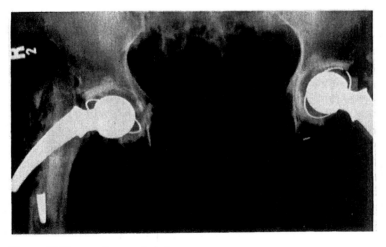

Figure 51 Fractured cemented stem.

tion Organization (ISO) have test methods for femoral stems that support the distal stem and leave the proximal stem unsupported. Although noncemented stems rarely have this type of failure mode, these stems are often tested with this test method. The disadvantage of the method is that if the stem is designed to pass the test, it encourages a bulky and stiff design. This is the opposite of what is needed for maintenance of bone strain and what is desired to combat bone resorption due to stress shielding. An alternative test method that has been reported utilizes proximal fixation with a free distal stem except for a point load on the lateral stem. Both ASTM and ISO are developing test methods to be used with low-stiffness stems. Similar fatigue tests have been developed for other joints such as the knee. Loading typically is at high frequency and at loads higher than expected in service. Ten million cycles has been chosen as representing a run-out; that is, the load is probably below the endurance limit.

V. SOCIAL–ECONOMIC CONSIDERATION

There is no debate on the fact that cost is becoming more and more an influence on the decision process for medical treatments and on product development programs.

A. The Current Health Care Environment

The health care environment includes the following important characteristics:
- Enormous duplication of services
- Competition among providers
- Technology that changes faster than clinical practice
- Pressure from payers for less costly service
- Pressure on providers to deliver care in a capitated environment
- Vertical Integration and consolidation
- Pressure for information on the value of new approaches

B. Factors Influencing Adoption of New Technology

Several factors are involved in adoption of new technology:
- Method of financing the initial cost
- Method of recovering operating costs
- Level of regulation
- Degree of competition
- Institutional capacity for technology assessment
- Organizational relationships: shared risk means slower adoption

C. Implications for Developers

Developers need to consider the following:
- Move from better medicine to better medical economics
- *New* is not synonymous with *improved*
- Expect a bumpy ride in an increasingly volatile market
- Focus product development
- "In God We Trust. All others bring data."

VI. IMMEDIATE FUTURE TRENDS AND PRODUCTS

Use of modularity in the acetabulum has contributed to significant debris generation problems (Fig. 52) [4,9]. This trend is slowly reversing and it is predicted that developers will go back to preassembled, metal-backed, porous-coated devices with molded polyethylene inserts rather than machined. One such ideal design would have the following characteristics:

- Hemispherical shape
- Sintered, porous beads for ingrowth
- Polyethylene, compression molded directly to metal shell
- Peripheral screw holes for adjunct fixation with no dome screw holes and/or a capping mechanism to seal the holes
- Neutral poly liner (no offsets)

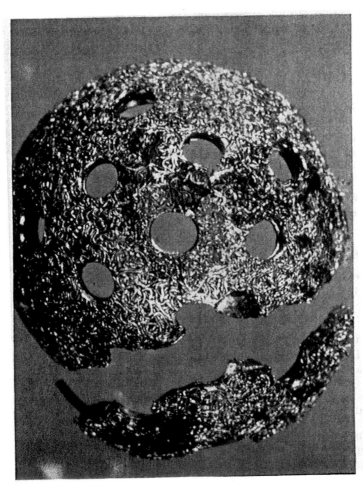

Figure 52 Failed porous mesh cementless cup.

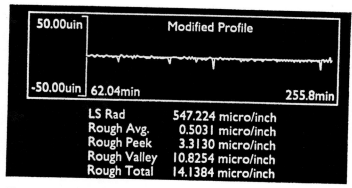

LS Rad	547.224 micro/inch
Rough Avg.	0.5031 micro/inch
Rough Peek	3.3130 micro/inch
Rough Valley	10.8254 micro/inch
Rough Total	14.1384 micro/inch

Figure 53 Surface finish for ceramic femoral head.

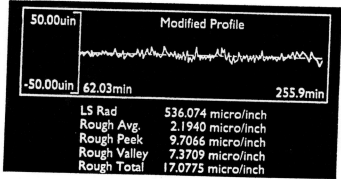

LS Rad	536.074 micro/inch
Rough Avg.	2.1940 micro/inch
Rough Peek	9.7066 micro/inch
Rough Valley	7.3709 micro/inch
Rough Total	17.0775 micro/inch

Figure 54 Surface finish for CoCr femoral head.

VII.   NEAR FUTURE PRODUCTS

Ceramics have characteristics that are very desirable for use in sliding, rotating, and articulating bearing surfaces (Figs. 53 and 54). In addition to high compressive strength, they exhibit high wear and corrosion resistance with relatively low frictional movements. However, use of such ceramic materials in bearing systems has been inhibited because such materials are susceptible to fracture due to their relatively low tensile and shear strengths. This weakness is one reason why metal and/or polymeric materials have been used for many bearing surfaces. Compared to bearing ceramics, bearing metals and polymers typically have lower wear and corrosion resistance and higher frictional movements.

In bearing systems where ceramics have been used, their low tensile and shear strengths often force the adoption of costly design compromises. Thus, one design compromise has been to make the entire bearing component, rather than just a portion thereof, out of solid ceramic, effectively increasing the structural strength of the bearing surface. Such a solid ceramic bearing component can be larger and bulkier than its metal and/or

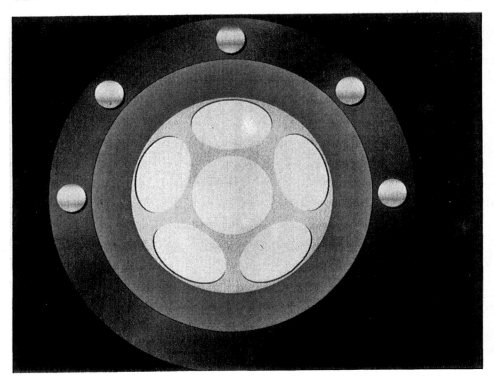

Figure 55 Segmented ceramic cup.

polymeric counterpart.

Making an entire bearing component such as the acetabular cup out of solid ceramic helps to compensate for the relatively poor tensile and shear strength typically found with ceramics. Also, because bearing ceramics are typically inflexible, additional manufacturing quality control of the geometry of both articular surfaces must be maintained in order to maximize the contact area between the two surfaces. If tight control is not maintained, point contact may develop between the bearing surfaces. As the contact area between two bearing surfaces decreases, the stress that is transmitted between the surfaces increases. This can result in greater wear and can increase the possibility of fracture of one or both surfaces [35,64].

In an attempt to address these problems, a segmented, ceramic bearing system has been developed [53] (Fig. 55). The segmented bearing system provides ceramic surfaces for mechanical bearings that would apply loads over a greater bearing area, resulting in reduced bearing stresses and would, in turn, reduce creep, wear, and the likelihood of fracture of the bearing surfaces.

The acetabular component is designed with ceramic articular segments that are backed and held in a predetermined pattern and configuration by either polyetheretherketone or polyethylene. Both of these materials have a lower elastic modulus than the segmented ceramic material. In addition, the polymeric material is reduced in height so that only the

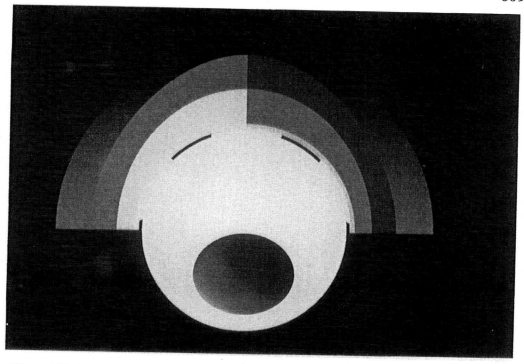

Figure 56 Lubrication channels in segmented cup.

segmented ceramic material articulates with a ceramic femoral head.

Because of its resilience and lower elastic modulus, the polymeric material flexes as loads are transmitted between bearing surfaces while the shape of the surfaces of the segments remain relatively unchanged. This freedom of movement of the segments, under an applied load, allows for greater contact area between bearing surfaces because the segments as a group are able to conform to the geometry of the opposing bearing surface. Thus, rather than having the highly localized stress concentrations typically occurring in bearing systems, any applied load is shared by a number of segments, which results in lower stress being applied to the bearing surface and each segment.

An additional feature of this design is the formation of channels generated by locating the polymeric material slightly below the surface of the ceramic segments for lubrication and for allowing debris that finds its way into the bearing to either pass between the segments or be trapped into the polymeric material (Fig. 56).

This design allows for the segmented composite insert to be used with cemented hemispherical designs or cementless acetabular components. This highly innovative design provides for an alternative bearing surface that is cost-effective while it reduces or eliminates the generation of articulated polymeric or metallic debris. This design should have a tremendous positive effect on the overall reduction of particulate debris, resulting in increased longevity of total hip arthroplasty.

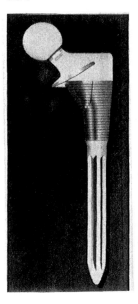

Figure 57 Unibody stem.

VIII. NEW DESIGN CONCEPT

In light of all that has been discussed, this section provides a review and current description of a new cementless total hip system. This system is a comprehensive system designed for primary and revision total hip replacement arthroplasty.

Patients face a variety of problems and solutions must be tailored to their individual needs.

A. Unibody Stem

This stem is a geometric design that features a proximal anterior flare that works in tandem with a 30° proximal conical flare collar. These two specific features aid in axial and torsional stability while providing increased surface geometry, resulting in increased compressive stress to the proximal femur. The neck shaft angle is 135° with 10° of antevision. Lateral displacement of the femoral head is 40 mm.

The proximal conical collar allows for settling of the implant resulting in increased surface contact throughout the entire proximal stem geometry. In addition, the conical shape acts as a step in transferring hoop stress into compressive loads.

While providing improved fit and fill, the proximal conical shape provides a seal occluding wear debris from entering the femoral canal (Fig. 57).

B. Bibody Modular Stem

This stem's design incorporates a proximal, modular body that allows for correction of version, offset, and vertical height without disruption of the stem body. The two modular parts feature a double locking mechanism. The first is a trunion that engages in the stem

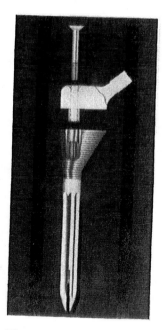

Figure 58 Bibody stem.

body by means of ratchet teeth. The specific design of these ratchet teeth allow for version adjustment in increments of 10°. The second locking feature is a set screw, which protects from disassembly.

The unique features of this design traps any debris that might be generated by the modularity and restricts this debris from interfacing with the host bone. In addition, once the bone has grown into the proximal porous area, polyethylene debris generated from normal wear is restricted from the distal stem area. Proximal bodies of different offsets, and vertical heights (Fig. 58) will allow for fine tuning hip joint biomechanics without removal of the stem.

IX. STEM DESIGN FEATURES

A. Material

This stem will utilize high-strength titanium alloy. Manufacture will utilize forgings.

B. Taper Head Neck

The neck will accept a chrome-cobalt or ceramic articulation. The neck diameter has been designed to maximize range of motion as compared to other designs.

C. Offset

In order to improve biomechanical function, offset has been increased in comparison to competitive stems.

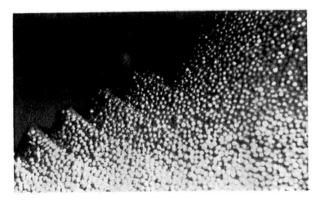

Figure 59 Stepped geometry with porous coating.

D. Surface Preparation

The stem is proximally porous coated utilizing a single, beaded porous coating of commercially pure titanium. This is sintered over a macrotextured design of horizontal steps, which helps to protect the beaded interface from shear forces and also helps in transferring hoop stresses to compression forces (Fig. 59). An additional option is a coating of HA which is plasma sprayed over the single, beaded porous surface. This single, beaded porous surface protects the HA in shear while also providing a backup for bony remodeling in case the HA is biochemically mobilized. Also, the nonporous surface has been treated with a proprietary microclean process that leaves a clean yet microrough surface [55].

E. Distal Bending Stiffness

The distal one third of the stem has been slotted in both the coronal and sagittal planes. These slots serve to reduce distal stem stiffness, allowing the stem to flex with the femur during normal daily activity. This feature has historically demonstrated re-

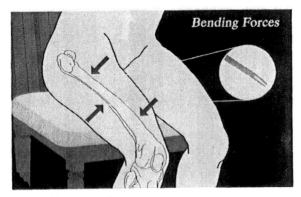

Figure 60 Bending forces.

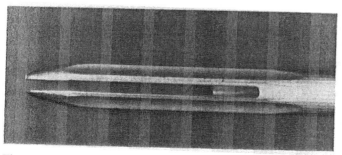

Figure 61 Distal slot design with flutes.

duced thigh pain (Fig. 60) [13]. In addition, it helps to reduce chances of intraoperative femoral fractures during stem insertion.

F. Distal Stability

To increase stem rotational stability, distal flutes have been incorporated into the stem design (Fig. 61). Rotational stability remains the primary concern of any femoral component.

G. Stem Tip

Bulleted geometry helps reduce distal point loading while creating a smooth transition zone for load transfer.

H. Instruments

Both stems — unibody and bibody — utilize the same instruments. Thus cost is reduced and there is also surgical ease in going from one stem to the next.

I. Acetabular Components

Two acetabular designs are offered in the system. The first is a standard ultra-high molecular weight (UHMWP) articulation that is compression molded to a hemispherical titanium alloy shell with CPT porous coating. This design will feature reduction in modularity with no angled offsets, which can result in decreased range of motion and can also result in increased chances of generation of particulate debris. The metal shell will feature peripheral screws for additional adjunct bony fixation, if indicated. This device will be indicated for, but not limited to the patient with a life expectancy of less than 15 years. It will also have significant cost savings over traditional systems.

The second design will have the same features; however, it will provide a ceramic articulation and will be indicated for, but not limited to the patient who has a life expectancy of more than 15 years.

X. SUMMARY

In view of the hundreds of thousands of total hip surgeries that have been performed since the surgery was introduced by Sir John Charnley over two decades ago, the small number of reported failures are not wholly unexpected. There is currently a great deal of debate over cement versus cementless indications. Initial concerns about wear rates of polyethylene have risen again due to the increased incidence of osteolysis induced by particulate debris.

Current methods of achieving implant fixation vary in concepts and techniques. Each method presents problems which must be addressed if cementless fixation is to survive long term. The justification for the continued use of cementless implants should be based on well-developed clinical and radiographic evidence.

In our opinion, everything possible should be done to reduce the generation of particulate debris. Continued research in surgical methodology, materials, and component design of total hip replacement can help to increase the longevity of implants and increase indications to a broader range of patients.

REFERENCES

1   Adler, E., Stuchin, A., and Kummer, F. J., Stability of press-fit acetabular cups, *J. Arthroplasty,* Vol. 7, No. 3, 1992.
2   Agins, H. J., Alcock, H. W., Bansal, M., Salvati, E. A., Wilson, P. D., Jr., Pellicci, P. M. , and Bullough, P. G., Metallic wear in failed titanium-alloy total hip replacements: A histological and quantitative analysis, *J. Bone Joint Surg.,* 70A, 347, 1988.
3   Bardos, D. I., Stainless steels in medical devices, in *Handbook of Stainless Steels* (Donald Peckner and I. M. Bernstein, eds.), 1977, p. 42.
4   Bartel, D.L., Burstein, A.H., Toda, M.D. Edwards, D.L.: The Effect of Conformity and Plastic Thickness on Contact Stresses in Metal-Backed Plastic Implants, *Journal of Biomechanical Engineering,* Vol. 107: 193-199, 1985.
5   Bechtol, C. O., Ferguson, A. B., and Laing, P. G., *Metals and Engineering in Bone and Joint Surgery,* Williams and Wilkins, Baltimore, MD, 1959.
6   Bechtol, C. O., Failure of femoral implant components in total hip replacement operations, *Ortho. Rev.,* Vol. 4, No. 11, 1975.
7   Black, J., Sherk, H., Bonini, J., Restoker, W. R., Schajowicz, F., and Galante, J. O., Metallosis associated with a stable titanium-alloy femoral component in total hip replacement: A case report, *J. Bone Joint Surg.,* 72A, 126-130, Jan. 1990.
8   Blum, H.J., Noble, P.C., Tullos, and H.S., Migration and rotation of cementless acetabular cups: Incidence, etiology and clinical significance, *Orthop. Trans.,* 14, 580, 1990.
9   Bobyn, J. D., Collier, J. P., Mayor, M. B., McTighe, T., Tanzer, M., and Vaughn, B. K., Particulate debris in total hip arthroplasty: Problems and solutions, Scientific Exhibit, AAOS Annual Meeting, 1993.
10 Boutin, P., Arthoplastie totale de la hanche par prothise en alumine fritie, Rev. *Clin. Orthop.,* 58, 229-246, 1972.

11 Boutin, P., Les protheses totale de la hanche en alumine, llancrage direct sans ciment dans 50 cas., Rev. *Clin. Orthop.*, 60, 233-245, 1974.

12 Callaghan, J. J., Dysart, S.H., and Savory, C.G., The incremented porous-coated anatomic total hip prosthesis, *J. Bone Joint Surg.*, 70A, 337, 1988.

13 Cameron, H.U., Trick, L.W., Shepherd, B.D., Turnbull, A., Noiles, D., McTighe, T., An international multi-center study on thigh pain in total hip replacements. Scientfific Exibit, AAOS Annual Meeting, 1990.

14 Cameron, H. U., Jung, Y-B., Noiles, D. G., McTighe, T., Design features and early clinical results with a modular proximally fixed low bending stiffness uncemented total hip replacement, Scientific Exhibit, AAOS Annual Meeting, 1988.

15 Chandler, H.P., Reineck, F.T., Wixson, R.L., and McCarthy, J.C., Total hip replacement in patients younger than thirty years old, *J. Bone Joint Surg.*, 63A, 1426, 1981.

16 Charnley, J., The long-term results of low-friction arthroplasty of the hip performed as a primary intervention, *J. Bone Joint Surg.*, 54B, 61, 1972.

17 Charnley, J., *Low Friction Arthroplasty of the Hip*, Springer-Verlag, 1978.

18 Charnley, J., Anchorage of the femoral head prosthesis to the shaft of the femur, *J. Bone Joint Surg.* (Br.), 42, 28, 1960.

19 Collier, J. P., Bauer, T., Bloebaum, R.D., et al., Results of implant retrieval from postmortem specimens in patients with well-functioning long-term THA, *Clin Orthop.*, 274, 68A, 97-112, 1992.

20 Collis, D.K., Cemented total hip replacement in patients who are less than fifty years old, *J. Bone Joint Surg.*, 66A, 353, 1984.

21 Cook, S. D., Clinical radiographic and histologic evaluation of retrieved human non-cement porous-coated implants, *J. Long Term Effect Med. Implants*, 1, 11-51, 1991.

22 Cook, S. D., Barrack, R. L., Thomas, K. A., and Haddad, R. J., Quantitative analysis of tissue growth into human porous total hip components, *J. Arthroplasty*, 3, 249-262, 1988.

23 Cook, S. D., Thomas, K. A., Barrack, R. L., and Whitecloud, T. S., Tissue growth into porous-coated acetabular components in 42 patients: Effects of adjunct fixation, *Clin. Orthop.*, 283, 163-170, 1992.

24 Cook, S. D., Kester, M. A., Dong, N. G., Evaluation of Wear in a Modular Sleeve/Stem Hip System, Poster Exhibit, Annual ORS Meeting, 1991.

25 Cooke, F. W., Ceramics in orthopedic surgery, Clin. Orthop., 135, 143, 1992.

26 Cornell, C.W., and Rannawatt, C.S., Survivorship analysis of total hip replacement: Results in a series of active patients who were less than fifty-five years old, *J. Bone Joint Surg.*, 68A, 1430, 1986

27 De Lee, J.G., and Charnley, J., Radiologic demarcation of cemented sockets in total hip replacement, *Clin. Orthop.*, 121, 20, 1976.

28 Denham, R. A., Hip mechanics, *J. Bone Joint Surg.*, 41B, 550, 1959.

29 Dorr, L.D., Takei, G.K., and Conaty, J.P., Total hip arthroplasties in patients less than forty-five years old, *J. Bone Joint Surg.*, 65A, 474, 1983.

30 Eggers, E., and McTighe, T., *Is intraoperative identification and fabrication a viable option for cementless TA?* Paper presented at the 6th Annual International Society for the Study of Custom Made Prosthesis, 1993.

31 Engh, C. A., and Bobyn, J. D., The influence of stem size and extent of porous-

coating on femoral resorption after primary cementless hip arthroplasty, Clin. Orthop., 231, 7-28, 1988.

32 Frankel, V. H., and Nordin, M., Basic Biomechanics of the Skeletal System, Lea and Febiger, 1980.

33 Greenwald, A.S., and Haynes, D.W., Weight-bearing areas in the human hip joint, *J. Bone Joint Surg.* (Br. Vol.), 54, 163, 1972.

34 Harris, W. H., Advances in total hip arthroplasty, *Clin. Orthop.,* Vol. 183, 1984.

35 Holmer, P., and Nielsen, P. T., Fracture of ceramic femoral heads in total hip arthroplasty, *J. Arthroplasty,* Vol. 8, No. 6, 1993.

36 Howie, D. W., Tissue response in relation to type of wear particles around failed hip arthroplasties, *J. Arthop.,* 5, 337, 1991.

37 Inman, V. T., Functional aspects of the abductor muscles of the hip, *J. Bone Joint Surg.,* 29, 607, 1947.

38 Jansons, H. A., The development of endoprostheses in the U.S.S.R., *Critical Review in Biocompatibility,* Vol. 3, Issue 2, 1987.

39 Judet, R., Total Huftencloprothesen aus Posometall ohne zement Verankerung, Z. Orthop., 113, 828-829, 1975.

40 Keating, E. M., Ritter, M. A., and Faris, P. M., Structures at risk from medially placed acetabular screws, *J. Bone Joint Surg.,* 72A, 509-511, April 1990.

41 Krygier, J. J., Bobyn, J. D., Dujovne, A. R., Young, D. L., Brooke, L. E., Strength, Stability and Wear Analysis of a Modular Titanium Femoral Hip Prosthesis Tested in Fatigue. Technical Monograph, Montreal General Hosp., McGill University, 1991.

42 Krushell, R. J., Burke, D. W., and Harris, W. H., Range of motion in contemporary total hip arthroplasty, *J. Arthrop.,* Vol. 6, No. 2, 1991.

43 Kurtz, S. M., Gabriel, S. M., and Bartel, D. L., The effect of non-conformity between metal-backing and polyethylene inserts in acetabular components for total hip arthroplasty, *Trans. 39th Ann. Meet. Orthop.* Res. Soc., San Francisco, 1993.

44 Livermore, J., Ilstrup, D., and Morrey, B., Effect of femoral head size on wear of the polyethylene acetabular component, *J. Bone Joint Surg.,* 72A, 518, 1990.

45 Longo, J. A., McTighe, T., Koeneman, J. B., Gealer, R. L., Torsional Stability of Uncemented Revision Hip Stems, Poster Exhibit Annual ORS Meeting 1992.

46 Lord, O., Bancel, P., The Madreporic cementless total hip arthroplasty: New experimental data and a seven-year clinical follow-up study. *Clin. Orthop.,* 1983; 176:67.

47 Mattingly, D., McCarthy, J., Bierbaum, B. E., Chandler, H. P., Turner, R. H., Cameron, H. U., and McTighe, T., Revising the deficient proximal femur, Scientific Exhibit, Annual AAOS meeting, 1991

48 McCarthy, D. S., White, S. E., Whiteside, L. A., Rotational Stability of Noncemented Total Hip Femoral Components. Scientific Exhibit AAOS Annual Meeting, 1993.

49 McKee, G. K., Development of total prosthetic replacement of the hip, *Clin. Orthop.,* 72, 85-103, 1970.

50 McKee, G. K., and Watson-Farrar, J., Replacement of arthritic hips by the McKee-Farrar prosthesis, *J. Bone Joint Surg.* (Br.), 42, 245-259, 1966.

51 McTighe, T., Threaded acetabular component design concepts, Joint Medical Product Corp. Reconstructive Review, 1986.

52　McTighe, T., Introduction, update news, *Joint Implant Surgery and Research Foundation,* April 1992

53　McTighe, T., New approach to bearing surfaces for total hip arthroplasty, Poster Exhibit, AAOS Annual Meeting, 1994.

54　McTighe, T., A historical review of metal backed acetabular components, *Reconstructive Review, Joint Medical Products Corp. Newsletter,* 1985.

55　McTighe, T., Hastings, R., Vaughn, B. K., Vise, G. T., Surface Finishes for Titanium Cementless Stems, A Poster Exhibit AAOS Annual Meeting 1993.

56　Mittelmeier, H., Five years clinical experience with alumina-ceramic hip prostheses, *First World Biomaterials Congress,* Baden near Vienna, Austria, 1980, p. 1.1.

57　Mittelmeier, H., Ceramic prosthetic devices, in The Hip: *Proceedings of the 12th Open Scientific Meeting of the Hip Society* (R. B. Welch, ed.), C. V. Mosby, St. Louis, 1984.

58　Mittelmeier, H., Cementless revisions of failed total hip replacement: Ceramic autophor prosthesis. In: Welch, R. B. (ed): Proceedings of the Hip Society, St. Louis, C. V. Mosby Co., 1984, p. 321, p. 146.

59　Pauwels, F., *Biomecanique de la hanche saine et pathologique,* Springer Verlag, Berlin, 1977, p. 277.

60　Perona, P. G., Lawrence, J., Paprosky, W. G., Patwardhan, A. G., and Sartori, M., Acetabular micromotion as a measure of initial implant stability in primary hip arthroplasty, *J. Arthroplasty,* Vol. 7, No. 4, 1992.

61　Pidhorz, L. E., Urban, R. M., Jacobs, J. J., Sumner, D. R., and Galante, J. O., A quantitative study of bone and soft tissue in cementless porous coated acetabular components retrieved at autopsy, *J. Arthroplasty in press.*

62　Pugh, J., *Biomechanics of the Hip. Part 2: Total Hip Replacement,* Orthopedic Surgery Update Series, Vol. 3, Lesson 27, 1984.

63　Pugh, J., Averill, R., Pachtman, W., Bartel, D., and Jaffe, W., Prosthesis surface design to resist loosening, *Transactions of the 27th Annual Meeting ORS,* 1981, p. 189.

64　Riska, E. B., Ceramic endoprosthesis in total hip arthroplasty, *Clin. Orthop.,* No. 297, 1993, pp. 87-94.

65　Rothman, R. H., Hearn, S. L., Eng, K. O., and Hozack, W. J., The effect of varying femoral offset on component fixation in cemented total hip arthroplasty, Scientific Exhibit, Annual AAOS Meeting, 1993.

66　Schmalzied, T. P., Justy, M., and Harris, W. H., Periprosthetic bone loss in TA, *J. Bone Joint Surg.,* 74A, 849, 1992.

67　Shepherd, B. D., Walter, W., Sherry, E., Cameron, H. U., and McTighe, T., Difficult hip replacement surgery: Problems and solutions, Scientific Exhibit, AAOS Annual Meeting, 1989.

68　Sivash, K. M., *Arthroplasty of the Hip Joint,* Medicina, Moscow, 1967.

69　Smith Nephew Richards, Porous-coated Femoral Component Mechanical Testing, Technical Monograph, 1993.

70　Teinturier, P., Terver, S., and Jaramillo, C.V., Rev. *Chir. Orthop.,* Suppl. II, 1984.

71　Tradonsky, S., Postak, P. D., Froimson, M. I., and Greenwald, A. S., Performance characteristics of two-piece acetabular cups, *Scientific Exhibit AAOS,* 1991, p. 246.

72　Urist, M. R.: The principles of hip-socket arthroplasty. *J. Bone Joint Surg.* 39 AM: 786-1957.

73 Wasielewski, R. C., Cooperstein, L. A., Kruger, M. P., and Rubash, H. E.,
    Acetabular anatomy and the transacetabular fixation of stress in total hip
    arthroplasty, *J. Bone Joint Surg.,* 72A, 501-508, April 1990.

74 Wiles, P., The surgery of the osteoarthritic hip, *Br. J. Surg.,* 45, 488, 1959.

75 Willert, H. G., and Semlitsch, M., Reactions of the articular capsule to wear
    products of artificial joint prostheses, *J. Biomed. Mater. Res.,* 11, 157, 1977.

76 Wright, T. M., and Rimnac, C. M., Ultra-high-molecular-weight polyethylene, in
    Joint Replacement Arthroplasty (B. F. Morrey, ed.), Churchill Livingstone, New
    York, 1991, pp. 37-45.

21

Polyethylene Wear in Orthopedics

Keith W. Greer, John V. Hamilton, and Edward J. Cheal
Johnson & Johnson Professional, Inc.
Raynham, Massachusetts

I. INTRODUCTION

Wear of the ultrahigh molecular weight polyethylene (UHMWPE) components of conventional hip and knee replacement prostheses is the subject of many clinical and laboratory research studies. The laboratory studies include traditional wear experiments, such as pin-on-disk and reciprocating motion analyses, as well as more complex hip and knee joint simulator experiments. Unfortunately it is difficult to predict the long-term *in vivo* wear performance of total joint replacements using only the results of laboratory studies; many factors, including patient activity, body weight, anatomy, and surgical technique, can affect the actual wear performance. The specific objectives of this chapter are to discuss: (1) general background information on polymers, polyethylene, and UHMWPE in particular; (2) the mechanical properties of UHMWPE; (3) the material and design issues related to UHMWPE wear; (4) the possible biological consequences of UHMWPE wear debris, especially osteolysis; and (5) the potential improvements to the wear performance of total joint replacement prostheses under current investigation.

A. Definition of Polymers

Polymers are long molecules made up of repeated units, known as *mers*. The mers in polyethylene are ethylene molecules that consist of two carbon atoms and four hydrogen atoms. Polyethylene grades are described by density and/or molecular weight of the polymer (Miller, 1990; Stein, 1988). Polymer chains can be considered to be made up of two components: side groups and a backbone. The size and number of the side groups determine if the polymer can be categorized as either a linear or a branched polymer. Polymers with a linear structure have the mers joined together predominately in a straight line with minimal side groups branching from the polymer backbone. Polymers with a branched structure also have a linear backbone, but the side groups are more complex, longer, and more numerous than the side groups of linear polymers.

The morphology or arrangement of a polymer chain is categorized as amorphous or crystalline. In the amorphous state, the polymer chain is randomly oriented. In the crystalline state, the polymer chain has a large degree of orientation, often folded over on itself. Polymers are categorized as either amorphous or semicrystalline. In an amorphous polymer, the polymer chain is completely in the amorphous state. In a semicrystalline polymer, the polymer chain has both amorphous and crystalline regions (Fig. 1). This is the usual condition for UHMWPE.

1. *Polyethylene as a Polymer*

Polyethylene is a very commonly used polymer and comes in a variety of grades (Fig. 2). Polyethylene is usually categorized by density, except UHMWPE, which is categorized by molecular weight. The major differences between the grades of polyethylene are the degree of branching, the molecular weight, and the density (Miller, 1990; Stein, 1988). The highly branched polyethylenes are typically low molecular weight and low density. Low-density polyethylene (LDPE) falls into this category. LDPE is commonly used as a film in food packaging. The linear materials have a higher molecular weight and density. High-density polyethylene (HDPE) and UHMWPE are examples of linear polymers. UHMWPE has a molecular weight 12 to 15 times greater than that of HDPE. However, UHMWPE has a lower density than HDPE due to increased chain entanglements that restrict the degree of crystallinity.

2. *History of UHMWPE in Orthopedics*

UHMWPE is not the first plastic to be used as an articulating surface in joint replacements. In the 1950s, acrylics were used for surface replacements. However, this material performed poorly, often failing after only several months in service. Sir John Charnley first used polytetrafluorethylene (PTFE, similar to Teflon®) as the cup material in total hip arthroplasties. The initial clinical results were encouraging, but severe wear problems developed after several years. Several materials were evaluated as replacements for PTFE. These included polyacetal, polyethylene terephthalate (PET), and UHMWPE. UHMWPE has proven to be the most successful and has been used in total joint arthroplasty for the last 30 years (Charnley, 1979; Dumbleton, 1983).

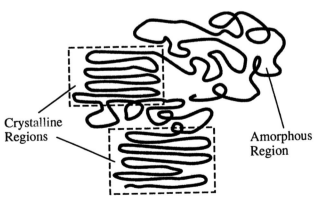

Figure 1   Diagram of a semi-crystalline polymer, showing the crystalline and amorphous regions.

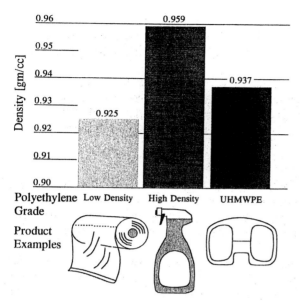

Figure 2   Density and example products for each grade of polyethylene.

3.   Biocompatibility of UHMWPE

UHMWPE in bulk form has excellent biocompatibility and is used as a control for biocompatibility testing of other materials. However, the very small wear debris particles that can be produced by articulating joints (Lee et al., 1992), especially the particles that are less than 1 μm in size, while nontoxic chemically, can lead to osteolytic lesions in the vicinity of the joint replacement components. The mechanisms by which this occurs are discussed in a later section.

B.   Production of UHMWPE Components

Producing UHMWPE components is a three-step process consisting of polymerization, consolidation, and machining. Polymerization is the process of transforming the ethylene molecules into UHMWPE in a powder form. Ethylene gas is fed into a reactor where temperature, pressure, and proprietary catalysts produce polyethylene. The processing conditions in the reactor determine the average molecular weight and its distribution, and the powder particle size and shape. The description of the particle size and shape is known as the particle *morphology*.

Hoechst Celanese (Texas) and Hoechst (Germany) are the only manufacturers of UHMWPE powder that meets the current ASTM standards for medical implants. These two companies produce two grades of UHMWPE powder, with the major difference between the two grades being the molecular weight of the polyethylene. The material produced in Germany is marketed as Chirulen P or RCH 1000. The Texas company markets both GUR 412, which is similar to RCH 1000, and GUR 415; GUR 415 has a higher molecular weight than GUR 412, but both materials meet the requirements of American Society for Testing and Materials, ASTM F648 (ASTM, 1984). Hercules (Wilmington, DE) is another manufacturer of UHMWPE. The trade name of their material is Himont 1900, which has been used in the past for some orthopedic applications. Currently, it is not marketed by Hercules for medical applications. However, Biomet, Inc. (Warsaw, IN) apparently is using Himont 1900 in their compression-molding processes.

The consistency of UHMWPE from lot to lot is controlled through the use of material specifications. The baseline specification for UHMWPE used by all orthopedic companies is ASTM Standard F648 (ASTM, 1984). Most importantly, all UHMWPE powder sold today as medical-grade material comes from only two sources, Hoechst and Hoechst Celanese.

1. Consolidation of UHMWPE

The extremely high molecular weight that is responsible for the superior wear properties of UHMWPE also limits the options available for converting this material from a powder to a final product. More specifically, the extremely high molecular weight reduces the ability of the material to flow, thus limiting the processing options available to orthopedic device manufacturers.

The two methods available at present for converting the powder to a solid material are referred to as *ram extrusion* and *compression molding* (Fig. 3). In the ram extrusion process, the powder is continuously compacted while pushing the powder through a die with sufficient force and heat to fuse the powder particles into a solid. Circular rods are typical intermediate products from this process, and these rods are later machined into final products. In the compression-molding process, the UHMWPE powder is placed in a mold, and then compacted and heated to fuse the powder into a solid. Compression molding is the more flexible approach, allowing a wide variety of forms to be produced, with shapes ranging from large sheets to nearly finished parts. In most cases the compacted powder, whether it be in rod form (from ram extrusion) or blocks (from compression molding), is machined and polished to produce the final part.

2. Quality Control

Throughout the entire manufacturing process, all UHMWPE parts are checked to ensure that they meet both the industry standards, ASTM Standard F648 (ASTM, 1984) and International Standards Organization (ISO) Standard 5834 Parts 1 and 2 (ISO, 1985a,

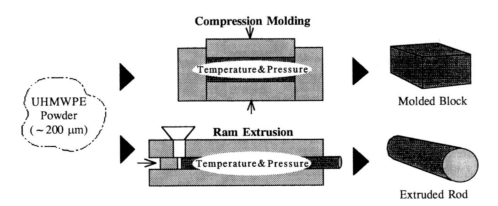

Figure 3   The second stage of production: formation of stock materials from the UHMWPE powder.

1985b), and the implant manufacturer's standards. The powder is checked to ensure that it meets the requirements for molecular weight, chemistry, and cleanliness. After compaction, the material is checked for mechanical properties, density, and contamination that may have occurred during the compaction process. Finally, after the machining process, the parts are inspected to ensure that there are no visible contaminates. The dimensions of the finished part are also checked against the engineering drawings to ensure proper fit and performance.

3. Sterilization of UHMWPE Components

Gamma radiation is the standard method for sterilization of UHMWPE implants. Dose levels typically range from about 2.5 to 5.0 Mrad. The potential effects of radiation sterilization on the wear behavior are discussed below.

II. MECHANICAL PROPERTIES OF UHMWPE

The mechanical properties of UHMWPE are a function of the raw material (molecular weight, crystallinity, etc.) and the processing. The measured properties are also a function of the sample size and shape, the gauge length, and the loading or displacement rate used in the particular test. Thus, when the final UHMWPE bar or sheet is fabricated, test samples are made from that material, and the properties are measured using standardized methods. In general, the fabricator performs these tests and provides the results to the customer (the orthopedic device manufacturer). The fabricator certifies the material to the industry and/or customer specifications and provides the test results on the certification to ensure that the properties meet the requirements of the customer.

A. Test Methods

1. Tensile Properties

Tensile properties are measured using a test bar that is pulled apart using a tensile load (Fig. 4). Some of the primary mechanical properties used to describe UHMWPE are the tensile properties of yield strength, ultimate tensile strength, ultimate elongation, and elastic modulus (Fig. 5). Elastic modulus is often used to describe the material but is currently not part of the ASTM or ISO specifications. In a polymer such is UHMWPE, elastic modulus is difficult to measure because the material, even below the yield strength, will exhibit some permanent deformation after removal of the load. The elastic region is also strongly influenced by sample size, configuration, and strain rate.

2. Compressive Creep

Compressive creep is a measure of the response of a material to a constant compressive load as a function of the time loaded and unloaded. It is a test required by ASTM (1984) but not ISO (1985b). In this test, an UHMWPE sample is loaded with a constant

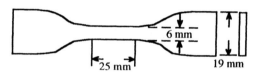

Figure 4   Tensile test bar for UHMWPE per ASTM Standard D638, Type IV.

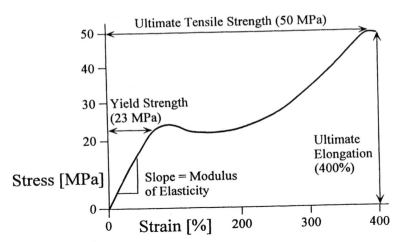

Figure 5   Typical stress–strain curve for UHMWPE tested in tension showing the uield strength, ultimate tensile strength, elastic modulus, and ultimate elongation.

compressive stress of 6.89 MPa for 24 h, then the stress is removed for 90 min and the amount of permanent deformation is measured (Fig. 6).

3. Impact

Impact is a direct measure of toughness of the polymer. The typical impact test used for UHMWPE is the Izod test in which a rectangular bar sample is produced having either one or two very sharp 15° notches (Fig. 7). One end of the sample is gripped tightly in a vise while the free end is impacted by a "hammer" of known weight falling from a known height and thus striking the sample with a known impact force. When the sample is broken, the amount of energy absorbed by the sample divided by the failed area is recorded as the impact strength of the sample. However, because of the superior tough-

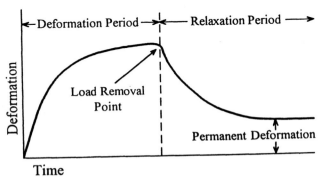

Figure 6   Typical compressive creep curve for UHMWPE. The deformation (i.e., creep) of the sample increases with time under a constant load until the load is removed, and then the deformation decreases. The permanent deformation that exists after 90 minutes of relaxation reflects the amount of creep for that sample.

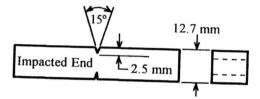

Figure 7 Double-notched Izod impact sample used for testing UHMWPE.

ness of UHMWPE, in almost all cases with a single notch the impact will not cause the sample to break into two separate pieces. If this occurs, it is recorded as a "nonbreak," which means that the impact strength exceeded the minimum impact strength requirement, even though the test samples have not broken into two distinct pieces. Poorly consolidated material or material with a molecular weight below the specification limits would have a lower toughness and would fail this test.

B. UHMWPE Properties

1. Material Certification

To evaluate the consistency of UHMWPE sold as medical-grade material, we compiled the material certification data from 5 lots of GUR 412 plate stock and 11 lots of GUR 415 rod stock that were purchased recently. The yield strength, ultimate tensile strength, and ultimate elongation were then compared to the minimum values from the ASTM and ISO standards (Fig. 8). In all cases, the mean values exceeded the specification minimum values. The creep and impact values for the purchased rod and plate materials were also

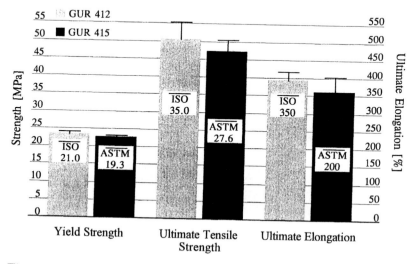

Figure 8 Mean (± 1 SD) values for yield strength, ultimate tensile strength, and ultimate elongation from certifications for GUR 412 plate (5 lots) and GUR 415 rod (11 lots) materials. Relevant ISO or ASTM minimum value noted on each bar.

Table 1   Average Values of Creep and Impact Versus Vendor Specifications

	Creep	Impact
Extruded rod (GUR 415), $n = 11$	0.73%	No break (> 140 mJ/mm^2)
ASTM specification	Less than 2%	140 mJ/mm^2 minimum
Molded sheet (GUR 412), $n = 5$	Not reported	161 mJ/mm^2
ISO specification	Not required	140 mJ/mm^2 minimum

compared to the corresponding ASTM and ISO specifications (Table 1). For impact, using the ISO units of measurement, both the ASTM and ISO require an impact strength of greater than 140 mJ/mm^2. For creep, the ASTM specification requires the creep to be less than 2% while ISO does not require a creep test. The supplied materials had impact values in excess of the ASTM and ISO specifications and creep values below the ASTM maximum value for the extruded rod material. The creep value for the plate material was not reported by the vendor because it is not required by the ISO.

The mechanical properties obtained from the multiple lots of material indicated the consistency of the UHMWPE material utilized in the production of orthopedic devices (Table 2). For both plate and bar materials, the yield strength was 12% to 18% greater than the specification minimum while the standard deviation was only 1.7% to 2.2% of the mean. There was slightly more variation in the ultimate elongation and ultimate tensile strength values, but the mean values exceeded the specification minimum by at least 12% and 44%, respectively.

Consistency of material has also been addressed by Westlake Plastics Company (Lenni, PA), a vendor that purchases the UHMWPE powder and extrudes bars that are then purchased by orthopedic manufacturers. A recent technical report by Westlake (Serwatka and Ploskonka, 1993) indicates the consistency of properties from 22 separate UHMWPE lots, including the properties of yield strength, ultimate tensile strength, ultimate elongation, Izod impact strength, compressive creep, and hardness (Table 3).

2.   Comparison of Molded Sheet and Extruded Rod

Recently some comments have been made about the "superiority" of GUR 415 material over GUR 412 material because of higher molecular weight. Although there is a molecular weight difference, other factors and properties must also be considered. Because of the

Table 2   Mechanical Properties of GUR 412 and GUR 415 Relative to the Specifications

Material	Property	Specification minimum	Mean value	% greater than minimum	SD, % of mean
GUR 412 plate	Yield strength	21 MPa	23.4 MPa	12%	2.2%
GUR 412 plate	UTS[a]	35 MPa	50.3 MPa	44%	9.9%
GUR 412 plate	Ultimate elongation	350%	393%	12%	6.0%
GUR 415 rod	Yield strength	19.3 MPa	22.7 MPa	18%	1.7%
GUR 415 rod	UTS	27.5 MPa	47.0 MPa	71%	7.4%
GUR 415 rod	Ultimate elongation	200%	360%	80%	11.9%

[a]UTS = ultimate tensile strength

Table 3   Mechanical Properties of 22 Lots of GUR 415 UHMWPE

Property	Units	Mean	SD	ASTM F648 requirement
Tensile yield strength	MPa	22.4	0.66	19.3 min
Ultimate tensile strength	MPa	46.3	4.28	27.6 min
Ultimate elongation	%	347	32	200% min
Izod impact strength	mJ/mm^2	No break	NA	140 min
Deformation under load	%	0.92	0.11	2% max
Hardness	Shore D	68.7	0.97	60 min

Source: Serwatka and Ploskonka (1993)

higher molecular weight, the GUR 415 material is more difficult to process, and thus the crystallinity and degree of consolidation may be lower. Most importantly, the mechanical properties of the materials should be compared, as well as the molecular weight. From the certification data given above (Tables 1 and 2), it appears that there is no major difference in the mechanical properties of the two materials (bar and molded sheet); however, these materials were tested by different vendors, and thus important differences may have been masked by different test methods, including different sample sizes, test speeds, surface finishes, or gauge lengths. For this reason, we chose to evaluate extruded rod material (GUR 415) from two different vendors and compare it to sheet material (GUR 412) molded by two different vendors, using consistent test methods for both materials (Table 4). Two material lots from each vendor were included, thus giving four lots of extruded rod and four lots of molded sheet. The measured properties included yield strength, ultimate tensile strength, ultimate elongation, and Izod impact strength. Note that the Izod impact specimens were triple notched, and thus the impact strengths appear lower and should not be compared to the ASTM and ISO standards, since those standards call for double-notched specimens. The third notch was used to guide the fracture path and thus produce more consistent results for each material.

Our tests indicated that, despite the higher molecular weight of GUR 415, the GUR 412 materials had higher tensile and impact properties than the GUR 415 materials (Figs. 9 and 10). However, the differences were statistically significant only for the ultimate elongation and the Izod impact strength (Fig. 10). Overall, there were no marked differences between the different vendors of the same material form.

Table 4   Mechanical Properties of Molded Sheet (GUR 412) and Extruded Rod (GUR 415) UHMWPE

Property	Units	Molded sheet		Extruded rod	
		Mean	SD	Mean	SD
Yield strength	MPa	24.9	1.3	24.2	0.50
UTS[a]	MPa	54.1	9.4	46.8	4.8
Ultimate elongation	%	465	58	379	25
Izod impact	mJ/mm^2	68.6	7.7	49.5	4.5

[a]UTS = ultimate tensile strength

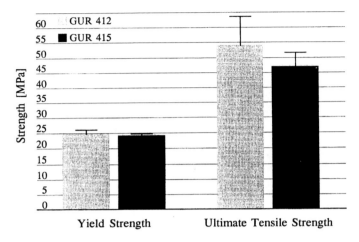

Figure 9 Mean (±1 SD) yield strength and ultimate tensile strength for four lots each of GUR 412 plate and GUR 415 rod material.

3. Significance of Mechanical Properties

In general, the ideal UHMWPE for orthopedic applications would have a very high strength, as reflected by the yield, impact, and ultimate tensile strengths, and high creep resistance, while having a relatively low elastic modulus. Presumably, the high strength would make the material wear resistant, while the low modulus would make the material conformable and thus minimize the mechanical stresses. Unfortunately, strength and modulus generally are positively related, and thus as the strength of UHMWPE is increased, the modulus is also increased. In regard to the specific strength parameters, yield strength and ultimate tensile strength of UHMWPE have not been shown to be directly

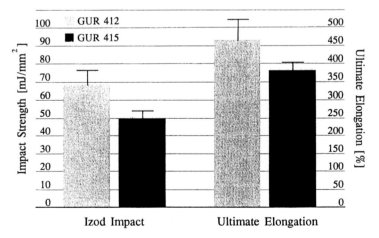

Figure 10 Mean (±1 SD) Izod impact strength (triple-notched) and ultimate elongation for four lots each of GUR 412 plate and GUR 415 rod material.

related to wear properties or to fatigue strength. Ultimate elongation as a measure of the brittleness may be a more important parameter. However, for materials having elongation higher than the minimum required by ASTM and ISO, there is no known correlation with wear or fatigue properties. In summary, it can be very misleading to focus on one or two material properties, since the wear performance of the material is dependent on all of these interrelated properties in a complex manner. Most importantly, our measurements of the mechanical and physical properties of processed medical-grade UHMWPE indicate that the process controls and quality assurance testing in place today result in a material that is consistent from batch to batch, and that is mechanically similar with regard to extruded rod and molded sheet.

III. WEAR OF POLYETHYLENE

The objective of this section is to discuss the various mechanisms of wear of UHMWPE and the ways in which wear is affected by the design of the implants and the properties of the materials. Some notable clinical failures are also briefly discussed in light of these material and design considerations.

A. Wear Mechanisms

There are several mechanisms by which UHMWPE bearing surfaces can wear and thus form distinct wear particles with which the body will interact. These wear mechanisms have been described based on the appearance of retrieved devices. It is obvious from the literature that a variety of wear mechanisms exist for UHMWPE. Any one total joint may show some or all of these wear mechanisms and with different levels of severity depending on various factors relating to the material, loading, design, and so on.

The most common wear mechanisms reported in the literature are adhesive, abrasive, and fatigue wear. Within these three major areas, many different wear descriptions and terms have been used; thus Hood et al. (1983) chose to define seven different modes of surface damage, of which five can be directly considered as wear modes (burnishing, abrasion, scratching, delamination, and pitting) and are included in the descriptions below. The other two modes, surface deformation and embedded acrylic debris, are surface damage modes related to creep and hardness, rather than wear, while acrylic debris is also related to third-body wear (abrasion). Retrieval studies indicate that wear mechanisms are different in total hip replacements as compared to total knee replacements, as discussed below. It is thus likely that the optimal material combination for total knee replacements is different from the optimal combination for total hip replacements.

1. Adhesive Wear

Adhesive wear is a process that generates fine particles due to the adhesion of the UHM-WPE to the mating metallic or other material on a microscopic basis. This occurs even under lubricated conditions, where the microscopic roughness peaks of the two materials come in contact with high enough loads to result in removal of the weaker UHMWPE material (Fig. 11). Burnishing is a wear mechanism in which the UHMWPE surface attains a highly polished appearance. It probably is the result of creep combined with adhesive wear caused by a polished counterface. Adhesive wear is considered a major component of the wear of hip sockets. However, in knee replacements, the adhesive wear component is often overshadowed by fatigue or delamination wear.

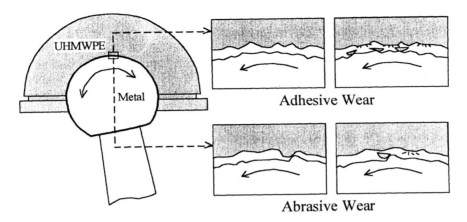

Figure 11 Adhesive and abrasive wear mechanisms. Adhesive wear: as the two surfaces move in relation to each other, the actual points of contact have high stresses, and thus small particles of UHMWPE adhere to the metallic component and are removed from the UHMWPE component. Abrasive wear: as the two surfaces move in relation to each other, a sharp surface feature on the metallic component shears off a particle of UHMWPE.

2. Abrasive Wear

Abrasive wear is a process of wear in which sharp particles abrade either of the two bearing surfaces (Fig. 11). The particles are often third-body abrasive particles such as bone cement, bone chips, or debris from a failed coating such as hydroxyapatite or porous metals. In some cases, the abrasion may be caused by very rough metal surface features or by bone that has not been fully removed far enough away from the articulating portion of the metal or ceramic component. Abrasive wear is reported as a component of both knee and hip prosthesis wear. In cases of third-body debris, it can lead to rapid loss of the material.

In addition to abrasive wear of the bearing surface, abrasion can occur in metal-backed components between the acetabular shell or tibial tray and the UHMWPE liner or insert. Burnishing and surface deformation can also occur at this interface. The magnitude of the abrasive wear depends on the fit and finish of the components, and the relative motion between the components under cyclic loading.

Scratching can be considered a form of abrasive wear; the term describes a long and/or deep wear path that would have been caused by the action of a single abrasive particle or sharp abrasive surface feature.

3. Fatigue Wear

Fatigue wear is a process of wear in which stresses in the UHMWPE material at and below the surface exceed the fatigue properties of the UHMWPE and cause subsurface cracking to occur after repeated loading and unloading of the material. These subsurface cracks can intersect cracks growing perpendicular to the surface and thus generate large wear particles (Fig. 12). Delamination wear is a wear mechanism in which large sheets of UHMWPE are separated from the bulk of the material. This appears to be a form of fatigue wear, and in some publications these two mechanisms are not differentiated.

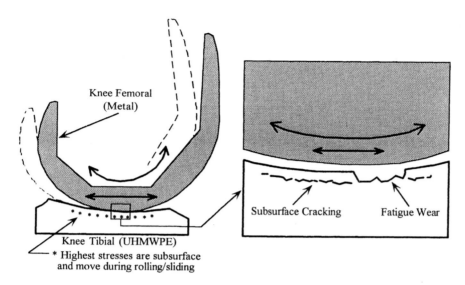

Figure 12 Fatigue wear mechanism. After many cycles, subsurface cracks are formed that may connect with the surface, resulting in fatigue wear (pitting or delamination).

Pitting wear is a wear mechanism in which small pits are formed in the articulating surface of a component. These pits may be due to the release of UHMWPE powder particles or they may be due to a fatigue damage mechanism.

Fatigue wear appears to be a major component of knee prosthesis wear. It may also play a role in hip prosthesis wear, although the typically lower hip joint stresses probably make it less of a factor than adhesive or abrasive wear.

4. Wear Particles

Once UHMWPE wear particles are generated during the wear process, the tissues of the body will interact with these particles in various ways depending on their size, shape, chemistry, and surface properties. Larger wear particles are treated as foreign bodies and thus are surrounded by fibrous tissue and giant cells. These particles are relatively easy to see in tissue cross sections. The most damaging particles appear to be the very fine ones (less than 1 μm) that are small enough to be taken into the cells (macrophages). These small particles can only be seen by techniques such as transmission electron microscopy. At some point, the cells containing these particles may produce substances that lead to bone resorption (i.e., osteolysis). Osteolysis is discussed at greater length in a separate section below.

B. Design Considerations

The wear of UHMWPE can be affected by the design features of the total joint replacement components (Engh et al., 1992). Designers can improve wear by providing designs that result in lower stresses on the material or improved lubrication, thus reducing the friction. In the case of total hip replacements, recent publications have indicated that 22 mm and 28 mm diameter hip heads provide less wear debris per year of service than 32 mm diameter hip heads (Kabo et al., 1993; Livermore et al., 1990). Two other important design parameters are the conformity between the mating components and the thickness of the UHMWPE components (Bartel et al., 1986).

1. Conformity

Improvements in conformity of mating components can lead to a reduction in stresses within the UHMWPE and thus lower the wear rate. For total hip replacements, conformity generally is high because of the ball-and-socket nature of the joint. With such conformity, the loads are spread over a relatively large contact area and the contact stresses are lower. For total knee replacements, the conformity is less than in total hip replacements and the conformity must be balanced with the level of geometric constraint of the design. A knee prosthesis design with high constraint (e.g., cruciate sacrificing) can be designed with more conformity since the cruciate ligaments will not be present to force the motion (kinematics) of the device. A knee prosthesis design with less constraint (e.g., cruciate retaining) cannot be designed with as much conformity because of the kinematic motions that the design must allow due to the retained soft tissues.

The issue of conformity has been raised by many researchers. Bartel et al. (1985, 1986) used a finite element model to estimate the increase in stresses that occur as the mismatch between the curvature of the mating components is increased. The contact areas between various knee replacement designs, with varying degrees of conformity, have been reported by a number of investigators (Collier et al., 1991; Hayes et al., 1993; Postak et al., 1993; Sommerich et al., 1992; Statler et al., 1992).

2. *Thickness*

As the thickness of UHMWPE components is decreased, the stresses in the material are increased, and thus the wear rate of the UHMWPE presumably is increased (Bartel et al., 1985, 1986). Based on their linear elastic finite element analyses, Bartel et al. (1991) currently recommend a minimum UHMWPE thickness of 8 mm for tibial inserts and 6 mm for acetabular components. Unfortunately, selecting a component for minimum wear (i.e., maximizing thickness) is at odds with the surgical objective of minimizing the amount of bone resection; thus, there must be a compromise between these conflicting objectives. Also, while finite element analysis techniques are good at predicting trends, they typically provide only an estimate of stress magnitudes and are very dependent on the assumptions and particular solution techniques employed. For example, DeHeer and Hillberry (1992) have shown that linear elastic finite element models overestimate the stress magnitudes in UHMWPE by as much as 40% relative to more realistic models that include nonlinear material behavior. Finally, while the stress levels in the UHMWPE are clearly important, it is not possible to directly relate these stress levels to actual *in vivo* wear rates due to the many other contributing factors.

3. *Surface Finish*

The wear of UHMWPE is affected by the surface finish of the mating component. The highly polished finish on orthopedic devices is for the purpose of providing improved wear behavior. As the surface finish becomes rougher, the wear mechanism will be related more to abrasion than to adhesion. Several laboratory studies (Dowson et al., 1985; McKellop et al., 1978, 1981) have shown that improving the surface finish will decrease the wear of UHMWPE. Our evaluations of knee tibial components from various manufacturers indicated that polishing of knee prosthesis components results in surface finishes ranging from about 0.013 μm to 0.051 μm; however, a much larger variation in surface finish exists on nonpolished surfaces, such as the inside of tibial trays.

4. Scratching

Scratching of metallic bearing surfaces can have an impact on wear behavior. Small scratches can affect wear by creating a rougher surface finish, while large scratches can act like a large cutting or abrasive particle and thus have a large impact on the wear behavior. Embedded bone cement or other particles are detrimental because they can lead to scratches in the surface finish of the metallic component. In particular, the barium sulfate or zirconium oxide radio-opaque particles within bone cement may be responsible for scratching the metallic components (Isaac et al., 1986).

5. Ceramic Mating Surfaces

The use of ceramic heads in total hip replacement bearing against UHMWPE has been shown to decrease the polyethylene wear by both *in vitro* wear tests and radiographic evaluation of implanted devices in patients (Saikko et al., 1993; Saito et al., 1992; Semlitsch et al., 1977; Zichner and Willert, 1992). Alumina (i.e., aluminum oxide) has been the ceramic of choice in the past. However, zirconia (zirconium oxide) is beginning to be used because of its improved toughness which decreases the chance for fracture of the ceramic head during assembly or use. Ceramics also have higher hardness than metals and are more resistant to scratching or roughening *in vivo*, thus probably providing better wear properties. Although a limited number of ceramic knee femoral components have been produced and implanted (Oonishi et al., 1992), the use of ceramics in knee femoral components is currently not feasible either technically (e.g., strength, reliability) or economically.

C. Material and Fabrication

Another factor in the wear of UHMWPE is the material itself and the degree of consolidation of the powder particles. The impact of these variables on wear has been difficult to establish because of the unique molecular nature of UHMWPE, the difficulty in characterizing it fully, and the limited amount of process research and development work that has been published. These are areas in which much work is underway to try to further understand UHMWPE and to optimize the material processing.

1. Molecular Weight

The molecular weight of polyethylene materials has been shown to influence their abrasion resistance in tests where polyethylene samples are rotated in a slurry of sand and water. Thus, some companies have made the statement that higher molecular weight means greater wear resistance. However, a higher molecular weight can also lead to more difficulty in processing the material and can affect the consolidation of the powder particles. Since sand slurry testing does not evaluate other wear mechanisms such as adhesive wear or fatigue wear, it is incorrect to conclude that higher molecular weight, by itself, correlates with improved wear properties for a device in clinical use.

2. Crystallinity

The importance of increased crystallinity to the wear of UHMWPE has not been established at this time. Increased crystallinity will lead to a stiffer material with a higher modulus, which will in turn decrease contact area and increase stresses in the wear area.

For increased crystallinity to improve wear, the stiffer material must have a sufficiently increased strength to compensate for the higher stresses.

Hylamer™ (DePuy–Dupont Orthopaedics, Warsaw, IN) is an UHMWPE material that has been developed with an increased crystallinity. Several wear tests have been reported in the literature comparing Hylamer™ with standard UHMWPE. In those published studies, the wear properties of both materials have been shown to be not significantly different (McKellop et al., 1992).

3. Consolidation

The presence of UHMWPE powder particles that are not fully bonded during the fabrication process (extrusion or molding) would lead to a weaker particle-to-particle interface that could be more susceptible to wear mechanisms such as fatigue or pitting. These wear mechanisms have been reported primarily in knee prosthesis evaluations. A recent study has also pointed to the possible connection between these "fusion defects" and the appearance of the UHMWPE wear surfaces of retrieved knee components (Blunn et al., 1992).

D. Other Considerations

1. Sterilization

The effect of various sterilization processes on the wear of UHMWPE is controversial. Free radicals created during sterilization react with either the polymer itself or absorbed oxygen (Jahan et al., 1991). Reactions within the polymer can produce crosslinks throughout the material and thus increase the elastic modulus and reduce the ductility of the material (Nusbaum and Rose, 1979; Roe et al., 1981). Reactions with oxygen can produce an increase in the density and crystallinity of the subsurface (Eyerer et al., 1987; Shinde and Salovey, 1985). How these changes affect the wear of UHMWPE is not well understood at present. The process of gamma irradiation at low doses such as 2.5 Mrad has been shown to both increase and decrease the wear rate over nonirradiated material (Kurth and Eyerer, 1991; McKellop et al., 1981; Rose et al., 1984). Research into the effects of irradiation on mechanical properties is also underway.

2. Material Aging

Aging of UHMWPE, especially in regard to progressive oxidative degradation, has been raised as a concern for the wear performance of the material (Grood et al., 1982). It is known that the degree of oxidation can increase with time during storage in air after irradiation sterilization (Streicher, 1991). However, the effects of oxidation on the wear performance are not clear. Also, a recent study in which wear test samples were made from retrieved acetabular cups showed that the wear resistance of UHMWPE did not change with time *in vivo*, even after implantation times of up to 17.5 years (Weightman et al., 1991). This finding suggests that the oxidation that does occur *in vivo* may not measurably affect the wear resistance of the UHMWPE.

3. Surgical and Patient Factors

There are several surgical and patient factors that can influence the wear of UHMWPE. Poor alignment in the knee typically results in higher stresses on one condyle and sometimes articulation that is too far anterior or posterior, in which case the areas of high stress during flexion or extension may not be the areas designed to provide the best wear resistance.

Many retrieval studies have pointed out the wear damage done by third-body debris such as bone cement. Careful cleaning of the tissues around the joint and removal of third-body wear particles are necessary to provide the best opportunity for satisfactory wear behavior.

The weight and activity level of the patient are also important factors in the wear of the implant. Higher weight leads to higher stresses while more activity provides more fatigue cycles and usually higher peak stresses. Both of these factors can lead to increased wear of UHMWPE.

E. Clinical Failures

1. Carbon Fiber Reinforcement

In the late 1970s, a composite of carbon fibers in an UHMWPE matrix was developed as an improved wear material for total joint replacements (Poly Two™ Carbon Polyethylene Composite; Zimmer, Inc., Warsaw, IN). Laboratory testing indicated the material had higher strength and modulus, and lower creep and wear than UHMWPE (Wright et al., 1981; Zimmer, 1977). However, clinical experience has shown instances of poor wear performance (Wright et al., 1988), and this material was taken off the market. The primary cause for failure of the material was probably due to the lack of bonding between the carbon fibers and the UHMWPE powder and a difficulty in getting an even mixture of powder and fiber, which led to clumps of fibers with no powder to bond them together. In either case, defects were created in the material that made it weaker and susceptible to failure during use (Stern et al., 1991; Wright and Rimnac, 1991). This material also had a higher elastic modulus, and thus higher predicted contact stresses (Bartel et al., 1986).

2. Heat-Pressed Polyethylene

The process of heat pressing was utilized in the PCA™, knee tibial component (Howmedica, Rutherford, NJ) for the purpose of providing a superior UHMWPE surface finish. Based on the clinical performance, this turned out to be a negative wear factor instead of a positive one (Jones et al., 1992; Mintz et al., 1991). Heat pressing the UHMWPE creates a thin layer of altered material and a relatively weak interface below the articular surface. This interface could then fail due to the repetitive loads to which the material is subjected, resulting in fatigue failure and delamination. The design of this prosthesis may also have contributed to the clinical failures, including nonconforming articular surfaces and thin UHMWPE components (Wright et al., 1992). This experience points out the interconnection of the factors involved—including surface finish, material, fabrication, and design—and the need to consider all aspects of the wear process and not simply a single one, such as surface finish or molecular weight.

3. Metal-Backed Patellae

The clinical failures exhibited by many metal-backed patella designs have been well documented in the literature. Retrieved, failed devices often show major areas of creep (cold flow), delamination, and pitting as well as fracture of the UHMWPE or the metal backing (Bayley et al., 1988; Lombardi et al., 1988). The patella component can be subjected to very high loads, especially when the range of motion is greater than 100–105°. In the case of metal-backed patellae, these stresses led to creep, fatigue, or delamination of the UHMWPE component, followed by separation of the UHMWPE from the metal backing. These failures point out the importance of potential high mechanical stresses in the determination of wear behavior.

4. *Titanium Articular Surfaces*

Titanium alloy (Ti–6Al–4V) has been used as an articulating surface in both total hip and knee replacements. Although there have been some reports of success in hip heads when third-body abrasive particles were not present, it has not been as good a material when used in knee prosthesis femoral components or in the presence of abrasive particles (Lombardi et al., 1989; Nasser et al., 1990). This was due to the known poor abrasion resistance of titanium; titanium is very susceptible to scratching, which then results in a rough surface and leads to greater abrasive wear of the UHMWPE.

Ion implantation and other surface treatments may improve the wear performance of titanium because these treatments harden the surface and improve the abrasion resistance (Matthews et al., 1986; Rostlund et al., 1989). These treatments also may affect the wettability of the surface and thus decrease adhesive wear. However, there are still questions about the longevity of these surface treatments since they may be only 0.1 to 0.2 μm in depth (Matthews et al., 1986).

IV. OSTEOLYSIS

Osteolysis is the pathological resorption of bone that has been observed with varying frequency in the vicinity of joint replacement components. The objective of this section is to briefly review the current state of knowledge regarding the incidence of osteolytic lesions and the relationship to UHMWPE wear debris.

A. Clinical Observations

Suggestions that UHMWPE wear debris could result in osteolytic lesions in the surrounding bone were made in the literature as early as 1977 (Black, 1978; Revell et al., 1978; Willert and Semlitsch, 1977). However, recognition of the frequency and potential severity of this phenomenon is more recent (Cooper et al., 1992; Huddleston, 1988; Maloney et al., 1990b; Tanzer et al., 1992). More specifically, for total hip replacements, Mulroy and Harris (1990) reported a 7% incidence of aggressive osteolytic lesions with cemented femoral components and a minimum 10-year follow-up, and Maloney et al. (1990a) reported a 13% incidence with uncemented femoral components and a minimum 2-year follow-up. UHMWPE wear debris has been implicated in the loosening of cemented acetabular components of total hip replacements, based on autopsy-retrieved specimens (Schmalzried et al., 1992b). Osteolytic lesions have also been reported around total knee replacements (Gross and Lennox, 1992; Nolan and Bucknill, 1992). Peters et al. (1992) reported a 16% incidence of osteolysis associated with uncemented total knee replacements, with a minimum 1 year follow-up; 56% of those arthroplasties (the 16% with diagnosed osteolysis) were revised at an average of 45 months after implantation.

There is evidence that particles of PMMA bone cement can also result in osteolytic lesions (Jasty et al., 1986; Willert et al., 1990). This problem has largely been addressed by improved cement techniques and by improvements in implant design, such as the elimination of sharp corners at cement interfaces (Harris and McGann, 1986; Russotti et al., 1988). However, particles of bone cement can accelerate the wear of UHMWPE by acting as a third body (Isaac et al., 1991; Winkler-Gniewek and Ungethum, 1991).

B. Biological Processes

Examination of retrieved tissues from osteolytic lesions around total joint replacements has revealed particles of PMMA bone cement, metal, and UHMWPE. The larger particles are generally surrounded by fibrous tissue or foreign-body giant cells while the smaller particles (less than 1 μm in size) are associated with macrophages (Goodman et al., 1991; Revell et al., 1978; Santavirta et al., 1990; Schmalzried et al., 1992a). Based on tissue culture studies, macrophages release a number of cytokines and proteolytic enzymes following ingestion of these small particles, including prostaglandin-E2, interleukin-1, and tumor necrosis factor (Goldring et al., 1988; Murray and Rushton, 1990). While bone resorption is a complex process, these factors are known to recruit and/or stimulate osteoclasts, the cells that resorb bone (Vaes, 1988).

Recently, it has been shown that the UHMWPE particles in macrophages and foreign-body giant cells are not directly cytotoxic (Benz et al., 1994). These cells display a normal ultrastructure in close proximity to the UHMWPE particles on examination by transmission electron microscopy. It also appears that the risk of cancer from particles of UHMWPE is minimal based on experimental carcinogenicity studies (Brand, 1991).

It is clear that the extremely fine particulate debris that can result from the wear of UHMWPE orthopedic implants can lead to osteolytic lesions in the surrounding bone. Fortunately, these particles do not appear to be cytotoxic (the cells that ingest these particles are not damaged) or carcinogenic. However, little is known at present about the transport and distribution of these particles throughout the body and the end-organ effects. The current research and development goal is to minimize, or even eliminate, the generation of this debris through improvements in design, materials, and surgical instrumentation.

V. POTENTIAL FUTURE ALTERNATIVES

The objective of this section is to describe some of the options being discussed in the scientific literature to improve the wear performance of total joint replacements. These approaches include changes to the sterilization and storage procedures for UHMWPE components, modifications to the UHMWPE material, and alternative materials and material combinations, including polymers, ceramics, and metal-on-metal.

A. Sterilization and Storage

Several alternative sterilization processes are currently under evaluation. These include electron beam, modified atmosphere, gas, and gas plasma sterilization. The common objective of these approaches is to minimize changes to the polymer, especially oxidative degradation.

Electron beam sterilization offers two significant potential advantages over gamma irradiation. The first advantage is that it is substantially faster, and thus the free radicals that are formed within the polymer are more likely to result in crosslinking of the chains, rather than oxidative chain scission. The second advantage is that the process can be controlled with more precision than gamma sterilization, minimizing the amount of free radicals formed (Kurth and Eyerer, 1991).

Sterilization in an inert atmosphere or vacuum also favors the crosslinking reaction over oxidative chain scission. In addition, excluding oxygen available to the free radicals during storage can further minimize oxidation. Oxygen-free storage alone cannot eliminate the oxidative chain scission process, but it can delay the process until after the component is implanted (Streicher, 1991).

Gas-based sterilization techniques are available or are currently under development. These include ethylene oxide using non-CFC carrier gases and vapor-phase hydrogen peroxide. These processes do not form free radicals; however, there are several problems that must be overcome. One problem is the lack of dosimetric release for monitoring purposes; sample components must be incubated and evaluated to ensure sterility, increasing the cost of the product. Another problem is that the toxic ethylene oxide gas is absorbed into the polymer, requiring lengthy out-gassing procedures before release of the product (Jordy, 1991).

Gas plasma is another alternative sterilization technique currently under investigation. This process uses an ionized gas to sterilize the device. At the present time the effects of gas plasma on UHMWPE are unknown. Initial applications being considered for this approach include surgical instruments and medical packaging.

B. Modifications of UHMWPE

It is possible to alter the wear behavior of UHMWPE through changes to the material and/or part fabrication processes. The fundamental processing parameters include the time, temperature, and pressure to which the UHMWPE powder is subjected during consolidation. Hylamer™ (DePuy–Dupont Orthopaedics, Warsaw, IN) is an example in which the consolidation process was modified so as to produce a higher-crystalline material. However, as discussed above, the wear behavior of UHMWPE is dependent on the interaction of a number of material properties. This interaction is not well understood at present, and the only method available to evaluate this behavior is extensive testing on joint simulators.

Another approach currently under investigation is a surface modification of polymers via ion implantation (Lee et al., 1991). The ion implantation process consists of bombarding the material with high-energy ions such as nitrogen, boron, or argon. The ions penetrate the polymer to a depth of 1 to 5 μm. Measured changes in properties include an increase in hardness and a decrease in the coefficient of friction. The mechanisms by which these changes occur are not well understood at this time, but they are thought to be related to an increase in the crosslinking of the polymer. Wear testing of nitrogen-implanted UHMWPE has shown an improvement in wear over nonimplanted material (Rieu et al., 1991). However, one major concern with this process is that an interface is created, perhaps analogous to the effects of heat pressing, and that degeneration of this interface may lead to delamination and failure under long-term cyclic loading. Additional tests at higher loads and cycle counts typical of orthopedic applications are needed before this process could be implemented.

C. Alternative Materials

There are two major requirements that must be met for a new material to be considered as an articulating surface: superior wear resistance and biocompatibility. As discussed above, extensive tests on joint simulators are required to establish superior wear resistance. However, any new material must also go through a series of studies to establish biocompatibility, including tests of tissue compatibility, mutagenicity, and carcinogenicity. These studies can take many years, with the potential for making introduction of a new material unfeasible due to economic constraints.

Polyaryletherketones are a group of polymers that offer theoretical improvements over UHMWPE. These polymers have greater resistance to free-radical generation from the aromatic components, improved mechanical properties, and coefficients of friction that are comparable to UHMWPE. Wear test results to date are encouraging, but tests that are more specific to orthopedic applications are still needed (Yoo and Eiss, 1993).

Ceramic materials have been used since the early 1970s in total hip replacements in both ceramic-on-UHMWPE and ceramic-on-ceramic articulations. Ceramic-on-ceramic (alumina-on-alumina) appeared promising due to the high abrasion resistance and low coefficient of friction of the material. However, clinical complications related to loosening of the components, fracture of the acetabular cup, and pain, have prevented wide acceptance of this approach (Clarke, 1992).

Metal-on-metal hip replacements are currently being reevaluated. The best-known example of this approach is the McKee–Farrar total hip replacement. Developed in the late 1950s and early '60s, it was considered an alternative to the Charnley "low friction" hip replacement. Unfortunately, the narrow medial and lateral surfaces, curved stem, and large neck all contributed to clinical complications that resulted in the device falling into disfavor when compared to the Charnley. However, some retrieved devices have shown excellent wear performance in the long term (August et al., 1986; Jacobsson et al., 1990; Schmalzried, 1993). These encouraging results have been attributed to improved finishes and tolerances between the head and the cup. Several groups are currently reevaluating metal-on-metal articulations using modern stem designs.

VI. CONCLUSION

The potential for wear of UHMWPE joint replacement components is a primary concern to orthopedic surgeons today. This concern is largely due to the many clinical and research studies focused on UHMWPE wear, with results and recommendations reported in the scientific literature that are sometimes confusing and/or conflicting. Based on these studies, it is clear that the fine particulate debris that can be produced, especially by adhesive and abrasive wear mechanisms, can result in osteolytic lesions in the surrounding bone. While these lesions may not necessarily lead to failure of the joint replacement, revision surgery is sometimes needed.

There are a number of possibilities for implant manufacturers to reduce the potential for UHMWPE wear, including refinements of the material properties and implant designs. Unfortunately, the wear performance of UHMWPE is dependent on multiple interrelated material properties, and thus it is insufficient to focus on one or two properties of the material for improved wear resistance. At the present time, it is most important to ensure consistent material quality with minimal inclusions and defects. However, there are some design parameters that are clear, including the need for sufficient conformity and thickness of the components. Improved laboratory experiments and computer-aided design and manufacturing, along with past clinical experience, have resulted in marked improvements in the total hip and knee replacement prostheses that are available today. Finally, improved wear performance through alternative sterilization and storage methods, and perhaps substitution of alternative materials, may be possibilities in the near future.

REFERENCES

ASTM (1984). Standard specification for ultra-high-molecular-weight polyethylene powder and fabricated form for surgical implants. ASTM Standard F648, American Society for Testing and Materials.

August, A. C., Aldam, C. H. and Pynsent, P. B. (1986). The McKee–Farrar hip arthroplasty. A long-term study. *J. Bone Joint Surg. [Br.], 68*, 520–527.

Bartel, D. L., Burstein, A. H., Toda, M. D. and Edwards, D. L. (1985). The effect of conformity and plastic thickness on contact stress in metal-backed plastic implants. *J. Biomech. Eng., 107*, 193–199.

Bartel, D. L., Bicknell, V. L. and Wright, T. M. (1986). The effect of conformity, thickness, and material on stresses in ultra-high molecular weight components for total joint replacement. *J. Bone Joint Surg. [Am.], 68*, 1041–1051.

Bartel, D. L., Rimnac, C. M. and Wright, T. M. (1991). Evaluation and design of the articular surface. In *Controversies of Total Knee Arthroplasty* (Goldberg, V. M., ed.), pp. 61–73. Raven Press, New York.

Bayley, J. C., Scott, R. D., Ewald, F. C. and Holmes, G. B. (1988). Failure of the metal-backed patellar component after total knee replacement. *J. Bone Joint Surg. [Am.], 70*, 668–674.

Benz, E. B., Federman, M., Godleski, J. J., Bierbaum, B. E., Thomhill, T. S., Sledge, C. B. and Spector, M. (1994). Ultrastructure of cells that have phagocytosed polyethylene particles in peri-implant tissue from revision arthroplasty. *Trans. Orthop. Res. Soc., 19*, 200.

Black, J. (1978). The future of polyethylene. *J. Bone Joint Surg. [Br.], 60*, 303–306.

Blunn, G. W., Joshi, A. B., Lilley, P. A., Engelbrecht, E., Ryd, L., Lidgren, L., Hardinge, K., Nieder, E., and Walker, P. S. (1992). Polyethylene wear in unicondylar knee prostheses. *Acta Orthop. Scand., 63*, 247–255.

Brand, G. (1991). Cancer risk through foreign body implants. In *Ultra-High Molecular Weight Polyethylene as Biomaterial in Orthopaedic Surgery* (Willert, H.-G., Buchhom, G. H. and Eyerer, P., eds.), pp. 107–110. Hogrefe & Huber Publishers, Toronto.

Charnley, J. (1979). *Low Friction Arthroplasty of the Hip. Theory and Practice.* Springer-Verlag, New York.

Clarke, I. C. (1992). Role of ceramic implants. *Clin. Orthop., 282*, 19–30.

Collier, J. P., Mayor, M. B., McNamara, J. L., Surprenant, V. A. and Jensen, R. L. (1991). Analysis of the failure of 122 polyethylene inserts from uncemented tibial knee components. *Clin. Orthop., 273*, 232–242.

Cooper, R. A., McAllister, C. M., Borden, L. S., and Bauer, T. W. (1992). Polyethylene debris-induced osteolysis and loosening in uncemented total hip arthroplasty. A cause of late failure. *J. Arthroplasty, 7*, 285–290.

DeHeer, D. C., and Hillberry, B. M. (1992). The effect of thickness and nonlinear material behavior on contact stresses in polyethylene tibial components. *Trans. Orthop. Res. Soc., 17*, 327.

Dowson, D., Diab, E.-H., Gillis, B. J. and Atkinson, J. R. (1985). Influence of counterface topography on the wear of ultra high molecular weight polyethylene under wet or dry conditions. *Am. Chem. Soc. Ser., 287*, 171–187.

Dumbleton, J. G. (1983). Prosthesis materials and devices – A review. In *Biocompatible Polymers, Metals, and Composites* (Szycher, M., ed.), pp. 427–460. Technomic Publishing, Lancaster.

Engh, G. A., Dwyer, K. A., and Hanes, C. K. (1992). Polyethylene wear of metal-backed tibial components in total and unicompartmental knee prostheses. *J. Bone Joint Surg. [Br.], 74*, 9–17.

Eyerer, P., Kurth, M., McKellup, H. A., and Mittlmeier, T. (1987). Characterization of UHM-WPE hip cups run on joint simulators. *J. Biomed. Mater. Res., 21*, 275–291.

Goldring, S. R., Jasty, M., Roelke, M., Petrison, K. K., Bringhurst, F. R., Schiller, A. L., and Harris, W. H. (1988). Biological factors that influence the development of a bone-cement membrane. In *Non-Cemented Total Hip Arthroplasty* (Fitzgerald, R. H., Jr., ed.), pp. 35–39. Raven Press, New York.

Goodman, S. B., Fornasier, V. L. and Kei, J. (1991). Quantitative comparison of the histological effects of particulate polymethylmethacrylate versus polyethylene in the rabbit tibia. *Arch. Orthop. Trauma Surg., 110*, 123–126.

Grood, E. S., Shasta, R. and Hopson, C. N. (1982). Analysis of retrieved implants: crystallinity changes in ultrahigh molecular weight polyethylene. *J. Biomed. Mater. Res., 16*, 399–405.

Gross, T. P., and Lennox, D. W. (1992). Osteolytic cyst-like area associated with polyethylene and metallic debris after total knee replacement with an uncemented vitallium prosthesis. A case report. *J. Bone Joint Surg. [Am.], 74*, 1096–1101.

Harris, W. H., and McGann, W. A. (1986). Loosening of the femoral component after use of the medullary-plug cementing technique: Follow-up note with a minimum five-year follow-up. *J. Bone Joint Surg. [Am.], 68*, 1064–1066.

Hayes, W. C., Lathi, V. K., Takeuchi, T. Y., Hipp, J. A., Myers, E. R. and Dennis, D. A. (1993). Patello-femoral contact pressures exceed the compressive yield strength of UHMWPE in total knee replacements. *Trans. Orthop. Res. Soc., 18*, 421.

Hood, R. W., Wright, T. M., and Burstein, A. H. (1983). Retrieval analysis of total knee prostheses: A method and its application to 48 total condylar prostheses. *J. Biomed. Mater. Res., 17*, 829–842.

Huddleston, H. D. (1988). Femoral lysis after cemented hip arthroplasty. *J. Arthroplasty, 3*, 285–297.

Isaac, G.H., Atkinson, G.R., Dowson, D. and Wroblewski, B. M. (1986). The role of cement in the long term performance and premature failure of the Charnley low-friction arthroplasties. *Eng. Med., 15*, 19–22.

Isaac, G. H., Atkinson, J. R., Dowson, D., and Wroblewski, B. M. (1991). The role of acrylic cement in determining the penetration rate of the femoral heads in the polyethylene sockets of Charnley hip prostheses. In *Ultra-High Molecular Weight Polyethylene as Biomaterial in Orthopaedic Surgery* (Willert, H.-G., Buchhorn, G. H., and Eyerer, P., eds.), pp. 128–136. Hogrefe & Huber Publishers, Toronto.

ISO (1985a). Implants for surgery—Ultra-high molecular weight polyethylene—Part 1: Powder form. ISO Standard 5834/1, International Organization for Standardization.

ISO (1985b). Implants for surgery—Ultra-high molecular weight polyethylene—Part 2: Moulded forms. ISO Standard 5834/2, International Organization for Standardization.

Jacobsson, S.-A., Djerf, K., and Wahistrom, O. (1990). A comparative study between McKee-Farrar and Charnley arthroplasty with long-term follow-up periods. *J. Arthroplasty, 5*, 9–14.

Jahan, M. S., Wang, C., Schwartz, G., and Davidson, J. A. (1991). Combined chemical and mechanical effects on free radicals in UHMWPE joints during implantation. *J. Biomed. Mater. Res., 25*, 1005–1017.

Jasty, M. J., Floyd, W. E., III, Schiller, A. L., Goldring, S. R., and Harris, W. H. (1986). Localized osteolysis in stable, non-septic total hip replacement. *J. Bone Joint Surg. [Am.], 68*, 912–919.

Jones, S. M. G., Paider, I. M., Moran, C. G., and Malcolm, A. J. (1992). Polyethylene wear in uncemented knee replacements. *J. Bone Joint Surg. [Br.], 74*, 18–22.

Jordy, A. (1991). Influence of sterilization procedures and packing material on the desorption reaction of UHMWPE after sterilization with ethylene oxide (EO). In *Ultra-High Molecular Weight Polyethylene as Biomaterial in Orthopaedic Surgery* (Willert, H.-G., Buchhom, G. H. and Eyerer, P., eds.), pp. 74–79. Hogrefe & Huber Publishers, Toronto.

Kabo, J. M., Gebhard, J. S., Loren, G., and Amstutz, H. C. (1993). *In vivo* wear of polyethylene acetabular components. *J. Bone Joint Surg. [Br.], 75*, 254–258.

Kurth, M., and Eyerer, P. (1991). Effects of radiation sterilization on UHMWPE. In *Ultra-High Molecular Weight Polyethylene as Biomaterial in Orthopaedic Surgery* (Willert, H.-G., Buchhom, G. H., and Eyerer, P., eds.), pp. 82–88. Hogrefe & Huber Publishers, Toronto.

Lee, E. H., Lewis, M. B., Blau, P. J., and Mansur, L. K. (1991). Improved surface properties of polymer materials by multiple ion beam treatment. *J. Mater. Res., 6*, 610–628.

Lee, J.-M., Salvati, E. A., Betts, F., DiCarlo, E. F., Doty, S. B., and Bullough, P. G. (1992). Size of metallic and polyethylene debris particles in failed cemented total hip replacements. *J. Bone Joint Surg. [Br.], 74*, 380–384.

Livermore, J., Ilstrup, D., and Moffey, B. (1990). Effect of femoral head size on wear of the polyethylene acetabular component. *J. Bone Joint Surg. [Am.], 72*, 518–528.

Lombardi, A. V., Jr., Engh, G. A., Volz, R. G., Albrigo, J. L., and Brainard, B. J. (1988). Fracture/dissociation of the polyethylene in metal-backed patellar components in total knee arthroplasty. *J. Bone Joint Surg. [Am.], 70*, 675–679.

Lombardi, A. V., Jr., Mallory, T. H., Vaughn, B. K. and, Drouillard, P. (1989). Aseptic loosening in total hip arthroplasty secondary to osteolysis induced by wear debris from titanium-alloy modular femoral heads. *J. Bone Joint Surg. [Am.], 71*, 1337–1342.

Maloney, W. J., Jasty, M., Harris, W. H., Galante, J. O., and Callaghan, J. J. (1990a). Endosteal erosion in association with stable uncemented femoral components. *J. Bone Joint Surg. [Am.], 72*, 1025–1034.

Maloney, W. J., Jasty, M., Rosenberg, A., and Harris, W. H. (1990b). Bone lysis in well-fixed cemented femoral components. *J. Bone Joint Surg. [Br.], 72*, 966–970.

Matthews, F. D., Greer, K. W., and Armstrong, D. L. (1986). The effect of nitrogen ion implantation on the abrasive wear resistance of the Ti-6Al-4V/UHMWPE couple. In *Biomedical Materials* (Williams, J. M., Nichols, M. F., and Zingg, W., eds.), pp. 243–252. Materials Research Society, Pittsburgh.

McKellop, H., Clarke, I. C., Markolf, K. L., and Amstutz, H. C. (1978). Wear characteristics of UHMWPE polyethylene: A method for accurately measuring extremely low wear rates. *J. Biomed. Mater. Res., 12*, 895–927.

McKellop, H., Clarke, I., Markolf, K., and Amstutz, H. (1981). Friction and wear properties of polymer, metal, and ceramic prosthetic joint materials evaluated on a multichannel screening device. *J. Biomed. Mater. Res., 15*, 619–653.

McKellop, H., Lu, B., and Li, S. (1992). Wear of acetabular cups of conventional and modified UHMWPE polyethylenes compared on a hip joint simulator. *Trans. Orthop. Res. Soc., 17*, 356.

Miller, R. C. (1990). UHMWPE polyethylene. In *Modern Plastics Encyclopedia*, pp. 76–78. McGraw Hill, New York.

Mintz, L., Tsao, A. K., McCrae, C. R., Stulberg, S. D. and Wright, T. (1991). The arthroscopic evaluation and characteristics of severe polyethylene wear in total knee arthroplasty. *Clin. Orthop., 273*, 215–222.

Mulroy, R. D., and Harris, W. H. (1990). The effect of improved cementing techniques on component loosening in total hip replacements: an 11-year radiographic review. *J. Bone Joint Surg. [Br.], 72*, 757–760.

Murray, D. W., and Rushton, N. (1990). Macrophages stimulate bone resorption when they phagocytose particles. *J. Bone Joint Surg. [Br.], 72*, 988–992.

Nasser, S., Campbell, P. A., Kilgus, D., Kossovsky, N., and Amstutz, H. C. (1990). Cementless total joint arthroplasty prostheses with titanium-alloy articular surfaces. A human retrieval analysis. *Clin. Orthop., 261*, 171–185.

Nolan, J. F., and Bucknill, T. M. (1992). Aggressive granulomatosis from polyethylene failure in an uncemented knee replacement. *J. Bone Joint Surg. [Br.], 74*, 23–24.

Nusbaum, H. J., and Rose, R. M. (1979). The effects of radiation sterilization on the properties of ultrahigh molecular weight polyethylene. *J. Biomed. Mater. Res., 13*, 557–576.

Oonishi, H., Aono, M., Murata, N., and Kushitani, S. (1992). Alumina versus polyethylene in total knee arthroplasty. *Clin. Orthop., 282*, 95–104.

Peters, P. C., Jr., Engh, G. A., Dwyer, K. A., and Vinh, T. N. (1992). Osteolysis after total knee arthroplasty without cement. *J. Bone Joint Surg. [Am.], 74*, 864–876.

Postak, P. D., Steubben, C. M., and Greenwald, A.S. (1993). *Tibial Plateau Surface Stress in TKA: A Factor in Clinical Failure*. The Mt. Sinai Medical Center, Case Western Reserve University.

Revell, P. A., Weightman, B., Freeman, M. A. R., and Vernon-Roberts, B. (1978). The production and biology of polyethylene wear debris. *Arch. Orth. Traum. Surg., 91*, 167–181.

Rieu, J., Pichat, A., Rabbe, L.-M., Rambert, A., Chabrol, C., and Robelet, M. (1991). Ion implantation effects on friction and wear of joint prosthesis materials. *Biomaterials, 12,* 139–143.

Roe, R.-J., Grood, E. S., Shastri, R., Gosselin, C. A., and Noyes, F. R. (1981). Effect of radiation sterilization and aging on ultrahigh molecular weight polyethylene. *J. Biomed. Mater. Res., 15,* 209–230.

Rose, R. M., Goldfarb, E. V., Ellis, E., and Crugnola, A. N. (1984). Radiation sterilization and the wear rate of polyethylene. *J. Orthop. Res., 2,* 393–400.

Rostlund, T., Albrektsson, B., Albrektsson, T., and McKellop, H. (1989). Wear of ion-implanted pure titanium against UHMWPE. *Biomaterials, 10,* 176–181.

Russotti, G. M., Coventry, M. B., and Stauffer, R. N. (1988). Cemented total hip arthroplasty with contemporary techniques. A five-year minimum follow-up study. *Clin. Orthop., 235,* 141–147.

Saikko, V. O., Paavolainen, P. O., and Slatis, P. (1993). Wear of the polyethylene acetabular cup. Metallic and ceramic heads compared in a hip simulator. *Acta Orthop. Scand., 64,* 391–402.

Saito, M., Saito, S., Ohzono, K., Takaoka, K., and Ono, K. (1992). Efficacy of alumina ceramic heads for cemented total hip arthroplasty. *Clin. Orthop., 283,* 171–177.

Santavirta, S., Konttinen, Y. T., Hoikka, V. and Eskola, A. (1990). Aggressive granulomatous lesions associated with hip arthroplasty. *J. Bone Joint Surg. [Am.], 72,* 252–257.

Schmalzried, T. P., Jasty, M., and Harris, W. H. (1992a). Periprosthetic bone loss in total hip arthroplasty. Polyethylene wear debris and the concept of the effective joint space. *J. Bone Joint Surg. [Am.], 74,* 849–863.

Schmalzried, T. P., Kwong, L. M., Jasty, M., Sedlacek, R. C., Haire, T. C., O'Connor, D. O., Bragdon, C. R., Kabo, J. M., Malcolm, A. J., and Harris, W. H. (1992b). The mechanism of loosening of cemented acetabular components in total hip arthroplasty. Analysis of specimens retrieved at autopsy. *Clin. Orthop., 274,* 60–78.

Schmalzried, T. P. (1993). *What about metal on metal articulations?* 23rd Annual Hip Course, Boston, MA.

Semlitsch, M., Letimann, M., Weber, H., Doeffe, E., and Willert, H.-G. (1977). New prospects for a prolonged functional life-span of artificial hip joints by using the material combination polyethylene/aluminium oxide ceramic/metal. *J. Biomed. Mater. Res., 11,* 537–552.

Serwatka, J. S., and Polskonka, J. J. (1993). *A Statistical Study of the Mechanical Properties of Ram Extruded Lennite® Ultra High Molecular Weight Polyethylene.* Westlake Plastics Company, Lenni, PA.

Shinde, A., and Salovey, R. (1985). Irradiation of ultrahigh-molecular-weight polyethylene. *J. Polym. Sci., 23,* 1681–1689.

Sommerich, R. M., Corbo, A. M., and Zalenski, E. B. (1992). *A Comparison of Femoral-Tibial Contact Areas for Various Knee Replacement Systems.* Johnson & Johnson Orthopaedics, Inc., Raynham, MA.

Statler, K. D., Werner, F. W., Ayers, D. C. and Murray, D. G. (1992). Contact surface areas in cruciate sparing knee replacements. *Trans. Orthop. Res. Soc., 17,* 331.

Stein, H. L. (1988). Ultrahigh molecular weight polyethylenes (UHMWPE). *Engineering Plastics* (ASM International, Metals Park, OH), pp. 167–171.

Stern, L. S., Manley, M. T., Parr, J. E., Stulberg, B. N., Price, H., and Ries, M. (1991). Wear properties of retrieved carbon-reinforced and UHMWPE tibial components. In *Ultra-High, Molecular Weight Polyethylene as Biomaterial in Orthopaedic Surgery* (Willert, H.-G., Buchhom, G. H., and Eyerer, P., eds.), pp. 258–261. Hogrefe & Huber Publishers, Toronto.

Streicher, R. M. (1991). The behavior of UHMWPE when subjected to sterilization by ionizing radiation. In *Ultra-High Molecular Weight Polyethylene as Biomaterial in Orthopaedic Surgery* (Willert, H.-G., Buchhom, G. H., and Eyerer, P., eds.), pp. 66–73. Hogrefe & Huber Publishers, Toronto.

Tanzer, M., Maloney, W. J., Jasty, M., and Harris, W. H. (1992). The progression of femoral cortical osteolysis in association with total hip arthroplasty without cement. *J. Bone Joint Surg. [Am.], 74*, 404–410.

Vaes, G. (1988). Cellular biology and biochemical mechanism of bone resorption: A review of recent developments on the formation, activation, and mode of action of osteoclasts. *Clin. Orthop., 231*, 239–271.

Weightman, B., Swanson, S. A. V., Isaac, G. H., and Wroblewski, B. M. (1991). Polyethylene wear from retrieved acetabular cups. *J. Bone Joint Surg. [Br.], 73*, 806–810.

Willert, H.-G., and Semlitsch, M. (1977). Reactions of articular capsule to wear products of artificial joint prostheses. *J. Biomed. Mater. Res., 11*, 157–164.

Willert, H. G., Bertram, H., and Buchhorn, G. H. (1990). Osteolysis in alloarthroplasty of the hip. The role of bone cement fragmentation. *Clin. Orthop., 258*, 108–121.

Winkler-Gniewek, W., and Ungethum, M. (1991). Wear phenomena due to cement deposits on UHMWPE bearing surfaces in clinical application. In *Ultra-High Molecular Weight Polyethylene as Biomaterial in Orthopaedic Surgery* (Willert, H.-G., Buchhorn, G. H., and Eyerer, P., eds.), pp. 137–142. Hogrefe & Huber Publishers, Toronto.

Wright, T. M., Fukubayashi, T., and Burstein, A. H. (1981). The effect of carbon fiber reinforcement on contact area, contact pressure and time dependent deformation in polyethylene tibial components. *J. Biomed. Mater Res., 15*, 719–730.

Wright, T. M., Astion, D. J., Bansal, M., Rimnac, C. M., Green, T., Insall, J. N., and Robinson, R. P. (1988). Failure of carbon fiber-reinforced polyethylene total knee-replacement components. A report of two cases. *J. Bone Joint Surg. [Am.], 70*, 926–932.

Wright, T. M., and Pimnac, C. M. (1991). Analysis of retrieved polyethylene components from total joint replacements. In *Ultra-High Molecular Weight Polyethylene as Biomaterial in Orthopaedic Surgery* (Willert, H.-G., Buchbom, G. H., and Eyerer, P., eds.), pp. 202–207. Hogrefe & Huber Publishers, Toronto.

Wright, T. M., Rinmac, C .M., Stulberg, S. D., Mintz, L., Tsao, A. K., Klein, R. W., and McCrae, C. (1992). Wear of polyethylene in total joint replacements. Observations from retrieved PCA knee implants. *Clin. Orthop., 276*, 126–134.

Yoo, J. H., and Eiss, N. S., Jr. (1993). Tribological behavior of blends of polyether ether ketone and polyether imide. *Wear, 162*, 418–425.

Zichner, L. P., and Willert, H.-G. (1992). Comparison of alumina–polyethylene and metal–polyethylene in clinical trials. *Clin. Orthop., 282*, 86–94.

Zimmer, Inc. (1977). *Poly Two^TM carbon polyethylene composite.* Technical Report, Zimmer, Inc., Warsaw, IN.

22
Bone Substitution and Bone Repair in Trauma Surgery

Peter Patka, Henk J. Th. M. Haarman, and Maarten van der Elst

Free University Hospital
Amsterdam, The Netherlands

I. BONE SUBSTITUTION

A. Introduction on Substitution

The management of traumatic defects in long bones has become an increasing problem in surgery of trauma. Repair of bone defects has resulted in a growing need for a suitable bone tissue replacement material. This also applies to defects caused by malignant disease and to the necessity of bone augmentation in several surgical specialities. Many materials have been used and improved in the past [1].

An ideal bone substitute has to mimic the tissue it replaces in size, shape, consistency, and function. It should not be predisposed to infection and it should not evoke a healing response that would alter its characteristics. As it disappears it has to acquire qualities of the tissue it replaced or augmented. Finally, if it does not disappear, it has to be tolerated permanently.

The best material for bone defect repair seems to be an autograft. However, the available quantity is limited, and obtaining the autograft itself may cause a higher morbidity [1,2]. Therefore, it may turn out that the best bone substitute will be allografts, and that, as the host rejection phenomenon is overcome, permanent incorporation of transplanted allografts might become possible. The influence of genetic incompatibility resulting in rejection of an allograft at present can be reduced but not fully eliminated by treating these grafts by special procedures [3]. However, these procedures influence not only the biological but also the mechanical properties of an allograft.

Within the scope of these problems there is a continuing search for an ideal material for surgical bone repair that combines total biological inertness with adequate mechanical properties.

Research on biocompatibility has brought to light some ceramic materials that may be suitable for permanent bone tissue replacement. Ceramics made from the calcium phosphate system have a unique biological profile. In particular hydroxyapatite seems to be useful as a permanent bone substitute. This biomaterial exhibits an excellent biocompatibility with respect to bone tissue. Earlier studies on the use of hydroxyapatite as a hard tissue implant showed this material to be suitable for small-volume implantation in cases where applied mechanical stress is either minimal or restricted to compressive physiological loads. More recently data have been reported on the use of apatite ceramics for repair of large defects.

B. Natural Bone Tissue

Bone is a specialized type of connective tissue, characterized by the presence of cells with long branching processes (osteocytes) that occupy cavities (lacunae) and fine canals (canaliculi) in a hard, dense matrix consisting of bundles of collagenous fibers in an amorphous ground substance (cement) impregnated with calcium phosphate complexes. The osteocytes as well as the osteoblasts and osteoclasts are derived by differentiation from mesenchymal cells. The osteoblasts, precursors of osteocytes, lay down the organic matrix of new bone, which subsequently is mineralized. In forming new bone, osteoblasts secrete collagen, usually apposed to a preexisting calcified surface. The osteoclast is a multinucleated giant cell responsible for the dissolution and removal of matrix and mineral. In the steady state this process occurs virtually simultaneously. The origin of the osteoclast is still the subject of discussion.

The bone matrix contains collagen, ground substances, and bone mineral (calcium phosphate complexes). Collagen is fibrillar in nature, having a definite arrangement of amino acid groups in a particular crystal structure. The collagen fibers demonstrate frequent cross-linkages. Between the fibers there is a material referred to as *ground substance* (cement), which is composed of protein mucopolysaccharides. The collagen supports the mineral component within the ground substance. The bone mineral contains complexes of calcium phosphate in amorphous and crystalline fractions. With aging the crystalline fraction increases related to the amorphous fraction. The major mineral bone component is hydroxyapatite: $Ca_{10}(PO_4)_6(OH)_2$. This calcium phosphate salt is nonstoichiometric and has a calcium/phosphorus ratio of 9 : 6, in contrast to a stoichiometric salt, which has a ratio of 10 : 6. Hydroxyapatite has a hexagonal crystal structure (Fig. 1). The largest crystal dimension does not exceed 60 nm.

The main part of apatite crystals in bone is elongated along the crystallographic *c* axis and is oriented parallel to the collagen fibers. Besides plate-like crystallites, needle-like apatite crystallites have been demonstrated [5]. The crystals first appear within the substance of the collagen fibers and then additional crystals form around the peripheries of these fibers. The final product, bone, consists mainly of collagen fibers and hydroxyapa-

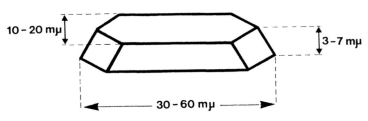

Figure 1   A diagrammatic picture of bone mineral crystal according to Robinson and Watson [4].

tite crystals. Other calcium phosphates present in small quantities in bone are octacalcium phosphate, calcium pyrophosphate, and brushite.

There are two basic types of bone structure found in mammals: woven and lamellar bone. The bone cells (osteocytes) surrounded by calcified matrix are concentrically oriented to central canaliculi occupied by a capillary vessel. They form solid cylinders (osteons) around the central, longitudinally situated canals (Haversian systems). The bone is built up with osteon units [6].

Osteogenesis, or ossification, is the normal manner in which bone growth occurs in the body. There are four different types of osteogenesis:

- Enchondral osteogenesis
- Appositional osteogenesis
- Remodeling of bone
- Fracture healing

Enchondral ossification is indirect bone ingrowth. Indirect bone formation means that bone is formed after and from the primary formation of cartilage. Direct bone formation by-passes the intermediate stage of cartilage formation. Appositional bone growth and bone remodeling are both examples of direct bone growth.

Healing of bone fractures involves direct and indirect bone formation. The potency of regeneration and self-repair of bone tissue in cases of fracture or other bone tissue damage has been recognized but the mechanism of osteogeneic induction in cases of bone tissue self-repair is controversial [7]. Following a fracture, the bone structure will be restored through several stages consisting of fibrous tissue and cartilage (callus), and finally by remodeling through simultaneous osteoblastic and osteoclastic activity. As is generally known, this process can be disrupted by many factors [8]. In cases of proper reposition, fixation, and compression of a fracture with no bone tissue defect, only direct bone formation (primary osteogenesis) occurs. The bone responds to mechanical stress by placing or displacing bone elements in the direction of the applied forces, and increases or decreases in mass reflect the level of these forces. The mechanism by which mechanical forces affect the activity of the osteogenic cells is unknown [7]. In the course of time, further thickening and reorientation of trabeculae along the lines of stress ceases and the remodeling process gradually decreases to the skeleton's normal rate of physiological turnover.

Bone remains elastic up to about three quarters of its breaking strain. The study of stress and strain in bones has been of major interest to many investigators and they produced an extensive bibliography of elastic moduli of bone tissue [9]. However, a wide variation of the modulus of elasticity (Young's modulus) can be observed in experimental models [10]. Young's modulus of elasticity has been found to be about $14\text{--}21 \times 10^9$ $N \cdot m^{-2}$ for human bone. The stress resistance capacity and elasticity of natural bone depends upon the individual methods of loading, the test conditions, the freshness of the test specimen, and the age of the specimen at death [11]. Characteristics of human bone material properties are summarized in Table 1.

If one endeavors to take into account all the biological, chemical, and physical properties now known to be either mandatory or desirable in an artificial bone replacement material, then the design and production of such a material is still fraught with difficulties. At the present time biomaterials, and especially some of the ceramics, show some of the qualities of natural bone tissue and are the subject of experimental and clinical studies [1,12].

Table 1 Mechanical Properties of the Human Femur

	Average or range ($N \cdot m^{-2}$)
Tensile strength	$90–110 \cdot 10^6$
Flexural strength	$80 \cdot 10^6$
Compressive strength	$130–170 \cdot 16^6$
Shear strength parallel to longitudinal axis	$110 \cdot 10^6$
Shear strength parallel to transverse axis	$40–90 \cdot 10^6$
Break stress of twisting	$70 \cdot 10^6$
Modulus of elasticity (Young)	$14–21 \cdot 10^9$

C. History of Bone Defect Repair

The oldest evidence of bone defect repair is seen in remains of trephined prehistoric skulls [13]. There is a report on a rather large defect in a bronze age skull that was evidently closed by reimplanting the removed fragment as an orthotopic bone autograft. In the specimen, the cut margin shows no sign of healing, so the operation may have been fatal.

The first successful bone defect repair was recorded by the Dutch surgeon Job van Meek'ren in 1668 (Fig. 2) [14]. He described the filling of a defect in a soldier's cranium

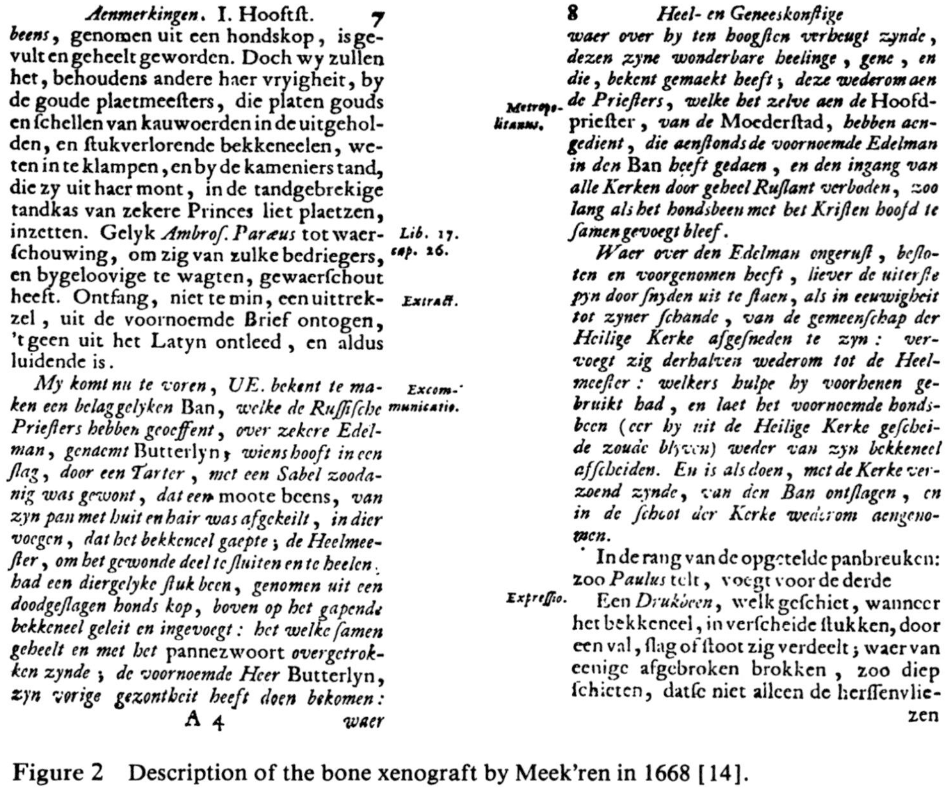

Aenmerkingen. I. Hooftſt. 7

beens, genomen uit een hondskop, is gevult en geheelt geworden. Doch wy zullen het, behoudens andere haer vryigheit, by de goude plaetmeeſters, die platen gouds en ſchellen van kauwoerden in de uitgeholden, en ſtukverlorende bekkeneelen, weten in te klampen, en by de kameniers tand, die zy uit haer mont, in de tandgebrekige tandkas van zekere Princes liet plaetzen, inzetten. Gelyk Ambroſ. Paræus tot waerſchouwing, om zig van zulke bedriegers, en bygeloovige te wagten, gewaerſchout heeft. Ontfang, niet te min, een uittrekzel, uit de voornoemde Brief ontogen, 't geen uit het Latyn ontleed, en aldus luidende is. *Lib. 17. cap. 26.* *Extract.*

My komt nu te voren, UE. bekent te maken een belaggelyken Ban, welke de Ruſſiſche Prieſters hebben geoeffent, over zekere Edelman, genaemt Butterlyn, wiens hooft in een ſlag, door een Tarter, met een Sabel zoodanig was gewont, dat een moote beens, van zyn pan met huit en hair was afgekeilt, in dier voegen, dat het bekkeneel gaepte; de Heelmeeſter, om het gewonde deel te ſluiten en te heelen, had een diergelyke ſtuk been, genomen uit een doodgeſlagen honds kop, boven op het gapende bekkeneel geleit en ingevoegt: het welke ſamen geheelt en met het pannezwoort overgetrokken zynde; de voornoemde Heer Butterlyn, zyn vorige gezontheit heeft doen bekomen: *Excommunicatio.*

A 4 waer

8 Heel- en Geneeskonſtige

waer over by ten hoogſten verheugt zynde, dezen zyne wonderbare heelinge, gene, en die, bekent gemaekt heeft; deze wederom aen de Prieſters, welke het zelve aen de Hoofdprieſter, van de Moederſtad, hebben aengedient, die aenſtonds de voornoemde Edelman in den Ban heeft gedaen, en den ingang van alle Kerken door geheel Ruſlant verboden, zoo lang als het hondsbeen met het Kriſten hoofd te ſamen gevoegt bleef. *Metropolitanus.*

Waer over den Edelman ongeruſt, beſloten en voorgenomen heeft, liever de uiterſte pyn door ſnyden uit te ſtaen, als in eeuwigheit tot zyner ſchande, van de gemeenſchap der Heilige Kerke afgeſneden te zyn: vervoegt zig derhalven wederom tot de Heelmeeſter: welkers hulpe hy voorhenen gebruikt had, en laet het voornoemde hondsbeen (eer hy uit de Heilige Kerke geſcheide zoude blyven) weder van zyn bekkeneel afſcheiden. En is als doen, met de Kerke verzoend zynde, van den Ban ontſlagen, en in de ſchoot der Kerke wederom aengenomen.

In de rang van de opgetelde panbreuken: zoo Paulus telt, voegt voor de derde

Een Drukbeen, welk geſchiet, wanneer het bekkeneel, in verſcheide ſtukken, door een val, ſlag of ſtoot zig verdeelt; waer van eenige afgebroken brokken, zoo diep ſchieten, datſe niet alleen de herſſenvliezen *Expreſſio.*

Figure 2 Description of the bone xenograft by Meek'ren in 1668 [14].

with a piece of dog skull. This bone xenograft had to be removed 2 years later on the patient's wish, since after the transplantation he was excommunicated and he wanted to return to the good graces of the Church.

The scientific approach to the problem of osteogenesis and bone transplantation was started by du Hamel in 1739 [15]. However, it took almost 200 years before anyone was able to report large series of patients with an autogenous bone transplant. The problems of humoral and cellular immune response to bone allografts remain unsolved until this very day [3].

Bone is transplanted more often nowadays than any other tissue with the possible exception of skin and blood. During the period 1977–1979 more than 12,000 bone-grafting procedures were performed in the Netherlands alone. The yearly increase is almost 10%. Today it is estimated that in a single year in the United States over 100,000 procedures are performed involving bone grafts or implants [16].

Bone transplants are used to unite fractures, to fuse joints, and to repair skeletal defects only in those cases where they can satisfy the criteria of mechanical stability and host incorporation without complications. The acquisition of autogenous bone transplant material is not without consequences for the patient, which can include:

- Additional surgical incision
- Weakened bone at the donor site
- Increased postoperative morbidity [2]

Not only is the amount of autogenous bone restricted, but furthermore, the bone graft may have insufficient mechanical, biological, and physiological properties.

Because of the limited availability of appropriate bone replacement materials, many artificial materials for bone substitution have been developed [1,17–19]. Some of them are clearly related to bone tissue. In that case the term *transplant* as well as *implant* can be used.

According to the genetic relationship between donor and recipient, there are four classes of bone transplants:

1. *Autogenous bone graft* (autograft): donor and recipient are the same individual
2. *Isogenous bone graft* (isograft): donor and recipient are genetically identical individuals of the same species (monozygotic twins, animals of highly inbred strain)
3. *Allogenous bone graft* (allograft): donor and recipient are genetically dissimilar individuals of the same species
4. *Xenogenous bone graft* (xenograft): donor and recipient are individuals of different species

Transplantation generally does not include the use of prostheses, synthetic materials, or artificial implants that may be fixed within or attached to the body but that do not comprise human or animal cells or tissues. However, the materials could coincidentally be of similar composition to living tissue or even be produced by living organs. An example of such a material is the porous calcium carbonate and hydroxyapatite skeletal structure of some marine invertebrates. In this context, the xenograft may encompass artificial implants.

According to the site of implantation, transplants are termed *orthotopic* when the transplantation site and donor site are the same, and *heterotopic* when these sites are different.

Grafts may be viable or nonviable when implanted.

1. Autogenous Bone Graft

Autogenous bone graft possesses maximum biocompatibility. Therefore autogenous cancellous bone is generally considered to be the best material available for bone grafting [1]. Cancellous grafts are more rapidly and completely revascularized than cortical grafts.

Fundamentally both cancellous and cortical bone are incorporated by the same process including apposition and resorption, but there is a difference in the rate of apposition and resorption. The substitution of a cancellous bone graft first involves a phase of appositional bone formation and secondarily a resorptive phase, whereas a cortical bone graft undergoes a process sometimes described as *creeping substitution* and in most cases remains as an admixture of necrotic and viable bone [20].

The mechanical strengths of cancellous and cortical autogenous bone grafts may be correlated with their respective repair processes. Cancellous bone autografts tend to become strong first, whereas cortical grafts lose strength in the beginning. This weakening of cortical transplant is a function of its internal porosity. This is caused by the cumulative effects of increased osteoclastic and decreased osteoblastic activities and illustrates the creeping substitution [21]. Experimental cortical bone transplants were shown to be approximately 40-50% weaker than normal bone from 6 weeks to 6 months after transplantation. Cortical bone strength was regained in approximately 1-2 years as the internal porosity approached that of normal bone. The "segmental" autogenous cortical bone transplant has to be protected when the resorptive phase has outstripped the appositional phase. It is not precisely known when these critical phases occur in humans.

The active osteogenesis by the living cells of an autogenous bone transplant, in contrast to the inductive properties of the noncellular organic and inorganic elements of the graft, is the main advantage of autogenous bone grafting. It is not known how much of the final incorporation of the transplant is due to the tissue of the host and how much is due to the remaining living cells of the graft.

Transplant failure occurs in 15-25% of autogenous segmental cortical transplants: Most of them have failed principally because they did not satisfy the necessary biological, physiological, and mechanical requirements [21]. Adequate fixation of the graft following its insertion is essential, "as study of various means for these ends in such work as tree grafting will show" [22]. The revascularization of bone autograft by microvascular anastomoses has been the subject of experimental studies and may become of practical importance in bone grafting [23-25]. As early as 1923 Albee pointed out the following requirements for bone grafting from his experience of 3000 grafts:

1. The graft should be autogenous.
2. The marrow of the graft should be in contact with the marrow of the host bone.
3. The graft should be the internal fixation agent, within limits. Use of metal plates or other foreign material is not recommended.
4. The graft should consist of all four bone layers, namely periosteum, complete thickness of cortex, endosteum, and marrow.
5. The graft should be inserted so that corresponding cambium layers come in close contact.
6. The graft should be strong enough so that it will resist fracture during and after the period of artificial external support, until osteogenesis occurs to a sufficient degree.

Despite the excellent biocompatibility, the limited availability and the higher morbidity associated with obtaining the autograft remain disadvantages of autogenous bone graft [2,26]. Therefore many bone-saving procedures, such as the use of boiled or frozen orthotopic bone autograft, have been developed in traumatology for the repair of massive loss of bone, and in oncological surgery after eradication of malignant or benign bone tumors [27,28]. The insertion of a prosthesis to repair the continuity of bone is only a good treatment for patients with bone tumors of low-grade malignancy. Even a massive tumorous bone segment can be resected, autoclaved, and replaced to reconstruct bone continuity. However, addition of free, fresh autogenous bone chips and a rigid fixation with long-term stability would be necessary. The benign but locally destructive bone tumor can be treated by freezing. The osteogenetic potential and the mechanical properties of bone transplants treated this way are not the same as those of autogenous bone.

The advantages of boiled or frozen autograft can be summarized as follows:

- The immediate availability of bone tissue.
- The graft is a "good fit."
- Sufficient stability.
- Extensive use of bone from donor sites is not required.
- Reconstruction of large bone defects is possible.

However, it is not always possible to save or obtain autogenous bone for bone defect repair. The defect may be too large to be filled by an autogenous bone graft alone. The operation required for obtaining pieces of autogenous bone graft may be an unnecessary additional stress for the patient [2,26]. In cases of facial bone defects as well as in cases of reconstructive middle ear surgery, additional difficulties in the shaping and restoration of the normal and symmetrical facial contour may be encountered when bone chips are used. The same applies in middle ear reconstructive surgery. In such cases some other hard tissue substitute material is needed [20].

The alternative for repair of bone defects by transplantation of autogenous tissue, such as free non- or revascularized autogenous periosteum, has been reported in experimental studies. However the lack of stability and the long period of time needed for bone formation from periosteum are the main problems in the clinical use of periosteal transplant in cases of massive loss of bone.

2. Isogenous Bone Graft

Isogenous bone graft is only of theoretical importance in human bone defect repair because of the low incidence (1 : 250 pregnancies) of monozygotic twins. There is no literature concerning this subject in the field of bone transplantation.

3. Allogenous Bone Graft

Skeletal surgery, especially bone tumor surgery, often requires additional supplies of bone, which may not be obtained in sufficient quantity and quality from the host without unacceptable risks [2,22,26]. Therefore, allogenous and even xenogenous grafts and, more recently, artificial materials have been considered as alternatives to autogenous bone grafts.

Allogenous bone grafts became a relatively popular alternative to autogenous bone. However, allogenous bone grafts present an immunological problem. Transplants of fresh allogenous bone follow the immunological principles of other tissue allografts. The main disadvantages of allografting is elicitation of the immunological host response, resulting in graft rejection. Because of this allograft property, the bone autograft, even if difficult to obtain, is still preferable in bone tissue replacement [23–25].

The histocompatibility antigens of bone allografts are presumably proteins or glycoproteins on cell surfaces, although it is not certain if the bone matrix itself is able to elicit the immunological host response [21]. The rejection of bone allografts is considered to be a cellular rather than a humoral mechanism. The graft rejection is expressed by the disruption of vessels, an inflammatory reaction dominated by lymphocytes, fibrous encapsulation, peripheral graft resorption, callus bridging, nonunions, and fatigue fractures. The remodeling of allografted bone is a long-term process. This also includes the possibility of late rejection of bone allografts.

Many techniques have been suggested to minimize the antigenic differences between the donor and the recipient of a bone allograft. Destruction of the antigens within the bone allograft, blocking the host's immune response and recently, tissue typing have been suggested as means of minimizing antigenic differences [26]. Bone allografts that are treated to destroy their antigenicity prior to implantation lack viable cells and become implants. The treatment of allografts by chemical procedures, heating or freezing, and by ionizing radiation energy causes changes in the physical and biological properties of the graft.

One of the oldest methods is boiling the bone graft [27]. Boiling destroys the antigens of the bone, but boiled bone is less successfully incorporated in the recipient because the cells are destroyed and the proteins are denatured. Its inductive repair capacity has been negated. Despite loss of bone induction, some excellent clinical results have been claimed in boiled allogenous bone implants [28,29].

Frozen bone grafts have frequently been used as a substitute material for autografts because they are considered to be almost nonantigenic. However, the experimental and clinical findings demonstrate that bone immunogenicity is partially retained. Freeze-dried bone allografts have been used for the clinical packing of small defects or the bridging of large defects [28,29]. The final evaluation of freeze-dried bone grafting is incomplete. Long-term evaluation suggests complications similar to those found with frozen grafts [21].

Treatment of an allogenous bone graft by chemicals may involve deproteinization, decalcification, and lipophilization. Deproteinized bone implants were obtained by ethylenediamine extraction or glycerol-ashing, but they were mechanically quite fragile and therefore not suitable as supportive skeletal struts [30,31]. Organic decalcified bone allografts heal a skeletal defect more successfully than inorganic implants do. Cortical bone matrix decalcified in hydrochloric or ethylene diaminetetra-acetic (EDTA) or formic–citric acids, in contrast to decalcifying agents such as nitric acid, provide the local conditions for histotypic and organotypic formation of new bone according to several investigators [28,32,33]. Partially decalcified allogenous bone used to bridge large osteoperiosteal defects has been reported to retain its repairing capacity [34].

Irradiation has been used for destroying the antigens contained within the bone. The irradiated implants can still induce osteogenesis in the host [35]. However, they may contain activated tissue and produce mutagenic radicals. The effect of irradiation on the physiological integrity of the tissue and problems concerning sterilization constitute additional disadvantages of this method. Therefore, the irradiated bone graft has, in practice, been little used in bone augmentation surgery.

The temporary immunosuppression of the host, while the allograft undergoes creeping substitution and depletion of transplantation antigens, has not been fully investigated yet. This concept seems to be of limited practical value because of the need for long-term immunosuppression and its concomitant side effects. Histocompatibility tissue typing improves acceptance of bone allografts in experimental studies and may be of value in clinical situations. However, the difficulties with tissue typing procedures are still not solved [26,36].

As an allogenous tissue, bone is antigenically active [37–39]. Although many methods have been used to reduce or avoid this antigenicity, none of them has so far gained widespread acceptance. Conflicting reports regarding the bone-forming efficiency of allogenous bone -matrix may be due to the chemical, physical, and biological treatment of bone matrix before implantation [40]. We cannot exclude the possibility that such treatment preceding implantation may in fact render a tissue of such poor quality as to confer no particular advantage over a purely artificial substance [41–43]. The conclusion may be drawn that an allogenous bone graft is not a suitable aid for restoring the continuity of a bone in adults [44]. Bone allografts can also transmit human immunodeficiency virus (HIV).

4. Xenogenous Bone Graft

Xenogenous (hetero) grafts can be divided into two main groups: cross-species bone grafts and artificial material implants.

Cross-Species Bone Grafts. The cross-species (mostly bovine) bone grafts have to be specially treated because of genetic incompatibility, but this must be done without changing its structural characteristics [45]. The organic fraction (antigens, fats, mucopolysaccharides, etc.) has to be removed to allow the host's acceptance of this so-called Os Purum [36]. Ethylenediamine-treated anorganic bone has been a widely used material in bone replacement [39]. Defatted, decalcified, xenogenous bone impregnated with fresh autologous marrow has been used in experimental bridging of large cortical defects. However, reports on the use of this bone material have given conflicting results. Bone-inducing properties have been reported by some but denied by others. Defatted calcified bovine graft (Kiel bone) has been used in spinal fusion [47]. Frozen bone xenografts were used in so-called bone-banks but were eventually discarded because of problems arising from their genetic incompatibility.

Artificial Material Implants. The artificial (mostly anorganic) materials (xenoimplants) constitute a large group of metals, plastic polymers, ceramics, and composite materials. Even wooden implants have been proposed for bone tissue replacement [48].

Biocompatibility. The development and application of surgical and orthopedic implants made it necessary to give increasing attention to the materials used for the manufacture of such implants. These materials, which are also referred to as *biomaterials* have to meet certain chemical, physical, and biological requirements in order to ensure optimum and lasting function of the implant and success of the implantation procedure. The chemical and physical requirements include such properties as strength, wearing friction behavior, and corrosion resistance, as well as workability and sterilizability. Acceptance by living tissues and stability within the body constitute important biological requirements.

Biocompatibility is determined by the extent of chemical and biological interaction between host and implant, and the stability (mechanical integrity) of the implant [49]. Rapid and inexpensive *in vitro* techniques can be used to predict the quantity and cytotoxicity of moieties released by an implant. These techniques can also be used to predict changes in mechanical properties of a material during implantation. This can be important in selection of materials as candidates for definitive preclinical animal experimental and clinical studies.

A compatible implant would have no effect on the adjacent tissue, the nearby cells would show no abnormalities, no variant cell types would appear, there would be no inflammatory reactions, and there would be no cell necrosis. The histology of the tissue surrounding the implant would be altogether normal [50].

The implant recognized by the recipient as a foreign body will be isolated by encapsulation. Commonly, the thickness of the encapsulating fibrous tissue membrane is often taken as a measure of the compatibility of the implant in relation to the surrounding tissue. The thinner the membrane, the better the compatibility of the implant [51,52].

Animal studies of biocompatibility are necessary because of the complexity of chemical, biological, and physical (mechanical) implant–host interactions. Strong dependence of the tissue response on the biomechanical conditions along the interfaces has been demonstrated in experimental studies. The amount of motion between the implant and the adjacent tissues contributes greatly to the biological response. Any histological evaluation of a biomaterial for bone replacement must be accompanied by a careful description of the load and changes that have been applied to the bone–implant interface. The portion of the interface from which the histological sample was taken has to be noted [53].

Unfortunately, methods of determination of compatibility are not standardized. This complicates any comparison of different studies of a specific implant material. Sometimes it makes it impossible. Therefore it has been proposed to establish a rigid system in determining material biocompatibility by standardized test controls [51,54,55]. Implant materials should be subjected to biological tests in a stepwise standardized procedure. As is well known, no general agreement on this has yet been reached. In general, either a material has slowly evolved to fulfill a long-established clinical need or a new material has been tried on a somewhat arbitrary basis to explore clinical and commercial possibilities. Probably most biomaterials have become known to us in this fashion. This situation is less satisfactory than if a thoroughly scientific approach to the development of biocompatible materials had been adopted.

Biodegradability; Bioactive and Bioinert Material.   The terms *biodegradable, bioactive,* and *bioinert* are related to the biochemical response the implanted material provokes in the surrounding tissue and relates to the notion of *biocompatibility.* The tissue reactions caused by relative movement between the implant and the adjacent tissue are not covered by these terms [56]. The term *biodegradable* (bioresorbable) has been used for material that, after insertion into host tissue, is dissolved without provoking any adverse tissue reaction. Some of the calcium phosphate ceramics possess such a property [57].

The terms *bioactive* and *bioinert* are related to the biochemical response induced by the material at the site of implantation. The bioactive materials induce the same reaction as natural bone mineral would do at the same implant area while the bioinert materials cause no reaction at all. Bioactive ceramics can form a tight junction with the osseous tissue, analogous to the natural bone mineral. This seems to be a biochemical phenomenon, but there is still no explanation for this behavior of bioactive materials [50,57–60].

Metals.   Implants used in the repair of bone defects were already described by Peàn in 1894 [61]. Metal implants are currently widely used in prosthesiology (articular prostheses) and in surgery (internal or external support) for fractures. The use of metals for bone tissue replacement never succeeds because a metal implant of any composition placed in bone tissue will become surrounded by a fibrous tissue layer [62]. This fibrous tissue layer presents a weak point in the metal implant–bone fixation. There have been several attempts to provide better fixation of a metal implant in bone by means of a porous material. However, after rapid bone ingrowth in the pores had occurred, a thin layer of fibrous tissue was still seen surrounding individual metal fibers lying interposed between them and the bone trabeculae [63].

A metal implant is tolerated by but not incorporated into the living tissue. Corrosion or similar chemical degradation caused by the action of body fluids and tissues on the implant not only changes the physical properties of the implant, but moreover, the products so formed are often toxic, causing an allergenic and/or carcinogenic response and subsequent isolation and exposure of the foreign body [64,65]. Metal carcinogenesis has been postulated many times in the literature but has never been really proved by animal or clinical studies [65–71].

The new metal implants are more resistant to corrosion, are better tolerated by the body tissues, and possess better strength resistance capacity, and some of them even show better biocompatibility [72]. An example of such a metal is titanium, whose surface becomes ceramic through oxidation.

Nonetheless, the use of metals in bone defect repair will be limited to temporary support and fixation because of their low-grade biocompatibility.

Plastics. Plastic polymer implants are widely used as bone tissue replacements despite their inferior mechanical properties. The vast majority of polymers are used in a modified form after the admixture of one or more of a great variety of additives (plasticizers, fillers, heat stabilizers, ultraviolet light stabilizers, pigments, and lubricants).

The end product is usually called a *plastic*. The main additives for biomedical plastic are introduced to improve mechanical properties or inertness. Certain plastic materials, especially polyethylene, polyvinyl, acrylic compounds, and methylmethacrylate, in compact or porous form, have been used as a bone substitute material [73,74].

Mechanical properties of some plastic implants can be influenced and changed by body substances such as enzymes after implantation [73,75]. Low wear resistance gives rise to a pronounced foreign-body giant-cell reaction and to excessive fibrosis. The mechanical properties of newer plastic polymers are the subject of experimental studies. The modulus of elasticity influences the process of ingrowth of sprouting capillaries, perivascular tissue, and osteoprogenitor cells from the recipient bone bed into porous plastic materials. Better mechanical compatibility of new porous plastics results in ingrowth of bone that mimics normal bone repair. One can expect a better ingrowth of bone into the pores of porous plastic implants, because of their elasticity [76].

Plastic implants, like metal ones, are mostly surrounded by connective tissue. Some of them can even be toxic to living tissue. Apparent incompatibility can generally be traced to the presence of extractable materials (additives) that may give rise to toxic reactions [51]. Most experimental implantations of polymers are followed by an initial foreign-body reaction. Incidental reports indicate that polymers may be carcinogenic in animals [77,78].

An impressive number of plastic implants and even plastic bone tissue replacement materials have been developed during the last three decades. The most important disadvantage of plastics seems to be their lack of biocompatibility. However, with the development of new plastic materials in reconstructive surgery, new materials of better biocompatibility can be expected.

Ceramics. Ceramics comprise heterogeneous groups of related materials [57]. There is no universal classification for these materials. Therefore, it is not very useful for practical purposes to classify ceramics on the basis of their chemical structure, crystalline structure, or biocompatibility [52].

Most ceramic materials are crystalline in nature. However, there are amorphous or glassy ceramics, too. The distinction between those ceramics that are amorphous or glassy and some types of glass, which have high melting points, is somewhat difficult to draw.

Different ceramics—such as calcium phosphate ceramics; crystalline variants of bioglasses; and materials such as calcium aluminates, titanates, zirconates, and alumina

(Al$_2$O$_3$) and silica (SiO$_2$)—have been used for surgical implantation. Alumina, first, and hydroxyapatite later, became the most widely used ceramic implants [72,79]. Ceramics, in compact or porous form, offer an attractive alternative to metals as a bone tissue replacement material. They possess the following advantages.

- Many ceramic oxides are at their highest energy level and cannot be oxidized further.
- They are mostly insoluble in body fluids.
- They are highly inert and some of them are even bioactive [18,29,80].

The disadvantages, however, are that ceramics are known to be brittle materials possessing no ductility, and generally they have an extremely high modulus of elasticity and low flexural and tensile strength. They are also difficult to manufacture, as high temperatures are required, and they are difficult to mold in applicable forms. For these reasons, in the past very little serious consideration of ceramic materials proceeded further than the consideration of their mechanical properties. With the development of technology and instruments for designing ceramics in applicable forms and the development of new ceramics and composites, these disadvantages are being overcome.

In the absence of systematic guidelines, the history of the choice of ceramic materials for repair of bone defects has been one of trial and error. The first report of the use of ceramics to fill defects in bone came in 1892 from Trendelenburg's clinic in Bonn. Plaster of Paris (biodegradable calcium sulfate dihydrate: dihydrate 2CaSO$_4$) was used to fill bone cavities of different origins (tuberculosis, osteomyelitis, and enchondroma) in eight patients with satisfactory results [81]. Since then, plaster of Paris has been used in a limited number of experimental and clinical studies. It has never been used widely, due to its poor mechanical properties and because its resorption rate is too rapid to allow adequate bone ingrowth [82–85].

Only within the last few years have reports have appeared on the use of ceramic materials for internal prosthetic application and also on the repair of skeletal defects [86]. In 1963, almost 70 years after the first use of plaster of Paris to fill a bone defect, a porous ceramic material with a good tissue compatibility was proposed for bone replacement. Porous aluminate ceramic has been considered nontoxic and noncarcinogenic, and therefore useful as a bone tissue replacement material. Ossicular chain replacement in reconstructive middle ear surgery using aluminate ceramic material led to promising results in the experimental animals as well as in clinical cases. Jahnke performed more than 250 tympanoplasties with this material [29]. Extensive use of aluminum oxide ceramic in prosthesiology has been reported [87].

Since this success of aluminum oxide ceramic as a bone tissue replacement material, many other ceramic materials—such as calcium phosphates, calcium aluminates and calcium silicates, aluminum silicates and titanium oxide, and bioglass ceramics—have been developed and tested during the last two decades. The first applications of these materials were in dentistry and in oral and maxillofacial surgery. Later, various methods were used to replace bone with different ceramic materials in surgery and orthopedics. Ceramics have been injected as a solution or implanted as granules to stimulate osteogenesis; they have been used as a filler that is resorbed at approximately the same rate as new bone regenerates. They have also been used as a compact material in places of attrition or as a porous implant that would invite osseous proliferation into open pores. A most important observation has been the high degree of compatibility between the host bone and some of the ceramic materials [88–90].

The use of porous ceramics in soft tissue replacement, such as tracheal prostheses or in the cardiovascular system as valve replacement, have not been generally recommended because of the high infection rate and because of their severe thrombogenic activity when in direct contact with blood [91,92]. Still, dense ceramics such as vitreous carbon have found wide application in replacement of heart valves.

At the moment, the ceramics used as bone tissue replacement material show encouraging experimental and clinical results. The cell and tissue compatibility of many ceramic materials has been improved in recent studies. Particularly hydroxyapatite displays an attractive profile that features its excellent biocompatibility [90–92]. Porous ceramics, with a pore size greater than 100 μm show significant ingrowth of natural bone when these implants are in contact with host bone tissue [86] (Figs. 3 and 4). These ceramics have already been developed as commercially available implants (Fig. 5) and are used in clinical practice (Fig. 6). Reduced mechanical resilience appears to be the only disadvantage at the present time that might restrict its clinical application. The search continues for an ideal ceramic material for surgical implants that would combine complete biological inertness with adequate mechanical strength.

Composite Materials. A composite material is simply a combination of two or more different materials. In order to design a composite material having a certain set of properties, the following characteristics of the compounds have to be considered:

- The biodegradability
- The biocompatibility
- The elastic moduli
- The mechanical strength
- The binding tendencies between the components

These variables interact in a complex manner, and a detailed consideration of each is necessary to anticipate the behavior of various components when combined to form a composite material.

Modern composites are intended to imitate nature. Bone is a composite of the strong but soft protein collagen and the hard but brittle mineral hydroxyapatite. Modern composites try to achieve similar results by the combination of strong fibers of a material such as carbon in a soft matrix. The new materials provide strength, stiffness, and lightness, and are also inert.

Most composite materials include a ceramic component because of the biocompatibility and the biodegradability of ceramics. The other component can be metal or plastic. A familiar example is Cerosium (alumina and epoxy resin) and Fibreglass (fiber glass reinforced plastic). An unscratched ceramic can be very strong, but flaws enable it to be easily cracked. If the ceramic is divided into minute pieces, as in powder, any cracks that are present cannot find a continuous path through the material. For the particles, or more usually fibers, to form a useful structural material, they must be bound together in a matrix. The properties of the matrix are of great importance. The matrix must not scratch the fibers and introduce cracks. It must transmit stress to the fibers, be plastic and adhesive to immobilize the fibers securely, and, finally, it must deflect and control cracks within the composite. Under tensile load, virtually all the stress is carried by the fibers, so that the matrix makes a negligible contribution to the breaking strength of the composite.

Under stress, the fibers with cracks may break, but the soft matrix hinders propagation of the crack. The fibers do not fail at one plane, so that the progression of the crack completely across the material occurs only if the fibers are withdrawn from the matrix. If the adhesion between matrix and fibers is low, a crack that initially runs at right angles to

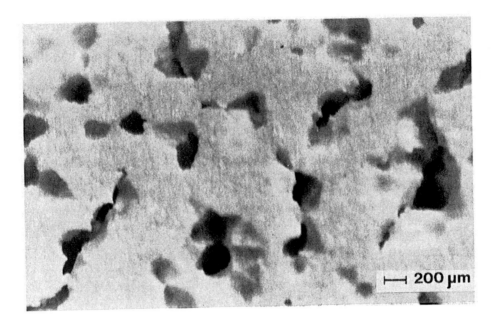

(a)

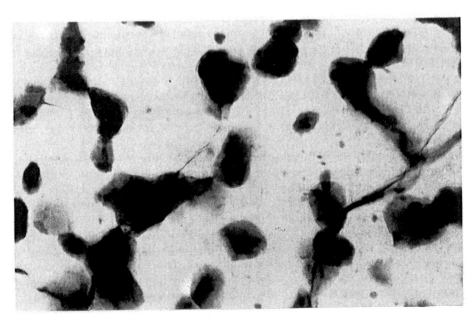

(b)

Figure 3   Photomicrograph of sintered hydroxyapatite of a total porosity of 45% (a) (magnified 25×); the same implant 6 months after implantation (b).

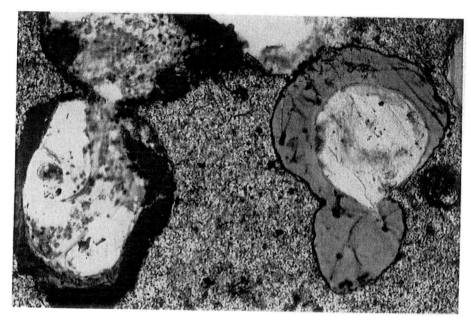

(a)

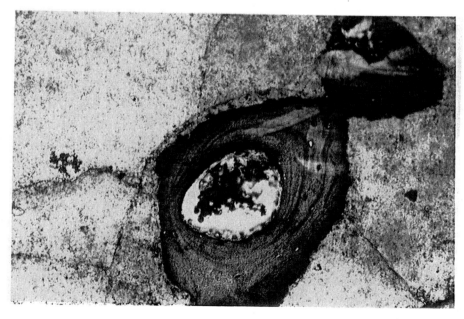

(b)

Figure 4 Microradiographs of a longitudinal section of a porous implant: (a) 6 months after implantation (magnified 80×) showing a starting bone ingrowth; (b) 2 years after implantation (magnified 80×) showing a completed bone filling.

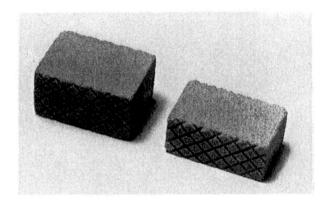

(a)

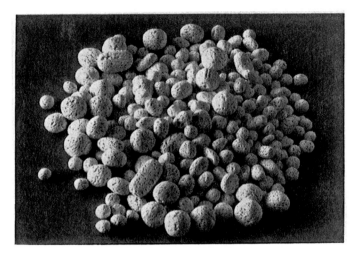

(b)

Figure 5   Commercially available porous hydroxyapatite bone implants: (a) Ceros 80®, developed by Robert Mathys Co. (magnified 1.5 ×); (b) porous hydroxyapatite granula (actual size).

the fibers will be deflected along the weak interface and be rendered harmless as far as the tensile strength of the composite is concerned. For resistance to tension, shear stress, and compression, multiple orientation of fibers provides moderate strength in many directions although the absolute strength in any axis will be compromised. For internal reconstruction of the skeleton, the absolute strength of the implant would be no advantage because it would be so different from that which is present in bone. To use rigid implant materials, some methods of providing a gradual transmission in stiffness across the bone–implant interface would be necessary. At present, composites are under consideration that may provide both superior metals and polymers for implantation [80,93,94].

Early composite materials for bone replacement were developed from plaster of

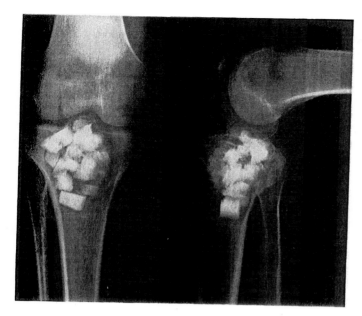

(a)

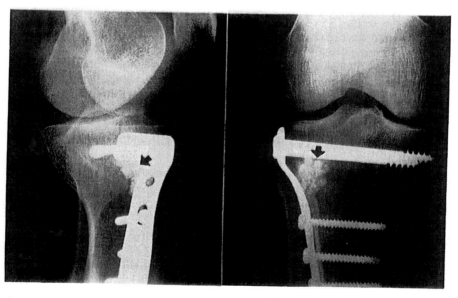

(b)

Figure 6 (a) Bone cavity of proximal tibia filled with hydroxyapatite blocks. (b) Lateral and antero-posterior radiograph of a lateral tibia plateau impression-fracture treated by fracture reduction, filling of bone defect with hydroxyapatite granulae, and using of metal hardware.

Paris. In 1960 plaster of Paris was mixed with epoxy resin to achieve better strength for the filling of large osseous defects. The epoxy resin, however, made this material incompatible with living tissue [83].

In 1963 Smith combined the advantages of a rigid, 48% porous ceramic composite of alumina, silica, potassium, and magnesium carbonates, with the resilience and elasticity of epoxy resin (diepoxide O type mixed with a hydroxyaliphatic amine hardener) in a composite material called "Cerosium" [95].

Cerosium had an elasticity comparable to bone. This porous material relied on close adherence of bone and tissue to external surface, but even so there was no ingrowth of bone into the pores of the material, since the pore size of 18–23 μm was too small to permit this. Besides, the pores were already filled with the epoxy resin. The epoxy resin was not completely stable and underwent degradation and resulted finally in a low biocompatibility. After the development of Cerosium many other combinations followed. Many of these were unsuccessful [96].

Metals such as aluminum or titanium or polymers provide the required mechanical attributes for a matrix. They are soft or weak in shear so that they do not scratch the fibers. Fiber-reinforced metals with graphite fibers have been studied, as have carbon fiber reinforced polyethylene. Fiber-reinforced carbon (carbon fiber reinforced carbon) appears to elicit a greater tissue response than does vitreous carbon. However, implants made from carbon fiber reinforced carbon as well as Proplast®, which is a composite of Teflon® and vitrous carbon, show fibrous tissue encapsulation. In the case of Proplast® there is histological evidence of breakdown of the implants [97]. Bioactivated bone cement (glass ceramics of vitreous fiber and polymethylmethacrylate) have the disadvantages of its plastic component.

The coating of a high-strength metal by a continuous physical barrier of biocompatible ceramic material eliminates many of the disadvantages, especially corrosion and toxicity, of metal implants [86]. Differences in elastic moduli, strength, and thermal expansion between the metal and the ceramic component at their interface result, however, in the ceramic coat chipping off when such an implant is subjected to severe stress.

Compositions of apatite powder and a collagen matrix with the same ratio of these components as exists in bone have been developed recently [80,98]. However, lack of mechanical stability still prevents the use of this material (Collapat®) in bone replacement surgery. This material, with its bone-like composition, may become an important bone substitute in the future. At the present time, there is still no synthetic composite material available possessing both biocompatibility and mechanical properties necessary for segmental bone replacement.

D. Concluding Remarks on Bone Substitution

A suitable material of proper quality that is readily available is still needed for surgical repair of bone defects. Some ceramics and some ceramic composite materials are being investigated because of their biocompatibility and similarity to normal bone.

Ceramics, as oxides, are not subject to the oxidative corrosion to which all metals are susceptible; neither do they evoke the tissue reaction characteristic of many polymers. The open porosity of these structures allows ingrowth of living tissues within the interstices of the material, thereby encouraging its active fixation. Furthermore, even osteoconductivity has been reported in the case of some ceramics.

Although the abrasion resistance may be comparable to that of metals, and strength in compression far superior, the tensile strength of conventional ceramics is far below the requirements for an implant material in bone tissue. Therefore the clinical use of ceramics is still limited to parts of the skeleton that are exposed only to compression forces. The possibility of impregnating a brittle ceramic material with a ductile and resilient material to improve its mechanical properties is the subject of many investigations. At this moment, the ideal combination has not yet been discovered.

II. BONE REPAIR

A. Introduction to Repair Techniques

Throughout history people have possessed a need to repair broken parts of the human body that have become nonfunctional. For hundreds of years crutches and wooden legs have been examples of simple yet meaningful attempts to improve body functions.

As our knowledge and technical skill increased, so did our ability to provide more sophisticated surgical procedures and even implants to aid the natural healing process. All kinds of materials have been used to provide support and immobility to damaged extremities or joints. Wood, clay, stones, and plaster components have been applied on the outer surface of injured limbs. Later, implants of different origins were designed and clinically tested.

B. Current Bone Repair Technology

Most implants currently used in traumatology for bone repair are of stainless steel, due to their satisfactory mechanical properties and availability. However, significant problems are associated with stainless steel implants for fracture fixation, such as stress shielding, the risk of infection, corrosion problems, even sensitivity, and mostly, the necessity of removal of implants [64,65].

Bioresorbable fracture fixation materials without these disadvantages and without the need for a removal operation could be very useful in fracture treatment [99]. Bioresorbable fracture fixation materials, derived from the resorbable suture materials developed in the 1960s, can be completely metabolized in a biological system. There is no need for an operation in removing these implants, which will give a medical, financial, and psychological advantage to the patient [100].

At present, the most important degradable implant materials are:

- Poly-L-lactic acid (PLLA)
- Poly-DL-lactic acid (PDLLA)
- Polyglycolic acid (PGA)
- Polydioxanone (PDS)
- Polyorthoester (POE)
- Poly-ε-caprolactone (PCL)

Different biodegradable materials for fracture fixation have been tested in the research laboratory and in a clinical setting. In a prospective randomized study on fractures of the ankle joint PLLA/PGA (Biofix®) biodegradable implants were tested in patients [101]. Forty-three patients with fracture dislocation on the ankle joint were treated by open reduction and fixation with either steel or biodegradable implants (Fig. 7). Results in both groups were favorable and the biodegradable material appears to be useful for some fracture fixations to obviate the need for a second operation.

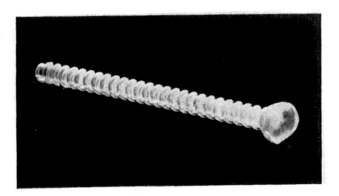

Figure 7   Poly-L-lactide screw.

The use of biodegradable implants is not, however, without problems. The most commonly occurring postoperative complication of these implants is the delayed inflammatory reaction resulting in a sterile sinus or a delayed wound swelling. The patient has no local or systemic signs of a problem within the wound in the immediate postoperative period. The main interval between fixation of the fracture and the clinical manifestation of the reaction is 12 weeks.

The histological characteristics of specimens obtained during debridement of the sinus tracts demonstrate a nonspecific foreign-body reaction with abundant giant cells phagocytosing the debris from the polymer [102]. This polymer debris possesses a high crystallinity.

In experimental studies several investigators have demonstrated that implants of polyglycolic acid, polylactic acid, or polyparadioxanone are completely absorbable within bone tissue. New bone is deposited on and within the implant as degradation proceeds (Fig. 8).

In the experimental laboratory large biodegradable implants for the fixation of femur fractures were recently tested in pigs. Polylactic acid, with a high mean molecular weight (260,000), a large degree of crystallinity, and a small amount of free monomers, was used. The tissue response to PLLA versus stainless steel intramedullary nails was studied after 1 and after 3 months of implantation. Fracture healing characteristics, and chemical and mechanical properties of the PLLA rods were studied after retrieval of an implant.

Mechanical properties deteriorated during implantation and chemical properties changed significantly in 1 and 3 months of implantation. PLLA and stainless steel implants induced similar tissue reactions. Both implants were completely surrounded by a fibrous tissue layer.

However, in another study, intramedullary implants of PLLA wire in rat tibiae were evaluated concerning the fracture healing processes and the tissue reaction on the PLLA in a fractured bone. The fracture healing after PLLA implantation was compared to that in the sham-operated animals. In all animals with intramedullary PLLA wire implantation newly formed bone formation was seen immediately against the implant 2 and 6 months after implantation (Fig. 8). None of the sham-operated animals showed newly formed intramedullary bone formation other than fracture healing callus and normal trabecular bone.

A burst phenomenon was simulated *in vivo* by implantation of a large amount of a

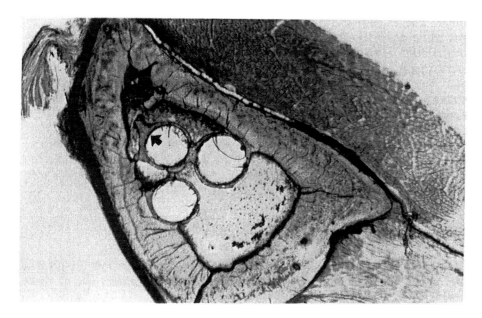

(a)

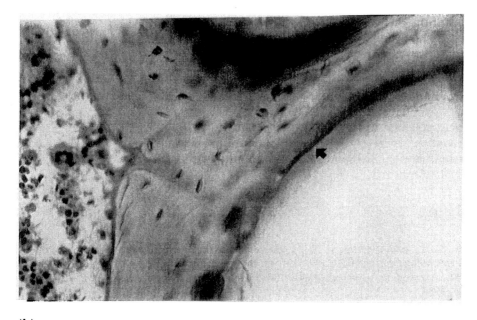

(b)

Figure 8   An intramedullary PLLA wire implant (3 cross sections) surrounded by new bone (boundary area marked by arrow): (a) magnified 20×; (b) magnified 80×.

PLLA monomer. The tissue reaction on the release of a large amount of depolymerized monomer showed no adverse reaction on bone tissue. This is important, because it was shown that degradation of a solid implant proceeds faster in the center than at the surface due to the increasing amount of degradation by-products. Thus after a certain interval there is an intact outer layer filled with a jelly-like mass of monomers of high crystallinity.

When breakage of the outer layer occurs the contents of this reservoir can be released in a short period of time: the burst phenomenon. To study this phenomenon PLLA interlocking nails were implanted in the femur of pigs after a midshaft osteotomy. After 4 weeks the pigs were reoperated. The PLLA rods were removed and a low molecular weight PLLA powder was inserted. After 4 weeks the animals were sacrificed and the femora were studied histologically and mechanically. Active bone remodeling was seen without an inflammatory response.

C. Concluding Remarks on Bone Repair

Resorbable implants are promising options for fixation of fractured bone in trauma surgery. However, some problems remain to be solved prior to general use of these implants in surgery.

Examples of these problems are:

1. The progress of the resorption process
2. The control of mechanical properties
3. The effect of the decreased pH
4. The burst phenomenon
5. The possibility of mutagenicity

The polymer chemist, the clinician, and the experimental worker will have to find ways to improve and evaluate biodegradability and biocompatibility of these new materials.

The clinical potential for the use of biodegradable osteosyntheses is enormous. The optimal degradation characteristics of an implant for tissue protection and for improving the tissue strength during the healing process of bone fractures still have to be found.

REFERENCES

1. Damien, C. J., and Parsons, J. R., Bone graft and bone graft substitutes: A review of current technology and applications, *J. Appl. Biomater., 2*, 187–208, 1991.
2. Grob, D., Autologous bone transplantation: Problems at the donor site, *Unfallchirurg, 89*, 339–345, 1986.
3. Dijk, B. A. van, Stassen, J., Kunst, V. A. J. M., Slooff, T. J. J. H., and Hoorn, J. R. van, Rhesus immunization after bone allografting, *Acta Orthop. Scand., 59*, 482, 1988.
4. Robinson, R. A., and Watson, M. L., Crystal collagen relationships in bone as observed in the electron microscope. III. Crystal and collagen morphology as a function of age, *Ann. New York Acad. Sci., 60*, 596–627, 1955.
5. Münzenberg, K. J., and Gebhardt, M., Brushite octacalcium phosphate and carbonate—containing apatite in bone, *Clin. Orthop. Rel. Res., 90*, 271-3, 1973.

6. Cohen, J., and Harris, W. H., The three−dimensional anatomy of haversian systems, *J. Bone Joint Surg.*, *40A*, 419–434, 1958.

7. Urist, M. R., Dowel, T. A., Hay, P. H., and Strates, B. S., Inductive substrates for bone formation, *Clin. Orthop.*, *59*, 59–96, 1968.

8. Strange, F. G. St. C., Union of fractures, *Lancet, 1*, 305–307, 1963.

9. Evans, P. G., *Mechanical Properties of Bone*, C. C. Thomas. Springfield, IL, 1973.

10. Bonfield, W., and Grynpas, M. D., Anisotropy of the Young's modulus of bone, *Nature, 270*, 453–454, 1977.

11. Hulbert, S. F., and Young, F. A., *Use of Ceramics in Surgical Implants*, Gordon and Breach Science Publishers, London, 1978.

12. Recum, A. F. von, The academic environment of biomaterials science and engineering, *J. Appl. Biomater.*, *3*, 63–71, 1992.

13. Parry, T. V., Trephination of the living human skull in prehistoric times, *Br. Med. J., 1*, 457–460, 1923.

14. Meek'ren, J., *Heel−en Geneeskonstige Aanmerkingen*, Casparus Commelijn, Amsterdam, 1668.

15. Hamel, M. du, Sur le developpement et la crue des os des animaux, *Mem. l'Acad. Roy Sci., Paris, 55*, 354–370, 1742.

16. Ray, R. D., Bone grafts and bone implants, *Otolaryngol. Clin. N. Am., 5*, 389–398, 1972.

17. Rubin, R. L., *Biomaterials in Reconstructive Surgery*, C. V. Mosby, London, 1983.

18. Patka, P., Otter, G. den, deGroot, K., and Driessen, A. A., Reconstruction of large bone defects with calcium phosphate ceramics; an experimental study, *Neth. J. Surg., 37*, 38–44, 1985.

19. Hollinger, J. O., Mark, D. E., Goco, P., et al., A comparison of four particulate bone derivates, *Clin. Orthop. Rel. Res., 267*, 255–263, 1991.

20. Enneking, W. F., Burchardt, H., Puhl, J. J., and Piotrowski, G., Physical and biological aspects of repair in dog cortical-bone transplants, *J. Bone Joint Surg., 57A*, 237–252, 1975.

21. Burchardt, H., and Enneking, W. F., Transplantation of bone, *Surg. Clin. N. Am., 58*, 403–427, 1978.

22. Albee, T., Fundamentals in bone transplantation. Experience in three thousand bone graft operations, *J. Am. Med. Assoc., 81*, 1429–1432, 1923.

23. Leung, P. C., Reconstruction of a large femoral defect using a vascular pedicle iliac graft, *J. Bone Joint Surg., 65A*, 1179–1180, 1983.

24. Lan, R. S. F., and Leung, P. C., Bone graft viability in vascularized bone graft transfer, *Br. J. Radiol., 55*, 325–329, 1982.

25. Moore, J. R., Weiland, A. J., and Daniel, R. K., Use of free vascularized bone grafts in the treatment of bone tumours, *Clin. Orthop. Rel. Res., 175*, 37–44, 1983.

26. Blakmore, M. E., Fractures at cancellous bone graft donor sites, *Injury, 14*, 519–522, 1983.

27. Kirkup, J. R., Traumatic femoral bone loss, *J. Bone Joint Surg., 47B*, 106–110, 1965.

28. Wilson, P. D., and Lance, E. M., Surgical reconstruction of the skeleton following segmental resection for bone tumours, *J. Bone Joint Surg., 47A*, 1629–1656, 1965.

29. Jahnke, K., and Plester, D., Bioinert ceramic implants in middle ear surgery, *Ann. Otol. Rhinol. Laryngol., 90*, 640–642, 1981.

30. Mankin, H. J., Doppelt, S. H., Robin, Sulivan T., and Tomford, W. W., Osteoarticular and intercalcary allograft transplantation in the management of malignant tumours of bone, *Cancer, 50*, 613–630, 1982.

31. Boyne, P. J., Induction of bone repair by various bonegrafting materials, *Assoc. Sci. Publ., 11*, 121–141, 1973.

32. Heiple, K. G., Chase, S. W., and Herdon, Ch. H., A comparative study of the healing process following different types of bone transplantation, *J. Bone Joint Surg., 45*, 1593–1616, 1963.

33. Williams, R. G., Comparison of living autogenous and homogenous grafts of cancellous bone heterotopically placed in rabbits, *Anat. Rec., 143*, 93–101, 1962.

34. Bos, G. D., Goldberg, U. M., Powell, A. E., Heiple, K. G., and Zika, J. M., The effect of histocompatibility matching on canine frozen bone allografts, *J. Bone Joint Surg., 65A*, 89–96, 1983.

35. Gallie, W. E., and Robertson, D. E., The transplantation of bone, *J. Am. Med. Assoc., 20*, 1134–1140, 1918.

36. Orell, S., Surgical bone grafting with "os purum", "os novum" and "boiled bone," *J. Bone Joint Surg., 19*, 873–885, 1937.

37. Williams, G., Experiences with boiled cadaveric cancellous bone for fractures of long bones, *J. Bone Joint Surg., 46B*, 398–403, 1964.

38. Hurley, L. A., Zeier, F. G., and Stinchfield, F. E., Anorganic bone grafting, *Am. J. Surg., 100*, 12–21, 1960.

39. Losee, F. L., and Hurley, L. A., Bone treated with ethylenediamine as a successful foundation material in cross species bone grafts, *Nature, 177*, 1032–1033, 1956.

40. Oikarinen, J., and Korhonen, L. K., The bone inductive capacity of various bone transplanting materials used for treatment of experimental bone defects, *Clin. Orthop., 40*, 208–215, 1979.

41. Urist, M. R., Dowell, T. A., Hay, P. H., and Strates, B. S., Inductive substrates for bone formation, *Clin. Orthop., 59*, 59–96, 1968.

42. Gupta, D., and Tuli, S. M., Osteoinductivity of partially decalcified alloimplants in healing of large osteoperiosteal defects, *Acta Orthop. Scand., 53*, 857–865, 1982.

43. Bassett, C. A. L., Hurley, L. A., and Stinchfield, F. E., The fate of long term anorganic bone implants, *Transplant Bull., 29*, 51–55, 1962.

44. Habal, M. B., and Reddi, A. H., *Bone Grafts and Bone Substitutes*, W. B. Saunders, London, 1992.

45. Karges, D. E., Anderson, K. J., and Dingwall, J. J., Experimental evaluation of processed heterogenous bone transplants, *Clin. Orthop., 29*, 230–247, 1963.

46. Anderson, K. J., Le Cocg, J. F., Akeson, W. H., and Harrington, P. R., End-point results of processed heterogenous, autogenous and homogenous bone transplants in the human: A histological study, *Clin. Orthop., 33*, 220–236, 1964.

47. Taheri, Z. E., Experience with calf bone in cervical interbody spinal fusion, *J. Neurosurg., 36*, 67–71, 1972.

48. Colville, J., Carbonised wood: An experimental bone implant, *J. Bone Joint Surg., 62B*, 259, 1980.

49. Hall, C. W., The need for biomaterials research, *J. Biomed. Mater. Res. Symp., 2*, 1–4, 1971.

50. Clark, A. E., Hench, L. L., and Paschall, H. A., The influence of surface chemistry on implant interface histology: A theoretical basis for implant materials selection, *J. Biomed. Mater. Res., 10*, 161–174, 1976.

51. Leininger, R. I., Polymers as surgical implants, *Crit. Rev. Bioeng., 3*, 333–381, 1972.

52. Mears, D. C., *Materials and Orthopaedic Surgery*, Williams & Wilkins, Baltimore, 1979.

53. Heimke, G., Griss, P., Werner, E., and Jentschura, G., The effects of mechanical factors on biocompatibility tests, *J. Biomed. Eng., 3*, 209–213, 1981.

54. Hegyeli, R. J., Limitations of current techniques for the evaluation of the biohazards and biocompatibility of new candidate materials, *J. Biomed. Mater. Res., 1*, 1–14, 1971.

55. Willert, H. G., Proposed guideline for the biological testing of orthopaedic implant materials and implants, *Biomaterials, 1*, 179–182, 1980.

56. Williams, D. F., *Definition in Biomaterials*, Elsevier, Amsterdam, 1987.

57. Ducheyne, P., and Lemons, J. E., Bioceramics: Material characteristics versus *in vivo* behavior, *Ann. NY Acad. Sci., 523*, 1988.

58. Osborn, J. F., and Newesely, H., The material science of calcium phosphate ceramics, *Biomaterials, 1*, 108–111, 1980.

59. Hench, L. L., and Paschall, H. A., Histochemical responses at a biomaterials interface, *J. Biomed. Mater. Res. Symp.*, 5, 49–64, 1974.

60. Hench, L. L., Splinter, R. J., and Allen, W. C., Bonding mechanisms at the interface of ceramic prosthetic materials, *J. Biomed. Mater. Res. Symp.*, 2, 117–141, 1971.

61. Peàn, J. E., Des moyens prosthetiques destinés a obtenir la reparation de parties ossueses, *Graz. de Jôp., Paris*, 67, 291–297, 1894.

62. Cameron, H. V., Macnab, I., and Pilliar, R. M., A porous metal system for joint replacement surgery, *Int. J. Artif. Organs*, 1, 104–109, 1978.

63. Galante, J., Rostoker, W., Lueck, R., and Ray, R. D., Sintered fibre metal composites as a basis for attachment of implants to bone, *J. Bone Joint Surg.*, 53A, 101–114, 1971.

64. Kummer, F. J., and Rose, R. M., Corrosion of titanium/cobalt–chromium alloy couples, *J. Bone Joint Surg.*, 65A, 1125–1126, 1983.

65. Harrison, J. W., McLain, D. L., Hohm, R. B., Willson, G. P., Chalman, J. A., and MacGowand, K. N., Osteosarcoma associated with metalic implants, *Clin. Orthop. Rel. Res.*, 116, 253–257, 1976.

66. Delgado, E. R., Sarcoma following a surgically treated fractured tibia, *Clin. Orthop.*, 12, 315–318, 1958.

67. Dube, V. E., and Fisher, D. E., Hemangioendothelioma of the leg following metalic fixation of the tibia, *Cancer*, 30, 1260–1266, 1972.

68. Sinibaldi, K., Rosen, H., Liu, S. K., and DeAngelis, M., Tumours associated with metalic implants in animals, *Clin. Orthop.*, 118, 257–266, 1976.

69. Sunderman, F. W., Metal carcinogenesis in experimental animals, *Food Cosmet. Toxicol.*, 9, 105–120, 1971.

70. Tayton, K. J. J., Ewing's sarcoma at the site of a metal plate, *Cancer*, 45, 413–415, 1980.

71. Gaechter, A., Alroy, J., Anderson, G. B. J., Galante, J., Rostoker, W., and Schajowicz, F., Metal carcinogenesis, *J. Bone Joint Surg.*, 59A, 622–624, 1977.

72. Park, J. B., and Lakes, R. S., *Biomaterials: An Introduction*, Plenum Press, New York, 1992.

73. Willert, H. G., Buchhorn, G. H., and Eyerer, P., *Ultra-High Molecular Weight Polyethylene as Biomaterial in Orthopedic Surgery*, Hogrefe & Huber, Toronto, 1991.

74. Rubin, L. R., *Biomaterials in Reconstructive Surgery*, C. V. Mosby, St. Louis, 1983.

75. Ungethüm, M., Kunststoffe in der Knochenchirurgie, *Kunststoffe*, 72, 647–651, 1982.

76. Oppenheimer, E. T., Willhite, M., Danishefski, I., and Stout, A. P., Observations on the effects of powdered polymer in the carcinogenic process, *Cancer Res.*, 21, 432–437, 1961.

77. Vincent, J. F. V., *Structural Biomaterials*, Macmillam Press Ltd., London, 1982.

78. Rigdon, R. H., Plastics and carcinogenesis, *Southern Med. J.*, 67, 1459–1465, 1974.

79. Engelhardt, A., Salzer, M., Zeibig, A., and Locke, H., Experiences with Al_2O_3 implantation in human to bridge resection defects, *J. Biomed. Mater. Res. Symp.*, 6, 227–232, 1975.

80. Clarke, K. I., Graves, S. E., Wong, A. T. C., Triffitt, J. T., Francis, M. J. O., and Czernuszka, J. F., Investigation into the formation and mechanical properties of a bioactive material based on collagen and calcium phosphate, *J. Mater. Sci. Mater. Med.*, 4, 107–110, 1993.

81. Dreesmann, H., Veber Knochenplombierung, *Beitr. Klin. Chir.*, 9, 804–810, 1892.

82. Frame, J. W., Porous calcium sulphate dihydrate as a biodegradable implant in bone, *J. Dentistry*, 3, 177–187, 1975.

83. Gourley, I. M. G., and Arnold, J. P., The experimental replacement of segmental defects in bone with a plaster of paris-epoxy resin mixture, *Am. J. Vet. Res.*, 21, 1119–1122, 1960.

84. Hulbert, S. F., Horrison, S. J., and Klawitter, J. J., Tissue reaction on three ceramics of porous and non-porous structures, *J. Biomed. Mater. Res.*, 6, 347–374, 1972.

85. Peltier, L. F., The use of plaster of paris to fill defects in bone, *Clin. Orthop.*, 21, 1–31, 1961.

86. Klawitter, J. J., and Hulbert, S. F., Application of porous ceramics for the attachment of load bearing internal orthopedic applications, *J. Biomed. Mater. Res.*, 2, 161–229, 1971.

87. Salzer, M., Knahr, K., Loeke, H., et al., A bioceramic endoprosthesis for the replacement of the proximal humerus, *Arch. Orthop. Traumat. Surg., 93*, 169–184, 1979.

88. Iwano, T., Kurosawa, H., Murase, K., Takeuchi, H., and Oh Kubo, J., Tissue reaction to collagen-coated porous hydroxyapatite, *Clin. Orthop. Rel. Res., 268*, 243–252, 1991.

89. Metsger, D. S., Dephilip, R. M., and Hayes, T. G., An autoradiographic study of calcium phosphate ceramic bone implants in turkeys, *Clin. Orthop. Rel. Res., 291*, 283–294, 1993.

90. Klein, C. A. P. T., Patka, P., and Hollander, den W., Macroporous calcium phosphate bioceramics in dog femora: A histological study of interface and biodegradation, *Biomaterials, 10*, 59–62, 1989.

91. Hulbert, S. F., Morrison, S. J., and Klawitter, J. J., Compatibility of porous ceramics with soft tissue: Application to tracheal prosthesis, *J. Biomed. Mater. Res. Symp., 2*, 269–279, 1971.

92. Vos, G. A., Patka, P., Klein, C. A. P. T., Hoitsma, H. F. W., and deGroot, K., Tracheal reconstruction with hydroxyapatite tracheal prosthesis, *Life Support Systems, 4*, 283–287, 1986.

93. Kocialkowski, A., Angus Wallace, W., and Prince, H. G., Clinical experience with a new artificial bone graft: Preliminary results of a prospective study, *Injury, 21*, 142–144, 1990.

94. Fitzer, E., and Schlichting, J., Fibre reinforced ceramics, *Sci. Cer., 10*, 71–82, 1980.

95. Smith, L., Ceramic-plastic material as a bone substitute, *Arch. Surg., 87*, 653–661, 1963.

96. Welsh, R. P., Pilliar, R. M., and MacNab, I., Surgical implants, *J. Bone Joint Surg., 53A*, 963–977, 1971.

97. Kerr, A. G., Proplast and Plastipore, *Clin. Otolaryngol., 6*, 187–191, 1981.

98. Mittelmeier, H., and Katthagen, B. D., Klinische Erfahrungen mit Collagen-Apatit-Implantation zur Localen Knochenregeneration, *Z. Orthop., 121*, 115–123, 1983.

99. Böstman, O., Vainionpää, S., Hirvensalo, E., Mäkelä, A., Vihtonen, K., Törmälä, P., and Rokkanen, P., Biodegradable internal fixation for malleolar fractures. A prospective randomised trial, *J. Bone Joint Surg., 69B*, 615–619, 1987.

100. Böstman, O., Current concepts review. Absorbable implants for the fixation of fractures, *J. Bone Joint Surg., 73A*, 148–153, 1991.

101. Dijkema, A. R. A., Elst, M. van der, Breederveld, R. S., Verspui, G., Patka, P., and Haarman, H. J. Th. M., Surgical treatment of fracture dislocations of the ankle joint with biodegradable implants: A prospective randomised study, *J. Trauma, 34*, 82–84, 1993.

102. Böstman, O., Hirvensalo, E., Vanionpää, S., Vihtonen, K., Törmälä, P., and Rokkanen, P., Degradable polyglycolide rods for the internal fixation of displaced bimalleolar fractures, *Int. Orthop., 14*, 1–8, 1990.

103. Hofman, G. O., Biodegradable implants in orthopaedic surgery, A review on the state of art, *Clin. Mater., 10*, 75–80, 1992.

23

UHMW Polyethylene in Total Joint Replacement: History and Current Technology

Dane A. Miller, Stephen M. Herrington,
Joel C. Higgins, and David W. Schroeder
Biomet, Inc.
Warsaw, Indiana

I. HISTORY OF ULTRAHIGH MOLECULAR WEIGHT POLYETHYLENE

Industrial and aerospace applications for ultrahigh molecular weight polyethylene (UHMWPE) precedes Sir John Charnley's use of this material in total hip replacements in the late 1960s. As process control and reagent chemical purity had gradually improved since World War II, the German and American polymer chemists were able to produce longer and longer molecular weight polyethylene of a linear type by the 1960s. This higher molecular weight polyethylene was recognized for its improved toughness and durability in commercial and aerospace applications; however, its miraculous performance in total joint replacement was never even imagined until Sir John Charnley's timely use. The first industrial applications for this tougher, more durable polyethylene were in heavy industries where abrasive deterioration of both metals and plastics often occurred. UHMWPE's most frequent applications were in mining and in industrial conveyor systems initially, but by the 1960s and '70s it was recognized for its excellent wear behavior as a lubricationless bearing in both aerospace and chemical processing environments. By the late 1960s UHMWPE was being used routinely by National Aeronautics and Space Administration engineers where hydrocarbon lubricants could not be used because of their tendency to evaporate in the vacuum environment of outer space.

Sir John Charnley, of Reddington, England, first used polytetrafluoroethylene (PTFE) in his first total hip design. Sir Charnley named this first procedure a low-friction arthroplasty due to the low friction behavior of polytetrafluoroethylene. Within 24 months, after a few hundred patients, Sir John Charnley fortunately chose UHMWPE to replace his worn PTFE sockets. Were it not for this fortunate decision, nearly 10 million total hip patients might not have walked or continued walking during the past quarter century. As you will see from the next few paragraphs, the use of PTFE would not be the

665

last incorrect solution for a misunderstood problem as it relates to UHMW polyethylene in total joint replacement.

In its early use as a material for articulating total joint components, the importance of ultrahigh molecular weight was not fully understood. Several manufacturers of total joint replacements produced early quantities of total hips from high-density, and not ultrahigh molecular weight, polyethylene. Fortunately in those early years of total joint replacement, total hips were only used on older patients where limited patient survival prevented catastrophic wear failure of their joints. By the early 1970s, a great deal of commercial and academic research was underway to produce more spherical heads with microscopically smoother surfaces. The primary articulating material, or femoral component material, was cast cobalt–chromium alloy produced by several manufacturers worldwide. Certain attempts on improved femoral head surface finish involved solution annealing of the femoral component. While there was considerable doubt in many research circles as to the importance of high surface finishes, it became evident clinically, by the mid-'70s that solution annealing had been a technical error. Solution annealing of the cast cobalt alloy femoral component caused severe reductions in mechanical characteristics of the cobalt chrome alloy and relatively high levels of fatigue fracture of femoral stems occurred.

At about the same time, research was underway to identify a better polymer than UHMW polyethylene for this application. During the late '70s, both polyesters and polyacetals were used in limited clinical application, with poor durability and relatively short-term clinical failure. Also, during the early application of UHMWPE in total joints, various metal-on-metal systems were used. While there continue to be anecdotal reports of long-term success with metal-on-metal articulation in total joint replacement, the broader body of clinical evidence clearly suggests that this is not a suitable wear couple in total joint applications.

By the late 1970s and early 1980s an alumina–ceramic wear couple found rapid market and clinical acceptance. It became apparent, however, after a few years of clinical use that these ceramic-on-ceramic total joints were not performing well clinically. While several explanations for this poor clinical performance have been proposed, the most coherent appears to relate to the absence of the shock-absorbing structure that polyethylene provides when rigid ceramic articulates against rigid ceramic.

In approximately the same time period, extensive research produced carbon fiber reinforced polyethylenes. The theory behind this carbon-reinforced polyethylene suggests that the articulation between the metallic components and the carbon-reinforced components allows for the load to be carried on the carbon fibers, generating very low levels of wear debris. In clinical practice, this clearly has not proven to be the case. Higher levels of wear debris were created by such reinforced polyethylene, leading to higher levels of local inflammatory tissue response and higher rates of reoperation.

One final miscue of the 1980s involved attempts to improve the surface finish of polyethylene articulating components through a heat-pressing or hot-stamping technique. This processing technique attempted to eliminate the surface asperities created in the machining of implant components from preformed bar stock. A high-temperature female form, after rough machining of the implant component, was used to compress the final form into the articulating surface. Clinical results from polyethylene components produced by this technique show a significantly higher level of polyethylene surface delamination due to the thermal damage of the surface layers [1].

Fortunately, with all these futile attempts to eliminate polyethylene wear from the total joint system, much has also been learned about the material and many techniques have been developed to improve consistency and quality of this miraculous polymer.

The remaining sections of this chapter detail improved techniques developed for the characterization and processing of UHMWPE for this life-saving application in medicine. We trust, as you read the remainder of this chapter, that you will agree with the authors that polyethylene has been truly a miracle material in orthopedics.

II. UHMWPE FOR MEDICAL APPLICATIONS

Ultrahigh molecular weight polyethylene (UHMWPE) is currently used extensively in the orthopedic industry as a bearing material. The components are produced using a variety of manufacturing methods, many which can have an effect on the longevity and performance of the device. Recently there has been extensive research into the causes of loosening of orthopedic devices. One area that has been targeted as a cause for loosening is reaction to particulate debris from these appliances [2–13]. As understanding of biological reactions to particulates improved, increased emphasis was placed on the quality of the UHMWPE used for orthopedic bearing surfaces. Due to this increased awareness, various manufacturing and quality control improvements have been made throughout the industry. The following text addresses various commercial methods for fabricating orthopedic bearings and possible effects on properties.

UHMWPE is converted from raw resin directly to final form or machined from block, sheet, or rod. All conversion processes rely on enough heat to be applied for the entire thickness of resin being formed to reach a fusion temperature and adequate pressure applied during heating and cooling to ensure full consolidation. The standard conversion processes include ram extrusion; compression molding of sheet or plate; isostatic, or uniform compression molding; and direct compression molding. Each of these processes has advantages and disadvantages, but the key to the manufacturing of orthopedic devices is to determine which process yields consistent and favorable mechanical properties while remaining economically feasible and commercially acceptable.

A. Ram Extrusion

Ram extrusion is a continuous process that produces UHMWPE bar stock of different cross sections. The most widely used cross sections in orthopedic bearing manufacturing are round and rectangular. A schematic of a ram extruder is shown in Fig. 1. The ram extruder operates by forcing resin into a heated die that is several feet long and has the same cross section as that of the rod to be formed. Resin is fed from a hopper into a chamber where an oscillating ram forces the material into the die. As the powder is moved through the open-ended die, heat is applied. The resin melts from the surface to the center of the die forming a cone of nonmelted material that extends into the die. This is depicted in Fig. 2. Nonconsolidated regions can result in the center of the extrusion if the cone of nonmelted material extends beyond the heated zone of the die. An example of a nonconsolidated center is shown in Fig. 3.

In the ram extruder, pressure is applied to the melted resin by the friction of the resin against the die and thermal expansion resisting the force being applied by the ram. The greatest pressures are generated near the ram and at the edges of the die. The applied pressure tapers off down the die and toward the center of the bar. This implies that the last part of the bar to melt also sees the least amount of pressure. It is also important to

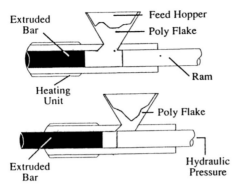

Figure 1 Schematic of ram extruder.

note that the pressure applied is not constant but varies. These variations are due to the oscillation of the ram (on/off pressure) as well as the differences between dynamic and sliding friction as the bar is extruded.

The major advantages of ram extrusion are derived from reduced cost of manufacturing as well as volume of output due to the continuous nature of the extrusion process. Also, the capital expenditure required for a ram extruder is much less than that required for a press to make sheet stock. The cost advantage of ram-extruded material is also realized by the orthopedic device manufacturer by the volume of output from machining devices versus molding the bearings one at a time. Ram-extruded material can be used to manufacture components that have tight tolerances (± 0.005 to 0.001 inches) because it is typically purchased in the annealed (i.e., thermally stress relieved) form from a converter. The cross-sectional shape of extruded material can be tailored to meet the end use of the product.

B.   Sheet Molding

Sheet molding is a form of compression molding used to manufacture large sheets of material. Sheet molding utilizes presses with multiple daylight openings. The platens on these presses often exceed 30 ft^2. To form these sheets, resin is poured onto the platen and the resin is leveled with a strike bar so that a uniform resin height is maintained. Once the presses are loaded with resin, the platens are brought together and heat is applied. Some fabricators may also incorporate a bump cycle prior to heating to remove any trapped gases [14,15]. After a specified heating cycle has been completed, the pressure is increased to the desired set point and the material is allowed to cool under pressure. An

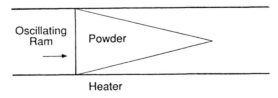

Figure 2 Powder cone that forms during extrusion of a bar.

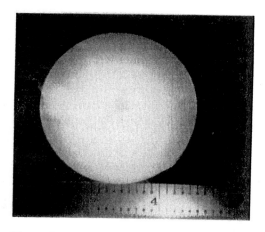

Figure 3 Cross section of an extruded bar with a nonconsolidated center.

exploded view of sheet-molding platens is shown in Fig. 4. The sheet formed can be of varied thickness, based upon the quantity of resin loaded between the platens. The sheet that is removed from the press is usually skived to remove any surface discoloration and oxidized material, and it is then sent to the end user, where the final shapes are machined from the sheet [15].

Sheet molding allows for greater pressures to be applied during the final consolidation phase compared to ram extrusion. This may result in a more uniform product than ram extrusion, although areas of varying density and mechanical properties from surface to center of the sheet may form if proper pressures are not applied. Another disadvantage of sheet forming is that variance in bulk density of the resin can lead to inconsistency in the amount of powder in one region of the sheet versus another. This will result in pressure differentials during forming from one area of the sheet to another, thus resulting in property differences.

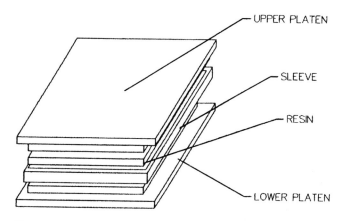

Figure 4 Schematic of sheet molding press.

C. Direct Compression Molding

The direct compression molding process is used to form the finished component from raw resin. The concept of the process is similar to block or sheet forming except on a smaller scale. Instead of using flat platens, the plungers have the contour of the components being formed. The plungers are contained in a sleeve that has the same internal diameter (ID) geometry as the outside contour of the component being formed. Figure 5 shows a metal mold tool and a finished component. The tooling may also allow for an insert to be molded into the component.

To mold a component, the bottom plunger is placed into the sleeve and a known weight of resin is poured into the mold. The top plunger is then placed into the mold. This is typically done in a controlled atmosphere. The mold with the resin is then placed into a press and cycled through a specified pressure and temperature profile. Once the component has cooled under pressure, it is removed from the mold and any flash is trimmed. The component is essentially finished at this point.

This process has many advantages over the other processing methods. These advantages include control over bearing surface roughness, control over resin quality, optimization of applied heat and pressure for each component configuration, and reduction in capital equipment necessary to produce a component. The bearing surface finish is controlled by the roughness of the plungers used to produce the component. Better initial surface finishes can reduce the amount of debris generated during the break-in period. By consolidating the resin using an inhouse process, the orthopedic device manufacturer avoids dependence on resin converters and is able to choose only the highest quality lots of resin. Since the area of the mold is much smaller than a sheet-forming press, higher pressures and more uniform heat can economically be applied to counteract the differences in powder height. The capital equipment required to produce direct compression molded components is less than that required to produce sheet or round stock. In addition

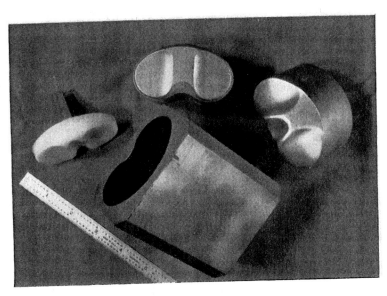

Figure 5   Direct compression molding tool and finished component.

to reduction in capital costs, the components do not usually require additional machining.

The disadvantages of compression molding are the initial cost of tooling, the difficulty of fabricating the mold tooling, and the time required to manufacture a component. The mold tooling usually requires a large quantity of components to be fabricated to justify the initial costs. Also, the tooling is limited to the production of one specific component shape. In addition, the cycle time required to fabricate a component can be quite extensive, thus limiting the amount of components that can be produced for a given work period across limited tooling.

D. Uniform Compression Molding

One of the major causes of high wear rates has been identified as incomplete consolidation of the UHMWPE [3,4,6,16–18]. In an attempt to improve consolidation, the uniform compression molding process was developed. This method of compression molding uses powder metal techniques to form bar stock, or completed or semicompleted components. The technique centers around isostatic pressing technology. The process consists of cold compaction into shape followed by vacuum sealing in a non-gas permeable container, then hot isostatically pressing the "canned" cold compact to fuse the resin. The major advantages of this process are uniform application of heat and pressure over irregular shapes and thicknesses, and the ability to apply a known amount of pressure during the cool-down cycle to all surfaces. Schematics of the process are shown in Figs. 6 and 7. The mechanical strength of this material is equal to or superior to material produced by the other methods discussed. In addition to mechanical strength, the material has been shown in laboratory testing to have superior wear characteristics to material consolidated by other methods. Also, the heated resin is never exposed to oxygen during processing, thereby eliminating a possible source of oxidative degradation.

This process allows for specification of resin for each individual bar fabricated since it is a noncontinuous process. Also, resins with very high molecular weights can be processed by this method without stearates or the degradation experienced with other methods [1,3,4,19–21]. It is also important to note this process is not shape dependent, which allows low-cost fabrication of difficult-to-machine components as well as components that are too large to machine from commercially available stock. Since the material is formed using pressure from all directions, the final product has dimensional stability equal to annealed ram-extruded bar.

These various manufacturing processes can yield quite different products. Table 1 compares the differences in mechanical properties of UHMWPE processed using various methods.

There can be large variations in the properties of the UHMWPE used to fabricate orthopedic bearings as well. This has led to the development of alternative manufacturing processes and quality control methods. Two recently commercialized manufacturing processes are pressure crystallization and uniform compression molding (hot isostatically molding). Pressure crystallization is a method of postprocessing ram-extruded bar by exposing the material to high pressures (approximately 40,000 psi) and thermal cycles to change the crystalline structures of the material [22–28]. The induced microstructural modifications translate into changes in the mechanical properties. Values from the literature are also shown in Table 1 for pressure-crystallized material. The most notable changes are in the yield strength, percent strain, and elastic modulus. The effects of these changes are further addressed in other sections of this chapter.

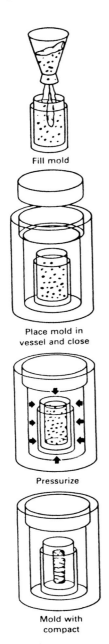

Fill mold

Place mold in
vessel and close

Pressurize

Mold with
compact

Figure 6   Schematic of cold compaction in cold isostatic press [29].

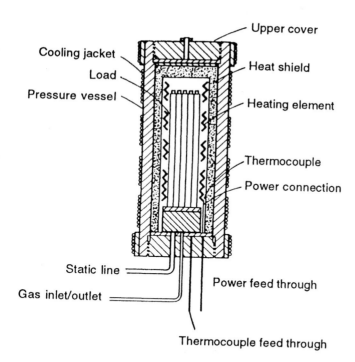

Figure 7 Schematic of hot isostatic press [29].

Table 1 Property Comparison of UHMWPe Processed by Different Methods

Processing technique	U.T.S. psi	Yield psi	Elonga-tion % strain	Defor-mation %	Hard-ness shore D	Crystal-linity %	Density gm/cc	Impact ft-lb
Ram extrusion	4949	3590	537	2.18	66	52.7	0.9377	no break
Direct compres-sion molded	7140	3626	474	1.34	66	53	0.9373	no break
Isostatically molded	6985	3895	539	1.6	66	55.2	0.9401	no break
Pressure crystal-lized*	6000**	4082	230	0.7	66	70	0.9555	no break
Test method	D-638	D-638	D-638	D-621	Duro-meter	DSC	D-1505	D-256

*Values from Ref. 27
**Value from Ref. 13

The quality control methods recently implemented by converters and orthopedic manufacturers include ultrasonic evaluation and laser candling. These methods are typically used in tandem, much the way magnetic particle and ultrasound are used in other industrial applications. Ultrasonic inspection is typically used to identify nonconsolidated regions or debris in the consolidated stock. This method is limited to defects below the surface of the stock. Laser candling was developed to identify surface discontinuities. During this inspection process, light is passed through the bar by a laser. The amount of transmitted light is monitored by a photodiode on the opposite side of the component, the side being evaluated. Debris or areas of nonconsolidation absorb more light than properly consolidated material and this is reflected in the output of the diode. This process can also be used visually and is highly sensitive to defects or discontinuities near the surface.

In addition to resin consolidation processes, postprocessing can have a major effect on the quality of components produced. Some of the processes that have an effect on the quality of the finished product are machining, additional thermal cycles, and packaging environment.

The machined surface can have a significant effect on the wear properties of the device, not only in relation to the initial breaking-in of the bearing but also from the standpoint of subsurface and wear surface changes in the material [10]. In addition to the work presented by Cooper et al. [30,31], other studies on explants report cracks approximately 10–15 μm in length, spaced 3–5 μm apart and perpendicular to machine lines, after only 1–2 years of implantation. The origin of these cracks has not been verified but it is speculated to be an artifact of machining stress coupled with polyethylene of questionable quality.

Another postprocess that can affect the properties of the UHMWPE is the use of additional thermal cycles to modify the component surface or anneal the stock for improved dimensional stability. Both of these processes can have a detrimental effect on the UHMWPE. The most dramatic has been the effect of heat pressing the surface to improve the finish. This process creates a highly crystalline layer (with respect to the bulk of the component) on the bearing surface several millimeters in depth [1]. This leads to stress concentration at the interface between this layer and the bulk of the component. The result is delamination of the surface layer and early failure of the component where the contact stress is a maximum. Annealing can also degrade the component by increasing the degree of crystallinity, resulting in an increase in elastic modulus which can correlate to higher contact stresses. In addition, if the stock is annealed in an oxygen-containing environment, the dissolved oxygen content of the material can be increased, which leads to a greater amount of oxidation after irradiation.

E. Irradiation Effects

Most components used in the orthopedic industry are gamma irradiated with 2.5–4.0 Mrads delivered from a Co^{60} source to assure sterility. This amount of radiation can cause changes in a UHMWPE component. The most notable changes are degree or percent crystallinity, discoloration, and amount of oxidation [20,21,32–39]. The irradiation causes chain scission within the polymer, creating highly reactive free radicals. Depending upon the packaging environment and the type of processes used to manufacture the component, the results can be quite different. The two basic reactions that tend to occur preferentially in the amorphous region of the polymer are oxidative chain scission or crosslinking and possible recombination of the chains [40].

Oxidative chain scission usually results in shorter, more mobile polymer chains that can align more easily than long, highly entangled polymer segments, thus causing an increase in crystallinity [40]. As the polymer is oxidized, in addition to an increase in crystallinity, a change in color or a yellowing usually occurs. This oxidative reaction can continue while the components are on the shelf, raising the question of a possible shelf-life. There have been several instances where components that were subjected to an annealing in air, prior to machining, and then packaged and irradiated under ambient conditions, have shown surface cracking and breakage prior to implantation after setting on the shelf for a period of 7–9 years. But currently there is not enough published information to make a decision on the shelf life question.

The other possible reaction after chain scission is crosslinking of the polymer. Cross-linking results in possible elimination of the free radical, decrease of active sites for oxidation, and reduction in the tendency for *in vivo* oxidation of the polymer. It must be noted, however, that if the component is in a reactive environment during and after irradiation, the polymer free radicals will preferentially decay by oxidative chain scission versus crosslinking.

Possible solutions to this oxidative degradation are pressure crystallization of the polymer, which may have some negative effects on wear [24], or packaging and storage in an inert environment such as argon gas. Many authors [20,21,32–38] have evaluated inert packaging environments with varying degrees of favorable results, but all agree it should be an integral part in the manufacturing of orthopedic bearings. But it must be noted that, in order to maximize the effects of packaging in an inert environment, the consolidation and postprocessing techniques must be designed to limit dissolved oxygen in the polymer.

Tables 2 and 3 show the results of a study on the percent crosslinking and oxidation of some commercially available components. The percent crosslinking was determined using a hot xylene extraction according to a procedure outlined in Hoechst Celanese Test Method GUR TADS/Method 18 [41]. The oxidation peaks generated on microtomed samples in Fourier transform infrared spectroscopy (FT-IR) were analyzed for intensity and normalized for specimen thickness using the methylene deformation band at 1470 nm. As the UHMWPE is degraded, whether it be *in vivo* or as a manufacturing effect, the soluble constituents are increased. Table 2 shows the results of the solubility experi-

Table 2   Results from Xylene Extraction Experiment

Manufacturing process	Average percent nonsoluable	Standard deviation
Ram extruded nonsterile	63.45	7.59
Ram extruded irradiated in air	68.03	3.55
Ram extruded irradiated in argon	65.38	12.54
Isostatically molded nonsterile	72.59	2.85
Isostatically molded irradiated in air	79.33	10.70
Isostatically molded irradiated in argon	85.50	4.36
Plate molded nonsterile	36.00	1.61
Pressure crystallized irradiated in air	27.98	1.70

*All reported values are an average of three runs.

Table 3   Peak Intensity Results From FT-IR Evaluation*

Material	Depth				
	Surface	10 Microns	20 Microns	50 Microns	80 Microns
Pressure crystallized irradiated in air #1	0.0346	0.0249	0.0231	0.0227	0.0159
Pressure crystallized irradiated in air #2	0.0323	0.0151	0.0140	0.0135	0.0078
Isostatically molded irradiated in air	0.0062	0.0014	0.0062	0.0059	0.0000
Isostatically molded irradiated in argon	0.0000	0.0000	0.0000	0.0000	0.0000
Ram extruded irradiated air	0.0167	0.0020	0.0000	0.0050	0.0066
Ram extruded irradiated argon	0.0070	0.0000	0.0021	0.0000	0.0039

*1740 peak

ments done on materials processed using different manufacturing techniques. The samples were taken from the surface of commercially available components. Table 3 shows the results of an FT-IR experiment to confirm that the degradation was due to oxidation.

III.   DESIGN OF UHMWPE COMPONENTS

This section defines and discusses the implications of polyethylene stress and wear for the orthopedic design of implants. Several factors of wear are presented with special emphasis on polyethylene contact stress.

Contact stress arises when two bodies are pressed together. These stresses are thought to be the main contributor to polyethylene failure. Obviously, it is desirable to minimize the stress seen in orthopedic implants in order to maximize the life of the implant system.

Stress is defined as force per unit area. Since the designer cannot change the force in total joints, the goal of the designer becomes maximization of the contact area. Contact area is a function of load, Poisson's ratio, modulus, and geometry of the mating surfaces [42,43].

Geometry and modulus are the two main factors that can be significantly affected in the design of orthopedic implants. Modulus is a measure of the stiffness of the material (the higher the modulus, the stiffer the material). Because the material has a higher modulus, the contact area is smaller, which gives rise to higher stresses. With respect to geometry, more conforming surfaces give rise to lower stresses. This explains why a hip cup is expected to have a longer life than a tibial bearing. While the hip can have conforming surfaces, the knee requires laxity in order to function properly. This laxity normally requires nonconforming geometry, which increases the contact stress. Analytical modeling has shown that conformance (congruency) in the coronal plane has the greatest effect on reduction of contact stresses in the tibial bearing [44]. Figures 8 and 9 show the results of a stress calculation for a knee that exhibits congruency in the coronal plane. These charts show the increase in contact stress when only the modulus is increased. Note that the difference in contact stress is magnified when the load is increased.

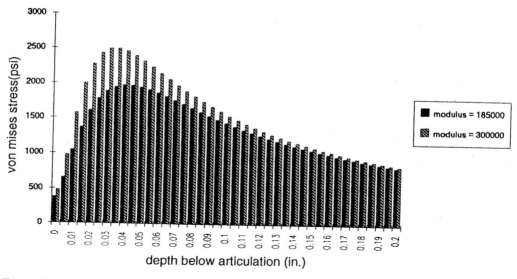

Figure 8   Contact stresses in UHMWPE tibial components with a 500 pound load.

Other factors that affect stress in polyethylene are the presence of screw holes and polyethylene thickness. It is desirable to eliminate screw holes in the metal in order to prevent cold flow into the holes, which would cause an effective reduction in thickness. It is also desirable to maintain a minimum thickness of more than 8–10 mm of polyethylene [44].

While high contact stress can contribute to polyethylene wear, it is not the only factor to consider. Component alignment, polyethylene quality, and polyethylene surface finish

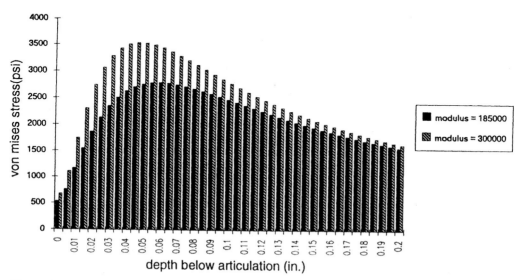

Figure 9   Contact stresses in UHMWPE tibial components with a 1000 pound load.

also play a role in polyethylene wear. These factors point to the need for good instrumentation systems and strict quality control measures. Surface finish is best addressed by having a molded articular surface versus a machined articular surface.

IV. WEAR

In order to better design components using UHMWPE or other polymers it is important to understand the mechanisms by which wear occurs. There are many theories on how UHMWPE wears in the body. However, as it is not possible to examine the bearing components at various time intervals when implanted into patients, the theoretical debate on how the UHMWPE wears in the body will continue. To this extent, the most prevalent theories on wear and wear testing are discussed in this section as they relate to polymers in general and specifically to UHMWPE.

A. Mechanisms of Wear

There are three main mechanisms of wear that occur with UHMWPE when used as a bearing surface for orthopedic implants: adhesive, abrasive, and fatigue. The importance of each of these mechanisms in determining the wear rate of UHMWPE is not completely understood at this time. Evaluation of retrieved implants show all three mechanisms to be active, but to different degrees. Quite often the three mechanisms interact with each other, which further complicates the analysis of the wear of UHMWPE.

Adhesive wear occurs when a hard, smooth counterface moves relative to a softer polymer surface, in this case UHMWPE. Thin layers of the polymer are transferred to the counterface and form a thin film on the counterface. This transfer occurs due to electrostatic forces, which are stronger between the UHMWPE and the counterface than within the bulk polymer itself. In many polymers this transfer continues until the transfer film fragments, generating wear debris. However, UHMWPE forms a unique transfer film that is stable and is responsible for its low wear rate. The UHMWPE transfer film is quite often on the order of 5–10 nm in thickness and the molecules are highly oriented in the direction of sliding [45]. The bulk polyethylene also produces a similar orientation on its surface. This combination of highly oriented molecules is responsible for the extremely low wear rates of UHMWPE as compared to other polymers.

Lubrication can have a very profound effect on the adhesive wear of UHMWPE. *In vivo* the synovial fluid appears to have very little effect on the adhesive mechanism of UHMWPE. However, *in vitro* tests can be highly affected by the lubricant used in the test. Certain lubricants (including water) are quite often associated with increased wear of polymers that form thin oriented films by disrupting the adhesion of the transfer layer to the counterface. This phenomenon is also dependent on the type of counterface present. For polymers bearing against other polymers and some ceramics, the lubricant does not have much effect, whereas with polymers bearing against metals, there can be orders of magnitude of difference in the wear rate of the polymer.

Abrasive wear in polymers is the wear of the polymer due to plastic displacement of the polymer. This is associated with a ploughing or cutting action. This can be caused by either a third-body abrasive, such as bone cement particles, or by rougher counterfaces. In the case of bone cement particles, wear of retrieved UHMWPE components appears to be significantly increased over components that do not have any entrapped bone cement particles. Third-body abrasive wear is very detrimental to UHMWPE.

One theory of the wear of UHMWPE is illustrated in Fig. 10. This theory incorporates abrasive wear mechanisms. This is seen by the occurrence of plastic deformation of the polymer surface, with subsequent plastic elongation and finally debris formation. Abrasive wear rates have a very good correlation with $1/s_u e_u$ where s_u and e_u are the ultimate tensile strength and elongation to failure of the polymer. This relationship is known as the Ratner–Lancaster correlation [45]. The product $s_u e_u$ is approximately proportional to the energy required to cause tensile rupture of a material. Therefore, optimizing these two properties for UHMWPE should reduce the wear rate of the UHMWPE. Direct compression molding of UHMWPE does optimize these properties, and clinical results from direct compression molding have been quite favorable [46].

Fatigue wear is the wear of a polymeric material caused by subsurface elastic deformation. Repeated elastic deformation causes cracks to form underneath the surface of the material. This is also due to the fact that the highest contact stress in UHMWPE bearings is beneath the surface of the material, as predicted by the Hertzian equation. The subsurface cracks then propagate during the cyclical loading of the component and eventually propagate to the surface of the component, generating wear debris. This mechanism is enhanced by the presence of voids, inclusions, or nonconsolidated areas in UHMWPE. These create stress concentrators and are initiation sites for cracks to form [3,4]. The amount of wear debris formed by fatigue wear is also dependent upon the fatigue crack growth rate of the material used. UHMWPE with a lower fatigue crack growth rate (or UHMWPE requiring higher stress to cause crack growth) should have a lower wear rate. This is because, for fatigue to cause wear, cracks must propagate. If a material has a slower crack growth rate (i.e., requires more energy for the crack to propagate), it will reduce the rate of wear and debris generation by fatigue. Figure 11 shows that isostatically molded UHMWPE has a lower crack growth rate (da/dN) than ram-extruded UHMWPE.

One other factor influencing the fatigue wear of UHMWPE is the elastic modulus of the material. UHMWPE with a higher elastic modulus (such as that formed by pressure crystallization) will have a higher contact stress [44]. Higher contact stress can increase the stress intensity increasing the fatigue crack growth rate and therefore the wear rate. Surface oxidation can also cause an increase in the modulus of elasticity at the surface of UHMWPE bearings [19]. Once again, this will increase the wear rate of the UHMWPE.

Fatigue wear has been proposed as one of the main mechanisms involved in the wear of UHMWPE tibial components for artificial knees; see Fig. 12. This is because the contact stresses in the knee are much higher than in the hip. Also contributing to the

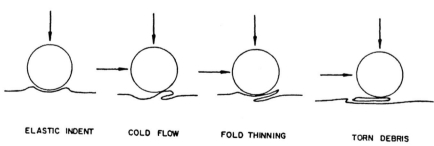

ELASTIC INDENT   COLD FLOW   FOLD THINNING   TORN DEBRIS

Figure 10   Abrasive wear mechanism for UHMWPE [47].

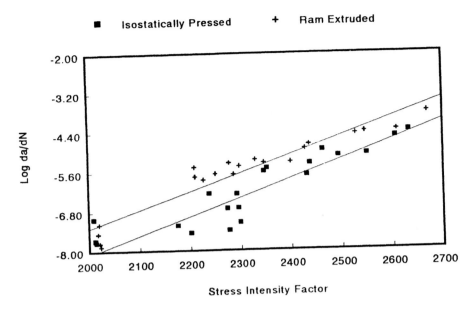

Figure 11   Crack growth rate vs. stress intensity factor.

fatigue wear mechanism in the knee is the constantly changing point of contact since the knee slides as well as rotates.

Pitting is another mechanism of fatigue wear of UHMWPE. Several retrieved tibial and acetabular components have shown pitting wear. Pitting wear is speculated to occur due to processing additives inclusions and nonconsolidated areas in UHMWPE. These stearate inclusions and nonconsolidated areas provide crack initiation sites and propagation paths, the two components needed for fatigue wear. Improved methods of manufacturing UHMWPE should reduce the amount of pitting that occurs in UHMWPE bearing components.

B.   Types of Wear Tests

Three main types of laboratory wear tests are widely used for evaluating materials for orthopedic applications. These tests vary in their complexity and their relationship to performance *in vivo*. However, they all try to determine the same thing, how to improve the wear resistance of bearings in orthopedic implants so that they generate less wear debris, and so that the debris is better tolerated by the body.

The pin-on-disk technique is the most readily understood and interpreted form of wear testing. In a pin-on-disk test, a load is applied to a spherical pin while the disk underneath the pin rotates unidirectionally. The parameters of this test include: the applied load (and therefore the contact stresses), the rotational speed of the disk, and the lubricant that the test is performed in. The wear is measured by measuring the amount of weight lost by the pin or the disk, or by measuring the depth of the wear groove by profilometry and calculating the volume of material removed. In addition to measuring

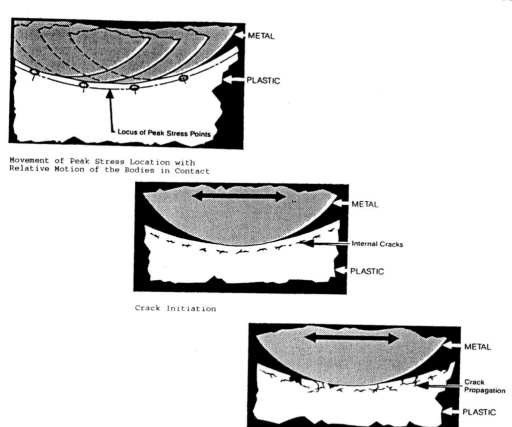

Figure 12 Fatigue wear in tibial components. (From Pappas et al., *Bio. Eng. Tech. Report*, No. 003, 1986.)

the wear of the materials, most commercially available pin-on-disk machines monitor the frictional force between the two components.

The pin-on-flat wear test is a modification of the pin-on-disk test that incorporates the wear mechanism of reciprocating motion. This reciprocating motion is thought to be important in the fatigue wear of UHMWPE. In this test a UHMWPE pin reciprocates on a flat counterface. Similar to the pin-on-disk test, the variables include the applied load, distance traveled, frequency, lubricant, and frictional forces. This test is slightly more relevant to orthopedic implants as most bearing surfaces have a reciprocating motion as opposed to an unidirectional motion. The standard method for this test is the American Society for Testing and Materials standard ASTM F-732.

Simulator tests attempt to match the *in vivo* forces and motions. Hip simulators are much more abundant than knee simulators due mainly to the larger complexity of the motion and forces involved in the knee. Hip simulator testing has been ongoing since the early 1960s with the Mk1 hip simulator at the University of London in Leeds [48]. The most well-known hip simulator is the USCATS at the University of Southern California, designed by McKellop and Clarke. In this simulator, the cup and head are inverted and the cup oscillates around the head at a 23° angle while the load is applied through the axis of the head. Other hip simulators have an anatomical position, 2° or 3° of motion, friction monitoring, etc. There are many designs of hip simulators. This has made comparing data from two laboratories very difficult since there is so much variability in the test procedure and the consequent data obtained. Clarke reviewed the status of all wear testing in 1982 and found that much information was available, but that it was all fragmentary and any correlations drawn in between two different tests were quite suspect [78]. He saw a need for a more standardized method of performing wear tests. Since that time, however, not much has changed. There are still no standards on simulator testing, and other wear testing is quite often run according to a researcher's preference.

Probably the most standard way of evaluating the wear of UHMWPE is by measuring the weight loss of the UHMWPE cup or sample. This is complicated by the fact that UHMWPE absorbs fluid. This problem can be corrected by presoaking the UHMWPE and using soak control specimens [80]. Other methods such as dimensional measurement and debris collection have been used, but these are slowly giving way to the gravimetric technique. Dimensional methods are suspect due to the creep of UHMWPE, while debris collection techniques are suspect due to the difficulty in collecting and separating the debris.

Figure 13 shows typical wear results on extruded UHMWPE and uniform compression molded UHMWPE, from a simulator similar to the one at USC. One of the important things to notice is the break-in phenomenon during the beginning of the test for about 500,000 to 750,000 cycles. During this break-in phase, there is a characteristic polishing of the machining lines in the area of contact. After this break-in phase, the wear rate appears to lessen and take on a linear rate for the remainder of the test. The other

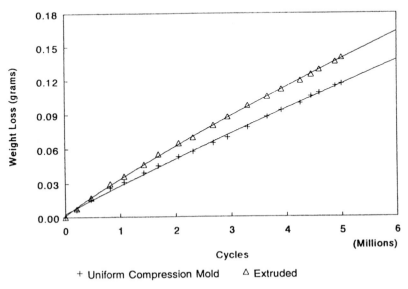

Figure 13   Hip simulator wear testing between extruded and isostatically molded UHMWPE.

interesting observation is that it sometimes takes over a million cycles to notice a difference in the wear rates of different material combinations.

The most significant problem presently encountered in the wear testing of UHMWPE is the lubricant in which the test is run. Three lubricants are commonly used today: bovine serum, distilled water, and saline [49–51]. There is currently much debate over which of these is the most relevant to evaluating the wear of UHMWPE. McKellop et al. showed that bovine serum reduced the tendency to form thick transfer films of UHMWPE on the metal counterfaces [80]. This is important as this thick transfer film is not seen on retrieved components [51]. However, serum has the problem of degrading quite rapidly during use. Its viscosity changes within hours after starting a test. Bactericides must be added to control bacterial growth during the test. However, even with these bactericides there is significant bacterial growth in the serum within 48 h [52]. Serum also makes analysis of the wear particles quite difficult and tedious. Distilled water and saline make analysis of the wear particles much easier; however, they tend to cause thick transfer films. The difference in the wear between serum and distilled water has been attributed theoretically to the lubrication of the metal counterface by proteins present in the serum. Another factor in the use of serum is the addition of a calcium-binding agent when testing ceramic components. Without this additive, calcium precipitates on the ceramic counterfaces, which then acts as a third-body abrasive not seen on retrieved components. One final example of serum and distilled water is a test done by Kumar et al. on a pin-on-flat test machine. In this test, it was noticed that the wear rates of zirconia and alumina were not affected by the choice of lubricant, whereas the 316 stainless steel had a 10 to 15 times higher wear rate in distilled water than in serum [53].

The problem of extrapolating *in vitro* testing to *in vivo* wear rates is quite complicated. One example of this is the use of Ti–6Al–4V as a bearing component. Various tests have been run to determine the suitability of Ti–6Al–4V, both ion implanted and non-ion implanted [49,54,55]. The results are as different as black and white. Some tests have shown very little wear whereas others have shown extremely high wear, to the point where the test was stopped. Clinically Ti–6Al–4V is now used very infrequently as a bearing surface.

Probably the most significant advance in the reduction of UHMWPE wear is the introduction of alumina and zirconia. These ceramic materials have shown anywhere from 2 to 10 times less wear than most metal alloys [49,53,54]. The only drawback to ceramics is the possibility of catastrophic failure. Most of these failures occurred early in the use of these materials and have been rectified by material and design improvements.

When evaluating new materials it is very important to evaluate the wear of these components. However, it should be recognized that no one test is more appropriate than another. In fact, all tests should be considered in order to evaluate new materials to see how these new materials or designs respond to different wear mechanisms. Until the wear mechanisms that occur *in vivo* are better understood and until a test is designed and agreed upon by researchers that simulates the wear mechanisms present in the body, the only true wear test will be the test of time in the human body.

V. FINAL REMARKS

It is the opinion of the authors that argon processing and packaging of compression-molded UHMW polyethylene can provide the optimum set of mechanical and wear properties for this polymer. It should be apparent to the reader that optimization of such properties in UHMWPE is extremely complex and, even after 30 years of clinical experience with this polymer in total joints, not fully understood. Through control of temperatures, pressures, processing environment, and manufacturing technique, it is possible to optimize molecular weight, crosslinking, and crystallinity to achieve the optimum polymer properties. Considering all of the miscues described in the initial paragraphs of this chapter, it now seems apparent that our best solution in reducing the wear problems associated with UHMWPE total joint components may be the precise control of these parameters and optimization of the miracle polymer that began total joint replacement approximately 30 years ago.

REFERENCES

1. Bloebaum, R. D., Nelson, K., Dorr, L. D., Hofmann, A. A., and Lyman, D. J., Investigation of early surface delamination observed in retrieved heat-pressed tibial inserts, *Clin. Orthop. Related Res.*, No. 269, August 1991, pp. 120–127.
2. Kummer, F. J., Jaffe, W. L., and Steiner, G. C., Wear caused failure of UHMWPE acetabular cup with associated granuloma: A case report, *Bull. Hosp. Joint Disease Orthop. Inst.*, *50*(2), 196–199 (1990).
3. Blunn, G. W., Joshi, A. B., Lilley, P. A., Engelbrecht, E., Ryd, L., Lidgren, L., Hardinge, K., Nieder, E., and Walker, P. S., Polyethylene wear in unicondylar knee prothesis, *Acta Orthop. Scand.*, *63*(3), 247–255 (1992).
4. Goodman, S., and Lidgren, L., Polyethylene wear in knee arthroplasty, *Acta Orthop. Scand.*, *63*(3), 358–364 (1992).
5. Collier, J. P., Mayor, M. B., McNamara, J. L., Surprenant, V. A., and Jensen, R. E., Analysis of the failure of 122 polyethylene inserts from uncemented tibial knee components, *Clin. Orthop. Related Res.*, No. 273, December 1991, pp. 232–242.
6. Landy, M. M., and Walker, P. S., Wear of ultra high molecular weight polyethylene component of 90 retrieved knee prostheses, *J. Arthroplasty*, October 1988, Suppl., pp. S73–S85.
7. Nolan, J. F., and Bucknill, T. M., Aggressive granulomatosis from polyethylene failure in an uncemented knee replacement, *J. Bone Joint Surg.*, *74-B*(1), 23–24 (January 1992).
8. Tsao, A., Mintz, L., McRae, C. R., Stulberg, S. D., and Wright, T., Failure of the porous-coated anatomic prosthesis in total knee arthroplasty due to severe polyethylene wear, *J. Bone Joint Surg.*, *75-A*(1), 19–26 (January 1993).
9. Kilgus, D. J., Funahashi, T. T., and Campbell, P. A., Massive femoral osteolysis and early disintegration of a polyethylene-bearing surface of a total knee replacement, *J. Bone Joint Surg.*, *74-A*(5), 770–774 (June 1992).
10. Weightman, B., Swanson, S. A. V., Isaac, G. H., and Wroblewski, B. M., Polyethylene wear from retrieved acetabular cups, *J. Bone Joint Surg.*, *73-B*(5), 806–810 (September 1991).
11. Rosner, B., Postak, P. D., Tradonsky, S., and Greenwald, A. S., *Cup/Liner Incongruity of Two Piece Acetabular Designs: A Factor in Clinical Failure?* Orthopaedic Research Laboratories, The Mt. Sinai Medical Center, Cleveland, OH, AAOS, 1993.
12. Kilgus, D. J., *The clinical aspects of wear: A problem in joint replacement today*, presented at UCLA Hip and Knee Meeting, October 1992.
13. Bobyn, J. D., Collier, J. P., Mayor, M. B., McTighe, T., Tanzer, M., and Vaughn, B. K., *Particulate debris in total hip arthroplasty: Problems and solutions*, Scientific Exhibit, AAOS Meeting, San Francisco, CA, 1993.
14. Himont Technical Information, *1900 ultrahigh molecular weight polymer compression molding techniques*, Bulletin HPE-102, June 1985.
15. *Hostalen GUR Technical Information Brochure*, Hoechst Plastics.
16. Collier, J. P., Mayor, M. B., Dauphinais, L. D., and Jensen, R. E., The biomechanical

problems of polyethylene as a bearing surface, *Clin. Orthop. Related Res.*, No. 261, December 1990.

17. Edelman, B., and Wright, T. M., UHMWPE varies, grade to grade, batch to batch, *Orthop. Today*, April 1992, p. 3.

18. Jensen, R. E., Collier, J. P., Mayor, M. B., and Surprenant, V. A., *The role of polyethylene uniformity and patient characteristics in the wear of tibial knee components*, presented at Implant Retrieval Symposium of the Society for Biomaterials, St. Charles, IL, September 17–20, 1992.

19. Eyerer, P., *Biodegradation of UHMWPE in joint endoprosthesis*, presented at 2nd World Congress on Biomaterials, 10th Annual Meeting of the Society for Biomaterial, Washington, DC, April 27–May 1, 1984.

20. Eyerer, P., et al., Polyethylene, in *Concise Encyclopedia of Medical and Dental Materials* (D. F. Williams, ed.), MIT Press, Cambridge, MA, 1990.

21. Eyerer, P., et al., Property changes of UHMWPE hip cup endoprostheses during implantation, *J. Biomed. Mater. Res., 18*, 1137–1151 (1984).

22. Li, S., and Howard, E. G., *Characterizations and Description of an Enhanced UHMWPE for Orthopedic Bearing Surfaces*, presented at 16th Annual Meeting of the Society for Biomaterials, Charleston, SC, May 20–23, 1990.

23. Kalkurni, K. M., Broutman, L. S., Kalpakjian, S., and Emery, D. B., High pressure non isothermal processing of linear polyethylenes, *Polym. Eng. Sci.*, Vol. 16, No. 1 (Jan. 1976).

24. Ellwanger, R., Eyerer, P., and Siegmann, A., *Very high pressure molding of UHMWPE*, presented at ANTEC 1987 Conference – Society of Plastics Engineers 45th Annual Technical Conference, Los Angeles, CA, May 4–7, 1987.

25. Li, S., and Howard, E. G., Jr., Process of manufacturing ultrahigh molecular weight linear polyethylene shaped articles, U.S. Pat. 5,037,928, August 6, 1991.

26. DePuy, Hylamer™ orthopaedic bearing polymer, *Innovations for Success*, Vol. 1, No. 2, 1990.

27. DePuy/DuPont, *A New Enhanced Ultra High Molecular Weight Polyethylene Orthopaedic Applications: A Technical Brief*, 1989.

28. DePuy, Hylamer-M™ Now Available in the AMK Knee, *Joint Efforts*, Vol. 2, No. 2, 1993.

29. *Metals Handbook*, 9th ed. Vol. 7, Powder Metallurgy, ASM, Metals Park, OH, 1984.

30. Cooper, J. R., Dawson, D., and Fisher, J., *Birefringent studies of polyethylene wear specimens and acetabular cups*, presented at ASME International Conference on Wear of Materials, April 7–11, 1991.

31. Cooper, J. R., Dowson, D., Fisher J., Isaac, G. H., and Wroblewski, B. M., *Observation of residual subsurface shear strains in the UHMWPE acetabular cups of Charnley hip prosthesis*, presented at Fourth World Biomaterials Congress, Berlin, April 24–28, 1992.

32. Streicher, R. M., Ionization irradiation for sterilization and modification of high molecular weight polyethylenes, *Plast. Rubber Process. Appl., 10*(4), 221–229 (1988).

33. Roe, R. J., et al., Effect of radiation sterilization and aging on UHMWPE, *J. Biomed. Mater. Res., 15*, 209–230 (1981).

34. Nusbaum, H. J., The effects of radiation sterilization on the properties of UHMWPE, *J. Biomed. Mater. Res., 13*, 557–576 (1979).

35. Kurth, M., Eyerer, P., and Cui, D., Effects of radiation sterilization on UHMWPE, *Annual Technical Conference – Society of Plastics Engineers, 45th*, 1987, pp. 1193–1197.

36. Streicher, R. M., Influence of ionizing irradiation in air and nitrogen for sterilization of surgical grade polyethylene for implants, *Radiat. Phys. Chem., 31*(4–6), 693–698 (1988).

37. Birkinshaw, C., Buggy, M., and White, J. J., Effect of sterilizing radiation on the properties of UHMW polyethylene, *Mater. Chem. Phys., 14*(6), 549–558 (June 1986).

38. Streicher, R. M., *Improving UHMWPE by ionizing irradiation crosslinking during sterilization*, presented at the 17th Annual Meeting of the Society for Biomaterials, Scottsdale, AZ, May 1–5, 1991.

39. Rimnac, C. M., Klein, R. W., Khanna, N., and Weintraub, J. T., *Post-irradiation aging of*

UHMWPE, presented at 19th Annual Meeting of the Society for Biomaterials, Birmingham, AL, April 28–May 2, 1993.

40. Parkinson, W. W., Radiation-resistant polymers, *EPST*, 1st ed., Oak Ridge National Laboratory Publication, pp. 783–809.

41. Hoechst Celanese Test Method, *Determination of percent crosslinking in polyethylene*, GUR TADS/Method 18.

42. Wright, T. M., *Design Principles of PE Joint Components*, Department of Biomechanics, The Hospital for Special Surgery, New York.

43. Pappas, J. J., Makrios, G., and Buechel, F. F., *Contact stresses in metal–plastic total knee replacements: A theoretical and experimental study*, Biomedical Engineering Technical Report, DePuy Report No. 003, January 23, 1986.

44. Bartel, D. L., Bicknell, V. L., and Wright, T. M., The effect of conformity, thickness, and material stresses on UHMWPE components for total joint replacement, *J. Bone Joint Surg.*, *68-A*(7), 1041–1051 (September 1986).

45. Hutchings, I. M., *Tribology; Friction and Wear of Engineering Materials*, CRC Press, Boca Raton, FL, 1992.

46. Bankston, A. B., Keating, E. M., Ranawat, C., Faris, P. M., and Ritter, M. A., *The comparison of polyethylene wear in machined vs. molded polyethylene*, presented at UCLA Hip and Knee Meeting, October 1992.

47. Rostoker, W., and Galante, J. O., Some new studies of the wear behavior of UHMWPE, *J. Biomed. Mater. Res.*, *10*, 303–310 (1976).

48. Wright, K. W. J., and Scales, J. T., Stanmore Hip Joint Simulators for the Study of Total Hip Joint Replacements. In *Evaluation of Artificial Joints*, edited by Dowson, D. and Wright, V., Biological Engineering Society, 1977.

49. Clarke, I. C., Wear-screening and joint simulation studies vs. materials selection and prosthesis design, *CRC Crit. Rev. Biomed. Eng.*, *8*(1), 29–91 (1992).

50. McKellop, H., Clark, I. C., Markolf, K. L., and Amstrutz, H. C., Wear characteristics of UHMWPE: A method for accurately measuring extremely low wear rates, *J. Biomed. Mater. Res.*, *12*, 895–927 (1978).

51. Cooper, J. R., Dowson, D., and Fisher, J., The effect of transfer film and surface roughness on the wear of lubricated ultra high molecular weight polyethylene, *Clin. Mater.*, *14*, 295–302 (1993).

52. Scales, J. T., and Wright, K. W. J., *The Evaluation of Six Stanmore MK3 Hip Joint Simulators*, Final Report to Department of Health and Social Security, Agreement No. 42/81 R/E 1049/162, 1985.

53. Kumar, P., et al., Low wear rate of UHMWPE against zirconia ceramic (Y-PSZ) in comparison to alumina ceramic and SUS 316L alloy, *J. Biomed. Mater. Res.*, *25*, 813–828 (1991).

54. Saikko, V., Paavolainen, P., and Slatis, P., Wear of the polyethylene acetabular cup: Metallic and ceramic heads compared in a hip simulator, *Acta Orthop. Scand.*, *64*(4), 391–402 (1993).

55. McKellop, H., and Rostlund, T., The wear behavior of ion-implanted Ti-6Al-4V against UHMW polyethylene, *J. Biomed. Mater. Res.*, *24*, 1413–1425 (1990).

BIBLIOGRAPHY

Boggan, R. S., Trieu, H. H., Richelsoph, K. C., Paxson, R. D., and Carroll, M. C., *The effect of radiation sterilization on the physical and mechanical properties of UHMWPE*, presented at 19th Annual Meeting of the Society of Biomaterials, Birmingham, AL, April 28–May 2, 1993.

Chillag, K. J., and Barth, E., An analysis of polyethylene thickness in modular total knee components, *Clin. Orthop. Related Res.*, No. 273, December 1991, pp. 261–263.

Cigada, A., Brunella, M. F., and Pezzi, D., *Wear and creep of UHMWPE by hip joint simulator tests*, presented at 19th Annual Meeting of the Society for Biomaterials, Birmingham, AL, April 28–May 2, 1993.

Connelly, G. C., Rimnac, C. M., Wright, T. M., Hertzburg, R. W., and Munson, J. A., Fatigue crack propagation behavior of UHMWPE, *J. Orthop. Res.*, *2*(2), 119–125 (1984).

Cooper, J. R., Dowson, D., and Fisher, J., *Wear mechanisms of UHMWPE under unidirectional sliding*, presented at Fourth World Biomaterials Congress, Berlin, April 24–28, 1992.

Crugnola, A. M., Radin, E. L., Rose, R. M., Paul, I. L., Simon, S. R., and Berry, M. B., UHMWPE as used in articular prostheses (a molecular weight distribution study), *J. Appl. Polym. Sci.*, *20*, 809–812 (1976).

DePuy, Ultra high molecular weight polyethylene, Part 1: The physical mechanical and manufacturing properties of UHMWPE, *Curr. Iss. Orthop.*, Vol. 1, No. 3-A, 1990.

Eyerer, P., Degradation of UHMWPE for joint endoprostheses, *Materials Sciences and Implant Orthopedic Surgery*, Martinus Nijhoff, Dordrecht, 1986, pp. 345–354.

Eyerer, P., Property changes of UHMWPE during implantation—First hints for Development of an alternative polyethylene, in *Advances in Biomaterials*, Technomic Publishing, Lancaster, PA, 1985, pp. 62–68.

Eyerer, P., Ellwanger, R., Maedler, H., and Federolf, H., Ultra high molecular weight polyethylene for joint replacement, *Kunstatoffe—German Plastics, 77*(6), 25–28 (1987).

Eyerer, P., and Kurth, M., *Material improvements of UHMWPE*, ANTEC 1986 Conference—Society of Plastics Engineers 44th Annual Technical Conference, Boston, MA, April 28–May 1, 1986.

Eyerer, P., Kurth, M., and Cui, D., Study of extraction method on measuring insolvable constituents of UHMWPE, *Adv. Polym. Technol.*, *7*(2), 169–176 (1987).

Eyerer, P., Kurth, M., McKellup, H. A., and Mittlmeier, T., Characterization of UHMWPE hip cups run on joint simulators, *J. Biomed. Mater. Res.*, *21*, 275–291 (1987).

Hoechst GUR, *Hoechst Plastics Technical Brief*, September 1982.

Jahan, M. S., Wang, C., Schwartz, G., and Davidson, J. A., Combined chemical and mechanical effects of free radicals in UHMWPE joints during implantation, *J. Biomed. Mater. Res., 25*, 1005–1017 (1991).

Jones, W. R., Jr., Hady, W. F., and Crugnola, A., Effect of irradiation on the friction and wear of ultrahigh molecular weight polyethylene, *Wear, 70*, 77–92 (1981).

Kurth, M., Eyerer, P., Ascherl, R., Dittel, K., and Holz, U., *An evaluation of retrieved UHMWPE hip joint cups*, presented at ANTEC 1986 Conference—Society of Plastics Engineers 44th Annual Technical Conference, Boston, MA, April 28–May 1, 1986.

Kusy, R. P., and Whitley, J. Q., Use of a sequential extraction technique to determine the MWD of bulk UHMWPE, *J. Appl. Polym. Sci.*, *32*(3), 4263–4269 (1986).

Mathot, V. B. F., and Fijpers, M. F. J., Heat capacity, enthalpy and crystallinity of polymers from DSC measurements and determination of the DSC peak base line, *Thermochim. Acta, 151*, 241–259 (1989).

McKellop, H., and Lu, B., Friction lubrication and wear of polyethylene/metal and polyethylene/ceramic hip prostheses on a joint simulator, presented at Fourth World Biomaterials Congress, Berlin, April 24–28, 1992.

McKellop, H., Lu, B., and Li, S., Effect of increased density and crystallinity on wear of UHWM polyethylene acetabular cups, presented at Fourth World Biomaterials Congress, Berlin, April 24–28, 1992.

McKellop, H., Lu, B., Lu, S., and Li, S., Wear of acetabular cups of conventional and modified UHMWPE compared on a hip joint simulator, presented at 38th Annual Meeting, Orthopaedic Research Society, Washington, DC, February 17–20, 1992.

McKenna, G. B., Crissman, J. M., and Khoury, F., Deformation and failure of ultra high molecular weight polyethylene, 39th Antec Proceeding SPE, Plastic-Creativity Value Through Innovation, Boston, MA, May 4–7, 1981, pp. 82–84.

Nagy, E. V., and Li, S., *A FT-IR technique for the evaluation of UHMWPE orthopaedic bearing material*, presented at 16th Annual Meeting of the Society for Biomaterials, Charleston, SC, May 20-23, 1990.

Nagy, E. V., and Li, S., Analysis of retrieved knee components via FT-IR, presented at 16th Annual Meeting of the Society for Biomaterials, Charleston, SC, May 20-23, 1990.

Rimnac, C. M., Klein, R. W., Burstein, A. H., and Wright, T. M., In vitro *chemical and mechanical degradation of UHMWPE: Three month results*, presented at 19th Annual Meeting of the Society for Biomaterials, Birmingham, AL, April 28-May 2, 1993.

Rostoker, W., Chao, E. Y. S., and Galante, J. O., The appearances of wear on polyethylene—A comparison of *in vivo* and *in vitro* wear surfaces, *J. Biomed. Mater. Res., 12*, 317-335 (1978).

Siegmann, A., Raiter, I., Narkis, M., and Eyerer, P., Effect of powder particle morphology on the sintering behavior of polymers, *J. Mater. Sci., 21*(4), 1180-1186 (April 1986).

Thomas, B. J., *Materials and design for total knee arthroplasty*, presented at UCLA Hip and Knee Meeting, October 1992.

Yusuniwa, M., Yamaquchi, M., Nakamuru, A., and Tsubakihara, S., Melting and crystallization of solution crystallized UHMWPE under high pressure, *Polym. J., 22*(5), 411-415 (1990).

24

All-Polymer Articulation: Experience with a Total Knee

Gary W. Bradley
Orthopedic Specialists of Santa Barbara
Santa Barbara, California
Michael A. R. Freeman and David J. Moore
Royal London Hospital Medical College
London, England
Michael A. Tuke
Finsbury Instruments Ltd.
Chessington, Surrey, England

I. INTRODUCTION

The first successful and widely used total joint arthroplasty was a cup arthroplasty developed and first performed by Smith-Peterson in the United States in 1939 [1]. This procedure used a single Vitallium component placed between the prepared femoral head and acetabulum, articulating with both but attached to neither. Various other endoprostheses and partial replacements were subsequently developed, mainly for the hip; and were used relatively widely [2-4].

These developments culminated in the pivotal work of Sir John Charnley in England in the late 1950s and early 1960s. Sir John first utilized a stainless steel stem and ball articulating against a polytetrafluoroethylene (PTFE) socket [5,6]. The unsatisfactory *in vivo* wear characteristics of PTFE soon became apparent and, ultimately, polyethylene (PE) was successfully introduced. Of equal importance and also developed by Sir John was the use of a cold-curing acrylic cement, poly(methylmethacrylate) (PMMA), for immediate implant fixation to the skeleton [6].

Over the past three decades large total joint arthroplasties have evolved so that chrome, cobalt, or titanium are used more commonly than stainless steel; ultrahigh molecular weight polyethylene remains the standard concave bearing surface for hips, knees, and other large joints. Various ceramic components also have been used, mainly in place of the metallic sphere, for the femoral component of a total hip. Ceramic components show some promise but have significant limitations.

A variety of other polymers have also been used in various applications in orthopedics. Polyacetal has been the most utilized polymer next to polyethylene. Certain characteristics of polyacetal are especially attractive: It has an approximately tenfold greater resistance to creep deformation and a fivefold greater hardness than polyethylene. Additionally, its elastic modulus much more closely approaches that of bone than does polyethylene.

Our interest in polyacetal grew with the early successful use of an all-polyacetal, "isoelastic" femoral component stem utilized for total hip replacements. This was developed by Morscher in the late 1970s. His experience, furthermore, demonstrated good tissue tolerance, at least in the short term [7–9].

In Scandinavia the Christiansen total hip, introduced in the early 1970s, consisted of a metal stem and separate metal ball with an interposed trunion of polyacetal. The metal ball then articulated against a polyacetal acetabular socket. Although this particular hip functioned well in the short term, it did not stand up well in the intermediate and long term [10].

These separate experiences suggested that polyacetal does not wear well against metal, but in block form (as in a femoral stem) it can be used in large joint arthroplasties. We further felt that an all-polymer total joint arthroplasty might demonstrate the following advantages over the more standard metal–polymer designs:

1. Because of relatively similar elastic moduli, a more "isoelastic" implant might be developed, possibly reducing micromotion at the bone–prosthesis interface as well as decreasing stress shielding.
2. There would be no release of potentially harmful metal debris or ions.
3. Radiolucency (not noted above but another feature of polymers) would provide for better longitudinal evaluation of the bone–implant interface.
4. Decreased cost.

In subsequent studies we also learned of the potential wear advantages of an all-polymer configuration. These findings are summarized in the following section.

II. MATERIALS

In the early 1980s we performed simple pin-on-disk and roller-in-trough studies using the two candidate polymers in a normal saline lubricant. These crude evaluations suggested that an all-polymer bearing configuration consisting of polyacetal versus polyethylene might have some merit.

Subsequently, Harry McKellop et al., at USC, performed formal wear testing using congruous surfaces, concave ultrahigh molecular polyethylene (UHMWPE) and convex polyacetal in a hip wear simulator. These results have been presented and published elsewhere: 41-mm balls were bathed in bovine serum and run under oscillating loads as described by Paul [11] for 1 million cycles. Polyacetal balls versus UHMWPE were compared to chrome-cobalt balls versus UHMWPE. The results from this study were:

1. Frictional target maximum load was approximately 17% lower for the polyacetal-polyethylene combination as compared to the chrome–cobalt/polyethylene combination (1.21 N/m vs. 1.45 N/m).
2. The polyethylene wear rate against polyacetal was nearly 40% lower than the wear rate of polyethylene against chrome–cobalt.
3. The total volume of wear produced with the polyethylene-polyacetal combination was approximately 20% lower than the volume of polyethylene wear produced in the metal-on-plastic configuration (ignoring any metal wear) [12,13].

Since polyacetal might, under certain conditions, degrade to form formaldehyde, the lubricant serum was evaluated for formaldehyde. Trace amounts of formaldehyde were found in 21 of 32 samples tested [12].

III. THE CLINICAL WEAR STUDY

Between 1980 and 1983 a series of all-polymer total knee replacements were performed. The design was based on a Freeman–Samuelson semiconstrained total knee replacement. Polyacetal was used for the convex femoral component and ultrahigh molecular weight polyethylene was utilized for the tibial and patellar components. All components, including the polyacetal femoral components, had polyethylene condylar fixation pegs; a few of the components had other intramedullary stem devices. All components could be press fit, but cement fixation could also be utilized. The articular surfaces provided area contact with the consequent advantage of relatively low interface stresses.

Between May of 1980 and July of 1983 a total of 64 total knee replacements were performed in 54 patients. The majority of these individuals resided in the United Kingdom but some lived in France ($N = 11$) and Sweden ($N = 6$). These all-polymer implants represent a relatively small number from a larger series of total knee replacements using conventional metal femoral components made of chrome–cobalt that were performed at about the same time. Concurrent with the development of this new design was a set of instruments specific to this total knee.

There were slightly more females than males; the diagnosis mix was nearly equal between osteoarthritis and rheumatoid arthritis, which is somewhat unusual as most series of knee replacements are weighted toward the diagnosis of osteoarthritis. The mean age was 61, with a range of 25–80. See Table 1.

The majority of the prostheses were press fit; polymethylmethacrylate cement was not utilized. Three tibial components were fixed using a full PMMA interface, and 12 tibial components were basically press fit but PMMA was used in bone defects. In only 3 patellae was PMMA utilized. Six femoral components had a full PMMA interface and 7 additional femoral components were press fit but PMMA was used in defects. Eighteen of the 49 uncemented knees received a bone graft.

Significantly, this series was not preselected. A number of the knees, as above, did have defects significant enough to require bone grafting. Eight knees had undergone previous operations.

Prospective follow-up was performed of all patients with clinical and radiographic

Table 1   Study Profile

Knees (N)	64
Patients (N)	54
Male (n)	15
Female (n)	39
Diagnosis (n)	
Osteoarthritis	28
Rheumatoid arthritis	25
Age (years)	
Mean	61
Range	25–80

Table 2   Follow-up Population

Reviewed at 10 years (N)	26
By examination (n)	15
By telephone (n)	11
Died, but with examination/ review longer than 5 years (mean: 5.5 years) (N)	10
Lost (N)	15
Revised (N)	13

evaluations at 6 weeks, 6 months, and 1 year. Evaluations were then also performed at each subsequent year. Preoperatively and at each follow-up evaluation a detailed protocol form was completed and computerized. Table 2 provides a summary on the patients available for long-term evaluation. At the 10-year follow-up, 11 of the patients had a telephone review as these individuals were prevented by various medical problems from attending a regular follow-up visit.

Radiologic evaluation included anteroposterior x-rays, lateral x-rays, and a skyline view of the patella (see Fig. 1). X-rays were all evaluated subjectively for changes in bone density or quality. They were also measured for angulatory changes or subsidence of components. Bone reaction around the pegs and at all interfaces was evaluated for resorption and sclerosis. More detail on the technique of x-ray analysis has been given elsewhere [14,15].

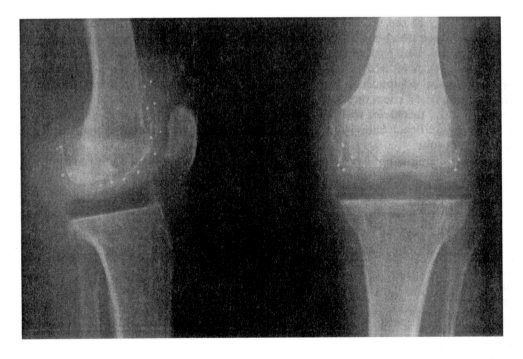

Figure 1   Lateral and anteroposterior x-rays of uncemented all-polymer total knee arthroplasty.

A total of 15 knees completed clinical and radiological follow-up at a minimum 10 years from the time of their operation. An additional 11 knees, in patients who were unable to travel, had a 10-year follow-up performed via telephone review.

An additional 10 knees (in 8 patients) were functioning satisfactorily at death; the average time was 5.5 years from operation.

Eleven knees were lost to follow-up within the 10-year period; none of these knees were known to have undergone revision surgery. Four knees were not satisfactorily followed because patients moved and could not be relocated.

A total of 13 knees were known to have been revised during the study period. The mode of failure was aseptic loosening in 3 knees. Ten knees developed deep infection; 7 of these knees were revised. In 3 of these knees an irrigation and open debridement was performed with salvage of the implant *in situ*. All of the infected knees were treated with antibiotics.

Most of the septic failures took place in knees that had been replaced within a relatively short time. It was belatedly learned that the vacuum used in the course of ethylene oxide sterilization of these all polymer components produced microbursts in the covering of the femoral component and a consequent loss of sterility. It is our belief that these septic failures were related to an inadequate sterilization technique, not to the use of polyacetal as a femoral component. Excluding septic failures, the loosening rate is consistent with other series of mainly uncemented knee replacements.

Histology was obtained from failed implants as well as from one nonfailed postmortem specimen (at 9 years following implantation). No differences were noted between the polyethylene and the polyacetal interfaces, nor was any qualitative difference noted in these tissue specimens compared to specimens from other conventional types of knee replacement failures. No evidence of severe wear was present on the implants removed from failed knees. There was slight burnishing or polishing of some of the polyethylene tibial components; no significant changes were visible on the polyacetal femoral components.

The clinical results in knees still functioning were comparable to a similar population treated with the same prosthesis but with a metal femoral component. Approximately one third of the knees had mild pain (requiring occasional nonnarcotic analgesia) and 5% of the knees had moderate pain (requiring occasional narcotic analgesia). Average flexion was over 95°. Ten percent of the knees lacked full extension, with the maximum deficit being 10°. Walking ability was more likely to be limited by factors other than the knee.

In x-ray evaluation, angulatory changes less than 3° and subsidence less than 3 mm cannot be accurately detected [14]. Within these limitations there was no significant subsidence nor angulatory change in these knees at final evaluation.

IV. DISCUSSION

The most common cause of long-term failure in large joint arthroplasty is aseptic loosening. This is believed to be related to a variety of factors but most implicated is bone resorption secondary to debris produced by otherwise normal wear. Other factors might include stress shielding from a large, relatively rigid (usually metallic) implant and the "normal" remodeling seen in aging bone [16].

Whenever two materials are rubbed together the softer of the two materials will be preferentially worn, but the harder material may also produce wear debris. Thus it is not surprising that in histologic evaluation of nonfailed as well as failed total joint interfaces, large amounts of polyethylene wear debris are seen. It is well known that smaller amounts of metallic debris can also be found [17–19].

Any bearing combination that reduces wear and, therefore, reduces the production of wear debris should have a beneficial effect on long-term implant fixation. Although at this time it appears to be much less of a factor, it is also probable that an implant causing less stress shielding should also have a better long-term outlook. The relationship, in the long term, between stress shielding and the bone remodeling that has been described in normal aging is unclear.

Returning to the subject of wear debris, there has been concern over the long-term effect of metal ions. Studies have demonstrated elevated metal concentration in tissues remote from as well as local to replaced joints [20–22]. Additionally, the serum and urine of patients with conventional cemented chrome–cobalt/polyethylene total joint replacements have been shown to have elevated metal concentrations [20,21]. The relationship of these increased metal concentrations to malignancy is not directly known, but it is known that sarcomatous degeneration has been associated with total joint replacement [23–25].

Gillespie et al. have also demonstrated a 70% increase in the incidence of tumors of lymphatic and hemopoietic tissue occurring at sites distant from an implant in patients with total hip replacements [26].

Regardless of any hypothetical advantage to avoidance of metal debris, our experience suggests that an all-polymer joint articulation can be used with success comparable to that of a conventional metal-on-polymer large joint replacement. We have found no specific untoward clinical effects after up to 10 years follow-up using an all-polymer configuration. Formal wear testing has demonstrated improved wear characteristics of this combination.

Based on the experience of others, we do not recommend using implants having a direct bone–plastic interface. We recognize that the long-term advantages to all-polymer total joint replacement remain to be seen and are not established by this small study. We do feel that we have demonstrated the feasibility of an all-polymer implant combination and that further investigations into the use of this type of large joint replacement should be considered.

REFERENCES

1. Smith-Peterson, M. N., Arthroplasty of the hip: A new method, *J. Bone Joint Surg., 21,* 269–88 (1939).
2. Moore, A. T., and Bohlman, H. R., Metal hip-joint: A case report, *J. Bone Joint Surg., 25,* 688–92 (1943).
3. Judet, J., and Judet, R., The use of an artificial femoral head for arthroplasty of the hip joint, *J. Bone Joint Surg., 32B,* 166–73 (1950).
4. King, D. E., Straub, L. R., and Lambert, C. N., Final report of the Committee for the Study of Femoral Head Prostheses, *J. Bone Joint Surg., 41A,* 883–886 (1959).
5. Charnley, J., *Low Friction Arthroplasty of the Hip,* Springer-Verlag, Berlin, 1979, pp. 6, 34.
6. Charnley, J., Anchorage of the femoral head prosthesis to the shaft of the femur, *J. Bone Joint Surg., 42B,* 28–30 (1960).
7. Bombelli, R., Gerundi, M., and Aronson, J., Early results of the RM-isoelastic cementless total hip prosthesis: 300 consecutive cases with 2 year follow-up, in *The Hip: Proceedings of the Twelfth Open Scientific Meeting of the Hip Society,* C. V. Mosby, St. Louis, MO, 1984, p. 133.

8. Jakim, I., Barlin, C., and Sweet, M. B. E., RM isoelastic total hip arthroplasty: A review of 34 cases, *J. Arthroplasty, 3,* 191–199 (1988).
9. Morscher, E. W., and Dick, W., Cementless fixation of "isoelastic" hip endoprosthesis manufactured from plastic materials, *Clin. Orthop., 176,* 177–187 (1983).
10. Goldie, I. F., and Raner, C., Total hip replacement with a trunion bearing prosthesis, *Acta Orthop. Scand., 50,* 205–216 (1979).
11. Paul, J. P., Force transmitted by joints in the human body, *Proc. Inst. Mech. Eng., 181,* 8–15 (1967).
12. McKellop, H., et al., Superior wear properties of an all-polymer hip prosthesis, *Trans. ORS 31st Annual Meeting,* Las Vegas, NV, 1986, p. 322.
13. McKellop, H. A., Rostlund, T., and Bradley, G. W., Evaluation of wear in an all-polymer total knee replacement: Part 1: Laboratory testing of polyethylene on polyacetal bearing surfaces, *Clin. Mater., 14,* 177–126 (1993).
14. Blaha, J. D., Insler, H. P., Freeman, M. A. R., et al., The fixation of a proximal tibial polyethylene prosthesis without cement, *J. Bone Joint Surg., 64B,* 326–335 (1982).
15. Bradley, G. W., et al., All polymer total knee replacement, *Am. J. Knee Surg., 5,* 3–8 (1992).
16. Martin, R. B., Pickett, J. C., and Zinaich, S., Studies of skeletal remodeling in aging men, *Clin. Orthop., 149,* 268–282 (1980).
17. Betts, B., Hansuaj, M., Bansal, M., and Wright, T. W., Metal release from cobalt–chrome prostheses: Analysis of tissues from revision total hip replacement, *Trans. 15th Annual Meeting Society for Biomaterials,* Lake Buena Vista, FL, April 28–May 2, 1989, p. 145.
18. Mirra, J. M., Marden, R. A., and Amstutz, H. C., The pathology of failed total joint arthroscopy, *Clin. Orthop., 170,* 175–183 (1982).
19. Willert, H. G., and Semlitsch, M., Problems associated with the anchorage of artificial joints, in *Advances in Artificial Hip and Knee Technology* (M. Chaldach and D. Hoffman, eds.), Springer-Verlag, Berlin, 1976, pp. 325–346.
20. Black, J., Editorial: Does corrosion matter? *J. Bone Joint Surg., 70(B),* 517–520 (1985).
21. Bartolozzi, A., and Black, J., Chromium concentration in serum, blood clot and urine from patients following total hip arthroplasty, *Biomaterials, 6,* 2–8 (1985).
22. Cracchiolo, A., and Revell, P., Metal concentration in synovial fluids of patients with prosthetic knee arthroplasty, *Clin. Orthop., 170,* 169–174 (1984).
23. Bago-Granell, J., et al., Malignant fibrous histiocytoma of bone at the site of total hip arthroplasty. A case report, *J. Bone Joint Surg., 66(B),* 38–40 (1984).
24. Penman, H. G., and Ring, P. A., Osteosarcoma in association with total hip replacement, *J. Bone Joint Surg., 66(B),* 632–634 (1984).
25. Swann, M., Malignant soft tissue tumor at the site of a total hip replacement, *J. Bone Joint Surg., 66(B),* 629–631 (1984).
26. Gillespie, W. I., Framptom, C. M. A., Henderson, R. I., and Ryan, P. M., The incidence of cancer following total hip replacement, *J. Bone Joint Surg., 70B,* 1–80 (1988).

V
TISSUE RESPONSE AND GROWTH

25

Tissue Engineered Biomaterials: Biological and Mechanical Characteristics

Lucie Germain and François A. Auger

Hôpital du Saint-Sacrement and
Laval University, Sainte-Foy, Québec, Canada

I. INTRODUCTION*

One must see a severely burned patient in an emergency ward to fully grasp the severity and the multisystemic nature of this trauma. Depending on the age and previous medical condition of these burn victims, the definition of severe may vary. However, most burn specialists agree that, when more than 20–30% of the total body surface has been injured with third-degree and/or second-degree burns, the consequences far exceed the local lesions to the skin [1–5]. These notions of multiple insults on different organs of the body go well beyond the scope of the present chapter of this encyclopedia. However, it must be understood that the diagnosis and treatment of burn wounds, with all their complications, demand the interaction and cooperation of various specialists: burn surgeons, burn nurses, chest specialists, infectious diseases specialists, anesthetists, cardiologists, internists, etc.

One must also envision the formidable surgical task that has to be accomplished during the next weeks after the trauma. The larger the body area involved, the more difficult and complex will this surgical approach be. These clinical facts can be summed up in a simple statement since the only definitive classic therapy for burn wound coverage is the patient's own skin taken from spared sites (called *donor sites*): The more a patient is burned, the fewer donor sites there are for long-term remedy [6–9]. Consequently, burn survival is, among other parameters, directly related to the total wound surface [7,10,11]. The clinical situation described by this statement used to be of a particularly ominous nature when the burned area was over 70% of the total body surface.

The preceding sentences can explain quite readily the need for an additional therapeutic option such as the one offered by tissue engineered epidermis. However, other less

---

*Please refer to explanatory note on page 724.

evident advantages of such a tissue reconstruction approach are expanded upon later in this chapter (see Sec. II.C).

One must also be aware of the very complex nature of the healing processes involved in the recovery of these patients. Thus, the treatment of burn patients cannot be seen as a simple mechanical coverage, but as a complicated biological phenomenon that is always imperfect. In other words, although minor skin injuries will heal with a minimum of defects such as scarring, large burn wounds are invariably accompanied by many disruptive phenomena, which seem to have most of their origin in the dermal cells [12–16]. Thus, the pattern of normal healing in these large wounds frequently leads to hypertrophic scarring and contracture [2–4,12–14]. These quite mechanical events must be countered by what is also a very physical approach: pressure garments. Carefully fitted garments are the only method for minimizing these inappropriate healing processes, which otherwise may lead to unsightly scars [13,17]. This unfortunate sequence of events is also another reason for trying to find new therapeutic modalities.

Tissue engineering of epidermis and skin seems to offer such valid therapeutic options. However, each of these tissue engineered organs has its advantages and pitfalls as we shall submit to the reader in the following paragraphs. Also, in response to the previously described clinical concerns related to wound coverage and appropriate healing processes, it can be stated immediately that the tissue engineered skin equivalent should be a better therapeutic option. However, this logical affirmation may have to be tempered by some sobering clinical conditions and evaluation, as we describe in this chapter.

II. TISSUE-ENGINEERED EPIDERMIS FOR WOUND COVERAGE

The growth and expansion of epithelial cells is not a new endeavor since the first references to this process can be found more than three decades ago [19–28]. Furthermore, skin epidermal cells have been shown over two decades to be dependent on "dermal factors" and "anchorage factors" (such as collagen) for successful growth [19–21,28–37]. However, only in the past 15 years have those techniques been successfully applied to the treatment of burn patients [38–50]. Many thousands of square centimeters of tissue engineered epidermis (TEE) can thus be obtained in the form of organized and stratified epithelium, from an initial biopsy of 1 to 6 cm^2 [29,39,51]. These results have opened the door to the present field of tissue engineering [52,53].

A. Why Is It Done?

The preceding paragraphs have shed some light on the most evident reasons for the use of tissue engineering in burn patients. Severely burned patients have such a shortage of donor sites that the contribution of cultured epidermal sheets can be thought of as life saving. This conclusion is in keeping with the clinical approach of rapidly covering large burn wounds in order to increase the survival rates of such patients [4,54,55]. For large burn wounds, recent clinical experience supports this aggressive approach [40]. However, without enough autografts, this approach is confronted with the unavailability of grafts unless epidermal tissue engineering is used. Cadaver skin grafts are only a temporary solution since graft rejection always ensues [56]. Furthermore, they now are subjected to very stringent microbiological control in order to obviate any infectious risks [57]. Moreover, the delay in permanent coverage will be deleterious to the patient, either by bringing about eventual infectious episodes and additional surgical procedures, or by exposing the patient to many foreign skin antigens. This last drawback has never been thoroughly studied but may have a significant impact on the already affected cellular immunological system of these trauma patients.

Another aspect of the rationale behind these cultured epidermal sheets is related to the very nature of the harvesting process of autologous skin grafts from these patients. These sites are "cropped" with a special knife, called a "dermatome", which inflicts a trauma similar to a second-degree burn. Not only does this entail pain and bleeding, but such harvesting of skin can rarely be done more than twice. Thus, a site that has been cropped three times will either heal quite slowly, become infected, or heal with vicious scarring. Thereafter, the solution may result in an additional problem since then the risk of a full thickness wound looms quite distinctly over the surgeon's shoulder. Any additional wounds have a negative impact on survival.

This tissue-engineering technique has a few applications in other areas. The treatment of giant nevi has been well explained [58,59]. These patients, very often children, are born with giant melanotic lesions. As in burn patients, when these lesions cover over 50% of the total body surface, the usual grafting process is quite difficult to carry through. A small initial biopsy allows the culture of many square centimeters of epidermis that can be transplanted at a slower pace than in the burn trauma situation. The only use for allogeneic cultured epidermal grafts (i.e., between nonimmunologically related individuals) has been in chronic skin ulcers [59–63]. The coverage is then temporary since these cells are always rejected, as we and others have shown [64–66].

B. How Is It Done? (Green's Method)

The following provides a description of a step-by-step approach to the reconstruction of epidermal tissue according to the method first described by Green [51]. The epidermis is the superficial layer of the skin and has important functional properties: It is a barrier for water loss and bacterial entry. The epidermis is formed by multiple layers of keratinocytes attached together by desmosomes. *In vivo*, the epidermis rests upon the dermis, which is an extracellular matrix (Type I and Type III collagens, fibronectin, elastin, proteoglycan) containing dispersed mesenchymal cells (fibroblasts).

1. Epidermal Cell Isolation

Keratinocyte culture is initiated from a small biopsy of the patient's skin. For burn patients, it is preferable to harvest the skin biopsy from a spared site, as early as possible after admission in the burn unit. A 1- to 6-cm^2 full-thickness skin biopsy is excised; placed aseptically into sterile transport medium [Dulbecco–Vogt modification of Eagles medium (DME) with Ham's F-12, Flow Labs, Mississauga, Ontario, Canada] in a 3 : 1 proportion (DME-Fl2), supplemented with 24.3 μg/ml adenine, 10% fetal calf serum (FCS, Flow Labs), 100 IU/ml penicillin G (PEN), 25 μg/ml gentamicine (GEN, Schering Canada Inc.), and 0.5 μg/ml amphotericin B (SQUIBB Canada, Montréal); sent to the culture laboratory; and processed immediately or kept at 4°C. The cell isolation procedure is initiated within 24 h following the harvesting.

The following procedures are performed under a sterile air flow hood. The skin biopsy is inverted in 2 ml of phosphate-buffered saline (PBS: 8 g NaCl + 0.2 g KCl + 1.15 g Na$_2$HPO$_4$ + 0.2 g KH$_2$PO$_4$ per liter of H$_2$O, PEN, GEN, and 0.5 μg/ml amphotericin B) into a 100-mm petri dish and the dermis is carefully excised with iris scissors. The dermis-poor biopsy is then placed into a 50-ml tube and strongly agitated in 20 ml of PBS containing antibiotics. The procedure is repeated 4 times with new PBS. The dermis-poor biopsy is then cut into very fine pieces (less than 1 mm^3) with the same scissors, in 2 ml of trypsin (0.1% in PBS containing PEN, GEN), into a 100-mm petri dish. The pieces are transferred to the trypsinization unit (single sidearms Celstir, Wheaton 356533, Millville, NJ) in 15 ml of trypsin–EDTA (1 : 1 trypsin 0.1% : EDTA 0.02% in PBS containing PEN, GEN). The trypsinization unit is placed onto a magnetic stirrer for gentle agitation during 30 min (120 rev/min, at 37°C). The skin pieces are allowed to settle (1 min) and the supernatant containing dissociated cells is transferred into a 50-ml tube and centrifuged at 300 $\times$ g, for 10 min (see next section). In the trypsinization unit, 20 ml of trypsin–EDTA is added to the pieces, which are returned to 37°C for 30 min under agitation. This serial digestion is performed 5 to 6 times.

2. Epidermal Cell Culture

After centrifugation of the supernatant, cells are resuspended in culture medium, counted, and plated at 2 to 5 $\times$ 10^6 cells per 75 cm^2 culture flasks in 25 ml of culture medium. The culture flasks are preseeded with 1 $\times$ 10^6 irradiated fibroblasts as feeder cells (see below). Then the flasks are transferred and kept in an incubator with an atmosphere containing 8% CO_2, at 37°C and 100% humidity.

The feeder layer is necessary to increase the keratinocyte ability to form colonies and to restrain human fibroblast overgrowth [29]. Mouse NIH Swiss 3T3 fibroblast cell line is maintained in culture in DME containing 10% FCS and routinely passaged by trypsinization. When needed, 3T3 are irradiated directly in culture flasks or in suspension (after trypsinization) with 6000 rad (^{60}Co source) to inhibit further growth, and plated in 75 cm^2 flasks 1 to 48 h before keratinocyte seeding.

The keratinocyte culture medium consists of DME-Fl2 (see transport medium, Section II.B.1), supplemented with 24.3 μg/ml adenine, 5 μg/ml bovine crystallized insulin, 5 μg/ml human transferrin, 2 $\times$ 10^{-9} M 3,3′,5′,triiodo-L-thyronine (Sigma Chemicals), 0.4 μg/ml hydrocortisone (Calbiochem, La Jolla, CA), 1 $\times$ 10^{-10} M cholera toxin (Schwarz/Mann, Cleveland, OH), 10% FCS (Flow Labs), PEN, and GEN. Human epidermal growth factor (EGF, Chiron Corp., Emeryville, CA), 10 ng/ml, is added on the third day after plating. The culture medium is changed 3 times a week.

These culture conditions favors keratinocyte proliferation and differentiation [29, 51,52,67,68]. Keratinocytes colonies begin to be visible about 4 days after seeding and confluent cultures are produced in 10 to 20 days. These flasks are then trypsinized for subculturing as follows: After removal of the culture medium, the flasks are rinsed with 2 ml of trypsin–EDTA. Ten milliliters of trypsin–EDTA are then added to each flask and they are incubated at 37°C until keratinocytes detach (10 to 20 min, depending on the confluence). The enzyme is inhibited with 7 ml of culture medium added directly to the flasks. The cells are well suspended by pipetting and then centrifuged at 300 $\times$ g, 10 min. The keratinocyte pellet is resuspended in keratinocyte culture medium and seeded on a 3T3 feeder layer at a concentration of 2 to 9 $\times$ 10^5 cells/75 cm^2 flask. After trypsinization, one flask yields 15 to 25 $\times$ 10^6 cells that can be further divided into 30 to 125 flasks. Depending on the seeding concentration used, confluent keratinocyte cultures are obtained after 9 to 15 days. The subculturing process can be repeated several times. The number of passages that can be done varies with the age of the donor.

3. EDTA Removal of Contaminating Human Fibroblasts

The growth of human fibroblast is restrained by the mouse fibroblast feeder layer. After several days in culture, irradiated mouse fibroblasts detach from the culture flask and are eliminated during subsequent media changes. If keratinocytes are not confluent by this time, contaminating human fibroblasts can then grow. The fibroblast growth potential in culture makes these cells undesirable contaminants. Moreover they limit the expansion and the fusion of keratinocyte colonies, two processes necessary for the formation of an organized epidermal sheet. Therefore, human fibroblasts must be removed as soon as possible when they are detected. The ability of fibroblasts to detach faster than keratinocytes when incubated with EDTA can be used to eliminate them. As some keratinocytes may be removed with this technique, it should not be performed before keratinocyte colonies are visible (4–5 days after plating). The culture medium of the flasks, contaminated with fibroblasts, is removed and 1 ml of EDTA (0.02% in PBS with PEN, GEN) is added. The flasks are then returned to the incubator (37°C for 2 to 5 min). The cultured cells are observed under a phase-contrast inverted microscope to ascertain fibroblast detachment. Careful monitoring is necessary to keep the EDTA for a minimum time in order to detach fibroblast without keratinocyte removal. The cultures are then rinsed 2 times with 5 ml PBS, and fresh culture medium is added along with mouse 3T3 fibroblasts since they are also removed by the EDTA treatment.

4. Epidermal Sheet Production

Epidermal sheets for transplantation are produced from keratinocyte cultures, 24 to 72 h post-confluence. Usually, 30 to 50 "peel away type" flasks of 75 cm^2 (Ezin^{TM} flask, Nuncion 171110, Roskilde, Denmark) are prepared together. Two days before grafting, the sterility of each flask is ascertained by seeding 1 ml of the culture medium, into thioglycolate broths (Quélab, Montréal, Canada). These cultures are kept at 37°C for 24 to 48 h. The day preceding the transplantation, the culture medium of each flask is changed for a medium devoid of cholera toxin. On transplantation day, the thioglycolate broths are verified and any presumptive positive culture is indicated by an abnormal turbidity. If this is the case, the corresponding epidermal culture flasks are discarded. The keratinocyte sheets are detached from the flasks with an enzyme (dispase) that breaks attachment between cell and plastic but not cell-cell links (desmosomes). This enzymatic specificity allows the whole culture to be obtained en bloc as a tissue sheet. Each flask is rinsed twice with 10 ml of serum-free DME-Fl2 medium containing PEN, GEN. Ten milliliters of the same medium containing 2.5 mg/ml dispase is then added to the flasks, which are incubated at 37°C for 40 to 60 min, until the sheets detach from the flask's border. The dispase is then removed and the flasks are rinsed twice with 10 ml of medium. The top of the flask is peeled away. Two milliliters of medium are added on the sheet to obviate dessication. A Vaseline-impregnated gauze, previously cut into a slightly smaller rectangle than the sheet dimension (25 cm^2), is deposited to facilitate the ensuing manipulations. The sheet borders are then brought back onto the gauze using a rubber "policeman." The gauze is smoothly pressed on the epidermal sheet with the same policeman while holding the gauze and cell sheet together with forceps. The epithelial sheet, now attached to the gauze, is turned over in the dish. Fourteen ligaclips (Ligaclip extra, Ethicon, Inc., Somerville, NJ) are added to secure the sheet onto the gauze. The gauze sheets are then transferred with forceps into sterile petri dishes (100 mm in diameter), and 15 ml of serum-free medium are added to cover the sheet, which is facing up. The petri dishes are placed into a mobile incubator filled with an atmosphere containing 8% CO$_2$, and transported to the surgery room.

For transplantation, the gauze sheet is taken with forceps from the petri dishes and deposited onto the wound, with the epithelium facing downward. The basal cell layer, which was attached to the culture flask, is now in direct contact with the wound bed while the differentiated layers are more superficial and the gauze protects them.

C. What Is Right?

Beyond the evident advantages that were alluded to in the introduction to this chapter, some specific aspects of the success of this technique are examined in the following sections.

1. Engraftment Level

It is unquestionable that these grafts do result in a *take* when transplanted. However, rates of success vary widely between various sites in the same patient, different patients, and different burn centers [38–50,59,69–71]. The exact reasons for these discrepancies are beyond the scope of this chapter, but they are similar to the problems in classical skin grafts. These parameters include wound bed, surgical preparation, microbial wound colonization or infection, nutritional status of the patient, and various systemic imbalances [70,71]. In our own institution, the take level averages 60% (with a range of 10–100%). The best results are obtained on a clean wound with some preserved dermis and in a patient who is recovering nicely: The take level is then approximately 80–90%.

2. Aspect of Graft

These grafts, after a successful take, steadily evolve to present a full-thickness epidermis with a normal stratum corneum. These wounds are then efficaciously and permanently covered with a self-regenerating living tissue [38,41,72–74). The self-repair properties of these grafts have also been demonstrated: They heal after wounding [59].

Furthermore, on a long-term basis, these grafts have given some very good results without excessive shrinking or scarring, as some had predicted [45,72]. A thorough histological study, over a 5-year follow-up for some patients in Boston, has shown some advantageous results compared to classically grafted sites on the same patients. The tissue-engineered epidermis had some seemingly positive modulatory effect over time on the reappearance of organized, although imperfect, dermis [72]. It should be pointed out that most of these cases were in a pediatric population, and some additional evaluation in older patients is certainly warranted.

3. Lowering Morbidity at Donor Sites

At times, in our burn unit, we have used this tissue-engineered epidermis to graft donor sites that had been harvested previously. As stated previously, these sites heal more slowly because recropping has been done. We have noted that TEE reverses this trend with a rapid and uneventful healing.

D. What Is Wrong?

1. Delay of Grafting

The culturing process for TEE can vary between 3 and 5 weeks for the first set of grafts. This is a rather long delay in severely wounded patients, where a rapid treatment is of utmost importance. The older the patient, the longer this delay usually will be.

2. Low Graft Take

In certain situations, the graft take of TEE has been very low (0–20%). The following conditions could be construed as a worst-case scenario: a bad wound bed such as fat, an infected site, movement of the grafts over the graft site (shearing effect), and finally, desiccation due to inappropriate dressing. Since these grafts are quite thin and fragile, extreme care must be given to the wound bed and infection control. Furthermore, displacement of grafts over the wound can have some deleterious effect on the basal cells. Desiccation will destroy all the graft.

3. Abnormal Dermoepidermal Junction

We have, as others, rapidly realized that some of our TEE-transplanted patient had a "blebbing" phenomenon occurring a few days to a few weeks after grafting. The probable cause for this was identified as the abnormal formation of anchoring fibers [69, 75]. At times, these blebs demand retransplantation, but they will heal spontaneously if their diameter is less than 1 cm. These abnormalities will eventually disappear with the reappearance of normal dermoepidermal junction structures after a few months [72,73].

4. Absence of a Dermal Layer

Even though a remodeling of a neodermal tissue occurs after TEE grafting, this process is long and may be fraught with abnormal healing events. Thus, some authors had previously demonstrated the importance of preventing severe *contracture* by dermal tissue [76,77]. This contracture phenomenon, as the term implies, is a form of abnormal healing that occurs when an inordinate level of contraction is brought about by dermal cells [13,14]. On the other hand, our clinical experience has not shown contractures to be excessive when TEE is used [40].

However, it seems that the addition of a dermal component may have some advantages related to the more rapid and physiological tissue repair that ensues. Thus, the immediate addition of the dermal layer adds many mechanical qualities such as resistance and suppleness [79–83]. In this regard, the series of studies by Cuono and others [84–88] are an indication of the importance of the dermal component in determining the final results. These investigators have sequentially transplanted appropriately treated (allogeneic) cadaver skin to their patients, then "shaved off" the epidermis after a few days to finally allow TEE transplantation. The result is thus a two-step approach to bilayered skin grafts: allogeneic dermis followed by autologous TEE. These authors claim excellent take levels (>80%) with superior macroscopic and microscopic (histologic) results.

E. What Do We Do About It?

1. Delay of Grafting Procedure

We have used a three-pronged approach to this problem.

Improved Isolation Method with Thermolysin and Trypsin.   First, we have established a new protocol for the enzymatic digestion of the initial biopsy from which the epidermal cells are extracted [89]. The sequential use of thermolysin and trypsin has not only allowed a much better yield of epidermal cells, but has also demonstrated, in a very significant way, the reduction of contamination by dermal fibroblasts (Figs. 1–3). The fibroblasts that were not eliminated by the standard procedure already described (Sec. II.B) can contaminate the TEE sheets. The elimination of these fibroblasts entails a harsh EDTA treatment for keratinocytes. This is also a time-consuming process as every day is important in burn treatment.

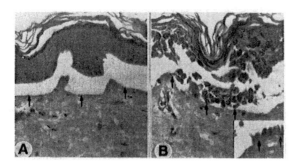

Figure 1   Skin digestion with thermolysin or trypsin. Hematoxylin, phloxine, and saffron staining of human skin digested with thermolysin (A) or trypsin (B) for 2 h 30 incubation at 37°C to separate the dermo-epidermal junction. Note that the dissociation of the epidermis from the dermis is complete when thermolysin is used (A). In contrast several cells from the basal layer are still attached to the dermal side when trypsin is used (B). Moreover, thermolysin does not break the cell–cell junctions (desmosomes), allowing the separation of the whole epidermis from the dermis. In addition to the disaggregation of epidermal cells, trypsin also liberate fibroblasts (×150). (From Germain et al., Ref. 89. Courtesy of *Burns*.)

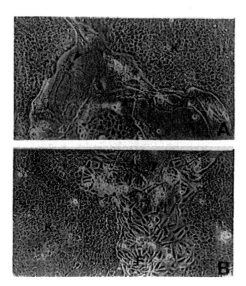

Figure 2   Fibroblast contamination in keratinocyte culture. Phase-contrast micrographs of cutaneous cell cultures. (A) Cells were isolated by the thermolysin and trypsin method (see Sec. II.E.1) or by the trypsin method (see Sec. II.B.1) and subcultured once. Note the presence of irridiated mouse mouse fibroblasts (arrowheads) between keratinocyte colonies (K) in cells dissociated by both methods, and the presence of human fibroblasts (F) only in the cell population isolated by the trypsin method (B) (×50). (From Germain et al., Ref. 89. Courtesy of *Burns*.)

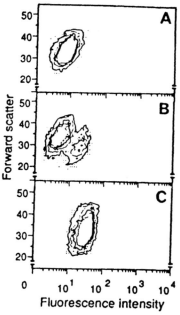
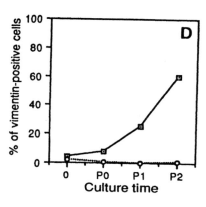

Figure 3 Fibroblast contamination of epidermal cell populations isolated with the thermolysin and trypsin method or the trypsin method. The presence of fibroblasts in epidermal cell cultures was assessed by labeling with vimentin, a marker specific for mesenchymal cells (fibroblasts). Dual parameter cytofluorimetric analysis for forward scatter and vimentin labeling (green fluorescence). Cells were isolated (A) by the thermolysin and trypsin method (see Sec. II.E.1) or (B) by the trypsin method (see Sec. II.B.1) and subcultured once (passage 1). In order to be able to assess for the presence of human fibroblasts, keratinocytes were cultured in the absence of 3T3 feeder layer. Positive control with pure human fibroblast population appears in panel (C). (D), Epidermal cell populations—freshly isolated (0) or after various time in culture [primary culture (p0), passage 1 (P1) and passage 2 (P2)]—were analyzed for their content of fibroblasts. The percentage of vimentin-positive cells was determined on contour graphs [for example, see (A) and (B)]. The dotted line represents epidermal cells dissociated by the thermolysin and trypsin method (see Sec. II.E.1). The solid line represents epidermal cells dissociated by the trypsin method (see Sec. II.B.1). Note that fibroblast and keratinocyte populations can be easily distinguished on these contour graphs (A–C). Fibroblasts are absent from epidermal cell population isolated with the thermolysin and trypsin method (A) whereas they are present in those isolated with the trypsin method (B), and their proportions increase with culture time (D). (From Germain et al., Ref 89. Courtesy of *Burns.*)

Furthermore, our extraction method is also advantageous in obtaining more cells that are rapidly replicating: The colony-forming efficiency level is higher [89]. This translates into a shorter time period necessary in order to obtain TEE sheets. The overall advantage may translate into a 10% to 20% reduction of the usual culture time; 2–4 days are saved in a situation where rapidity is the essence of the solution.

Briefly, this cell isolation procedure is designed to cleave the dermoepidermal junction with thermolysin (Fig. 1) and remove the dermis prior to epidermal cell dissociation with trypsin. The dermal layer is trimmed in order to reduce the skin thickness. Skin fragments (5 mm × 5 mm) are then floated on 500 μg/ml of thermolysin (Sigma Chemicals, St. Louis, MO) in 4-(2-hydroxyethyl)-1-piperazine ethane–sulfonic acid (HEPES) buffer (6.7 mM KCl : 142 mM NaCl : 10 mM HEPES : 1 mM CaCl$_2$: 0.45 mM NaOH, pH 7.4) for 2 h at 37°C. The epidermis is separated from the dermis with forceps, cut into small pieces, and further incubated with 0.05% trypsin–0.1% EDTA in PBS for 30 min at 37°C. Cells are then centrifuged and cultured as previously described (see Sec. II.B). The resulting cell population is free of fibroblasts (Figs. 2 and 3).

Conditioned Culture Media.   Investigators in our group are presently evaluating various conditioned media that have a stimulatory effect on the growth of keratinocytes. A further culture time decrease will probably ensue [90].

Autologous and Allogeneic Chimeric Grafts.   Lastly, as a third solution, we have evaluated a radical new approach. If allogeneic grafts were done, then either skin banks or cell banks could solve the delay problem: Grafting of previously prepared allogeneic epidermal sheets [56,91–94] could be accomplished as fast as the excision surgery proceeds. But many authors have commented on the rejection of such skin grafts, especially because skin transplantation studies are the very origin of transplantation immunology, with some landmark experiences by Medawar [95–97]. Furthermore, allogeneic TEE grafts have been shown to be rejected both in a clinical setting and in our laboratory with an animal model [64–66,96,98–106] (Figs. 4–6).

However, we have devised a unique type of chimeric graft by combining allogeneic and autologous epidermal cells *in vitro.* We have shown in an animal model that such chimeric TEE will give rise to a totally autologous epidermis a few days after transplantation. Thus, allogeneic cells were eliminated without an aggressive rejection phenomenon. These results may give fascinating possibilities for human therapy [106].

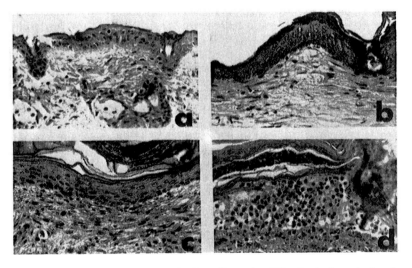

Figure 4   Rejection process of TEE allografts. Histological analysis of normal murine skin (a), compared to mouse TEE isografts (b) and allografts (c) and (d) harvested 11 (c) and 14 days post-transplantation [(b) and (d)]. The syngeneic and allogeneic TEE implants were obtained after a 3-day culture period of the newborn mice epidermal cells. Note the presence of a nice epidermis following isograft transplantation whereas allografting results in a leukocyte infiltration starting on the 11th day postgrafting and becoming intense on the 14th day postgrafting, indicating that the TEE allografts are rejected. Magnification ×250. (From Rouabhia et al., Ref. 64. Courtesy of *Transplantation.*)

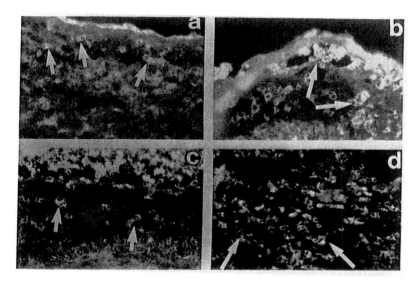

Figure 5 Identification of the cellular infiltrate in the TEE allografts. The allogeneic TEE implants were obtained after a 3-day culture period of newborn mice epidermal cells. Eleven and 14 days postgrafting, allograft biopsies were stained with anti-CD4 [(a) and (c)] and anti-MAC-1 [(b) and (d)] monoclonal antibodies. Note that the immuno-staining shows the presence of monocytes and lymphocytes in the cellular infiltrate accelerating the allograft rejection. Magnification ×250. (From Rouabhia et al., Ref. 64. Courtesy of *Transplantation*.)

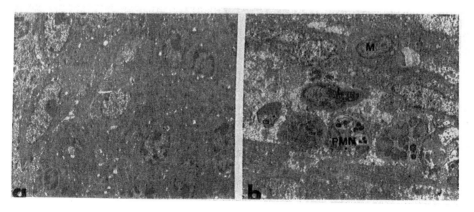

Figure 6 Electron microscopy analysis of TEE isografts and allografts. TEE were obtained and grafted as described in Fig. 4. Biopsies were taken from host dorsum 20 days after isografting (a) and 14 days after allografting (b) of mouse TEE. For the isografts, note the presence of multilayers of keratinocytes (a). However, for the allografts, note the detachment of the allograft from its grafting bed with the presence of monocytes (M), lymphocytes (L), and polymorphonulear (PMN) infiltration, demonstrating the activation of the rejection process. Magnification ×3200. (From Rouabhia et al., Ref. 64. Courtesy of *Transplantation*.)

2. Take Level

Once again, we have taken a multiple approach to this problem. First, with a particularly vigilant pregraft bacterial culture surveillance protocol [107], we do superficial swabs at prepared graft sites at least 48 h prior to surgery. We then adjust the systemic antibiotics to reduce the infectious risk for the exact microorganisms that were cultured. Antibiotics are given until 5–7 days after grafting.

Furthermore, we have also shown that a tissue glue has a positive effect on graft take levels [108]. This is probably due to an enhanced adhesion, allowing the immediate diffusion of nutrients without interposition of seromas or hematomas. This glue did not impede the usual sequence of human epidermal maturation (Figs. 7 and 8), and its transitory presence has no deleterious effect on the ensuing sequence of basement membrane formation (Figs. 9 and 10).

Lastly, a cautious use of topical antibiotics is warranted since we and others have shown many of these to be toxic for TEE [109–113]. Thus, the wound dressings are without any topical antibiotics whenever possible.

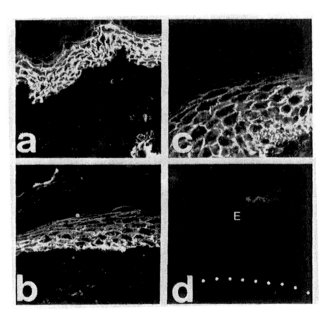

Figure 7 *In vivo* evolution of human TEE grafted onto athymic mice. Immunofluorescence microscopy of normal human skin (a) and of human TEE grafted on nude mice with previous Tisseel® (a tissue glue) application [(b) day 10 post-transplantation; (c) and (d), day 21] using mouse monoclonal antibodies to the major histocompatibility complex of human: anti-HLA-A,B,C [(a)–(c)]; or mouse anti-H$_2$D (d). Note that anti-HLA-A,B,C antibody labeled cell membrane of all stratum (except stratum corneum). The expression of human but not mouse major histocompatibility complex confirms the human nature of grafted epidermis (E). The dotted line (d) represents the epidermal–connective tissue junction (×180). (From Auger et al., Ref. 108. Courtesy of *Br. J. Plast. Surg.*)

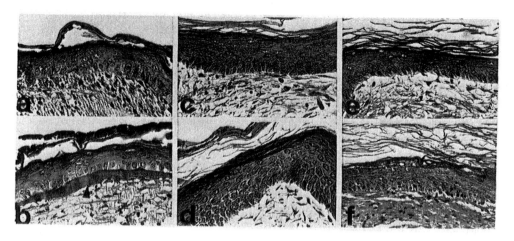

Figure 8 Transient observation of tissue glue after human TEE grafting . Hematoxylin, phloxine, and saffron staining of biopsies harvested 4 [(a), (b)], 10 [(c), (d)], and 21 [(e), (f)] days after transplantation of human TEE grafted on muscular graft bed without [(a), (c), (e)] or with previous application of Tisseel® [(b), (d), (f)]. Note that the tissue glue is observed at day 4 [(b), arrow] but not later on. The maturation of the epidermis and the formation of the stratum corneum was similar in the presence or absence of the glue ($\times$180). (From Auger et al., Ref. 108. Courtesy of *Br. J. Plast. Surg.*)

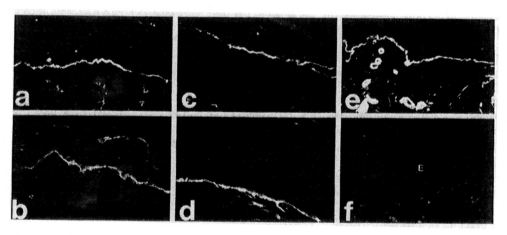

Figure 9 Basement membrane component expression after human TEE grafting with or without previous application of a tissue glue. Immunofluorescence staining with sheep polyclonal anti-human Type IV collagen antibodies of human TEE grafted on nude mice without Tisseel® [(a), day 4 post-transplantation; (c), day 21] or with previous Tisseel® application [(b), day 4 post-transplantation; (d), day 21]. Positive control of normal human skin (e). Negative control [primary antibody omitted, (f)]. Note the linear staining of the basement membrane. The fluorescence is slightly lower when Tisseel® was present at day 4 (b). This could be due to a masking of the Type IV collagen by tissue glue. However, the fluorescence intensity was comparable when biopsies were harvested later, suggesting that the tissue glue did not have any influence on the expression of basement membrane components 10 days or more after grafting. E, epidermis ($\times$180). (From Auger et al., Ref. 108. Courtesy of *Br. J. Plast. Surg.*)

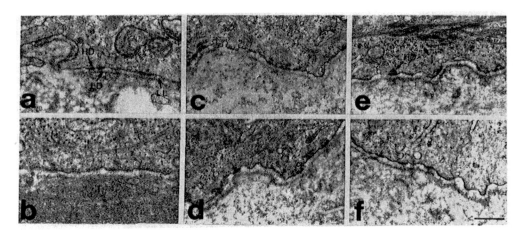

Figure 10 Ultrastructural analysis of basement membrane reformation after TEE grafting with or without a tissue glue. Transmission electron microscopy of cultured human epidermal sheets grafted on nude mice without Tisseel® [(a), day 4 post-transplantation; (c), day 10; (e), day 21] or with previous Tisseel® application [(b), day 4 post-transplantation; (d), day 10; (f), day 21]. The regions of the basement membrane zone, lamina lucida (LL) and lamina densa (LD) were already observed at day 4 post-transplantation in control group (a). Basal cell plasma membrane contained numerous electron dense plates characteristic of hemidesmosomes (HD). Note the presence of Tisseel® (T) at day 4 (b), which impedes the observation of lamina densa (LD). The ultrastructure of basement membrane is better defined 10 and 21 days post-transplantation and is similar for TEE grafted with or without tissue glue [(c), (d), (e), and (f)]. Bar represents 250 nm ($\times$ 29,000). (From Auger et al., Ref. 108. Courtesy of *Br. J. Plast. Surg.*)

III. TISSUE ENGINEERED SKIN

The preceding discussion has already given the reader some of the many reasons explaining the quest for a bilayered, dermal and epidermal equivalent. All of these and the following additional reasons are related to a clinical goal.

However, it must be stated that these tissue engineered skin (TES) equivalents have already proven their value for various experimental or *in vitro* purposes. Thus many studies in the fields of pharmacology, physiology, and physiopathology, as well as cosmetology, have been accomplished using various types of TES [114–123].

A. Why Is It Done?

Some of the reasons explaining the clinical need for a bilayered skin equivalent have been discussed in Sec. II.A. They relate to the theoretical and proven advantages of the dermal component in the healing of any skin graft. But there are also some more subtle reasons for initiating such a complex tissue engineering feat, such as the generation of a more complete dermoepidermal junction. The reasoning behind this expectation is that during the *in vitro* maturation of the TES, many of the components of the dermoepidermal junction would appear. Furthermore, the grafting process would not entail, as in the TEE sheets, a disruptive enzymatic maneuvre damaging this fragile structure. A few experimental and clinical results have already shown this sequence of events to be exact [124–129].

Moreover, the dermal layer may also be "tailored" to answer some of the expected and/or proven weaknesses of TES. It has been argued that various cytokines could be tagged onto the extracellular matrix of the dermal component to enhance either angiogenesis, wound healing, or both [130]. Other types of molecules such as antibiotics could also be added in order to reduce the frequent infection caused by the inescapable bacterial colonization of all burn wound surfaces [131,132].

Lastly, these composite grafts could treat burn lesions in a one-step surgical intervention. This is a significant advantage over the two-step technique described in Sec. II.D.4.

B. How Is It Done?

1. Production of TES (Bell's Method)

Fibroblast Culture. Human dermal fibroblasts are obtained from normal adult skin specimen removed during reductive breast surgery. Fibroblasts are isolated by collagenase digestion (200 IU/ml in DME, 20 h at 37°C) of the skin fragments. After centrifugation at 300 × g for 10 min, fibroblasts are plated in 75 cm^2 tissue culture flasks and grown in DME containing 10% fetal calf serum, as described above, at 37°C in a 8% CO_2, 92% air atmosphere. The culture medium is changed three times a week. Cells are routinely passaged by trypsinization with a solution of 0.01% EDTA and 0.05% trypsin in PBS (pH 7.45) before reaching confluence.

Keratinocyte Culture. Keratinocytes are obtained from normal adult skin specimens removed during reductive breast surgery and cultured according to the method described above (see Sec. II.E.1). Before plating on dermal equivalents, subconfluent keratinocyte cultures are trypsinized, and cells are counted and resuspended in keratinocyte culture medium.

Dermal Equivalent Preparation. Bell and colleagues [133–135] were the first to demonstrate that the incorporation of dermal fibroblasts within collagen gels leads to a matrix reorganization with a structure resembling human dermis. Various cell (5 × 10^3 to 5 × 10^5 cells/ml) and collagen (0.1 to 3 mg/ml) concentrations can be used. Typically, dermal equivalents are produced by mixing the following solutions into a 50-ml plastic centrifugation tube: 0.75 ml of 5 times concentrated DME medium containing 500 IU/ml PEN and 25 µg/ml GEN, 0.15 ml sodium bicarbonate (7.5%), 0.5 ml fetal calf serum, 0.7 ml distilled water, and 0.2 ml NaOH 0.1 N. Then, 2.5 ml of a 4.0 mg/ml acid-soluble, Type I collagen solution (Sigma type III, prepared by dissolution overnight at 4°C in 1 : 1000 acetic acid solution) is added to the tube and quickly mixed before and during the addition of 0.5 ml of fibroblast suspended in culture medium. The mixture is poured into a 60-mm plastic bacteriological petri dish (Fisher Scientific, Montréal, Québec, Canada). Dishes are incubated at 37°C in a 8% CO_2, 92% air atmosphere. Gelation begins a few minutes after incubation at 37°C, if the pH is optimal (7.4). The culture medium (DME containing 10% FCS, PEN, GEN) is changed every 2 days. The dermal equivalents do not attach to the dishes and form "floating" tissues that contract with time in culture.

TES Preparation. For keratinocyte seeding, the culture medium is removed until its level is just below the dermal equivalent surface. Half a milliliter of keratinocytes are added on top of the floating dermal equivalents at concentrations of 6 × 10^3 to 5 × 10^5 cells/cm^2 of dermal equivalent. After keratinocyte seeding, the dermal equivalents are transferred for 1 h at 37°C to allow the epithelial cells to attach to the dermal surface. Culture medium is then added and the equivalents are reincubated at 37°C in a 8% CO_2,

92% air atmosphere. The addition of keratinocytes onto the surface results in a bilayered dermoepidermal tissue [135–138].

It must be emphasized that this is not the only tissue-engineering method for the creation of TES. In the last decade, some authors have described other approaches that can be arranged in the two groups discussed in the following section (see also Sec. III.B.2).

2. Production of TES by Other Methods

Various Sponges Composed of Polymeric Biomaterials. Many polymers have been used, such as collagen, chitosan, and glycoseamino-glycan in various compositions and mixtures. These sponges can be seeded *in vitro* with either one or two cellular components: keratinocytes and fibroblasts [125,126,129,139–146]. Alternately, the infiltration and proliferation can occur after grafting with fibroblasts that creep into the pores of the sponge. Then, either classical skin grafts or TEE are deposited after a few days [147–153].

Scaffolding Meshes Made of Various Biomaterials. The growth of fibroblasts on a nylon mesh results in the formation of a dermal equivalent. After attachment to the mesh, fibroblasts secrete extracellular matrix that fills the interstices. Upon seeding of keratinocytes, a skin equivalent is produced with a differentiated epidermis laid on a structured basal lamina [122,128,154]. However, the production delay is very long: 26 days for the dermis and at least 1 more week for the epidermis [128].

C. What Is Right?

There is a flurry of encouraging animal grafting data concerning all types of TES. The levels of take and histological results are quite impressive [135,136,139,155–158]. Our group reproduced and expanded upon these animal results [159].

However, there is much less experience in human grafting [76,127,147,160–163]. The first results were positive but many questions remain unanswered. Some significant problems related to infections have been encountered but few of these results have found their way into the medical literature. But there are many ongoing trials with various types of grafts in the United States and a few in Europe. These studies should provide a clearer picture of the clinical value of these TES.

D. What Is Wrong?

Even though the clinical role of TES has not been clearly established, some drawbacks may already be commented upon. All of these comments are related to the technique described in Sec. III.B.1 and are less relevant when applied to the models briefly described in Secs. III.B.2 and B.3.

1. In Vitro *Shrinkage of TES*

Even though the first publications described the *in vitro* shrinkage phenomenon that occurs when fibroblasts are embedded into a collagen gel [133,136], this was not deemed to be a major issue. However, when the scale-up process is considered, it then becomes a serious drawback. All is well when the TES is only 5 to 10 cm^2 for *in vitro* studies and small animal grafts [135,136]. But when the goal is to produce many hundreds of TES sheets of around 30–50 cm^2, this shrinkage becomes a major hindrance.

When we strived to combine *in vitro* both cell types (fibroblasts and keratinocytes), we showed that "floating" TES will contract severely [164]. Furthermore, we have proven with an experimental design procedure that whatever the cell and/or collagen concentration, a severe shrinkage of TES will always occur. The final surface area was always 3% or less of the initial surface (Figs. 11 and 12, Table 1) [164]. This procedure was clearly inapplicable to the large-scale production necessary for human therapy. Some of our results were at odds with previous experiments by Bell [135]; they did not describe a further shrinkage due to the keratinocyte addition step. These discrepancies may be due to the fact that these investigators seemed to be adding freshly isolated keratinocytes and rapidly grafting their TES. We used subcultured keratinocytes (passages 1 to 4). It is important to emphasize that in human clinical production of TES, the keratinocytes will have to be subcultured a few times in order to obtain a sufficient seeding quantity for addition to the dermal equivalents.

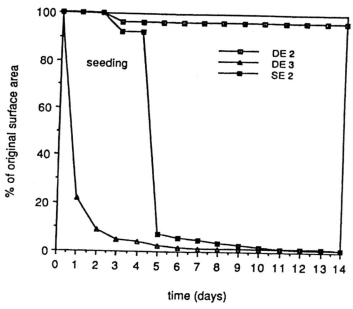

Figure 11 Influence of keratinocyte seeding on the contraction rate and final surface area of TES. TES were produced according to the method described in Sec. III.B. and cultured floating in bacterial petri dishes. The graph shows typical curves of the contraction of dermal and skin equivalents according to their composition. Dermal equivalent 2 (DE2) and skin equivalent 2 (SE2): 2.9 mg/ml collagen, 5×10^2 fibroblasts/ml, 2.5 mm thick (trial 2); DE3: 0.9 mg/ml collagen, 5×10^4 fibroblasts/ml, 2.5 mm thick. Direct comparison of the contraction of a dermal equivalent containing a high collagen and low cell concentrations (DE2) with the contraction of a dermal equivalent containing a low collagen and high cell concentrations (DE3) can be made. Until day 4, the contraction of duplicates of the dermal equivalent trial 2 is shown. Keratinocytes were seeded at day 4 on one of these samples to form skin equivalent (SE2). This sample SE2 rapidly contracted, resulting in a skin equivalent with 1.3% of the original surface area, while that of the corresponding dermal equivalent is 96.2% (From Rompré et al., Ref. 164. Courtesy of *In Vitro Cell Dev. Biol.*)

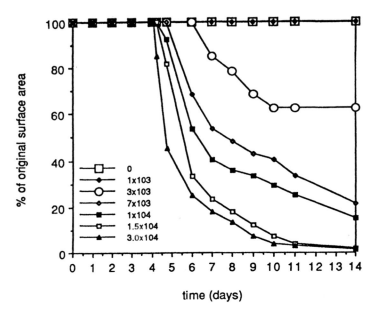

time (days)

Figure 12   Influence of keratinocyte seeding density on the contraction rate and final surface area of TES. Typical curves showing the contraction of TES in relation to the keratinocyte seeding densities. TES were produced according to the method described in Sec. III.B and cultured floating in bacterial petri dishes. The composition of the dermal portion of these skin equivalents was 2.9 mg/ml collagen, 5×10^2 fibroblasts/ml, 2.5 mm thick. Various concentrations of keratinocytes (indicated on the graph) were seeded at day 4 of dermal equivalent culture. Note that the extent of TES contraction is proportional to the concentration of keratinocytes. (From Rompré et al., Ref. 164. Courtesy of *In Vitro Cell Dev. Biol.*)

2. Delay Before Transplantation

As in tissue-engineered epidermis, the production of TES will necessitate, at least, a 3-week delay before the first transplantation. This is the time needed to obtain a sufficient amount of autologous cells and then prepare in sequence the dermal equivalents followed by keratinocyte seeding for the formation of TES. This delay is too long since the present trend of burn care calls for early wound excision over a maximum period of 2 weeks.

3. Engraftment Level

As was stated earlier, the animal transplantation studies have shown superb results [135,136,139,155–159]. However, the few clinical studies have only hinted at variable take levels. We feel that this situation is related to three rarely discussed problems in the field of tissue engineering.

Postgrafting Necrosis.   There seems to be at times, in TES, some level of necrosis after a few days of the overlying epidermis when grafts are bilayered. The exact causes are unknown but may well be related to the delay necessary for angiogenesis to proceed into the dermal layer and then allow diffusion of nutrients to the epidermis as in the normal physiological situation.

Table 1   Models for the Final Surface Areas of Dermal and Skin Equivalents

---

Dermal Equivalent

Model[a]

% original surface area $= 17.4 + 18.6X_1 - 42.8X_2 + 19.1X_2^2$
Statistical Tests
$R^2 = 0.92$
F test[b] $= 17.26$
Significance test on the variable[c] X_1 and X_2

Skin Equivalent

Model[a]

% original surface area $= 1.6 + 0.4X_1 + 0.3X_2 + 0.9X_3 - 0.3X_1^2 + 0.4X_1X_3 + 0.3X_2X_3$
Statistical Tests
$R^2 = 0.90$
F test[b] $= 0.51$
Significance test on the variable[c] X_1, X_2, and X_3

---

[a]A Box–Behnken analysis has been performed on floating dermal and skin equivalents to determine the optimal initial conditions of collagen concentrations (X_1), cell concentration (X_2, log scale), and gel thickness (X_3), resulting in equivalents with relatively large final surface area. The levels of the studied variables were as follows: $X_1 = 0.9, 1.9, 2.9$ mg/ml; $10^{X_2} = 2.7, 3.7, 4.7$ cells/ml; $X_3 = 1.3, 2.5, 3.7$ mm. The models are shown with statistically significant coefficients only (confidence level > 95%).
[b]F-test indicates if there is variation in the model not accounted for by random errors.
[c]Significance test on the variables is a joint test on all the parameters involving that variable. For example, the test for X_1 tests the hypothesis that the parameters for X_1, X_1X_1, and X_1X_2 are all zero.

Secretion of Collagenase.   The cells incorporated in the TES are secretors of a class of enzymes called, at large, the metalloproteinases [165–172]. In this group, the collagenases are well known for their role in tissue repair and rearrangement [173–182]. But if these cells secrete an inordinate amounts of collagenase, the grafts will be destroyed. Clinically, this will seem to be a liquefaction of the grafts.

4.   Infections

A similar situation can be encountered with infection of TES since bacteria are well-known secretors of various proteases including collagenases [183–185]. Furthermore, many other phenomena occur in the infections destruction of TES that are beyond the scope of this chapter.

E.   What Do We Do About It?

1.   In Vitro *Shrinkage of TES*

We have devised in our laboratory a particular method in order to prevent the inordinate amount of shrinkage caused by the contractile effect of cells [186]. A peripheral anchorage of porous material allows the attachment of the collagen matrix in the interstices, thus allowing the shrinkage of the dermal equivalent only along the thickness axis (Figs. 13 and 14). The final and the initial surfaces are thus constant under appropriate culture conditions, and the resulting surface area is not affected untowardly by the addition of keratinocytes [114,186,187]. Moreover, fibroblasts adopt a more physiological behavior in the anchored TES by aligning themselves parallel to the surface (Fig. 15), in contrast

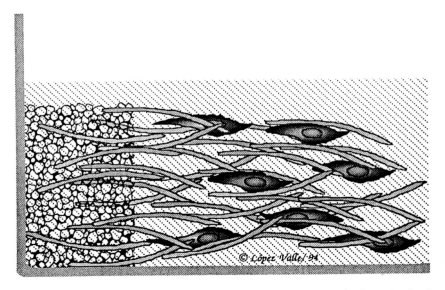

Figure 13   Schematic representation of anchored dermal equivalent. Anchoring dermal equiva-lents are produced by pouring the collagen and cell mixture in a petri dish containing a fiberglass ring. After gelation, the collagen is trapped in the filter paper and the surface area of the dermal equivalent does not diminish with culture time.

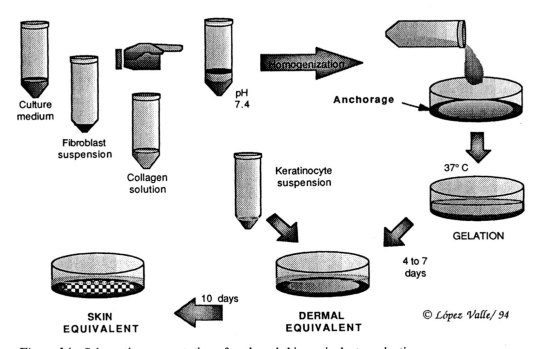

Figure 14   Schematic representation of anchored skin equivalent production.

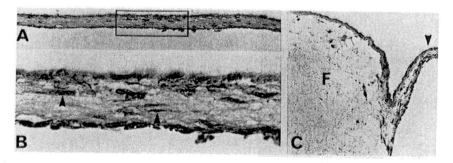

Figure 15 Histological analysis of anchored dermal equivalent. (A) Histological appearance of full thickness anchored dermal equivalent (ADE). Comparison with Fig. 16 shows that the ADE thickness resulting from the same initial conditions (intial cell and collagen concentrations) is smaller. Initial collagen concentration was 2.11 mg/ml and fibroblast number was 18,500/cm². Hematoxylin and eosin staining. Taken at 20× and enlarged photographically to 40×. (B) Enlargement of the indicated portion of Fig. 15A showing fibroblasts (arrowheads) and collagen fibers oriented longitudinally in relation to tissue length. Taken at 40× and enlarged photographically to 160×. (C) Histology of the fiberglass ring (F) interface with the ADE (arrowhead). Hematoxylin and eosin staining. Note that fibroblasts are absent from the fiberglass ring. Taken at 20× and enlarged photographically to 40×. (From López-Valle et al., Ref. 186. Courtesy of *Br. J. Dermatol.*)

to what is observed in the floating TES, where the orientation is perpendicular to the surface (Fig. 16).

Similar methods had been devised by the initial author (Bell) and others by pouring the collagen gel over a porous surface or cell monolayer [188–192]. Thus, all of the surface of these TES rests on various biomaterials and must then be severed if an *in vivo*

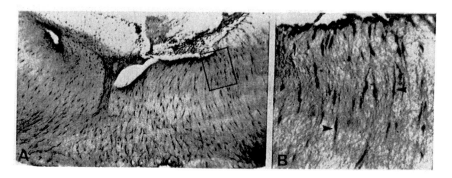

Figure 16 Histological analysis of floating dermal equivalents. (A) Histological appearance of full thickness floating dermal equivalents showing an envelope of fibroblasts mainly on the surface and one fold filled up by a colony of fibroblast (FC). Initial collagen concentration was 2.11 mg/ml and fibroblast number was 18,500/cm². Hematoxylin and eosin staining. Taken at 20× and enlarged photographically to 40×. (B) Enlargement of the indicated portion showing fibroblasts (arrowheads) and collagen fibers oriented perpendicularly in relation to tissue length. Taken at 80× and enlarged photographically to 160×. (From López-Valle et al., Ref. 186. Courtesy of *Br. J. Dermatol.*)

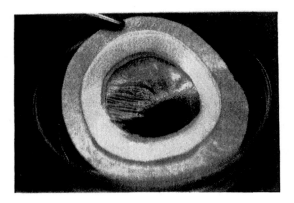

Figure 17 Anchored skin equivalents. Macroscopic view of anchored skin equivalents cultured at the air–liquid interface. Note the visual whitish aspect of the TES surface indicating the presence of a cornified layer.

transfer is envisioned, or also be eliminated in order to carry out some *in vitro* experiments [188–190].

The elegance of our methods obviates this type of manipulation by simply cutting out the TSE. This is then a true living skin tissue equivalent without intervening material (Fig. 17). We feel this to be a distinct advantage *in vitro* or *in vivo*. As a final note, upon

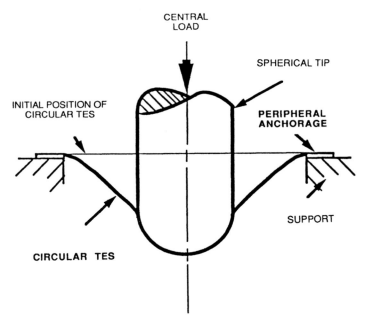

Figure 18 Basic principles for the evaluation of mechanical properties of anchored TES using the indentation apparatus. Diagram of a split front-view of deformed circular TES during indentation. The tensile properties are evaluated by measuring the central load on spherical tip and dermal equivalent deflection. (Courtesy of H. Lafrance, Ref. 195.)

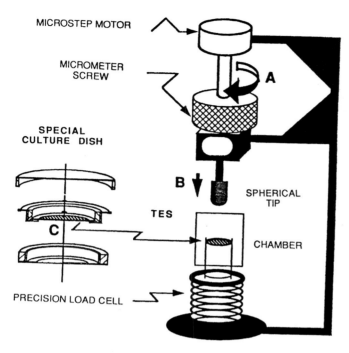

MICROSTEP MOTOR

MICROMETER
SCREW

SPECIAL
CULTURE DISH

A

B

SPHERICAL
TIP

TES

CHAMBER

C

PRECISION LOAD CELL

Figure 19 Diagram of a side-view of the indentation apparatus. The evaluation of tensile properties of anchored dermal equivalents or TES is realized with the indentation apparatus (right). Vertical displacement of the shperical tip induces axisymmetric tension within the equivalent. The resulting tension within the equivalent is measured by a precision load cell. The special culture dish is designed for adaptation to the indentation apparatus (left). At the end of the culture period, the circular anchored equivalent is removed from the dish with its support and mounted in the indentation apparatus. (Courtesy of H. Lafrance, Ref. 195.)

separating the fixed TSE from its anchorage, there is then very little surface shrinkage [186].

2. Delay Before Transplantation

Our approaches to this weakness have been closely related to our efforts for the TEE: thermolysin enzymatic separation, conditioned media, and eventually chimeric grafts (see Sec. II.E.1).

3. Engraftment Levels

This section of the present chapter is at the forefront of clinical application of skin tissue engineering. There are few published results, and some hypothesis have yet to be proven. But our approaches are in direct continuity with the various advantages that are sought, as explained in Sec. III.A.

4. Optimization of the TES

Our group has thus put forward a complete program in order to optimize the TES [114,138,159,164,186,187]. Furthermore, we have developed various analysis parameters to study the biological and mechanical optimization of our TES [114,193–195].

Biological Optimization.   Our descriptive analytical parameters in this field have been focused on light and electronic microscopic studies, and immunohistochemical studies of various molecules [114,138,187].

On the other hand, the functional analysis has been accomplished essentially through thymidine incorporation studies and dermatoabsorption methods [90,114]. The skin absorption studies may have more relevance to experimental purposes than clinical TES optimization purposes (burn therapy), but they still constitute a fascinating analysis end point.

Mechanical Optimization.   Our research group has thus embarked on a specific program in order to study the mechanical properties of our TES. This analysis has been accomplished with a team of biomedical engineers who have created a unique apparatus for the analysis of tensile strength and elasticity of our TES (Figs. 18–22) [194,195].

This goal was deemed to be important since this analysis allowed us to modulate the optimal parameter of TES production in order to create skin equivalents that had enough structural strength for clinical uses. Furthermore, this analytical device has enabled our group to obtain some comparative results. These results show a variation of the mechanical parameters as a function of fibroblast concentration and culture time of the anchored dermal equivalent [194,195].

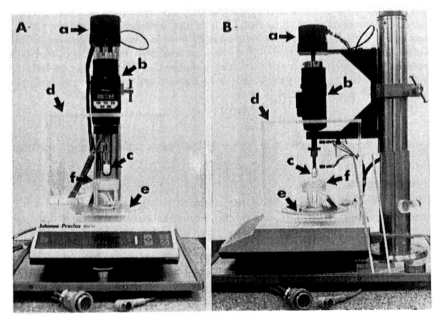

Figure 20   Photographs of the indentation apparatus for mechanical properties evaluation. (A) Face view showing the microstep motor, a; the micrometer, b; the spherical tip, c; the chamber, d; the precision load cell, e; and the anchored equivalent support. (B) Side view of the same components. (Courtesy of H. Lafrance, Ref. 195.)

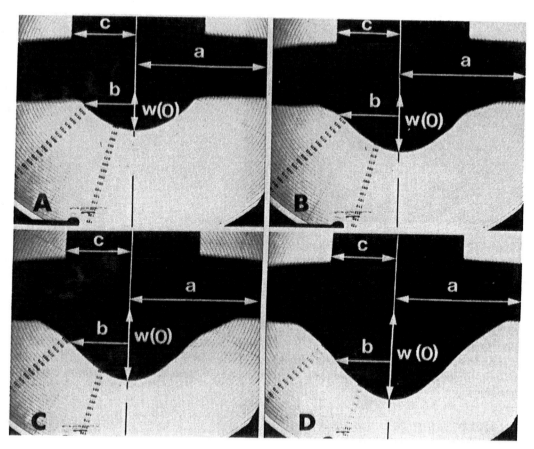

Figure 21 Optical comparator photographs of the dermal equivalent during a mechanical test. The movement of the spherical tip can be visualized and the variation of the deflection parameter, $w(0)$, can be evaluated [e.g., in panel (A), $w(0) = 3.2$ mm]. (Courtesy of H. Lafrance, Ref. 195.)

IV. CONCLUSION

The field of tissue engineering is progressing presently at a very fast rate. Wound coverage by TEE and TES happens to be the most advanced clinical project in this field. Furthermore, the scope and complexity of the present clinical studies are impressive.

These wound coverage studies should not only be of upmost importance for tissue engineering in general, but they may be a paradigm for all upcoming tissue-engineering applications. The future years shall be demanding and exciting.

ACKNOWLEDGMENTS

The authors are grateful to Drs. Francine Goulet and Mahmoud Rouabhia, and all members of the LOEX laboratory for their kind help, advice, and technical assistance in relation to the work presented in this review. The authors acknowledge the collaboration

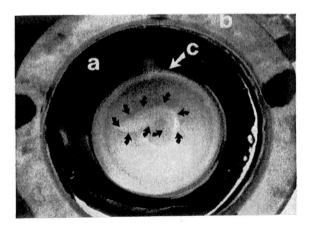

Figure 22 Macroscopic view of anchored dermal equivalent rupture during an indentation test. The dermal equivalent (a) anchored to the support; (b) has been ruptured by the spherical tip. Arrows point toward the rupture in the equivalent. (Courtesy of H. Lafrance, Ref. 195.)

of Dr. Michel Guillot and his group in the field of biomedical engineering, and also the plastic surgeons at the burn unit of the Hôpital du Saint-Sacrement. We also wish to thank Pierrette Roger for secretarial assistance, Lina Carrier and Brigitte Allard for their help in the preparation of figures and references, and Claude Marin for his photographic assistance.

ABBREVIATIONS

DME: Dulbecco–Vogt modification of Eagles medium
FCS: Fetal calf serum
GEN: Gentamicin
PBS: Phosphate-buffered saline
PEN: Penicillin
TEE: Tissue-engineered epidermis
TES: Tissue-engineered skin

EXPLANATORY NOTE

This chapter will be in keeping with the practical approach of this handbook. However, the reader must be warned that the tissue engineered skin organs presented here are of a different nature than what is usually defined as being a biomaterial. These biomaterials are living tissues, herein epidermis or living skin equivalent, from their inception since the various cells incorporated are not only actively dividing but also metabolically active. Furthermore, in the tissue engineered skin, the fibroblasts incorporated into the dermal component are also involved in the reorganization of the extracellular matrix. Nevertheless, we strove to present our clinical and experimental knowledge of these "organ equivalent" biomaterials in a step by step fashion. Thus, for both engineered tissues, epidermis and skin, a specific sequence of questions will be answered: Why is it done? How is it done? What is right? What is wrong? What do we do about it? Finally, in conclusion, we attempted to give the reader a brief outlook on the future of tissue engineering.

REFERENCES

1. Thomsen, M., and B. F. Alsbjorn, Development of the treatment of partial skin thickness burns since the Second World War: an overview, *Burns, 18* Suppl. 2, 11s–13s (1992).
2. Demling, R. H., and C. Lalonde, Burn trauma, in *Trauma Management*, Vol. 4 (Blaisdell and Trunkey, eds.), Thieme Medical Publishers, New York, 1989, pp. 1–318.
3. Polk, H. C., Jr., and H. H. Stone (eds.), *Contemporary Burn Management*, Little, Brown, Boston, 1971, pp. 1–444.
4. Dziewulski, P., Burn wound healing: James Ellsworth Laing memorial essay for 1991, *Burns, 18*, 466–478 (1992).
5. De Riel, S., Assessment of burn wound therapy systems, in *Burn Wound Coverings* (Donald L. Wise, ed.), CRC Press, Boca Raton, FL, 1984, pp. 1–37.
6. Tanner, J. C., J. Vandeput, and J. F. Olley, The mesh skin graft, *Plast. Reconstr. Surg., 34*, 287–292 (1964).
7. Demling, R. H., and C. Lalonde, Burn trauma, in *Trauma Management*, Vol. 4 (Blaisdell and Trunkey, eds.), Thieme Medical Publishers, New York, 1989, pp. 42–65.
8. Monafo, W. W., Tangential excision, in *Clinics in Plastic Surgery, Symposium on Burns*, Vol. 1 (J. A. Moncrief, ed.), W. B. Saunders, Philadelphia, 1974, pp. 591–601.
9. Shuck, J. M., Preparing and closing the burn wound, in *Clinics in Plastic Surgery, Symposium on Burns*, Vol. 1 (J. A. Moncrief, ed.), W. B. Saunders, Philadelphia, 1974, pp. 577–590.
10. Zöch, G., G. Meissl, S. Bayer, and E. Kyral, Reduction of the mortality rate in aged burn patients, *Burns, 18*, 153–156, (1992).
11. Scott-Conner, C. E. H., E. Meydrech, W. E. Wheeler, and J. A. Coil, Jr., Quantitation of rate of wound closure and the prediction of death following major burns, *Burns, 14*, 373–378 (1988).
12. Rudolph, R., Contraction and the control of contraction, *World J. Surg., 4*, 279 (1980).
13. Larson, D. L., S. Abston, B. Willis, H. Linares, M. Dobrkovsky, E. B. Evans, and S. R. Lewis, Contracture and scar formation in the burn patient, in *Clinics in Plastic Surgery, Symposium on Burns*, Vol. 1 (J. A. Moncrief, ed.), W. B. Saunders, Philadelphia, 1974, pp. 653–666.
14. Rudolph, R., J. Vande Berg, and H. P. Erlich, Wound contraction and scar contracture, in *Wound Healing: Biochemical and Clinical Aspects* (Cohen, Diegelmann, and Lindblad, eds.), W. B. Saunders, Philadelphia, 1992, pp. 96–114.
15. Sappino, A. P., W. Schurch, and G. Gabbiani, Differentiation repertoire of fibroblastic cells: Expression of cytoskeletal proteins as marker of phenotypic modulations, *Lab. Invest., 63*, 144–161 (1990).
16. Murray, J. C., and S. R. Pinnell, Keloids and excessive dermal scarring, in *Wound Healing: Biochemical and Clinical Aspects* (Cohen, Diegelmann, and Lindblad, eds.), W. B. Saunders, Philadelphia, 1992, pp. 500–509.
17. Boswick, J. A., Jr., The management of fresh burns of the hand and deformities resulting from burn injuries, in *Clinics in Plastic Surgery, Symposium on Burns*, Vol. 1 (J. A. Moncrief, ed.), W. B. Saunders, Philadelphia, 1974, pp. 621–631.
18. Puck, T. T., P. I. Marcus, and S. J. Ciectura, Growth characteristics of colonies from single HeLa cells with and without a "feeder layer": Clonal growth of mammalian cells *in vitro, J. Exp. Med., 103*, 273–289 (1956).
19. Karasek, M. A., Dermal factors affecting epidermal cells *in vitro, J. Invest. Dermatol, 59*, 99–106 (1972).

20. Melbye, S. W., and M. A. Karasek, Some characteristics of a factor stimulating skin epithelial cell growth *in vitro*, *Exp. Cell Res., 79*, 279–286 (1979).

21. Karasek, M. A., and M. E. Charlton, Growth of postembryonic skin epithelial cells on collagen gels, *J. Invest. Dermatol., 56*, 205–210 (1971).

22. Cruickshank, C. N. D., J. R. Cooper, and C. Hooper, The cultivation of cells from adult epidermis, *J. Invest. Dermatol., 34*, 339–342 (1960).

23. Flaxman, B. A., and R. A. Harper, Organ culture of human skin in chemically defined medium, *J. Invest. Dermatol., 64*, 96–99 (1975).

24. Freeman, A. E., H. I. Igel, B. J. Herman, and K. L. Kleinfeld, Growth and characterization of human skin epithelial cell cultures, *In Vitro, 12*, 352–362 (1976).

25. Karasek, M., *In vitro* growth and maturation of epithelial cells from postembryonic skin, *J. Invest. Dermatol., 65*, 60–66 (1975).

26. Levine, M., The growth of adult human skin *in vitro*, *Br. J. Dermatol., 86*, 481–490 (1972).

27. Pruniéras, M., C. Delescluse, and M. Régnier, Growth and differentiation of postembryonic mammalian epidermal keratinocytes in culture, *Front Matrix Biol., 3*, 52–76 (1976).

28. Holbrook, K. A., and H. Hennings, Phenotypic expression of epidermal cells *in vitro*: A review, *J. Invest. Dermatol., 81*, 11s–24s (1983).

29. Rheinwald, J. G., and H. Green, Serial cultivation of strains of human epidermal keratinocytes: The formation of keratinizing colonies from single cells, *Cell, 6*, 331–344 (1975).

30. Lillie, J. H., D. K. MacCallum, and A. Jepsen, Fine structure of subcultivated stratified squamous epithelium grown on collagen rafts, *Exp. Cell Res., 125*, 153–165 (1980).

31. Gilchrest, B. A., J. K. Calhoun, and T. Maciag, Attachment and growth of human keratinocytes in a serum-free environment, *J. Cell Physiol., 112*, 197–206 (1982).

32. Coulomb, B., C. Lebreton, and L. Dubertret, Influence of human dermal fibroblasts on epidermalization, *J. Invest. Dermatol., 92*, 122–125 (1990).

33. Lillie, J. H., D. K. MacCallum, and A. Jepsen, Growth of stratified squamous epithelium on reconstituted extracellular matrices: Long-term culture, *J. Invest. Dermatol., 90*, 100–109 (1988).

34. Rubin, J. S., H. Osada, P. W. Finch, W. G. Taylor, S. Rudikoff, and S. A. Aaronson, Purification and characterization of a newly identified growth factor specific for epithelial cells, *Proc. Natl. Acad. Sci., USA, 86*, 802–806 (1989).

35. Werner, S., K. G. Peters, M. T. Longaker, F. Fuller-Pace, M. J. Banda, and L. T. Williams, Large induction of keratinocyte growth factor expression in the dermis during wound healing, *Proc. Natl. Acad. Sci., USA, 89*. 6896–6900 (1992).

36. Ehrmann, R. L., and G. O. Gey, The growth of cells on a transparent gel of reconstituted rat-tail collagen, *J. Natl. Cancer Inst., 16*, 1375–1403 (1956).

37. Jones, P. H., and F. M. Watt, Separation of human epidermal stem cells from transit amplifying cells on the basis of differences in integrin function and expression, *Cell, 73*, 713–724 (1993).

38. Gallico, G. G., N. E. O'Connor, C. C. Compton, O. Kehinde, and H. Green, Permanent coverage of large burn wounds with autologous cultured human epithelium, *N. Engl. J. Med., 331*, 448–451 (1984).

39. Donati, L., G. Magliacani, M. Bormioli, M. Signorini, and F. W. Baruffaldi Preis, Clinical experiences with keratinocyte grafts, *Burns, 18*, Sl9–S26 (1992).

40. Auger, F., The role of cultured autologous human epithelium in large burn wound treatment, *Transplantation/Implantation Today, 5*, 21–26 (1988).

41. O'Connor, N. E., J. B. Mulliken, S. Banks-Schlegel, O. Kehinde, and H. Green, Grafting of burns with cultured epithelium prepared from autologous epidermal cells, *Lancet, 1*, 75–78 (1981).

42. De Luca, M., S. Bondanza, R. Cancedda, A. M. Tamisani, C. Di Noto, L. Muller, D. Dioguardi, E. Brienza, A. Calvario, R. Zermani, D. Di Mascio, and F. Papadia, Permanent coverage of full skin thickness burns with autologous cultured epidermis and re-

epithelization of partial skin thickness lesions induced by allogeneic cultured epidermis: A multicentre study in the treatment of children, *Burns, 18*, S16–S19 (1992).

43. Weekley, R., and R. Klein, Clinical nursing experience with cultured epidermal autografts, *J. Burn Care Rehab., 13*, 138–141 (1992).
44. Herzog, S. R., A. Meyer, D. Woodley, and H. D. Peterson, Wound coverage with cultured autologous keratinocytes: Use after burn wound excision, including biopsy follow-up, *J. Trauma, 28*, 195–198 (1988).
45. Kumagai, N., H. Nishina, H. Tanabe, T. Hosaka, H. Ishida, and Y. Ogino, Clinical application of autologous cultured epithelia for the treatment of burn wounds and burn scars, *Plast. Reconstr. Surg., 82*, 99–110 (1988).
46. Teepe, R. G. C., R. W. Kreis, E. J. Koebrugge, J. A. Kempenaar, A. F. P. M. Vloemans, R. P. Hermans, H. Boxma, J. Dokter, J. Hermans, M. Ponec, and B. J. Vermeer, The use of cultured autologous epidermis in the treatment of extensive burns, *J. Trauma, 30*, 269–275 (1990).
47. Hunyadi, J., B. Farkas, C. Bertényi, J. Oláh, and A. Dobozy, Keratinocyte grafting: A new means of transplantation for full-thickness wounds, *J. Dermatol Surg. Oncol., 14*, 75–78 (1988).
48. Clugston, P. A., C. F. T. Snelling, I. B. Macdonald, H. L. Maledy, J. C. Boyle, E. Germann, A. D. Courtemanche, P. Wirtz, D. J. Fitzpatrick, D. A. Kester, B. Foley, R. J. Warren, and N. J. Carr, Cultured epithelial autografts: Three years of clinical experience with eighteen patients, *J. Burn Care Rehab., 12*, 533–539 (1991).
49. Pittelkow, M. R., Cultured epidermal cells for skin replacement, *Perspect. Plast. Surg., 3*, 101–105 (1989).
50. De Luca, M., E. Albanese, S. Bondanza, M. Megna, L. Ugozzoli, F. Molina, R. Cancedda, P. L. Santi, M. Bormioli, M. Stella, and G. Magliacani, Multicentre experience in the treatment of burns, with autologous and allogeneic cultured epithelium, fresh or preserved in a frozen state, *Burns, 15*, 303–309 (1989).
51. Green, H., O. Kehinde, and J. Thomas, Growth of cultured human epidermal cells into multiple epithelia suitable for grafting, *Proc. Natl. Acad. Sci. USA, 76*, 5665–5668 (1979).
52. Green, H., and Y. Barrandon, Cultured epidermal cells and their use in the generation of epidermis, *News in Physiological Sciences, 3*, 53–56 (1988).
53. Langer, R., and J. P. Vacanti, Tissue engineering, *Science, 260*, 920–925 (1993).
54. Tompkins, R. G., J. P. Remensnyder, and J. F. Burke, Significant reductions in mortality for children with burn injuries through the use of prompt eschar excision, *Ann. Surg., 208*, 577–585 (1988).
55. Burke, L. F., W. C. Bondoc, and W. C. Quinby, Primary burn excision and immediate grafting: A method shortening illness, *J. Trauma, 14*, 389–395 (1974).
56. Salisbury, R. E., Thermal burns, in *Plastic Surgery* (J. G. McCarty, ed.), W. B. Saunders, Philadelphia, 1990, Chap. 23, pp. 804–832.
57. Clarke, J. A., HIV transmission and skin grafts, *Lancet, 1*, 983 (1987).
58. Gallico, G. G., N. E. O'Connor, C. C. Compton, J. P. Remensnyder, O. Kehinde, and H. Green, Cultured epithelial autografts for giant congenital nevi, *Plast. Reconstr. Surg., 84*, 1–9 (1989).
59. Carver, N., and I. M. Leigh, Keratinocyte grafts and skin equivalents, *Int. J. Dermatol., 30*, 540–551 (1991).
60. Teepe, R. C. G., E. J Koebrugge, M. Ponec, and B. J. Vermeer, Fresh versus cryopreserved cultured allografts for the treatment of chronic skin ulcers, *Br. J. Dermatol., 122*, 81–89 (1990).
61. Phillips, T. J., O. Kehinde, H. Green, and B. A. Gilchrest, Treatment of ulcers with cultured epidermal allografts, *J. Am. Acad. Dermatol., 21*, 191–199 (1989).
62. Beele, H., J. M. Naeyaert, M. Goeteyn, M. De Mil, and A. Kint, Repeated cultured epidermal allografts in the treatment of chronic leg ulcers of various origins, *Dermatologica, 183*, 31–35 (1991).

63. Leigh, J. M., P. E. Purkis, and H. A. Navsaria, Treatment of chronic venous ulcers with sheets of cultured allogeneic keratinocytes, *Br. J. Dermatol., 117,* 591–597 (1987).

64. Rouabhia, M., L. Germain, F. Bélanger, and F. A. Auger, Cultured epithelium allografts: Langerhans cell and thy-1[+] dendritic epidermal cell depletion effects on allograft rejection, *Transplantation, 56,* 259–264 (1993).

65. Auböck, J., E. Irschick, N. Romani, P. Kompatscher, R. Höpfl, M. Herold, G. Schuler, M. Bauer, C. Huber, and P. Fritsch, Rejection, after a slightly prolonged survival time, of Langerhans cell-depleted allogeneic cultured epidermis used for wound coverage in humans, *Transplantation, 45,* 730–737 (1988).

66. Phillips, T. J., Cultured epidermal allografts—A temporary or permanent solution? *Transplantation, 51,* 937–941 (1991).

67. Rheinwald, J. G., and H. Green, Epidermal growth factor and the multiplication of cultured human epidermal keratinocytes, *Nature, 265,* 421–424 (1977).

68. Simon, M., and H. Green, Enzymatic cross-linking of involucrin and other proteins by keratinocyte particulates *in vitro, Cell, 40,* 677–683 (1985).

69. Desai, M. H., J. M. Mlakar, R. L. McCauley, K. M. Abdullah, R. L. Rutan, J. P. Waymack, M. C. Robson, and D. H. Herndon, Lack of long-term durability of cultured keratinocyte burn-wound coverage: A case report, *J. Burn Care Rehab., 12,* 540–545 (1991).

70. Blight, A., E. M. Mountford, I. M. Cheshire, J. M. P. Clancy, and P. L. Levick, Treatment of full skin thickness burn injury using cultured epithelial grafts, *Burns, 17,* 495–498 (1991).

71. Woodley, D. T., Covering wounds with cultured keratinocytes, *J. Am. Med. Assoc., 262,* 2140–2141 (1989).

72. Compton, C. C., J. M. Gill, D. A. Bradford, S. Regauer, G. G. Gallico, and N. E. O'Connor, Skin regenerated from cultured epithelial autografts on full-thickness burn wounds from 6 days to 5 years after grafting. A light, electron microscopic and immunohistochemical study, *Lab. Invest., 60,* 600–612 (1989).

73. Mommaas, A. M., R. G. C. Teepe, I. R. Leigh, A. A. Mulder, E. J. Koegrugge, and B. J. Vermeer, Ontogenesis of the basement membrane zone after grafting cultured human epithelium: A morphologic and immunoelectron microscopic study, *J. Invest. Dermatol., 99,* 71–77 (1992).

74. Aihara, M., Ultrastructural study of grafted autologous cultured human epithelium, *Br. J. Plast. Surg., 42,* 35–42 (1989).

75. Woodley, D. T., H. D. Peterson, S. R. Herzog, G. P. Stricklin, R. E. Burgeson, R. A. Briggaman, D. J. Cronce, and E. J. O'Keefe, Burn wounds resurfaced by cultured epidermal autografts show abnormal reconstitution of anchoring fibrils, *J. Am. Med. Assoc., 259,* 2566–2571 (1988).

76. Gallico, G. G., Biologic skin substitutes, *Clin. Plast. Surg., 17,* 519–526 (1990).

77. Demarchez, M., D. J. Hartmann, M. Régnier, and D. Asselineau, The role of fibroblasts in dermal vascularization and remodeling of reconstructed human skin after transplantation onto the nude mouse, *Transplantation, 54,* 317–326 (1992).

78. Rudolf, R., and L. Klein, Healing processes in skin grafts, *Surg. Gynecol Obstet., 136,* 641–649 (1973).

79. Lanir, Y., A structural theory for the homogeneous biaxial stress–strain relationships in flat collagenous tissues, *J. Biomechanics, 12,* 423–436 (1979).

80. Daly, C. H., Biomechanical properties of dermis, *J. Invest. Dermatol., 79,* 17s–20s (1982).

81. Cook, T., H. Alexander, and M. Cohen, Experimental method for determining the 2-dimensional mechanical properties of living human skin, *Med. Biol. Eng. Comput., 15,* 381–390 (1977).

82. Tong, P., and Fung Y.-C., The stress–strain relationship for the skin, *J. Biomech., 9,* 649–657 (1976).

83. Kenedi, R. M., T. Gibson, and C. H. Daly, *Bioengineering studies of the human skin,* NATO advanced study course on connective tissue, St. Andrews, 1964.

84. Nave, M., Wound bed preparation: Approaches to replacement of dermis, *J. Burn Care Rehab., 13*, 147–153 (1992).

85. Cuono, C. B., R. Langdon, N. Birchall, S. Barttelbort, and J. McGuire, Composite autologous–allogeneic skin replacement: Development and clinical application, *Plast. Reconstr. Surg., 80*, 626–635 (1987).

86. Langdon, R. C., C. B. Cuono, N. Birchall, J. A. Madri, E. Kuklinska, J. McGuire, and G. E. Moellmann, Reconstitution of structure and cell function in human skin grafts derived from cryopreserved allogeneic dermis and autologous cultured keratinocytes, *J. Invest. Dermatol., 91*, 478–485 (1988).

87. Cuono, C., R. Langdon, and J. McGuire, Use of cultured epidermal autografts and dermal allografts as skin replacement after burn injury, *Lancet, 17*, 1123–1124 (1987).

88. Heck, E. L., P. R. Bergstresser, and C. R. Baxter, Composite skin graft: Frozen dermal allografts support the engraftment and expansion of autologous epidermis, *J. Trauma, 25*, 106–112 (1985).

89. Germain, L., M. Rouabhia, R. Guignard, L. Carrier, V. Bouvard, and F. A. Auger, Improvement of human keratinocyte isolation and culture using thermolysin, *Burns, 19*, 99–104 (1993).

90. Goulet, F., L. Germain, M. Rouabhia, A. Poitras, and F. A. Auger, Cellular cooperation between human keratinocytes and dermal fibroblasts through growth factor secretion *in vitro, J. Invest. Dermatol., 100*, 558 (1993).

91. Faure, M., G. Mauduit, A. Demidem, and J. Thivolet, Langerhans cell free epidermis used as permanent skin allografts in humans, *J. Invest. Dermatol., 86*, 474 (1986).

92. Hefton, J. M., M. R. Madden, J. L. Finkelstein, and G. T. Shires, Grafting of burn patients with allografts of cultured epidermis cells, *Lancet, 2*, 428–430 (1983).

93. Thivolet, J., M. Faure, A. Demiden, and F. Mauduit, Long term survival and immunological tolerance of human epidermal allografts produced in culture, *Transplantation, 42*, 274–280 (1986).

94. Hammond, E. G., R. L. Ng, M. A. Stanley, and A. G. Monro, Prolonged survival of cultured keratinocyte allografts in the nonimmunosuppressed mouse, *Transplantation, 44*, 106–112 (1987).

95. Billingham, R. E., L. Brent, and P. B. Medawar, Actively acquired tolerance to foreign cells, *Nature (Lond.), 172*, 606–609 (1953).

96. Auböck, J., and P. Fritsch, Epidermal allografts in humans: An unattainable dream?, *Dermatologica, 175*, 161–165 (1987).

97. Hutchinson, I. V., Cellular mechanisms of allograft rejection, *Curr. Opinion Immunol., 3*, 722–726 (1991).

98. Steinmuller, D., Survival of neonatal mouse epidermal allografts, *Transplantation, 50*, 1084–1085 (1990).

99. Auböck, J., E. Irschick, N. Romani, P. Kompatscher, R. Hopfi, M. Herold, G. Schuler, M. Bauer, C. Huber, and P. Fritsch, Rejection, after a slightly prolonged survival time, of Langerhans cell-free allogeneic cultured epidermis used for wound coverage in humans, *Transplantation, 45*, 730–737 (1988).

100. Gielen, V., M. Faure, G. Mauduit, and J. Thivolet, Progressive replacement of human cultured epithelial allografts by recipient cells as evidenced by HLA class I antigens expression, *Dermatologica, 175*, 166–170 (1987).

101. De Luca, M., E. Albanese, S. Bondanza, M. Megna, L. Ugozzoli, F. Molina, R. Cancedda, P. L. Santi, M. Bormioli, M. Stella, and G. Magliacani, Multicentre experience in the treatment of burns with autologous and allogeneic cultured epithelium, fresh or preserved in a frozen state, *Burns, 15*, 303–309 (1989).

102. Burt, A., C. D. Pallett, J. P. Sloane, M. J. O'Hare, K. F. Schafler, P. Yardeni, A. Eidad, J. A. Clarke, and B. A. Guterson, Survival of cultured allografts in patients with burns assessed with probe scientific for Y chromosome, *Br. Med. J., 298*, 915–917 (1989).

103. Brain, A., P. Purkis, P. Coates, M. Hackett, H. Navsaria, and I. Leigh, Survival of cultured allogeneic keratinocytes transplanted to deep dermal bed assessed with probe specific for Y chromosome, *Br. Med. J., 298*, 917–919 (1989).

104. Phillips, T. J., J. Bhawan, I. M. Leigh, H. J. Braun, and B. A. Gilchrest, Cultured epidermal autografts and allografts: A study of differentiation and allograft survival, *J. Am. Acad. Dermatol., 23*, 189–198 (1990).

105. Van der Merwe, A. E., F. J. Mattheyse, M. Bedford, P. D. Van Heiden, and D. J. Rossouw, Allografted keratinocytes used to accelerate the treatment of burn wounds are replaced by recipient cells, *Burns, 16*, 193–197 (1990).

106. Rouabhia, M., L. Germain, and F. A. Auger, Allogeneic-syngeneic cultured epithelia: A successful therapeutic option for skin regeneration, *Transplantation*, in press.

107. Auger, F. A., A. Roy, F. Roy, F. A. Tetu, N. Houle, and G. Hebert, Infection control factors implicated in a improved success rate of *in vitro* cultured autologous epithelial grafts for the therapy of burn patients, in *5th International Symposium on Infections in the Immunocompromised Host*, Noorwijkerhout, The Netherlands, June 5–8, 1988, p. 111.

108. Auger, F. A., R. Guignard, C. A. López-Valle, and L. Germain, Role and innocuity of Tisseel®, a tissue glue, in the grafting process and *in vivo* evolution of human cultured epidermis, *Br. J. Plast. Surg., 46*, 136–142 (1993).

109. Germain, L., R. Guignard, P. Jacques, S. Garceau, M. Gilbert, and F. A. Auger, Human epidermal culture model to evaluate the effect of topical antibiotics on keratinocyte growth, *Br. J. Dermatol., 129* (Suppl. 42), 22 (1993).

110. Cooper, M. L., S. T. Boyce, J. F. Hansbrough, T. J. Foreman, and D. H. Frank, Cytotoxicity to cultured human keratinocytes of topical antimicrobial agents, *J. Surg. Res., 48*, 190–195 (1990).

111. Boyce, S. T., and I. A. Holder, Selection of topical antimicrobial agents for cultured skin for burns by combined assessment of cellular cytotoxicity and antimicrobial activity, *Plast. Reconstr. Surg., 92*, 493–500 (1993).

112. Taylor, D., C. Whatting, J. N. Kearney, B. Matthews, and K. T. Holland, The effect of bacterial products on human fibroblast and keratinocyte detachment and viability, *Br. J. Dermatol., 122*, 23–28 (1990).

113. Damour, O., S. Z. Hua, F. Lasne, M. Villain, P. Rousselle, and C. Collombel, Cytotoxicity evaluation of antiseptics and antibiotics on cultured human fibroblasts and keratinocytes, *Burns, 18*, 479–485 (1992).

114. Michel, M., F. A. Auger, and L. Germain, Anchored skin equivalent cultured *in vitro*: A new tool for percutaneous absorption studies, *In Vitro Cell. Devel. Biol., 29A*, 834–837 (1993).

115. Slivka, S. R., L. K. Landeen, F. Zeigler, M. P. Zimber, and R. L. Bartel, Characterization, barrier function and drug metabolism of an *in vitro* skin model, *J. Invest. Dermatol., 100*, 40–46 (1993).

116. Parenteau, N. L., C. M. Nolte, P. Bilbo, M. Rosenberg, L. M. Wilkins, E. W. Johnson, S. Watson, V. S. Mason, and E. Bell, Epidermis generated *in vitro*: Practical considerations and applications, *J. Cell Biochem., 45*:245–251 (1991).

117. Ponec, M., P. J., J. Wauben-Penris, A. Burger, J. Kempenaar, and H. E. Bodde, Nitroglycerin and sucrose permeability as quality markers for reconstructed human epidermis, *Skin Pharmacol., 3*, 126–135 (1990).

118. Régnier, M., D. Caron, U. Reichert, and H. Schaefer, Barrier function of human skin and human reconstructed epidermis, *J. Pharm. Sci., 82*, 404–407 (1993).

119. Bell, E., N. Parenteau, R. Gay, C. Nolte, P. Kemp, P. Bilbo, B. Ekstein, and E. Johnson, The living skin equivalent: Its manufacture, its organotypic properties and its responses to irritants, *Toxicol. In Vitro, 5*, 591–596 (1991).

120. Gay, R. J., M. Swiderek, and D. Nelson, The living dermal equivalent as an *in vitro* model for predicting ocular irritation, *J. Toxicol. Cut. Ocular Toxicol., 11*, 47–68 (1992).

121. Ponec, M., *In vitro* cultured human skin cells as alternatives to animals for skin irritancy screening, *Int. J. Cosmet. Sci., 14,* 245–264 (1992).

122. Naughton, G. K., L. Jacob, and B. Naughton, A physiological skin model for in vitro toxicity studies, in *In Vitro Toxicity: New Directions* (A. Goldberg, ed.), Liebert, New York, 1989, Vol. 7, pp. 183–189.

123. Bilbo, P. R., C. M. Nolte, C. Tighe, and N. L. Parenteau, A highly differentiated organotypic skin model for dermatologic, pharmacologic, and toxicologic research, *J. Invest. Dermatol., 96,* 618 (1991).

124. Boyce, S., T. Foreman, and J. Hansbrough, Functional wound closure with dermal–epidermal skin substitutes prepared *in vitro, Tissue Eng.,* 1988, pp. 81–86.

125. Saintigny, G., M. Bonnard, O. Damour, and C. Collombel, Reconstruction of epidermis on a chitosan cross-linked collagen–GAG lattice: Effect of fibroblasts, *Acta Derm. Venereol. (Stockh), 73,* 175–180 (1993).

126. Hansbrough, H. F., Wound coverage with biologic dressings and cultured skin substitutes, *J. Invest. Dermatol., 101,* 892 (1993).

127. Hansbrough, J. F., S. T. Boyce, M. L. Cooper, and T. J. Foreman, Burn wound closure with cultured autologous keratinocytes and fibroblasts attached to a collagen–glycosaminoglycan substrate, *J. Am. Med. Assoc., 262,* 2125–2130 (1989).

128. Contard, P., R. L. Bartel, L. Jacobs II, J. S. Perlish, E. D. MacDonald II, L. Handler, D. Cone, and R. Fleischmajer, Culturing keratinocytes and fibroblasts in a three-dimensional mesh results in epidermal differentiation and formation of a basal lamina-anchoring zone, *J. Invest. Dermatol., 100,* 35–39 (1993).

129. Krejci, N. C., C. B. Cuono, R. C. Langdon, and J. McGuire, *In vitro* reconstitution of skin: Fibroblasts facilitate keratinocyte growth and differentiation on a cellular reticular dermis, *J. Invest. Dermatol., 97,* 843–848 (1991).

130. Stompro, B. E., S. T. Boyce, and J. F. Hansbrough, Attachment of peptide growth factors to implantable collagen, *J. Surg. Res., 46,* 413–421 (1989).

131. Boyce, S. T., B. E. Stompro, and J. F. Hansbrough, Biotinylation of implantable collagen for drug delivery, *J. Biomed. Mater. Res., 26,* 547–553 (1992).

132. Boyce, S. T., A. P. Supp, G. D. Warden, and I. A. Holder, Attachment of an aminoglycoside, amikacin, to implantable collagen for local delivery in wounds, *Antimicrob. Agents Chemother., 37,* 1890–1895 (1993).

133. Bell, E., C. Merrill, and D. Solomon, Characteristics of a tissue equivalent formed by fibroblasts cast in a collagen gel, *J. Cell Biol., 83,* 398A (1979).

134. Bell, E., B. Ivarssen, and C. Merrill, Production of a tissue-like structure by contraction of collagen lattices by human fibroblasts of different proliferative potential *in vitro, Proc. Natl. Acad. Sci. USA., 76,* 1274–1278 (1979).

135. Bell, E., H. P. Erhlich, D. J. Buttle, and T. Nakatsuji, A living tissue formed *in vitro* and accepted as a full thickness skin equivalent, *Science, 211,* 1042–1054 (1981).

136. Bell, E., S. Sher, B. Hull, C. Merrill, S. Rosen, A. Chamson, D. Asselineau, L. Dubertret, B. Coulomb, C. Lapière, B. Nusgens, and Y. Neveu, The reconstitution of living skin, *J. Invest. Dermatol., 81,* 2s–10s (1983).

137. Bell, E., P. Ehrlich, S. Sher, C. Merrill, R. Sarber, B. Hull, T. Nakatsuji, D. Church, and D. J. Buttle, Development and use of a living skin equivalent, *Plast Rec. Surg., 67,* 386–392 (1981).

138. Bouvard, V., L. Germain, P. Rompré, B. Roy, and F. A. Auger, Influence of dermal equivalent maturation on the development of a cultured skin equivalent, *Biochem. Cell Biol., 70,* 34–42 (1992).

139. Boyce, S. T., T. J. Foreman, K. B. English, N. Stayner, M. L. Cooper, S. Sakaby, and J. F. Hansbrough, Skin wound closure in athymic mice with cultured human cells, biopolymers, and growth factors, *Surgery, 110,* 866–876 (1991).

140. Boyce, S., and J. F. Hansbrough, Biologic attachment, growth, and differentiation of cul-

tured human epidermal keratinocytes on a graftable collagen and chondroitin-6-sulfate substrate, *Surgery, 103*, 421–431 (1988).

141. Berthod, F., D. Hayek, O. Damour, and C. Collombel, Collagen synthesis by fibroblasts cultured within a collagen sponge, *Biomaterials, 14*, 749–754 (1993).

142. Shahabeddin, L., F. Berthod, O. Damour, and C. Collombel, Characterization of skin reconstructed on a chitosan-cross-linked collagen–glycosaminoglycan matrix, *Skin Pharmacol., 3*, 107–114 (1990).

143. Collins, R. L. L., D. Christiansen, G. A. Zazanis, and F. H. Silver, Use of collagen film as a dural substitute: Preliminary animal studies, *J. Biomed. Mater. Res., 25*, 267–276 (1991).

144. Wasserman, A. J., C. J. Doillon, A. Glasgold, Y. P. Kato, D. Christiansen, A. Rizvi, E. Wong, J. Goldstein, and F. H. Silver, Clinical applications of electron microscopy in the analysis of collagenous biomaterials, *Scan. Microsc., 2*, 1635–1646 (1988).

145. Berthod, F., and O. Damour, *In vitro* models of reconstructed skin: Their manufacture, industrial developments *in vitro* and clinical applications, in *Primary and Secondary Burn Care*, European Burn Assocation Text Book, Masson Eds., Paris, in press.

146. Hansbrough, J. F., M. L. Cooper, R. Cohen, R. Spielvogel, G. Greenleaf, R. L. Bartel, and G. Naughton, Evaluation of a biodegradable matrix containing cultured human fibroblasts as a dermal replacement beneath meshed skin grafts on athymic mice, *Surgery, 111*, 438–446 (1992).

147. Burke, J. F., I. Yannas, C. Quinby, C. Bondoc, and W. K. Jung, Successful use of a physiologically acceptable artificial skin in treatment of extensive burn injury, *Ann. Surg., 194*, 413–428 (1981).

148. Damour, O., P. Y. Gueugniaud, M. Berthin, P. Rousselle, F. Berthod, and C. Collombel, A dermal substrate made of collagen–GAG–chitosan for deep burn coverage: First clinical uses, *Clin. Mater., 15*, 273–276 (1994).

149. Murphy, G. F., D. P. Orgill, and I. V. Yannas, Partial dermal regeneration is induced by biodegradable collagen–glycosaminoglycan grafts, *Lab. Invest., 63*, 305–313 (1990).

150. Heimbach, D., A. Luterman, J. Burke, A. Cram, D. Herndon, J. Hunt, M. Jordan, W. McManus, L. Solem, G. Warden, and B. Zawacki, Artificial dermis for major burns, *Ann. Surg., 208*, 313–320 (1988).

151. Yannas, I. V., and J. F. Burke, Design of an artificial skin. I. Basic design principles, *J. Biochem. Mater. Res., 14*, 65–81 (1980).

152. Yannas, I. V., J. F. Burke, P. L. Gordon, C. Huang, and R. H. Rubenstein, Design of an artificial skin. II. Control of chemical composition, *J. Biomed. Mater. Res., 14*, 107–131 (1980).

153. Yannas, I. V., J. F. Burke, D. P. Orgill, and E. M. Skrabut, Wound tissue can utilize a polymeric template to synthesize a functional extension of skin, *Science, 215*, 174–176 (1982).

154. Fleischmajer, R., P. Contard, E. Schwartz, E. D. MacDonald II, L. Jacobs II, and L. Y. Sakai, Elastin-associated microfibrils (10 nm) in a three-dimensional fibroblast culture, *J. Invest. Dermatol., 97*, 638–643 (1991).

155. Hull, B. E., S. E. Sher, S. Rosen, D. Church, and E. Bell, Structural integration of skin equivalents grafted to Lewis and Sprague–Dawley rats, *J. Invest Dermatol., 81*, 429–436 (1983).

156. Ramirez Bosca, A., E. Tinois, M. Faure, J. Kanitakis, and P. Roche, Epithelial differentiation of human skin equivalents after grafting onto nude mice, *J. Invest. Dermatol., 91*, 136–141 (1988).

157. Hansbrough, J. F., M. L. Coope, and R. Cohen, Evaluation of a biodegradable matrix containing cultured human fibroblasts as a dermal replacement beneath meshed skin grafts on athymic mice, *Surgery, 111*, 438–446 (1992).

158. Tinois, E., J. Tiollier, M. Gaucherand, H. Dumas, M. Tardy, and J. Thivolet, *In vitro* and post-transplantation differentiation of human keratinocytes grown on the human type IV collagen film of a bilayered dermal substitute, *Exp. Cell Res., 193*, 310–319 (1991).

159. López Valle, C. A., L. Germain, M. Rouabhia, F. Goulet, R. Guignard, and F. A. Auger, Cultured three-dimensional living skin equivalents for burn wound coverage: A tissue engineering issue, submitted for publication.

160. Nanchahal, J., W. R. Otto, R. Dover, and S. K. Dhital, Cultured composite skin grafts: Biological skin equivalents permitting massive expansion, *Lancet, 2,* 191 (1989).

161. Hansbrough, J. F., C. Doré, and W. B. Hansbrough, Clinical trials of a living dermal tissue replacement placed beneath meshed, split-thickness skin grafts on excised burn wounds, *J. Burn Care Rehabil., 13,* 519–529 (1992).

162. Boykin, J. V., Jr., and J. A. Molnar, Burn scar and skin equivalents, in *Wound Healing: Biochemical and Clinical Aspects* (Cohen, Diegelmann, and Lindblad, eds.), W. B. Saunders, Philadelphia, 1992, pp. 523–540.

163. Wassermann, D., M. Schlotterer, A. Toulon, C. Cazalet, M. Marien, B. Cherruau, and P. Jaffray, Preliminary clinical studies of a biological skin equivalent in burned patients, *Burns, 14,* 326–330 (1988).

164. Rompré, P., F. A. Auger, L. Germain, V. Bouvard, C. A. López-Valle, J. Thibault, and A. Le Duy, Influence of initial collagen and cellular concentrations on the final surface area of dermal and skin equivalents: A Box–Behnken analysis, *In Vitro Cell. Dev. Biol., 26,* 983–990 (1990).

165. Petersen, M. J., D. T. Woodley, G. P. Stricklin, and E. J. O'Keefe, Enhanced synthesis of collagenase by human keratinocytes cultured on type I or type IV collagen, *J. Invest. Dermatol, 94,* 341–346 (1990).

166. Bailly, C., S. Drèze, D. Asselineau, B. Nusgens, C. M. Lapière, and M. Darmon, Retinoic acid inhibits the production of collagenase by human epidermal keratinocytes, *J. Invest. Dermatol., 94,* 47–51 (1990).

167. Bauer, E. A., G. P. Stricklin, and J. J. Jeffrey, Collagenase production by human skin fibroblasts, *Biochem. Biophys. Res. Commun., 64,* 232–240 (1975).

168. Genever, P. G., E. J. Wood, and W. J. Cunliffe, Fibroblasts grown in attached and floating dermal equivalents differ in their level of collagenase production and responsiveness to epidermal growth factor, *J. Invest. Dermatol., 96,* 1021a (1991).

169. Lambert, C. A., E. P. Soudant, B. V. Nusgens, and C. M. Lapière, Pretranslational regulation of extracellular matrix macromolecules and collagenase expression in fibroblasts by mechanical forces, *Lab. Invest., 66,* 444–451 (1992).

170. Unemori, E. N., and Z. Werb, Reorganization of polymerized actin: A possible trigger for induction of procollagenase in fibroblasts cultured in and on collagen gels, *J. Cell Biol., 103,* 1021–1031 (1986).

171. Mauch, C., B. Adelmann-Grill, A. Hatamochi, and T. Krieg, Collagenase gene expression in fibroblasts is regulated by three-dimensional contact with collagen, *FEBS Lett., 250,* 301–305 (1989).

172. Karelina, T. V., G. J. Hruza, G. I. Goldberg, and A. Z. Eisen, Localization of 92-kDa type IV collagenase in human skin tumors: Comparison with normal human fetal and adult skin, *J. Invest. Dermatol., 100,* 159–165 (1993).

173. Porras-Reyes, B. H., H. C. Blair, J. J. Jeffrey, and T. A. Mustoe, Collagenase production at the border of granulation tissue in a healing wound: Macrophage and mesenchymal collagenase production *in vivo, Connect. Tissue Res., 27,* 63–71 (1991).

174. Oikarinen, A., M. Kylmaniemi, H. Autio-Harmainen, P. Autio, and T. Salo, Demonstration of 72-kDa and 92-kDa forms of type IV collagenase in human skin: Variable expression in various blistering diseases, inducing during re-epithelialization, and decrease by topical glucocorticoids, *J. Invest. Dermatol., 101,* 205–210 (1993).

175. Buckley-Sturrock, A., W. C. Woodward, R. M. Senior, G. L. Griffin, M. Klagsbrun, and J. M. Davidson, Differential stimulation of collagenase and chemotactic activity in fibroblasts derived from rat wound repair tissue and human skin by growth factors, *J. Cell Phys., 138,* 70–78 (1989).

176. Saarialho-Kere, U., E. S. Schang, H. G. Welgus, and W. C. Parks, Distinct localization of

collagenase and tissue inhibitor of metalloproteinases expression in wound healing associated with ulcerative pyogenic granuloma, *J. Clin. Invest, 90*, 1952-1957 (1992).

177. Agren, M. S., C. J. Taplin, J. F. Woessner, W. H. Eaglstein, and P. M. Mertz, Collagenase in wound healing: Effect of wound age and type, *J. Invest. Dermatol., 99*, 709-714 (1992).

178. Jeffrey J. J., The biological regulation of collagenase activity, in *Regulation of Matrix Accumulation* (R. P. Mecham, ed.), Academic Press, Orlando, FL, 1986, pp. 53-98.

179. Grillo, H. C., and J. Cross, Collagenolytic activity during mammalian wound repair, *Dev. Biol., 15*, 300-317 (1967).

180. Woessner, J. F. Jr., Matrix metalloproteinases and their inhibitors in connective tissue remodelling, *FASEB J., 5*, 2145-2154 (1991).

181. Mort, J. S., G. R. Dodge, P. J. Roughley, J. Liu, S. J. Finch, G. DiPasquale, and A. R. Poole, Direct evidence for active metalloproteinases mediating matrix degradation in interleukin 1-stimulated human articular cartilage, *Matrix, 13*, 95-102 (1993).

182. Porras-Reyes, B. H., H. C. Blair, J. J. Jeffrey, and T. A. Mustoe, Collagenase production at the border of granulation tissue in a healing wound: Macrophage and mesenchymal collagenase production *in vivo, Connect. Tissue Res., 27*, 63-71, (1991).

183. Mandell, G. L., R. G. Douglas, Jr., and J. E. Bennett (eds.), *Principles and Practice of Infectious Diseases*, 3rd ed., Churchill Livingstone, New York, 1990, p. 6.

184. Stadelmann, W., D. Greenwald, L. Stevens, S. Shumway, K. Leoni, and T. Krizek, Mechanical analysis of the effects of bacteria and aprotinin on skin wound healing in adult guinea pigs, *Wound Rep. Reg., 1*, 187-193 (1993).

185. Hoffmann, S., and F. Moesgaard, Bacterial lysis of fibrin seal *in vitro, Eur. Surg. Res., 20*, 75-81 (1989).

186. López-Valle, C. A., F. A. Auger, P. Rompré, V. Bouvard, and L. Germain, Peripheral anchorage of dermal equivalent, *Br. J. Dermatol., 127*, 365-371 (1992).

187. Auger, F. A., C. A. López-Valle, R. Guignard, N. Tremblay, B. Noel, F. Goulet, and L. Germain, Skin equivalent produced with human collagen, *In Vitro Cell. Devel. Biol.*, in press.

188. Parenteau, N. L., C. M. Nolte, P. Bilbo, M. Rosenberg, L. M. Wilkins, E. W. Johnson, S. Watson, V. S. Mason, and E. Bell, Epidermis generated *in vitro*: Practical considerations and applications, *J. Cell Biochem., 45*, 245-251 (1991).

189. Asselineau, D., B. A. Bernard, C. Bailly, M. Darmon, and M. Pruniéras, Human epidermis reconstructed by culture: Is it normal? *J. Invest. Dermatol., 86*, 181-186 (1986).

190. Lin, Y.-C., and F. Grinnell, Decreased level of PDGF-stimulated receptor autophosphorylation by fibroblasts in mechanically relaxed collagen matrices, *J. Cell Biol., 122*, 663-672 (1993).

191. Harriger, M. D., and B. E. Hull, Cornification and basement membrane formation in a bilayered human skin equivalent maintained at an air-liquid interface, *J. Burn Care Rehab., 13*, 187-193 (1992).

192. Lambert, C. A., E. P. Soudant, B. V. Nusgens, and C. M. Lapière, Pretranslational regulation of extracellular matrix macromolecules and collagenase expression in fibroblasts by mechanical forces, *Lab. Invest., 66*, 444-451 (1992).

193. Lafrance H., L'H. Yahia, M. Guillot, L. Germain, and F. A. Auger, Evaluation of tensile properties of anchored skin equivalents cultures *in vitro*, presented at 20th annual Meeting of the Society for Biomaterials, April 5-9, Boston, MA, 1994.

194. Lafrance, H., M. Guillot, L. Germain, and F. A. Auger, Method for the evaluation of tensile properties of skin equivalents, submitted for publication.

195. Lafrance, H., Analyse de la résistance mécanique d'équivalents cutanés cultivés, M.Sc. Thesis, Laval University, Québec, Canada, 1992, pp. 1-132.

26
Biological Resurfacing of Osteochondral Defects

Judith B. Ulreich and Donald P. Speer
University of Arizona College of Medicine
Tucson, Arizona

I. INTRODUCTION

Methods of restoring or replacing damaged joints represent a major contribution to medicine in the 20th century (Speer and Dahners, 1979). The major limiting factor in total joint arthroplasty is loosening of implants. While alterations in the geometry and composition of the implants and use of grouting materials have reduced loosening, the difficulty in interfacing materials of vastly different elastic moduli has not been substantially altered. This interface of a viscoelastic living tissue and a hard, stiff, nonliving substance eventually fills with fibrous tissue and loses its fixation to the underlying bone. The result is increasing pain and ultimately the need for surgical replacement of the implant. This chapter deals with development of clinically applicable methods of joint resurfacing that are designed to avoid "the interface problem" by approximating regeneration through biological means of resurfacing.

A. Regeneration of Adult Articular Cartilage

Biological resurfacing of a joint must approximate true regeneration of the joint surface as a functional organ. That adult articular cartilage is capable of such regeneration is indicated by several observations. Loose bodies of chondral or osteochondral fragments floating freely in an adult joint continue to grow an articular surface that has both the collagenous architecture and proteoglycan content of normal cartilage (Speer, 1982a). Osteophytes forming at the margin of degenerating joints include newly synthesized articular cartilage having a collagen fiber architecture and proteoglycan content similar to that of the original surface. The pathogenetic events at a pseudoarthrosis and a nonunion of a fracture include the formation of a synovial space and formation of fibrocartilaginous articulating surfaces with development of a subchondral bone surface manifested by sclerosis throughout the medullary canal of the nonunited bone fragment (Speer, 1982a).

735

While these pathological conditions do not result in fully normal articular surfaces, they do reflect formation and remodeling of articular cartilage with architectural and histochemical features of normal articular cartilage that may potentially provide a useful weight-bearing surface. Loosening and the interface problem can be avoided through use of living tissues that are capable of undergoing remodeling and repair in the face of functional strain.

B.   Limitations of Joint Transplantation

Transplantation of joints has been attempted in a variety of ways. Transplanting an entire bone end from the diametaphyseal portion of the bone to include the entire joint surface afforded the advantages of having ligamentous attachments plus a substantial bone stock to effect fixation of the transplant in the host. Such transplants have been achieved as partial (hemi) as well as total joint transplant arthroplasties. While enjoying a period of successful function associated with relief of pain, these transplants have undergone degenerative changes with use and have manifested rejection phenomena or failure of incorporation. Resurfacing procedures using transplanted "shells" of articular surfaces have been attempted with some success but even though articular cartilage has been called a "privileged" tissue from an immunologic point of view (Langer et al., 1978), the matrix of the transplanted cartilage eventually breaks down, permitting access of host cells to the transplant cells, and rejection phenomena occur. There has been extensive experience with bone homograft technology, but even with current treatments of homografts there is a major problem of marked delay or failure of incorporation of the graft at best and usually there are some mild rejection phenomena (Caffiniere et al., 1982; Gross et al., 1984; Jimenez and Brighton, 1984; Mankin, 1984; Meyers et al., 1984; Urist, 1980; Yablon and Shirahama, 1982; Yablon et al., 1977). Some workers have used autologous cartilage plugs to heal osteochondral defects (Hjertquist and Lemperg, 1972).

C.   Resurfacing of Osteochondral Defects

Many different approaches have been made in an attempt to regenerate or replace cartilage that has been damaged. Biological resurfacing has been used with success in our group using collagen sponge crosslinked with glutaraldehyde (Speer et al., 1979) and later with hexamethylene diisocyanate (Chvapil et al., 1983; Ulreich, 1990; Ulreich et al., 1985, 1986, 1987). Collagen sponge has been used for repair of osteochondral defects alone or in combination with autogenous chondrocytes or growth or attachment factors. Many of the numerous materials and methods used for eventual resurfacing of joints are categorized in Table 1. That articular cartilage is capable of regenerating in an adult animal is demonstrated by many of these experiments.

II.   CHARACTERISTICS OF AN IDEAL BIOLOGICAL JOINT RESURFACING MATERIAL

A fully satisfactory biological resurfacing material and methodology for synovial joints should have several features:

1.   Biocompatibility: The material should not provoke an inflammatory, foreign body, giant cell, or macrophage reaction and it should be nonantigenic, thus, not immunologically rejected.

Table 1   Materials Used to Study Cartilage Repair/Regeneration

A. Collagen

Collagen sponge/polyvinyl alcohol sponge	Holmes et al. (1975)
Collagen sponge–glutaraldehyde, crosslinked	Speer et al. (1979)
Collagen sponge–hexamethylene diisocyanate cross-linked/chondrocytes	Chvapil et al. (1983); Ulreich (1990); Ulreich et al. (1985, 1986, 1987)
Collagen implant/tricalcium phosphate	Hogervorst et al. (1992)
Collagen sponge	Maor et al. (1987)
Collagen–chondrocyte allografts/(collagen gel/collagen sponge)	Ben-Yishay et al. (1991)
Chondrocyte allografts/(collagen gel/fibrillar collagen matrix)/(fibrin glue or mussel adhesive)	Pitman et al. (1989)
Chondrocytes/gel matrix	Green (1977)

B. Other Polymers

Silastic sheet	Engkvist and Ekenstam (1982)
Expanded polytetrafluoroethylene	Hanff et al. (1990)
Biodegradable poly-L-lactide cups	Wedge et al. (1986)
Coralline hydroxyapatite/polylactide	Jamshidi et al. (1988)
Poly(vinyl alcohol) hydrogel	Naguchi et al. (1991)
Woven carbon fiber pads	Muckle and Minns (1990)
Carbon fiber mesh/hyaluronic acid-based delivery substance/chondrocyte enriched cultures from mesenchymal stem cells from bone marrow	Robinson et al. (1993)
Synthetic biodegradable polymers (polyglycolic acid, porous poly (L) lactic acid)/chondrocytes	Freed et al. (1993)
Synthetic biodegradable polymers/chondrocytes	Vacanti et al. (1991, 1993)
Xenogeneic embryonal chondrocytes/hyaluronic acid-based delivery system	Robinson et al. (1991)

C. Periosteum

Autogenous periosteal grafts	Moran et al. (1992)
Autogenous periosteal tibial grafts	O'Driscoll et al. (1986)
Autologous chondrocytes/periosteum	Grande et al. (1989)
Autologous periosteum/fibrin adhesive	Tsai et al. (1992)
Rib perichondrial autographs/bone core	Coutts et al. (1992)
Allogeneic demineralized bone/autogeneic perichondrium	Billings et al. (1990)

D. Allografts/Autografts

Cadaveric osteochondral shell	Kusnick et al. (1987)
Fresh osteochondral allografts	Meyers et al. (1989)
Sternal cartilage autografts	Vachon et al. (1992)
Allografts	Bentley (1992)
Autologous meniscus	Sung and Kim (1990)

2. Biodegradability: The graft material can ultimately be resorbed by the host just as normal "regenerated" tissues undergo remodeling in response to local stresses and host conditions.
3. Biomechanical competence: The graft must provide protection for cell and matrix ingrowth from the host. It must also promote restoration of the biomechanical properties of the normal tissue.
4. Conduction of cells: The porous architecture of the implant should provide a compatible surface for ingrowth of host cells and protection of new tissues. Surfaces must be hydrophilic and support cell proliferation, migration, and attachment.
5. Induction: Ideally, the graft should induce differentiation of local host mesenchymal cells into the desired cells or induce local cells to produce the desired matrix. While collagen sponge is not such an inducer, pretreatment with various factors may make it so.

A. Collagen Architecture

The spacial orientation of collagen fibers in articular cartilage is a major determinant of its biomechanical properties, particularly durability of the articular surface. The normal collagen fiber architecture of articular cartilage as well as its variation in different pathological conditions has been defined (Bohn et al., 1984; Speer, 1982a, 1982b, 1984; Speer and Dahners, 1979). In addition, in studies on biological resurfacing, the collagen fiber architecture restoration was studied and suggested as one of the criteria for the adequacy of biological resurfacing (Speer, 1979). Additional criteria include restoration of an adequate subchondral bone plate, resynthesis of matrix glycosaminoglycans and maintenance of the surface contour of the joint. In addition to restoration of the joint surface, the ingrowth of bone into the deeper layers of the sponge with restoration of the subchondral bone support for the overlying articular cartilage is important. It is critical, therefore, that the sponge be able to support ingrowth of surrounding bone. In previous studies, the arcade model of collagen fiber architecture of normal articular cartilage was confirmed by both scanning electron microscopy and polarized light microscopy (Speer et al., 1979). A significant and original finding in that study was that both the collagen fiber systems and the corresponding cellular (chondrocyte) distribution were anisotropic, showing both quantitative and qualitative differences when assessed parallel or perpendicular to the split line pattern of the joints. A criterion of adequacy of biological resurfacing of a joint surface is the degree to which the collagen fiber and associated chondrocyte cellular architecture and anisotropy are restored (Speer et al., 1979).

B. Collagen Matrices

Collagen approximates many of the ideal properties of a synthetic graft material (Table 2). It has the advantage of availability in large quantity, long shelf life, and easy "fitting" into defects or on joints at surgery. A high degree of crosslinking can render it resilient enough to support joint motion immediately following surgery. The crosslinking agent reduces the rate of biodegradation of the tissue-implanted collagen sponge, thus controlling the rate of resorption. This is important for maintenance of the mechanical strength of the implant as well as providing resilience and fluid absorbency (Chvapil, 1981). Rapid degradation of a collagenous implant may induce tissue reaction since collagen and its degradation products are chemotactic to inflammatory cells and fibroblasts (Chang and Houck, 1970; Postlethwaite, 1978). Collagen matrices can be fabricated to precise specifi-

Table 2   Characteristics of Collagen Used in the Construction of
Biomaterials

Physical
  High tensile strength
  Low extensibility
  Complex surface morphology
  Three-dimensional substrate for cell growth
    Sponge
    Fibers
    Sheets
    Fleece
Physical/chemical
  Controllable crosslinking regulating
    Solubility
    Swelling
    Resorption
    Antigenicity
Interaction with drugs, growth factors, nectins, etc.
Biological
  Low antigenicity (reduced by crosslinking)
  Chemotactic
  Adhesion sites for cells via nectins
  Platelet adhesion (effect on blood clotting)

---

cations. These include collagen type, fiber length, geometric orientation, nature and degree of crosslinking, porosity, and interaction with other materials. Collagen matrices have been used for burn dressings, artificial skin, biological resurfacing of joints, bone and cartilage graft substitutes, and drug delivery systems (Chvapil, 1980, 1981, 1982; Chvapil et al., 1973, 1983; Devore, 1973; Green, 1977; Gross et al., 1980; Hewitt et al., 1982; Nelson et al., 1977; Silverstein and Chvapil, 1981; Speer, 1981; Speer et al., 1979; Winter, 1973).

Most studies of articular cartilage deal with problems associated with degradation. In addition to the potential impact on clinically relevant aspects of joint reconstruction, collagen sponge used in healing of articular cartilage should provide basic information on repair or regeneration of cartilage. Treatment of joint disease based on manufactured prostheses could become obsolete if biological resurfacing proves feasible. The strength of the method lies in provision of highly crosslinked collagen matrices, the collagen architecture of which approximates that of normal cartilage. The matrix provides a scaffolding for regeneration of an articular surface with normal collagen architecture.

C.   Pretreatment of Matrices

Pretreatment of the collagen sponge with autologous chondrocytes reduces the time and improves the quality of host cell ingrowth and matrix synthesis. To be biomechanically competent, neoarticular cartilage must (1) contain safranin-O positive glycosaminoglycans, (2) have oriented collagen fiber systems, (3) be populated with live chondroblasts, and (4) maintain, through biological remodeling and turnover, a constant thickness of articular cartilage. The materials and methods used must result in the restoration of a subchondral bone plate of normal or near normal thickness to provide support and strain absorption for the overlying articular cartilage.

There is extensive literature on factors that, if used to pretreat matrices intended for use in repair of osteochondral defects or joints, might enhance the influx and growth of cells in such matrices and possibly induce in such cells differentiation and metabolic alterations beneficial to regeneration of the tissue involved. Fibronectin is discussed here as an example. In chondrogenesis, fibronectin (FN) is found associated with the cells early in the developmental sequence but later is present in reduced amounts, and exogenous FN may be inhibitory to further development. Weiss and Reddi (1980; Reddi, 1985), in studying mesenchymal cell proliferation in a collagenous matrix *in vivo*, have found that FN binds to the matrix early and accumulates during mesenchymal cell proliferation. At a later stage of chondrogenesis, FN is less conspicuous. As they differentiate *in vitro* and begin synthesizing their characteristic extracellular matrix, chondrocytes lose FN. Inhibition of differentiation by culture conditions (Dessau et al., 1978) or vitamin A (Hassell et al., 1979) leads to an accumulation of FN. Exogenous FN causes chondrocytes to flatten, reduce synthesis of proteoglycans and Type II collagen, and reacquire matrices of FN and Type I collagen (Pennypacker et al., 1979). It is postulated that diffusible matrix components such as FN may govern formation of chondrogenic primordia during limb development by promoting cell–cell aggregation, leading to chondrogenic nodules (Newman and Frisch, 1979). Hynes (1981) suggests that these hypotheses could be combined in sequence—the first stage of differentiation being one in which FN promotes cell–cell aggregation, followed by a stage where the cells no longer bind FN and are able to proceed with chondrogenic differentiation. By pretreating matrices prior to implantation or during *in vitro* studies of chondrocyte population of such matrices, enhancement might be achieved as a result of invasion by chondrogenic cells or (*in vivo*) induction of other cells to differentiate into chondroblasts that populate the matrix and produce cartilage matrix. Possibilities for further enhancement using various combinations of factors prior to implantation are numerous. Such factors may act (1) as chemotactic agents for chondroblasts, (2) as cell attachment factors to fix the cells in the sponge, and/or (3) as inducers of production of Type II collagen and glycosaminoglycans. Preimplantation population of matrices with autologous chondrocytes would provide neoarticular cartilage that has chondroblasts manufacturing matrix, which should render the implant more biomechanically competent. This would mean earlier movement of the resurfaced joint, especially where a large area or an entire joint has been resurfaced.

D. Antigenicity of Collagen Sponge

In order to test the antigenicity of our collagen matrices, New Zealand white rabbits (1.5–2.0 kg) received sensitizing injections of (1) Type I collagen, (2) Type I collagen in Freund's adjuvant, or (3) 0.05% acetic acid—sham control. Test rabbits received 1.2 ml collagen (prepared by soaking Type I collagen fleece in 70% alcohol and freezing in liquid nitrogen to disintegrate) in 0.05% acetic acid (10.75 mg/ml as determined by hydroxyproline analysis), injected alone or mixed with Freund's adjuvant. The material was injected intradermally into 14 sites on the back. Booster injections were given at 3 weeks in the same manner. Rabbits were bled from the ear at 7 and 10 weeks. Sera were stored at −70°C and assayed for antibodies to collagen by the ELISA (enzyme-linked immunosorbent assay) technique. There was no statistical difference between sham-injected controls and Type I collagen injected animals. Thus, no discernable antibodies were present under these experimental conditions. In the presence of Freund's adjuvant, antibodies to Type I collagen were formed.

Anticollagen antibodies have been produced in many species, generally with the use of Freund's complete adjuvant. The purity of the collagen is extremely important as the presence of contaminating acidic or serum proteins gives rise to antibodies. The nature of the immune response to collagen varies greatly, depending on the species of animal immunized and the origin of the collagen. Collagen-induced arthritis (by intradermal injection of native heterologous or homologous Type II collagen emulsified in adjuvant) results in a disease in some strains of mice and rats with both humoral and cellular immune responses. The pros and cons of this induced arthritis as a model for rheumatoid arthritis have been discussed (Trentham, 1982). The disease, however, usually does not occur in the absence of a relatively vigorous humoral immune response to Type II collagen. Staines et al. (1981) reported that bovine or porcine Type II collagen polymerized with glutaraldehyde and used in Freund's adjuvant to sensitize animals, showed some immunogenicity but was considerably less arthritogenic than soluble Type II collagen. Also, immunization with polymerized collagen conferred resistance to subsequent disease induction with soluble Type II collagen. Felts et al. (1981) report a lack of immunologic responsiveness to scleral allografts (primarily Type I collagen and small amounts of glycosaminoglycans) used in humans for periodontal therapy.

If a material can be rendered insoluble, antigenicity can be substantially reduced or eliminated. Materials that are insoluble at the time of implantation can be rendered soluble by naturally occurring enzymatic or chemical processes. It is believed that the introduction of sufficient crosslinks increases the stability and reduces the solubilization of the material, thus greatly reducing antigenicity (Carpentier et al., 1969). Some investigators have reported that crosslinkage of tissue proteins confers immunological inertness. However, there is evidence to suggest that glutaraldehyde-crosslinked tissues retain some measure of altered immunologic potential (Bajpai, 1983; Sallgaller and Bajpai, 1984). Despite this, heterograft bioprostheses such as glutaraldehyde-tanned porcine heart valves and bovine pericardium (for use as dura substitutes or heart valves) have been approved by the FDA and are in common use in humans.

For resurfacing of osteochondral defects, highly crosslinked collagen matrices are used. There is evidence that such insolubilized collagen is resistant to collagenase digestion (Harris and Farrell, 1972; Steven, 1976; Vater et al., 1979), thus, only slow resorption occurs with time (6–9 months). This rate of collagen degradation should not induce a significant immune response, and the implant should not be rejected but be replaced by invading chondrocytes and their products—endogenous Type II collagen and proteoglycans.

Serum levels of antibodies to collagen in sera of implanted animals are followed by the ELISA technique. An ELISA was developed for the detection of serum antibodies to insoluble collagen (Ulreich and Snider, 1992; Ulreich et al., 1991). Pulverized collagen sponge is used as the antigen to detect a humoral immune response. Furthermore, it has been shown that "partial hydrolysis" of collagen, as used by some investigators for achieving a more uniform coating of antigen in the ELISA plate, may destroy the epitopes recognized by the serum antibodies and lead to false-negative results (Ulreich and Snider, 1992; Ulreich et al., 1991).

III. BIOLOGICAL RESURFACING OF OSTEOCHONDRAL DEFECTS WITH COLLAGEN SPONGE

A. Surgical Technique

The following surgical technique was used for all studies cited in Sec. III.B–III.E. After administration of a general anesthetic, the animals were maintained in a supine position on the animal operating table. Both knee areas as well as the abdomen were shaved, prepped and draped in a sterile fashion. Lateral parapatellar incisions were used on both knees, dislocating the patella medially. This latter technique permitted immediate motion and ambulation following surgery. Using a drill of 3/16 in. diameter for the rabbits and a 1/4 in. drill plus a "punch cutter" for the dogs, defects were made in the central weight-bearing surface of the medial condyle of each femur. They were carried to a depth even with the coronal plane of the osteochondral margin of the joint, or about 1.2–1.4 cm in the dog (Fig. 1) and about 4–7 mm in the rabbit. The cancellous bone subjacent to the subchondral bone plate was curetted somewhat, giving a widened mortise for locking of the implant. In each instance, the test sponge material was placed in the defect in the right knee, and the left knee was maintained (1) as an untreated osteochondral defect for control or (2) as a location for a control sponge. The knees were closed in independent layers, closing the lateral capsule, the lateral retinaculum, and the skin with nonresorbable suture material. Unless otherwise specified, animals were allowed ambulatory activity immediately.

B. Polyvinyl Alcohol Sponge Versus Collagen Sponge

In this study collagen sponge was compared with polyvinyl alcohol sponge (PVA) and sham osteochondral defects in young (12 weeks) and adult (8 months) California white rabbits (Holmes et al., 1975). A defect 5 mm in diameter and 5 mm deep was aseptically created by a drill in the femur articular joint in the region adjacent to the patella. Defects were filled with sterile collagen sponge or with PVA, or left empty. The leg was immobilized with a cast for 3 weeks. Thirty-six rabbits 12 weeks old and 34 rabbits 8 months old were used. Histologic studies revealed rapid ingrowth of fibroblast-like cells with complete filling of both the collagen sponge and PVA sponge within 21 days. The PVA sponge was faster in its initial stages of fibroblastic ingrowth. However, with time, the collagen sponge showed osseous and cartilaginous metaplasia whereas the PVA group did not. Cells grew along the PVA sponge but did not adhere strongly to it. Rabbits with implanted collagen sponge at 6 weeks showed macroscopic and microscopic evidence of articular cartilage covering the original defect. By 12 weeks the resorption of the collagen sponge was complete. By 18 weeks the PVA group still showed no signs of osseous and cartilaginous metaplasia. The collagen sponge group, however, showed a cartilaginous surface in most cases. An experiment similar to that performed with young rabbits was carried out with adult rabbits, with similar results. The surface of the PVA sponge was coarse, sometimes coated with a thin fibrous membrane. The collagen sponge resorbed within 3 to 6 weeks and was replaced by bone and cartilage.

PVA sponge represented the most resilient matrix we have used in resurfacing of osteochondral defects. It did not collapse under the biomechanical conditions in the joint but, because it was not biodegradable, it sometimes wore through the surface of the defect. These results suggested that collagen sponge had greater potential then PVA sponge for bone repair and regeneration of articular cartilage.

C. Glutaraldehyde Versus Hexamethylene Diisocyanate Crosslinked Collagen Sponge

In our next study of biological resurfacing of synovial joints, 5 mm osteochondral defects were made in the medial femoral condyles of rabbits. The defects were filled with glutaraldehyde crosslinked sponges and the animals allowed immediate motion. These sponges supported the ingrowth of both bone and cartilage from the periphery, restoring neoarticular cartilage that was far superior to the control (unfilled) defects (Speer et al., 1979, 1981). In this study, residual glutaraldehyde-containing sponge was still present at 6 months and there were consistent though minimal giant-cell reactions to the implant material. Follow-up using tissue culture (Ulreich and Chvapil, 1983) confirmed the presence of glutaraldehyde and its role in inhibiting cell growth in proximity to the sponge (Fig. 2) (Speer et al., 1980). Fibroblast growth in tissue culture was inhibited 99% at concentrations of 3.0 ppm glutaraldehyde in the medium. It was shown that collagen tanned with glutaraldehyde retains the crosslinking agent, not only as part of the covalent cross link with the collagen molecule, but possibly as a different form, most likely that of a polymer, independent of or adsorbed to the collagen matrix. The rate of healing and cell infiltration into such a matrix used for resurfacing would be retarded by the cytotoxic effects of glutaraldehyde. We proposed that it was the polymerized glutaraldehyde retained within the collagen sponge that by slow, continuous hydrolysis released monomeric glutaraldehyde, that exerted its cytotoxic effect over time (Chvapil et al., 1983). A study with similar results was performed using glutaraldehyde crosslinked collagen sponge in dogs (Fig. 1). Figure 1a shows the collagen sponge filling the newly created defect in the femur. In the unfilled control defect [Fig. 1b] at 12 weeks, there is early osteophyte formation and joint degeneration. In the defect implanted with collagen sponge (Fig. 1c) at 12 weeks, there is resurfacing of the defect with cartilage having the proteoglycan content and collagen architecture of articular cartilage. Sponge manufacture was modified using hexamethylene diisocyanate as a crosslinking agent to avoid the toxic effects of glutaraldehyde. The characteristics of the collagen sponge are shown in Table 3. Subsequent biological resurfacing studies showed no giant-cell reaction and even better resurfacing of the joints studied (Speer et al., 1979). The maximum time interval studied was 6 months, and at that time there was no evidence of degenerative arthritis in the collagen sponge implanted joint while knees that received no implants were forming osteochondral margin osteophytes, indicating progressive degeneration. Furthermore, the surface contour of the joint was restored, with no exophytic proliferation of the regenerating surface.

D. Enhancement of Collagen Sponge Matrix with Chondronectin

A study was next performed to determine whether pretreatment of collagen sponge (Type I) with chondronectin, a 180-kDa glycoprotein that had been shown to be an adhesion factor specific for chondrocytes (Hewitt et al., 1982) (Bethesda Research Laboratories, Inc.), would enhance biological resurfacing of osteochondral defects in articular surfaces in rabbits (Ulreich et al., 1985). It was postulated that chondronectin would enhance the local ingrowth, attachment, and synthetic activity of chondrogenic cells in the local restoration of joint surfaces. Reconstituted collagen sponges (bovine Type I), tanned with diisocyanate, were pretreated with (1) saline (control); (2) soluble Type II collagen (2.5 μg/ml), which might produce a better substrate for chondrocytes that bind preferentially to Type II collagen); (3) chondronectin (100 ng/ml); or (4) Type II collagen followed by chondronectin (Type II collagen to try to improve binding of chondronectin

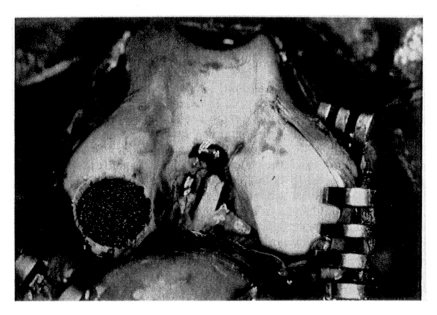

(a)

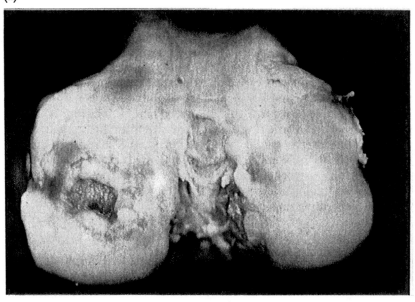

(b)

Figure 1   Resurfacing of canine osteochondral defect with collagen sponge crosslinked with glutaraldehyde. (a) Canine femoral condyle with freshly implanted collagen sponge filling the osteochondral defect. (b) Control at 12 weeks—in the absence of collagen sponge there is no filling of
the defect. Early osteophyte formation and joint degeneration are observed. (c) Experimental at
12 weeks following implantation of the sponge—resurfacing with cartilage having the collagen
architecture and proteoglycan content of articular cartilage is observed.

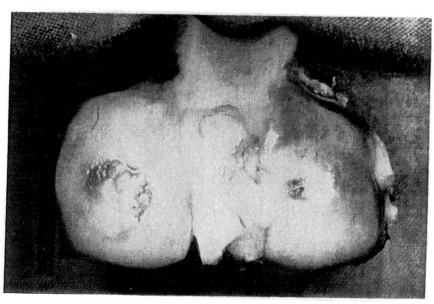

(c)

to the Type I collagen sponge). Osteochondral defects were made in the femoral condyles of 1-to 24-month-old New Zealand white rabbits for testing of control and chondronectin-pretreated sponges (Fig. 3a shows the osteochondral defect prior to sponge implantation and Fig. 3b shows the sponge in place). Control sponges were placed in the left knee and experimental sponges were placed in the right knee. The sponges were trimmed flush with the articular surface; the patella was relocated and the incision closed. Intermuscular pouches were created between the external and internal oblique musculature in the abdomen for comparative testing of all four sponge pretreatments. Collagen sponges (5 × 5 × 2 mm) were inserted and the incisions closed.

Animals were sacrificed at 3, 7, and 14 days after implantation. Distal femurs were removed, fixed in 10% buffered formalin, and cut sagittally in blocks that included the defect–implant zone. The bone was decalcified and prepared for histologic sectioning. Hematoxylin and eosin and safranin-O/fast green stained sections were cut at 5 μm. Sponges from intermuscular pouches were removed and prepared for histology (Fig. 4).

All experimental treatments of the sponge resulted in more rapid cell ingrowth into the sponges at both bony and intermuscular sites (Figs. 4c–4e). There was a corresponding enhancement of angiogenesis as reflected by ingrowth of capillary vasculature into the sponges. Proteoglycan synthesis and histologically apparent chondroidal tissue were observed at the joint surfaces to a greater extent and earlier in the treated sponges than in the untreated controls. At the bone–sponge interface there was fibrous, vascular, and bony ingrowth—no indication of "induction" of chondrogenic cell lines by the chondronectin or Type II collagen was noted.

In the osteochondral defects by 14 days there was substantial cartilaginous ingrowth into the chondronectin-pretreated sponge at the articular cartilage level, with complete coverage of neoarticular cartilage over the surface of the defect. Safranin-O stain showed faint positive areas of proteoglycan in association with cells that were large and round,

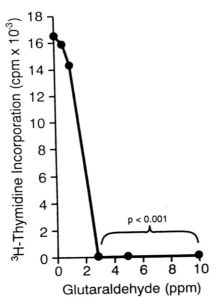

Figure 2   The effect of glutaraldehyde on incorporation of ³H-thymidine by log phase 3T3 fibro-blasts in 24-well tissue culture plates. At 3 ppm there is complete inhibition of division of the fibroblasts. (From Ulreich and Chvapil, 1981.)

having prominent nuclei and abundant cytoplasm (consistent with "chondroblasts"). Importantly, the restored surface of the joint was not recessed below the level of the surrounding articular cartilage and the bone–implant junction showed fibrous and vascular ingrowth at the subchondral and deeper bone levels. By comparison, the control implant at 14 days showed scant fibrous ingrowth at the articular surface and there were no safranin-O positive areas (Figs. 4a and 4b). At the bone–sponge interface there was fibrous ingrowth less deep than in the experimental sponge but without the degree of vascular ingrowth seen in the chondronectin-treated sponge. In general, the chondronec-

Table 3   Characteristics of Hexamethylene Diisocyanate Crosslinked Collagen Sponge

Crosslinking agent	Hexamethylene diisocyanate
Shrinkage temperature (degree of crosslinking)	65–70°C
Pore size (continuous channels)	50–120 μm
Composition	
Collagen	100% Type I collagen
Noncollagenous proteins	0%
Fluid binding capacity	43 g H_2O/g sponge (dry weight)
Resilience (load, in grams, compressing the sponge 50%)	25 g/cm²

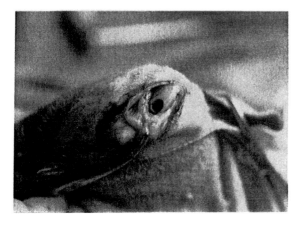

(a)

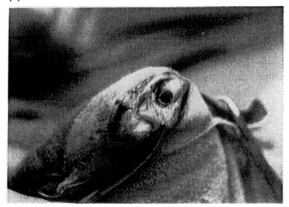

(b)

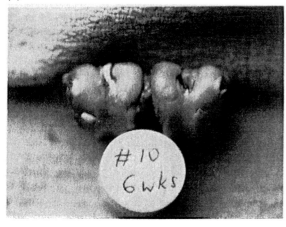

(c)

Figure 3 Freshly drilled 5 mm wide by 7 mm deep osteochondral defect in the medial condyle of the rabbit femur before (a) and after (b) filling the defect with collagen sponge. (c) Resurfaced defects at 6 weeks show complete coverage of the defects with cartilage.

tin-soaked sponges promoted faster cartilaginous ingrowth into the collagen sponge. The chondronectin-treated sponges not only improved cellular ingrowth but showed a greater degree of angiogenesis, with capillaries extending to a greater depth and in greater number than in the control, untreated sponges.

In the sponges implanted in the abdomen (Fig. 4f), the results showed that sponges treated with chondronectin, chondronectin + Type II collagen, or Type II collagen all showed a greater degree of fibrous and vascular ingrowth than was seen in the control sponges. Chondronectin alone was the most effective in terms of completeness of filling of the sponge with host cells. That is, addition of Type II collagen with or without chondronectin was not as effective as chondronectin alone.

At 7 days following intermuscular implantation, all three types of experimental sponge showed more fibrous ingrowth than controls but were not distinguished from one another with respect to the ingrowth of vessels or fibrous tissue. By 14 days, there was almost complete fibrous and vascular filling of the interstices of the collagen sponge treated with chondronectin. The sponges treated with Type II collagen or Type II collagen and chondronectin were similar to one another and showed less ingrowth of fibrous and vascular components at 14 days than did the sponges treated with chondronectin alone. They were, however, substantially better than control sponges. Pretreatment with Type II collagen may have moistened the collagen sponge so that in those sponges treated with Type II collagen and then chondronectin, there may have been reduced absorption/ binding of chondronectin, thus resulting in a less impressive improvement of the sponge matrix than treatment with chondronectin alone. The effect of the chondronectin may be more than one of adhesion–attachment–spreading. It may be a specific stimulus to synthesis of matrix components by host cells in addition to enhancing the migration and localization of the host cells in the sponge.

The study demonstrated the principle of manipulation of a synthetic graft material to

---

Figure 4   Ingrowth of host tissue into collagen sponge (±chondronection pre-treatment) at 14 days following implantation in a 5 mm wide and 7 mm deep defect in the rabbit femur. (Hematoxylin and Eosin stain.) Symbols: $\diamond$ = articular cartilage; $\triangle$ = neo-articular cartilage; $\bigcirc$ = skeletal muscle. (A) Control osteochondral defect showing junction of untreated collagen sponge with articular cartilage ($\diamond$) and subchondral bone. There is negligible ingrowth into the sponge, resulting in artifactual separation of the sponge from the defect wall (H&E ×10). (B) Same as (A) under polarizing light microscopy. The highly birefringent fibers of the collagen sponge are seen in the defect (×10). (C) Experimental osteochondral defect showing junction of chondronectin-impregnated sponge (at right) with articular cartilage and subchondral bone. Not only is there substantial ingrowth of cells into the sponge (arrow), but there is both morphologic and histochemical confirmation of production of neo-articular cartilage ($\triangle$) (H&E ×10). (D) Same as (C) under polarizing light microscopy. In addition to the birefringent fibers of the collagen sponge, there is a finer pattern of birefringence representing early orientation of new collagen fibers in the neo-articular cartilage matrix (×10). (E) High-power view of region about the arrow of (C) showing ingrowth and differentiation of chondroidal cells. The relationship of the cells and matrix of the neo-articular cartilage with the residual collagen sponge (arrow) is intimate, with no reactive inflammatory cells present (H&E ×10). (F) Collagen sponge impregnated with chondronectin and implanted in an abdominal muscle pouch ($\bigcirc$) in the rabbit. At 14 days following implantation there is significant cell/fibrous soft tissue ingrowth. Capillary ingrowth (arrow) is noted in greater profusion and depth than in controls in both the muscle pouch and osteochondral defect sponges (H&E ×10).

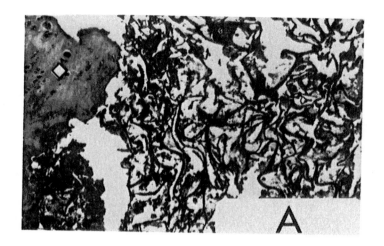

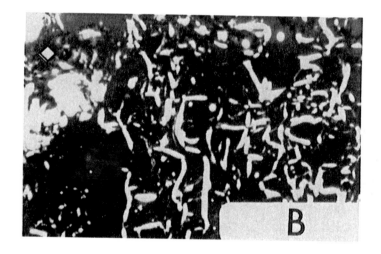

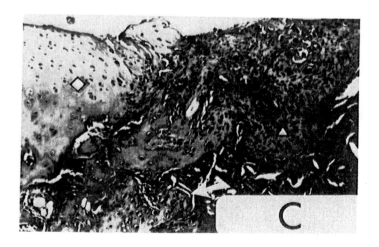

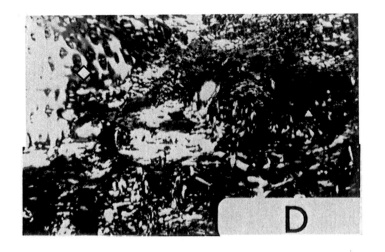

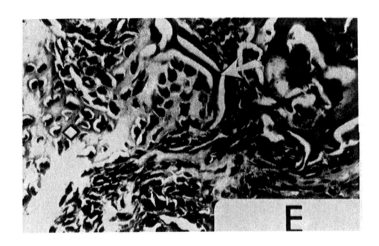

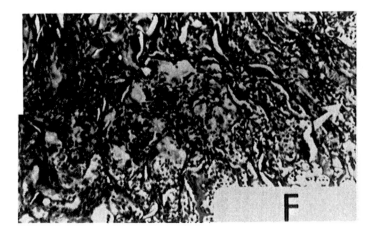

Figure 4 Continued.

enhance the regeneration of a defect in a host tissue by host cells. The graft met most of the theoretical criteria of an ideal material since it protected the early ingrowth of cells and disappeared with time. The model also showed the effectiveness of treatment of the graft material with chondronectin, which might have acted both as an attachment factor for cells and as a modulator of synthetic/differentiative activity.

E.   Seeding Collagen Sponge with Autologous Chondrocytes

In order to attempt to increase the speed of repopulation of the collagen sponge with cells *in vivo*, chondrocytes were isolated from proximal humerus cartilage of rabbits. The following day, these cells were injected into collagen sponge at the time of sponge placement in osteochondral defects. Animals were sacrificed at periods up to 3 weeks. Results showed that introduction of cells into the matrix produced a much faster resurfacing of the sponge, with a very thick surface layer of cells and collagen with good ingrowth of subchondral bone (Fig. 5). Long-term studies need to be undertaken to assess the quality of the surface with time. Continuous passive motion might be particularly appropriate in this model in order to "tighten up" the very thick resurfaced region.

IV.   *IN VITRO* CULTURE OF CHONDROCYTES ON COLLAGEN SPONGE

Rabbit articular chondrocytes were isolated by a modification of the method of Vetter et al. (1985) and introduced into Type I bovine skin collagen sponge (crosslinked with hexamethylene diisocyanate) by injection or by layering the cells on the sponge surface. Articular cartilage from rabbits was minced and incubated for 30 min at 37°C in Hams F-10, 0.25% trypsin, and 2 mg/ml collagenase. After stopping the reaction with FBS and pelleting the tissue, it was resuspended in Hams F-10, 10% FBS, glutamine (200 mM/L), and 2 mg/ml collagenase. After incubating at 37°C for 16 h, the tissue was pelleted, washed, and resuspended in Hams F-10, 10% FBS, penicillin, streptomycin, Fungizone, glutamine, and ascorbic acid (50 μg/ml). Cells were cultured on collagen sponge (cobalt irradiated and presoaked for 24 h in sterile Hams F-10). Cultures were maintained at 37°C in 5% CO_2/95% air. Media were changed twice weekly and sponges harvested at 15 min, 2 days, and 1, 2, 3, 4, 6, and 8 weeks. After placement in Karnovsky's fixative or snap freezing for immunofluorescence, the sponges were examined by scanning electron microscopy (Fig. 6) or bright-field microscopy (Figs. 7b–7d) of slides stained with H&E, trichrome, and safranin-O. Some sponges cultured for 2 weeks were incubated with ^{3}H-thymidine or $Na_2{}^{35}SO_4$ for 24 h prior to harvest. They were used for autoradiography (Fig. 7a) and stained with safranin-O (Ulreich, 1990; Ulreich et al., 1986, 1987). Results clearly showed the Type I collagen sponge to be an ideal substrate for the culture of chondrocytes that remain in a differentiated state. They rapidly divide and fill the interstices of the sponge both with cells and with a matrix rich in Type II collagen, as shown by trichrome stain and immunofluorescence with anti-collagen II primary antibody followed by a rhodamine-coupled second reagent (Fig. 8a). Figure 8b shows the absence of nonspecific staining of the Type I collagen sponge in the interior of the sponge, where only one small cluster of chondrocytes is present.

The three-dimensional porous collagen matrix combines several of the advantages of other methods of chondrocyte culture. Cells reach high density on a solid matrix while in an environment not unlike suspension culture with free access to nutrients. Once a high

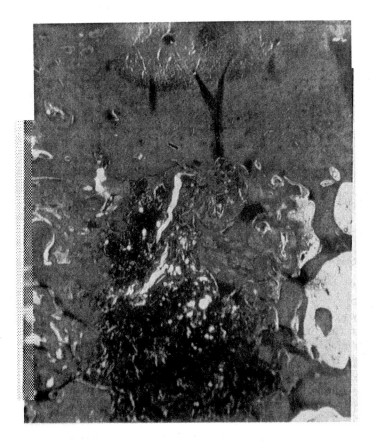

Figure 5   Collagen sponge was seeded with rabbit autologous chondrocytes at the time of implantation in a 5 mm wide, 7 mm deep osteochondral defect. After 2 weeks there is extensive deposition of collagen matrix by cells at the surface of the defect, and formation of a bony subchondral region. (Trichrome × 10).

cell density is reached on the sponge, it is similar to organ culture of a selected cell population.

A three-dimensional collagen matrix prepopulated with the animal's own cells should provide an ideal biological resurfacing material. The porosity allows rapid growth of bone at the bone sponge interface to cement the implant in place. The porosity can be increased by piercing the sponge.

V.   SUMMARY

In studies of biological resurfacing of synovial joints, we have demonstrated the efficacy of using collagen sponge in promoting healing of osteochondral defects. The desirable properties of collagen sponge include porosity, biodegradability, biocompatibility, ability

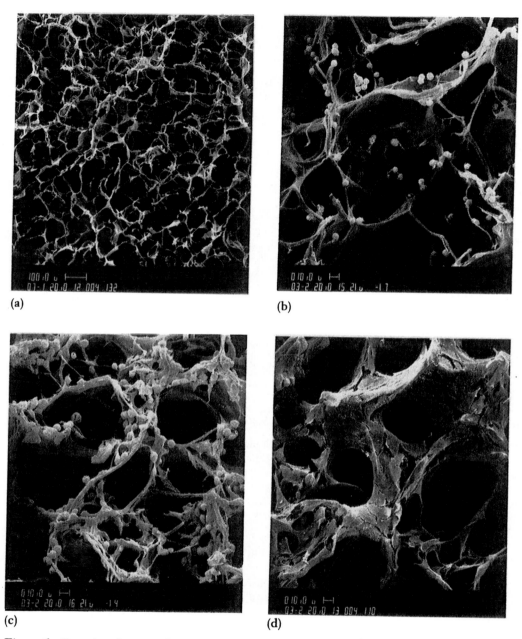

Figure 6   Scanning electron micrographs of collagen sponge seeded with rabbit articular chondrocytes and cultured *in vitro*. (a) "Virgin" collagen sponge prior to seeding with chondrocytes (× 70). Rabbit articular chondrocytes cultured *in vitro* on collagen sponge for 15 min (b), 2 days (c), or 14 days (d) (× 300).

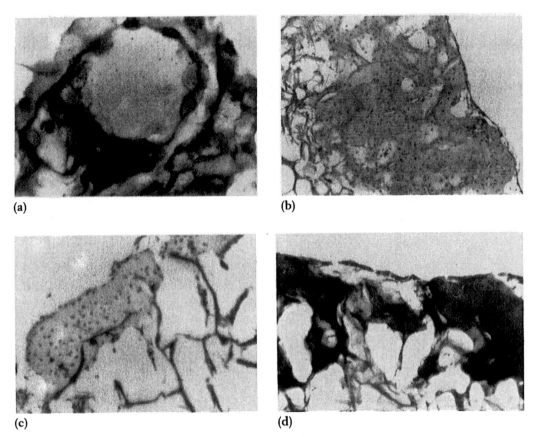

(a)   (b)

(c)   (d)

Figure 7 *In vitro* culture of rabbit articular chondrocytes in collagen sponge. After 2 weeks in culture, ^{3}H-thymidine autoradiography with safranin-O counterstain shows chondrocytes dividing within the collagen sponge and depositing proteoglycans (a) ($\times 100$). After 8 weeks in culture, the chondrocytes have grown down into the sponge (b) (H&E, $\times 25$) and deposited newly formed collagen matrix (c) (trichrome, $\times 10$). The chondrocytes have retained their differentiated state as shown by deposition of proteoglycans in the matrix. (d) (Safranin-O, $\times 10$).

to mechanically protect cells and matrix while directing cell ingrowth, and available chemical technology for modifying its biomedical and biological properties. In our hands, glutaraldehyde-crosslinked collagen sponge was superior to polyvinyl alcohol sponge because of its biodegradability. Hexamethylene diisocyanate-crosslinked collagen sponge was superior to glutaraldehyde-crosslinked sponge because it lacked the cytotoxicity from glutaraldehyde leaching from the matrix. Population of collagen sponge with autogenous chondrocytes prior to implantation provided more rapid resurfacing of osteochondral defects. Pretreatment of the collagen matrix with factors such as chondronectin also enhanced the rate of tissue ingrowth. Use of growth and attachment factors for chondrocytes constitutes the most exciting area for future research. The factors we believe are most critical to future studies are: (1) creation of osteochondral defects of sufficient diameter so that a true test of tissue regeneration can be performed and (2) drilling to a depth that includes the subchondral bone plate for more rapid vascularization and healing.

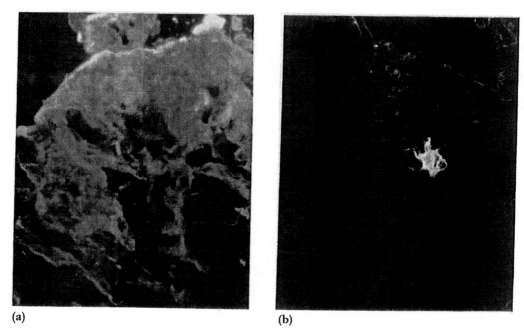

(a)   (b)

Figure 8 Rabbit articular chondrocytes cultured for 8 weeks on Type I collagen sponge demonstrate retention of phenotype. Immunofluorescent staining was with anti-Type II collagen primary antibody and a rhodamine-coupled secondary reagent. The surface of the collagen sponge populated with chondrocytes and matrix stains positively for Type II collagen (a). The internal area of the collagen sponge (b) serves as a negative control, with only a small cluster of chondrocytes staining positive for Type II collagen. The antibody does not stain the Type I collagen sponge nonspecifically.

In vitro collagen sponge provides an excellent three-dimensional matrix for the culture of chondrocytes. It incorporates several of the advantages of other methods employed to maintain the normal chondrocyte phenotype. Cells can be cultured at high density on a solid matrix that does not hinder access of macromolecular nutrients to the cells. Culture of chondrocytes in collagen sponge provides a useful model for study of the effects of various hormones and growth factors on the proliferation and differentiation of chondrocytes as well as providing a material for biological resurfacing of joints with living host cells capable of synthesizing biomechanically competent articular cartilage. The chondrocytes remain in a differentiated state. The cells continue to proliferate within the sponge over time, as shown by autoradiography, and produce a matrix rich in Type II collagen and proteoglycans. The chondrocyte-containing collagen sponge is remarkably similar to the physical model of articular cartilage constructed by Broom and Marra (1985). It is based on a system of deformable elements (hydrated proteoglycans) trapped within a three-dimensional network of tension-resisting fibrils (collagen).

ACKNOWLEDGMENTS

We wish to acknowledge M. Chvapil, M.D., Ph.D., D.Sc., for providing the collagen sponge and his expertise. Also, T. Chvapil, H. Holubec, B. J. Snider, and E. S. Frankel for excellent technical assistance.

REFERENCES

Bajpai, P. K. (1983). Antigenicity of glutaraldehyde-stabilized biological materials, in *Biomaterials in Reconstructive Surgery* (L. R. Rubin, ed.), C. V. Mosby, St. Louis, pp. 243–251.

Ben-Yishay, A., Grande, D. A., and Song, K. K. (1991). The use of a cartilage tissue analog for the repair of articular cartilage, *Proc. 17th Ann. Mtg. Soc. Biomater.*, p. 270.

Bentley, G. (1992). Articular tissue grafts, *Ann. Rheum. Dis., 51*, 292–296.

Billings, E. Jr., Von Schroeder, H. P., Mai, M. T., Aratow, M., Amiel, D., Woo, S. L.-Y., and Coutts R. D. (1990). Cartilage resurfacing of the rabbit knee: The use of an allogeneic demineralized bone matrix–autogenetic perichondrium composite implant, *Acta Orth. Scand., 61*, 201–206.

Bohn, W. W., Stein, R. M., Hsu, H. H. T., Morris, D. C., and Anderson, H. C. (1984). Isolation of a plasma membrane-enriched fraction from collagenase-suspended rachitic rat growth plate chondrocytes, *J. Orthop. Res., 1*, 319–324.

Broom, N. D., and Marra, D. L. (1985). New structural concepts of articular cartilage demonstrated with a physical model, *Connect. Tiss. Res., 14*, 1–8.

Broom, N. D. (1986). The collagenous architecture of articular cartilage — A synthesis of ultrastructure and mechanical functions, *J. Rheumatol., 13*, 142–152.

Caffiniere, J. Y., Martin E., Humbel, R., and Konsbruck, R. (1982). The importance of the bone in osteocartilaginous autografts of the rabbit knee, *Int. Orthop., 6*, 15–25.

Carpentier, A., Lemaigre, G., Robert, L., Carpentier, S., and Dubost, C. (1969). Biological factors affecting long-term results of valvular heterografts, *J. Thorac. Cardiovas. Surg., 58*, 467–483.

Chang, C., and Houck, J. (1970). Demonstration of the chemotactic properties of collagen, *Proc. Soc. Exp. Biol. Med., 134*, 22–26.

Chvapil, M. (1980, February 14). Method of manufacturing layers of collagen fibers in the form of felt or sponges. German Patent 1,811,290.

Chvapil, M. (1981). The fate of natural tissue prostheses, in *Fundamental Aspects of Biocompatibility*, Vol. 1 (D. F. Williams, ed.), CRC Press, Liverpool, pp. 88–104.

Chvapil, M. (1982). Considerations on manufacturing principles of a synthetic burn dressing: A review, *J. Biomed. Mater. Res., 16*, 245–263.

Chvapil, M., Kronethal, R. L., and Van Winkle, W., Jr. (1973). Medical and surgical applications of collagen, in *International Review of Connective Tissue Research* (D. A. Hall and D. S. Jackson, eds.), Academic Press, New York, pp. 1–61.

Chvapil, M., Speer, D. P., Mora, W., and Eskelson, C. (1983). Effect of tanning agent on tissue reaction to tissue implanted collagen sponge, *J. Surg. Res., 35*, 402–409.

Coutts, R. D., Woo S. L.-Y., Amiel, D., Von Schroeder, H. P., and Kwan, M. K. (1992). Rib perichondrial autografts in full-thickness articular cartilage defects in rabbits, *Clin. Orthop. Rel. Res., 275*, 263–273.

Dessau, W., Sasse, J., Timpl, R., Jilek, F., and von der Mark, K. (1978). Synthesis and extracellular deposition of fibronectin in chondrocyte cultures, *J. Cell Biol., 79*, 342–355.

DeVore, D. T. (1973). Collagen heterografts for bone replacement, *Dental Res., 36*, 609–615.

Engkvist, O., and Ekenstam, F. (1982). Joint cartilage formation by silastic sheet spacer, *Scand. J. Plast. Reconstr. Surg., 16*, 191–194.

Felts, C., Engel, D., Ammons, W., and Narayanan, A. S. (1981). Immunologic tolerance to collagen and glycosaminoglycan components of scleral allografts in humans: Evidence for T cell suppression, *J. Peridontol., 52*, 603–608.

Freed, L. E., Marquis, J. C., Nohria, A., Emmanual, J., Mikos, A. G., and Langer, R. (1993). Neocartilage formation *in vitro* and *in vivo* using cells cultured on synthetic biodegradable polymers, *J. Biomat. Mater. Res., 27*, 11–23.

Grande, D. A., Pitman, M. I., Peterson, L., Menche, D., and Klein, M. (1989). The repair of experimentally produced defects in rabbit articular cartilage by autologous chondrocyte transplantation, *J. Orthop. Res., 7*, 208–218.

Green, W. T., Jr. (1977). Behaviors of rabbit chondrocytes during tissue culture and subsequent allografting, *Clin. Orthop., 124*, 237–250.

Gross, A. E., McKee, N., Langer, F., and Pritzker, K. (1984). In *Reconstruction of Skeletal Deficits at the Knee. A Comprehensive Osteochondral Transplant Program* (G. E. Friedlaender, H. J. Mankin and K. W. Sell, eds.), Little, Brown, Boston, pp. 289–298.

Gross, B. D., Nevins, A., and Laporta, R. (1980). Bone-induction potential of mineralized collagen gel xenografts, *Oral Surg., Oral Med., Oral Pathol., 49*, 21–26.

Hanff, G., Sollermann, C., Abrahamson, S. O., and Lundborg, G. (1990). Repair of osteochondral defects in the rabbit knee with Goretex (expanded polytetrafluoroethylene), *Scand. J. Plast. Reconstr. Hand. Surg., 24*, 217–223.

Harris, E. D., and Farrell, M. E. (1972). Resistance to collagenase: A characteristic of collagen fibrils cross-linked by formaldehyde, *Biochim. Biophys. Acta, 278*, 133–141.

Hassell, J. R., Pennypacker, J. P., Kleinman, H. K., Pratt, R. M., and Yamada, K. M. (1979). Enhanced cellular fibronectin accumulation in chondrocytes treated with vitamin A, *Cell, 17*, 821–826.

Hewitt, A. T., Varner, H. H., Silver, M. H., Dessau, W., Wilkes, C. M., and Martin, G. R. (1982). The isolation and partial characterization of chondronectin, an attachment factor for chondrocytes, *J. Biol. Chem., 257*, 2330–2334.

Hjertquist, S.-O., and Lemperg, R. (1972). Long term observations on the articular cartilage and autologous costal cartilage transplanted to osteochondral defects on the femoral head, *Calc. Tiss. Res., 9*, 226–237.

Hogervorst, T., Meijer, D. W., and Klopper, P. J. (1992). The effect of TCP-collagen implant on the healing of articular cartilage defects in the rabbit knee joint, *J. Appl. Biomed., 3*, 251–258.

Holmes, M., Volz, R. G., and Chvapil, M. (1975). Collagen sponge as a matrix for articular cartilage regeneration, *Surg. Forum, 26*, 511–513.

Hynes, R. O. (1981). In *Cell Biology of Extracellular Matrix* (E. P. Hay, ed.), Plenum Press, New York, pp. 295–334.

Jamshidi, K., Shimizu, T., Usui, Y., Eberhart, R. C., and Mooney, V. (1988). Resorbable structured porous materials in the healing process of hard tissue defects, *ASAIO Transactions, 34*, 755–760.

Jimenez, S. A., and Brighton, C. T. (1984). In *Osteochondral Allografts* (G. E. Friedlaender, H. J. Mankin, and K. W. Sell, eds.), Little, Brown, Boston, pp. 73–79.

Kusnick, C., Hayward, I., Sartoris, D. J., et al. (1987). Radiographic evaluation of joints resurfaced with osteochondral shell allografts, *Am. J. Roentgenol., 149*, 743–748.

Langer, F. L., Gross, A. E., West, M., and Urovitz, E. P. (1978). The immunogenicity of allograft knee joint transplants, *Clin. Orthop., 132*, 155–162.

Mankin, H. J. (1984). In *Osteochondral Allografts* (G. E. Friedlaender, H. J. Mankin, and K. W. Sell, eds.), Little, Brown, Boston, pp. 59–72.

Maor, G., von der Mark, K., Reddi, H., Heinegard, D., Franzen, A., and Silbermann, M. (1987). Acceleration of cartilage and bone differentiation on collagenous substrata, *Coll. Rel. Res., 7*, 351–370.

Meyers, M. H., Akeson, W., and Convery, F. R. (1989). Resurfacing of the knee with fresh osteochondral allograft, *J. Bone Jt. Surg.*, Ser. A, *71*, 704–713.

Meyers, M. H., Bucholz, R. W., and Jones, R. E. (1984). In *Osteochondral Allografts* (G. E. Friedlaender, H. J. Mankin, and K. W. Sell, eds.), Little, Brown, Boston.

Moran, M. E., Kim, H. K., and Salter, R. B. (1992). Biological resurfacing of full-thickness defects in patellar articular cartilage of the rabbit: Investigation of autogenous periosteal grafts subjected to continuous passive motion, *J. Bone Jt. Surg. B, 74*, 659–667.

Muckel, D. S., and Minns, R. J. (1990). Biological response to woven carbon fibre pads in the knee, *J. Bone Jt. Surg., 72-B*, 60–62.

Naguchi, T., Yamamuro, T., Oka, M., Kumar, P., Kotoura, Y., Suong-Hyu, H., and Ikada, Y. (1991). Poly(vinyl alcohol) hydrogel as an artificial articular cartilage: Evaluation of biocompatibility, *J. Appl. Biomater., 2*, 101–107.

Nelson, J. W., Stanford, H. G., and Cutright, D. E. (1977). Evaluation and comparisons of biodegradable substances as osteogenic agents, *Oral Surg., Oral Med., Oral Pathol., 43*, 836–843.

Newman, S. A., and Frisch, H. L. (1979). Dynamic of skeletal pattern formation in developing chick limb, *Science, 205*, 662–668.

O'Driscoll, S. W., Keeley, F. W., and Salter, R. B. (1986). The chondrogenic potential of free autogenous periosteal grafts for biological resurfacing of major full-thickness defects in joint surfaces under the influence of continuous passive motion, *J. Bone Jt. Surg., 68-A*, 1017–1035.

Pennypacker, J. P., Hassell, J. R., Yamada, K. M., and Pratt, R. M. (1979). The influence of an adhesive cell surface protein on chondrogenic expression *in vitro, Exp. Cell Res., 121*, 411–415.

Pitman, M. I., Menche, D., Song, E.-K., Ben-Yishay, A., Gilbert, D., and Grande, D. A. (1989). The use of adhesives in chondrocyte transplantation surgery: *In vivo* studies, *Bull. Hosp. Joint. Dis. Orthop. Inst., 49*, 213–220.

Postlethwaite, A. E. (1978). Chemotactic attraction of human fibroblasts to type I, II, III collagens and collagen-derived peptides, *Proc. Natl. Acad. Sci., USA, 75*, 871–875.

Reddi, A. H. (1985). Implant-stimulated interface reactions during collagenous bone matrix-induced bone formation, *J. Biomed. Mater. Res., 19*, 233–239.

Robinson, D., Halperin, N., and Nevo, Z. (1991). Long-term follow-up of the fate of xenogeneic transplants of chondrocytes implanted into joint surfaces, *Transplantation, 51*, 380–383.

Robinson, D., Efrat, M., and Mendes, D. G. (1993). Implants composed of carbon fiber mesh and bone-marrow derived chondrocyte-enriched cultures for joint surface reconstruction, *Bull. Hosp. Jt. Dis., 53*, 75–82.

Sallgaller, M. L., and Bajpai, P. K. (1984). In *Proceedings of Second World Congress on Biomaterials*, Washington, DC, p. 194.

Silverstein, M. E., and Chvapil, M. (1981). Experimental and clinical experiences with collagen fleece as a hemostatic agent, *J. Trauma, 21*, 388–393.

Speer, D. P. (1979). Collagenous architecture of growth cartilage, perichondrial ossification groove, and perichondrial ring, *Trans. Orthop. Res. Soc., 4*, 220.

Speer, D. P. (1981). The pathogenesis of amputation stump overgrowth, *Clin. Orthop. Rel. Res., 159*, 294–307.

Speer, D. P. (1982a). Collagenous architecture of loose bodies and osteophytes: Neogenesis of articular cartilage, *Trans. Orthop. Res. Soc., 7*, 213.

Speer, D. P. (1982b). Collagenous architecture of the growth plate and perichondrial ossification groove, *J. Bone Jt. Surg., 64A*, 399–407.

Speer, D. P. (1984). Early pathogenesis of hemophilic arthropathy. Evolution of the subchondral cyst, *Clin. Orthop. Rel. Res., 185*, 250–265.

Speer, D. P., Chvapil, M., Volz, R. G., and Holmes, M. D. (1979). Enhancement of healing in osteochondral defects by collagen sponge implants, *Clin. Orthop., 144*, 326–335.

Speer, D. P., Chvapil, M., Eskelson, C. D., and Ulreich, J. (1980). Biological effects of residual glutaraldehyde in glutaraldehyde-tanned collagen biomaterials, *J. Biomed. Mater. Res., 14*, 753–764.

Speer, D. P., and Dahners, L. (1979). The collagenous architecture of articular cartilage, *Clin. Orthop., 139*, 267–275.

Speer, D. P., Peltier, L. F., and Chvapil, M. (1981). Synthetic bone graft for clinical use: Comparison of calcium sulfate and collagen sponge, *Trans. Orthop. Res. Soc., 6*, 111.

Staines, N. A., Hardingham, T., Smith, M., and Henderson, O. (1981). Collagen-induced arthritis in the rat: Modification of immune and arthritic responses by free collagen and immune anti-collagen antiserum, *Immunology, 44*, 737–744.

Steven, F. S. (1976). Polymeric collagen fibrils: An example of substrate-mediated steric obstruction of enzymic digestion, *Biochim. Biophys. Acta, 452*, 151–160.

Sung, J. M., and Kim, J. M. (1990). Histological changes of autotransplanted meniscus into articular cartilage defect, *J. Cathol. Med. Coll., 43*, 123–130.

Trentham, D. E. (1982). Collagen arthritis as a relevant model for rheumatoid arthritis: Evidence pro and con, *Arth. Rheum., 25*, 911–916.

Tsai, C. L., Liu, T. K., and Fu, S. L. (1992). Preliminary study of cartilage repair with autologous periosteum and fibrin adhesive system, *J. Formosan Med. Assoc., 91*(Suppl. 3), S239–S245.

Ulreich, J. B. (1990). Collagen matrices for culture of differentiated chondrocytes, *Trans. First Congress Asian–Pacific Organization for Cell Biology*, p. 315.

Ulreich, J. B., and Chvapil, M. (1981). A quantitative microassay for *in vitro* toxicity testing of biomaterials, *J. Biomed. Mater. Res., 15*, 913–922.

Ulreich, J. B., and Chvapil, M. (1983). *In vitro* toxicity testing: A quantitative microassay, in *Cell Culture Test Methods* (D. S. Brown, ed.), American Society for Testing and Materials, Philadelphia, PA, pp. 102–112.

Ulreich, J. B., Frankel, E. S., Chungi, V., and Purkait, B. (1991). ELISA for detection of serum antibodies to insoluble collagen/gelatin, *Trans. 17th Annual Mtg., Soc. Biomater.*, XIV, p. 234.

Ulreich, J. B., Holubec, H., Chvapil, M., and Speer, D. P. (1986). Chondrocytes maintain their phenotype when cultured on a three dimensional collagen matrix, *J. Cell Biol., 103*, 105a.

Ulreich, J. B., Holubec, H., Chvapil, M., and Speer, D. P. (1987). Collagen sponge—A three dimensional matrix for *in vitro* chondrocyte culture, in *Development and Diseases of Cartilage and Bone Matrix* (A. Sen and T. Thornhill, eds.), Alan R. Liss, New York, pp 107–113.

Ulreich, J. B., Paicius, R. M., Chvapil, M., and Speer, D. P. (1985). Chondronectin treated collagen sponge enhances osteochondral defect resurfacing, *J. Cell Biol., 101*, 96a.

Ulreich, J. B., and Snider, B. J. (1992). The effect of partial hydrolysis of insoluble collagen/gelatin biomaterials on ELISA analysis of antibodies, *Trans. 18th Annual Mtg., Soc. Biomater.*, XV, p. 585.

Urist, M. R. (1980). Bone transplants and implants, in *Fundamental and Clinical Bone Physiology* (M. R. Urist, ed.), JB Lippincott, Philadelphia, pp. 331–368,

Vacanti, C. A., Langer, R., Schloo, B., and Vacanti, J. P. (1991). Synthetic polymers seeded with chondrocytes provide a template for new cartilage formation, *Plas. Reconstr. Surg., 88*, 753–759.

Vacanti, C. A., Kim, W., Upton, J., Vacanti, M. P., Mooney, D., Schloo, B., and Vacanti, J. P. (1993). Tissue-engineered growth of bone and cartilage, *Transplant. Proc., 25*, 1019–1021.

Vachon, A. M., McIlwraith, C. W., Powers, B. E., McFadden, P. R., and Amiel, D. (1992). Morphologic and biochemical study of sternal cartilage autografts for resurfacing induced osteochondral defects in horses, *Am. J. Vet. Res., 53*, 1038–1047.

Vater, C. A., Harris, E. D., and Siegel, R. C. (1979). Native cross-links in collagen fibrils induce resistance to human synovial collagenase, *Biochemistry, 181*, 639–645.

Vetter, U., Helbing, G., Heit, W., Pirsig, W., and Sterzig, K. (1985). Clonal proliferation and cell density of chondrocytes isolated from human fetal epiphyseal, human adult articular and nasal septal cartilage. Influence of hormones and growth factors, *Growth, 49*, 229–245.

Wedge, J. H., Powell, J. N., Ulmer, B. G., and Reynolds, R. (1986). Biodegradable resurfacing of the hip in dogs, *Clin. Orthop., 208*, 76–80.

Weiss, R. E., and Reddi, A. H. (1980). Synthesis and localization of fibronectin during collagenous matrix–mesenchymal cell interaction and differentiation of cartilage and bone *in vivo*, *Proc. Natl. Acad. Sci. USA, 77*, 2074–2078.

Winter, G. D. (1973). Studies, using sponge implants, on the mechanism of osteogenesis, in *Biology of Fibroblasts* (E. Kulonen and J. Pikkarainen, eds.), Academic Press, pp. 103–105.

Yablon, I. G., Brandt, K. D., Delellis, R., and Covall, D. (1977). Destruction of joint homografts, *Arthritis and Rheumatism, 20*, 1526–1537.

Yablon, I. G., and Shirahama, T. (1982). *Orthopedics, 5*, 859–864.

27

Materials-Based Cell Differentiation: Osteoblastic Phenotype Expression on Bioactive Materials

Hajime Ohgushi, Motoaki Okumura, Yoshiko Dohi,
Susumu Tamai, and Shiro Tabata
Nara Medical University
Kashihara City, Nara, Japan

I. INTRODUCTION

Owen reported that there are two main cellular systems in the marrow cell population: hemopoietic stem cells and stromal stem cells, which are believed to differentiate into fibroblasts, adipocytes, reticular cells, and osteogenic cells [1]. A chemically bonded interface develops between calcium phosphate ceramics and bone [2]; and thus the ceramics are called *bioactive* [3]. We reevaluated the osteogenic differentiation of the marrow stromal stem cells in porous calcium phosphate ceramics to address the bone-bonding properties. The ceramics themselves did not produce bone formation in ectopic (intramuscular or subcutaneous) sites, whereas composites of the ceramics and marrow cells resulted in bone formation in the pore areas of the ceramics [4–9]. The bone formation process was intramembranous bone formation (cartilage did not appear) [4,5] and the bone attached directly to the ceramic surface without fibrous tissue interposition [7,8]. Thus bone formed in porous hydroxyapatite was viable and the bone–hydroxyapatite (HA) interface was stable even after 1 year postimplantation [9]. The osteogenic composite of marrow cells and porous calcium phosphate ceramics is able to show healing potential when applied in massive bone defects [10–12]. Interestingly, not only rat marrow cells but fresh and *in vitro* cultured human marrow cells showed osteogenic response in the bioactive porous hydroxyapatite ceramics [13,14]. These results were obtained using bioactive calcium phosphate ceramics; however, when we used nonbioactive materials, the bone formation was not consistent and the formation always started away from the material surface, resulting in fibrous tissue formation between the materials and thus formed bone [15–17]. All of these findings indicate the usefulness of our experimental protocol using subcutaneous implantation of a composite of porous materials and bone marrow cells to distinguish bioactive materials from nonbioactive materials. In this chapter, we describe the osteogenic composite of marrow cells and porous materials (especially bioactive hydroxyapatite) from the viewpoint of the biological reaction around the subcutaneously implanted materials, using biochemical and molecular biological approaches.

II. MATERIALS AND METHODS

A. Materials

The following materials were used in this study:

1. Kiel bone [15]: Partially deproteinized calf cancellous bone produced by Braun Melsungen, Germany.
2. True bone ceramic (TBC) [15] produced by Koken Co., Tokyo, Japan: Calf bone was treated in sodium hydroxide and hydrogen peroxide, then was sintered at 1450°C for 3–5 h.
3. Porous hydroxyapatite (HA) produced by Interpore International, Irvine, CA [18,19]: This material had macroporous architecture (pore volume of 50–60% and fully interconnected pores, measuring 190–230 μm in diameter). It was cut into disks, 5 mm in diameter and 2 mm thick.

B. Marrow Cell Preparation and Surgical Procedure

Detailed procedures for marrow cell preparation have been given previously [4–7]. Briefly, femurs and tibiae of five Fischer rats (male, 8 weeks old) were recovered and each diaphyseal portion was isolated by dissection. The marrow plugs from the diaphysis were then hydrostatically forced into a 2-ml centrifuge tube containing heparinized phosphate-buffered saline (PBS). The marrow was disaggregated by sequential passage through 18-G and then 20-G needles. It was centrifuged ($250 \times g$, 10 min) and the fat layer was removed to leave 200 μl of clear supernatant, then the tube containing the cell layer and 200 μl of the supernatant was disaggregated by vortex mixing. The porous materials were soaked in the disaggregated marrow cell suspension.

Syngeneic Fischer rats (8 weeks old) were anesthetized by intramuscular injection of pentobarbital (Nembutal, 3.5 mg/100 g BW) following light ether inhalation. For transplantation, four incisions (5 mm) were made on the back of the rat. Subcutaneous pouches were created by blunt dissection. Four materials were implanted: two without marrow and two with marrow (materials soaked in the disaggregated marrow suspension).

C. Northern Blot Analysis

After homogenization of the harvested implants, the guanidine isothiocyanate/cesium chloride density gradient method was used for preparation of total RNA. Total RNA from cancellous bone and bone marrow from 8-week-old rats was also prepared by this method. The denatured total RNA (10 μg) in 4-mm narrow slots was separated by electrophoresis with 1.1% agarose–formaldehyde gel and transferred to a nylon membrane (Immobilon N, Millipore Ltd., Japan). Prehybridization and hybridization of the blots with a ^{32}P-cDNA probe were carried out at 68°C in QuickHyb™ solution (Stratagene, CA, USA) for 20 and 120 min, respectively. Posthybridization washes in 2 × SSC, 0.1% SDS at room temperature and in 0.1 × SSC, 0.1% SDS at 60°C were performed. The membrane was exposed to Kodak X-Omat™ film (Eastman Kodak Co., Rochester, NY) at −80°C for 24 h with an intensifying screen.

D. DNA Probe for BGP

A complemental DNA probe for rat bone specific γ-carboxyglutamic acid protein (BGP, or osteocalcin) (363 base-pair Eco RI fragment of plasmid constructed from pUC 8) was kindly provided by Dr. P. A. Price. The DNA probe was labeled with ^{32}P by using a multirandom primer labeling kit (Amersham, Japan) and [α^{32}P]dCTP and used for the Northern blots. The cDNA was also inserted into pSP6/T7 plasmid DNA having SP6 and T7 promoters, then complemental RNA to the BGP cDNA was synthesized *in vitro* by SP6 RNA polymerase and used as a reference to quantify RNAs in Northern blot analysis. Using the synthesized RNA and radiolabeled 363 base-pair BGP cDNA, we found that at least 1 pg of the RNA could be detected using the Northern blotting.

E. DNA Probe for Alkaline Phosphatase (Cloning of Rat ALP cDNA)

Oligonucleotide primers corresponding to the regions of Leu^{-4}–Glu^4 and Glu^{325}–Leu^{332} of rat alkaline phosphatase (ALP) [20] were synthesized by a DNA synthesizer. These primers were used to amplify 1 kbp ALP DNA segment by polymerase chain reaction (PCR) as described later. Some original bases were changed to be cleaved by restriction enzymes of Eco RI and Hind III. The base changes were done because we intended to insert the amplified DNA into plasmid pcDNAII having multiple cloning sites (Eco RI, Hind III, etc.). Messenger RNA was purified from total rat cancellous bone RNA by oligo-dT immobilized latex beads and used for synthesizing a rat cancellous bone cDNA library by reverse transcriptase. The oligonucleotide primers for alkaline phosphatase and the rat cancellous bone cDNA library were then used to amplify a alkaline phosphatase cDNA probe corresponding to the region of Leu^{-4}–Leu^{332} by PCR. The amplified ALP cDNA was purified by agarose gel electrophoresis and digested with both Eco RI and Hind III, and then ligated to plasmid DNA (pcDNAII; 3 kbp length) having the multiple cloning sites in the LacZ DNA region. The ligated DNA was transformed into a competent cell (*E. coli* JM109, Toyobo, Japan) and cloned cells carrying the DNA were selected from the white colony (blue/white selection). Plasmid DNA extracted from the white colony showed 4 kbp length determined by agarose gel electrophoresis, and that from the blue colony showed 3 kbp length. Digestion of the DNA from the white colony with Eco RI and Hind III resulted in two DNA fragments of 3 kbp and 1 kbp, whereas the digestion of plasmid DNA from the blue colony did not affect the length of the DNA. Therefore, the restriction fragment pattern indicated that ALP cDNA(1 kbp) was inserted into the plasmid DNA (Fig. 1). To confirm this insertion, DNA sequencing was done using DNA sequencer (DSQ-1NE, Shimadzu, Japan). The DNA sequence determined by the DNA sequencer coincided with the DNA sequence of reported ALP DNA sequence except for the DNA region that we modified to be digested by Eco RI and Hind III restriction enzymes.

F. Histological Evaluation

For decalcified histological sections, the harvested implants were fixed in 10% buffered formalin and decalcified (K-CX solution, Falma Co., Tokyo) for about 16 h. Embedding was done in paraffin and the samples were cut parallel to the round face of the implant, stained with Hematoxyline and Eosin. For undecalcified sections, the implants were embedded in methylmethacrylate and cut into sections of 7 μm using a Jung Model K microtome. For scanning electron microscopy–electron probe microanalysis (SEM–

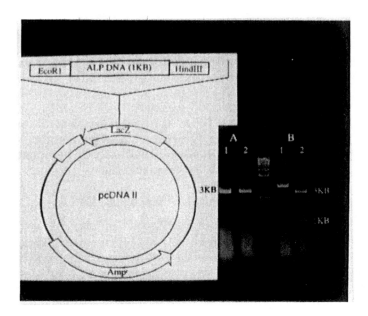

Figure 1   The amplified 1 kbp ALP cDNA having Eco RI and Hind III sites was ligated to plasmid DNA (pcDNAII; 3 kbp length). The plasmid DNA has multiple cloning sites in the LacZ region. The ligated DNA was transformed into a competent cell and cloned cells carrying the cDNA were selected from the white colony (blue/white selection). Plasmid DNA extracted from the white colony (lane B1) showed 4 kbp length determined by agarose gel electrophoresis, and that from the blue colony showed 3 kbp length (lanes A1 and A2). Digestion of the DNA from the white colony with Eco RI and Hind III resulted in two DNA fragments of 3 kbp and 1 kbp (lane B2), whereas digestion of plasmid DNA from the blue colony did not affect the length of the DNA (lane A2). Therefore, the restriction fragment pattern indicated that ALP cDNA (1 kbp) was inserted into the plasmid pc DNA II.

EPMA), the flat surface of the implant embedded in methylmethacrylate was prepared after surface coating with a thin layer of carbon. Details of these undecalcified section and SEM–EPMA analysis were presented previously [17,18].

III.   RESULTS AND DISCUSSION

Kiel bone (partially deproteinized bone substitute prepared from cancellous bone) has been used as a bone graft substitute in orthopedic surgery, and Salama et al. reported the usefulness of a composite of the patient's bone marrow and Kiel bone for the treatment of fractures and bone tumors [21].

Using our rat model, we combined the Kiel bone with rat marrow cells and implanted the composite subcutaneously. As shown in Fig. 2, some implants showed *de novo* bone formation in the pore regions of Kiel bone. However, appearance of the bone formation was not consistent when compared with bone formed in porous hydroxyapatite, and fibrous tissue interposition was seen between the newly formed bone and the surface of Kiel bone. Thus so-called distance osteogenesis (a characteristic feature of biotolerant implants concerning the bone dynamics) was detected in the composite of marrow cells and Kiel bone [15]. Therefore, Kiel bone is not a beneficial material for bone graft

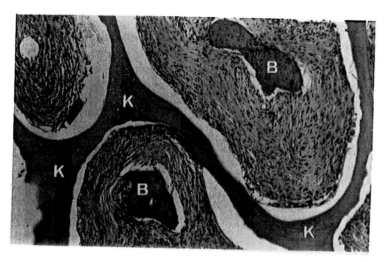

Figure 2 Kiel bone combined with marrow cells 4 weeks after subcutaneous implantation. Connective tissue interposition between Kiel bone (K) and newly formed bone (B) is found. Kiel bone having empty lacunae is easily distinguishable from the newly formed bone. H-E stain, ×100. (From Ref. 15.)

substitutes. Kiel bone contains calf-derived protein, which may cause a foreign-body reaction or an immunological reaction resulting in the distance osteogenesis. We can eliminate the protein moiety present in bone by a sintering procedure, resulting in the crystallization of bone minerals as hydroxyapatite, and such products made from calf bone are now commercially available (true bone ceramics—TBC, Koken Co., Tokyo, Japan). When TBC was combined with marrow cells and implanted subcutaneously, *de novo* bone formation was consistently seen, and as shown in Fig. 3, the backscattered

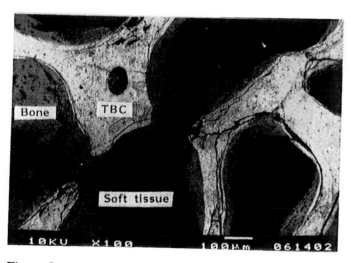

Figure 3 Backscattered electron image photograph of TBC with marrow cells 6 weeks after implantation. (From Ref. 15.)

electron image showed no intervening fibrous tissue between newly formed bone and TBC [15]. The appearance of the many cracks seen in the Fig. 3 was probably caused by the tissue preparation procedure; and interestingly, almost all cracks were not at the TBC–bone interface but in the TBC itself, thus firm bonding of the bone to TBC was suspected. The firm bonding was confirmed by continuous high levels of calcium and phosphorus content across the bone–TBC interface (Fig. 4). Also, bone dynamic experiments showed that the bone formation started on the surface of the TBC and progressed to the center of the pore regions, thus so-called bonding osteogenesis (a characteristic feature of bioactive implants) was seen [7,22]. Although the two implants (Kiel bone and TBC) were derived from calf cancellous bone (i.e., these implants have the same architecture of macroporosity and interconnection of the pores), these showed totally different bone formation processes in regard to bone dynamics; that is, Kiel bone is a biotolerant material whereas TBC is a bioactive material.

These results show that our subcutaneous implantation of a porous materials–marrow cell composite can clarify the material's properties regarding bone bioactivity. Another example is provided by our implantation of a composite of marrow cells and porous alumina ceramics, which are known to be bioinert materials; in that case, bone formation appeared away from the ceramic surface in the porous regions and proceeded bidirectionally both to the surface of the alumina and to the center of the pores [16,17]. Therefore, as seen in the newly formed bone in Kiel bone, the bone formation did not start on the implant surface; however hydroxyapatite coating on the alumina ceramics showed bone formation, which started on the surface of hydroxyapatite coated surface.

All of these results indicate the importance of hydroxyapatite surface in eliciting the firm bonding of the *de novo* bone to the material's surface. The bone marrow cell derived bone formation starts on the surface of hydroxyapatite at about 3 weeks postimplantation

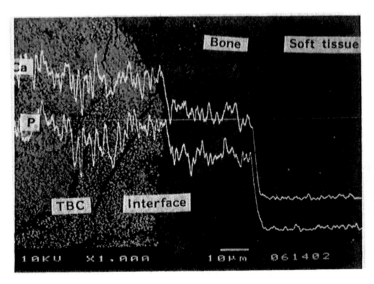

Figure 4   Higher magnification of Fig. 3. The pathway of the electron beam is indicated by the center white line. Simultaneous line analysis is shown by the upper (calcium, Ca) and lower (phosphorus, P) wave lines.

and the bone formation seems to be through the cascade of osteoblastic differentiation. As shown in Fig. 5, fibroblastic cells (undifferentiated cells) adhere on the hydroxyapatite surface, expand (preosteoblasts), and finally become cuboid- or polygonal-shaped cells (active osteoblasts) making bone matrix on the surface of hydroxyapatite. As we impregnated marrow cells in porous ceramics, our experimental model used an undifferentiated cell population (the term *undifferentiation* is used concerning the osteogenic phenotype) to evoke bone formation. Thus, histological findings of the osteoblasts *per se* imply osteogenic differentiation.

The differentiation was confirmed by biochemical and molecular biological findings. As shown in Fig. 6, biochemical analysis of ALP activities and BGP contents in the composite of marrow cells and porous hydroxyapatite showed that ALP began to appear at 2 weeks postimplantation, and that BGP began to appear at 3 weeks postimplantation, coinciding with the appearance of *de novo* bone, and BGP content increased thereafter [23,24]. In contrast, only traces of ALP and BGP could be detected in porous hydroxyapatite implants without marrow, which did not show bone formation. Though ALP is not specific for bone tissue, it is well known that osteoblasts show high ALP activity. BGP is one of the most abundant noncollagenous matrix proteins found in calcified tissues (bone and dentin) and is synthesized exclusively by osteoblasts [25,26]. Therefore, these biochemical data present the osteoblastic phenotype expression in the composite of marrow cells and porous hydroxyapatite ceramics. Further confirmation of the differentiation was done by a molecular biological approach (Northern blot analysis). Total RNAs were extracted from subcutaneously implanted porous hydroxyapatite with or without marrow cells, electrophoresed, and then transferred to a nylon membrane. The RNAs on the membrane were hybridized with ^{32}P-labeled ALP and BGP cDNAs to detect the

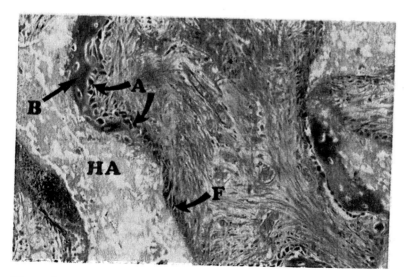

Figure 5   Bone formation on the surface of hydroxyapatite (HA). Decalcified section of marrow-hydroxyapatite composite at 3 weeks post implantation. Fibroblastic cells (F; undifferentiated cells) adhere on the hydroxyapatite surface, the cells expand (preosteoblasts), and finally become cuboid- or polygonal-shaped cells (A; active osteoblasts) making bone (B) on the surface of hydroxyapatite.

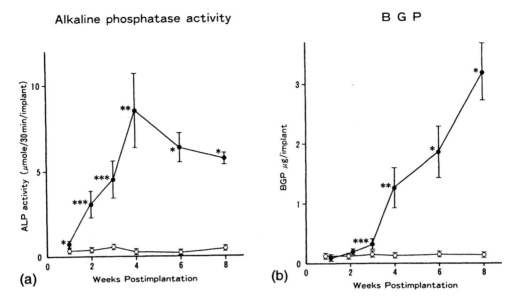

Figure 6 (a) Changes in ALP activity in hydroxyapatite ceramics after subcutaneous implantation. The activity in control (without marrow) ceramics, (open circles); and activity in ceramics with marrow cells, (closed circles). (From Ref. 23.) (b) Changes in BGP contents in ceramics after subcutaneous implantation. The contents in control (without marrow) ceramics, (open circles); and the contents in ceramics with marrow cells, (closed circles). (From Ref. 23.)

signals (mRNAS) of ALP and BGP genes. As shown in Fig. 7, these signals were clearly detected in the composite after 2 weeks subcutaneous implantation, whereas these signals were not detected in the hydroxyapatite implantation without marrow [27,28]. Again, these findings of Northern blot analysis confirm the osteoblastic differentiation in the composites.

    These results indicate the importance of the hydroxyapatite surface for differentiation of marrow stromal stem cells. Interestingly, other calcium phosphate materials such as β-tricalcium phosphate (TCP) [5,24] and HA/TCP composite [4] and calcium carbonate [29,30] also can support the osteoblastic differentiation on their surface. Though the mechanisms are not clear, we speculate that binding of biologically active molecules to the ceramic surface can activate the cell membrane receptors of stromal stem cells, resulting in the osteoblastic differentiation. This speculation is based on our recent findings of *in vitro* binding experiments using ^{125}I-labeled BGP. The experiments showed that extensive radioactivity was detected on the bioactive ceramic surface, whereas only a trace of the radioactivity was detected on the nonbioactive alumina surface, which cannot support osteoblastic differentiation of marrow cells [30]. Many workers have reported [3,31–34] that the surface of bioactive materials undergoes dissolution and precipitation from the biological fluids, resulting in carbonate apatite crystal formation on the surface. These phenomena on the surface of glass ceramics and calcium phosphate ceramics were well documented. And, recently, similar carbonate apatite formation on the surface of calcium carbonate (skeleton of marine coral) was reported [34]. The calcium carbonate (coral) was exactly the same material we used for subcutaneous implantation with mar-

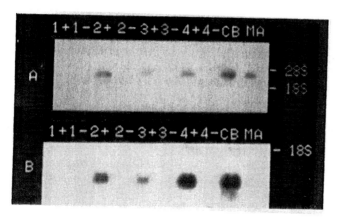

Figure 7   Northern blot analysis of mRNAs for alkaline phosphatase (A) and for bone Gla protein (B). Total RNA was extracted from HA without marrow (−) and HA with marrow (+) 1 to 4 weeks post-subcutaneous implantation. Numbers indicate the term of implantation. (e.g., 2+ means HA with marrow harvested at 2 weeks post-implantation). Total RNA was also extracted from marrow (MA) and cancellous bone (CB). These denatured RNAs (10 μg) were electrophoresed, stained with ethidium bromide, and transferred to a nylon membrane. Autoradiograms of Northern blots using ^{32}P-labeled cDNA probes of alkaline phosphatase (A) and bone Gla protein (B) are seen. Electrophoretic positions of 28S and 18S ribosomal RNAs are indicated as 28S and 18S, respectively.

row cells and was found to be categorized as a bioactive material [29]. Therefore, one conceivable mechanism of the bone bonding is that consolidation of the biological molecules on/in the carbonate apatite crystal triggers the cell differentiation and that epitaxy finally occurs between bone crystals produced by the differentiated osteoblasts and the apatite crystals formed on bioactive materials.

IV. CONCLUDING REMARKS

All of these results demonstrate that the surface of bioactive materials supports *de novo* bone formation by osteoblastic differentiation of marrow cells. The surface of biotolerant and bioinert materials, on the other hand, cannot support the differentiation. Therefore, we suppose that bioactive materials have the capability to differentiate a cell and cause the expression of its specific phenotype on the material surface. Such cellular events finally result in the integration of the material with surrounding new tissue.

ACKNOWLEDGMENTS

We wish to express our gratitude to Dr. Edwin C. Shors (Interpore International Corporation) for supplying the porous hydroxyapatite (Interpore 200), and Dr. Paul A. Price (University of California) for providing the DNA probe of rat BGP (Eco RI fragment of plasmid constructed from pUC 8). We also thank our colleagues at the Department of Orthopedics, Nara Medical University: Drs. T. Yoshikawa, K. Inoue, and N. Senpuku.

REFERENCES

1. Owen, M., Lineage of osteogenic cells and their relationship to the stromal system, in *Bone and Mineral Research*, Vol. 3 (W. A. Peck, ed.), Elsevier, 1985, pp. 1–25.

2. Jarcho, M., Calcium phosphate ceramics as hard tissue prosthetics, *Clin. Orthop., 157,* 259–278 (1981).

3. Hench, L. L., Surface reaction kinetics and adsorption of biological moieties, in *The Bone-Biomaterial Interface* (J. E. Davies, ed.), University of Toronto Press, 1991, pp. 33–48.

4. Ohgushi, H., Goldberg, V. M., and Caplan, A. I., Heterotopic osteogenesis in porous ceramic induced by marrow cells, *J. Orthop. Res., 7,* 568–578 (1989).

5. Ohgushi, H., Okumura, M., Tamai, S., and Shors, E., Marrow cell induced osteogenesis in porous hydroxyapatite and tricalcium phosphate, *J. Biomed. Mater. Res., 24,* 1563–1570 (1990).

6. Ohgushi, H., Okumura, M., Masuhara, K., Goldberg, V. M., Davy, D., and Caplan, A. I., Osteogenic potential of bone marrow sustained by porous calcium phosphate ceramics, in *Handbook of Bioactive Ceramics*, Vol. 2 (T. Yamamuro, L. L. Hench, and J. W. Hench, eds.), CRC Press, Boca Raton, FL, 1990, pp. 229–234.

7. Okumura, M., Ohgushi, H., and Tamai, S., Bonding osteogenesis in coralline hydroxyapatite combined with bone marrow cells, *Biomaterials, 12,* 411–416 (1991).

8. Okumura, M., Ohgushi, H., Tamai, S., and Shors, E. C., Primary bone formation in porous hydroxyapatite ceramic: A light and scanning electron microscopic study, *Cells Mater., 1,* 29–34 (1991).

9. Okumura, M., Ohgushi, H., Yoshikawa, T., and Tamai, S., Heterotopic osteogenesis in coralline hydroxyapatite induced by bone marrow cells, in *Ceramic in Substitutive and Reconstructive Surgery* (P. Viencenzini, ed.), Elsevier, 1991, pp. 353–361.

10. Ohgushi, H., Goldberg, V. M., and Caplan, A. I., Repair of bone defects with marrow and porous ceramic. Experiments in rats, *Acta Orthop. Scand., 60,* 334–339 (1989).

11. Ohgushi, H., Okumura, M., Masuhara, K., Goldberg, V. M., Davy, T., and Caplan, A. I., Calcium phosphate block ceramic with bone marow cells improves repair in a rat long bone defect, in *Handbook of Bioactive Ceramics*, Vol. 2 (T. Yamamuro, L. L. Hench, and J. W. Hench, eds.), CRC Press, Boca Raton, FL, 1990, pp. 235–238.

12. Ohgushi, H., Siomi, S., Simaya, M., Okumura, M., and Tamai, S., Treatment of depression fractures using composite of bone marrow cells and porous hydroxyapatite, in *Apatite*, Vol. 1 (H. Aoki, M. Akao, N. Nagai, and T. Tsuji, eds.), Japanese Association of Apatite Science, 1992, pp. 421–426.

13. Ohgushi, H., and Okumura, M., Osteogenic ability of rat and human marrow cells in porous ceramics, *Acta Orthop. Scand., 6*(5), 431–434 (1990).

14. Ohgushi, H., Okumura, M., Miyauchi, Y., Mii, Y., and Tamai, S., Composite grafts of human bone marrow cells and porous ceramics, in *Bioceramics*, Vol. 3 (J. E. Hulbert and S. F. Hulbert, eds.), Rose-Hulman Institute of Technology, 1992, pp. 279–286.

15. Okumura, M., Ohgushi, H., Yoshikawa, T., and Tamai, S., Heterotopic ossification in sintered bone ceramics and Kiel bone by using bone marrow, in *Bioceramics*, Vol. 2 (G. Heimke, ed.), German Ceramic Society, 1990, pp. 65–70.

16. Okumura, M., Van Blitterswijk, C. A., Koerten, H. K., and Ohgushi, H., Osteogenic response of rat bone marrow cells in porous alumina, in *Bioceramics*, Vol. 4 (W. Bonefield, W. Hastings, and K. E. Tanner, eds.), Butterworth-Heinemann, 1991, pp. 3–8.

17. Okumura, M., Ohgushi, H., Takakura, V., van Blitterswijk, C. A., and Koerten, H. K., Analysis of primary bone formation in porous alumina, *Bio-Med. Mater. Eng., 2,* 191–201 (1992).

18. White, E. W., and Shors, E. C., Biomaterial aspects of Interpore-200 porous hydroxyapatite, *Dent. Clin. N. Am., 30,* 49–67 (1986).

19. Shors, E. C., White, E. W., and Kopchok, G., Biocompatibility, osteoconduction and biodegradation of porous hydroxyapatite, tricalcium phosphate, sintered hydroxyapatite and calcium carbonate in rabbit bone defects, *Mater. Res. Soc. Symp. Proc., 110*, 211–218 (1989).

20. Misumi, V., Tashiro, K., Hattori, M., Sakaki, Y., and Ikehara, Y., Primary structure of rat liver alkaline phosphatase deduced from its cDNA, *Biochem. J., 249*, 661–668 (1988).

21. Salama, R., Burwell, R. G., and Dickson, I. R., Recombined grafts of bone and marrow, *J. Bone Jt. Surg., 55B*, 402–417 (1973).

22. Osborn, J. F., and Newsely, H., Bonding osteogenesis induced by calcium phosphate ceramic implants, in *Biomaterials 1980* (G. D. Winter, D. F. Gibbons, and H. Plenk, eds.), Wiley and Sons, 1982, pp. 51–58.

23. Yoshikawa, T., Ohgushi, H., Okumura, M., Tamai, S., Dohi, Y., and Moriyama, T., Biochemical and histoligigal sequences of membranous ossification in ectopic site, *Calcified Tissue Int., 50*, 184–188 (1992).

24. Yoshikawa, T., Ohgushi, H., Okumura, M., Tamai, S., Dohi, Y., and Moriyama, T., Biochemical sequence of bone formation in porous ceramics, in *Bioceramics*, Vol. 3 (J. E. Hulbert and S. F. Hulbert, eds.), Rose–Hulman Institute of Technology, 1992, pp. 157–162.

25. Price, P. A., Parthemore, J. G., and Detos, L. J., New biochemical marker for bone metabolism, *J. Clin. Invest., 66*, 878–883 (1980).

26. Price, P. A., Lothringer, J. W., Baukol, S. A., and Reddi, A. H., Developmental appearance of the vitamine K-dependent protein of bone during calcification: Analysis of mineralizing tissues in human calf and rat, *J. Biol. Chem, 256*, 3781–3784 (1981).

27. Ohgushi, H., Okumura, M., Yoshikawa, T., Inoue, K., Senpuku, N., and Tamai, S., Bone formation process in porous calcium carbonate and hydroxyapatite, *J. Biomed. Mater. Res., 26*, 885–896 (1992).

28. Ohgushi, H., Okumura, M., Yoshikawa, T., Senpuku, N., Inoue, K., and Tamai, S., Osteogenic capacity of hydroxyapatite coated porous calcium carbonate implants, in *Bioceramics*, Vol. 4 (W. Bonefield, W. Hastings, and K. E. Tanner, eds.), Butterworth–Heinemann, 1991, pp. 213–219.

29. Ohgushi, H., Okumura, M., Yoshikawa, T., Tamai, S., Tabata, S., and Dohi, Y., Regulation of bone development and the relationship to bioactivity: Osteoblastic phenotype expression of marrow stromal stem cells on the surface of bioactive materials, in *Bone-Bonding Biomaterials* (P. Ducheyne, T. Kokubo, and van Blitterswijk, eds.), Reed Healthcare Comm. Publ., The Netherlands, 1992, pp. 47–56.

30. Ohgushi, H., Dohi, Y., Tamai, S., and Tabata, S., Osteogenic differentiation of marrow stromal stem cells in porous hydroxyapatite ceramics, *J. Biomed. Mater. Res., 27*, 1401–1407 (1993).

31. LeGeros, R. G., Orly, I., Gregoire, M., and Daculsi, G., Substrate surface dissolution and interfacial biological mineralization, in *The Bone–Biomaterial Interface* (J. E. Davies, ed.), University of Toronto Press, 1991, pp. 76–88.

32. Kokubo, T., Ito, S., Huang, Z., Hayashi, T., Sakka, S., Kitsugi, T., and Yamamuro, I., Ca,P-rich layer formed on high-strength bioactive glass-ceramic A-W, *J. Biomed. Mater. Res., 24*, 331–343 (1990).

33. Radin, S. R., and Ducheyne, P., The effect of calcium phosphate ceramic composition and structure on *in vitro* behavior, *J. Biomed. Mater. Res., 27*, 35–45, 1993.

34. Ducheyne, P., Radin, S., and Ishikawa, K., The rate of calcium phosphate precipitation on metal and ceramics, and the relationship to bioactivity, in *Bone-Bonding Biomaterials*, (P. Ducheyne, T. Kokubo, and van Blitterswijk, eds.), Reed Healthcare Comm. Publ., The Netherlands, 1992, pp. 213–218.

28
Biology of Aseptic Loosening of the Cemented Arthroplasty

Sheila M. Algan and Stephen M. Horowitz
Hospital of the University of Pennsylvania
Philadelphia, Pennsylvania

I. INTRODUCTION

Aseptic loosening is defined as the failure of the bond between an implant and bone in the absence of infection. Prosthetic joint replacement is widely considered to be one of the most important contributions of orthopedics to society. Unfortunately, in large series of cemented hip replacements, the incidence of failure from aseptic loosening usually ranges from 10% to 30% at 15 years and then becomes dramatically worse. Because between 100 and 200 thousand hip replacements are performed each year in the United States, this represents a serious and commonly occurring health problem. It is so common that it is unusual for a week to go by in most orthopedic operating rooms without at least one patient having to undergo a revision for an aseptically loose prosthesis. Unfortunately, revision surgery is more difficult to perform than primary joint replacement and is associated with a much higher morbidity and higher aseptic loosening rate. In terms of numbers, aseptic loosening represents one of the most commonly occurring complications in the history of surgery. In addition, aseptic loosening is the main factor limiting the life span of the reconstructions and is the primary factor that limits the use of these reconstructive technologies in younger individuals. In this chapter, we concentrate on this problem, primarily on how it relates to cemented arthroplasty since this is the scenario for which we have the most information.

To understand the problem of aseptic loosening, it is necessary to appreciate the clinical process as well as the changes that occur on the cellular level. To accomplish this, this chapter is divided into four sections: clinical observations, retrieval studies, *in vivo* models, and *in vitro* studies.

II. CLINICAL OBSERVATIONS

The central issue in aseptic loosening involves the length of time it takes for the arthroplasty to fail. Early in the development of hip and knee reconstructions, problems such as infection or fatigue of the metals were prominent reasons for implant failure. As the technology and surgical technique improved, these problems became much less frequent. The primary factor that has emerged as limiting the longevity of the implants is maintaining the bond between the implant and the patient's bone. Aseptic loosening, which is the failure of the bond between implant and bone in the absence of infection, is the primary factor limiting the life span of these implants.

The problem of aseptic loosening has had far-reaching implications in the practice of orthopedic surgery. It is for this reason that patients who undergo hip arthroplasty are selected to be greater than 65 years of age so as to limit the amount of time the implant has to become loose. Unfortunately, many individuals younger than 65 also suffer from degenerative joint disease, and for these patients, there is no good reconstructive solution except for arthrodesis. An example of a patient in this group would be a young person who suffers a hip fracture, or fracture of the acetabulum, and then develops degenerative joint disease. Patients with poor bone quality are also considered to be at high risk for aseptic loosening. This would include a large group of individuals with rheumatoid arthritis and metabolic bone diseases such as osteomalacia, or patients on dialysis with renal osteodystrophy. It is the limited life span of the reconstruction secondary to aseptic loosening that limits the application of hip and knee replacement surgery in these patients.

The essential question is: how long can we expect the bond between the implant and bone to last? This is important because it will determine to which patients the use of this technology can be applied. There have been several studies in the literature that have attempted to determine the survival of cemented hip and knee reconstructions. Unfortunately, there are several problems inherent in all these studies. The first involves the direct issue of the length of time these reconstructions need to be observed to determine failure. For example, if 100 reconstructions were followed to determine longevity, it would take a certain number of years for the surgeon(s) to perform this surgery. Since the average prosthetic survival is probably around 15 years, these reconstructions would need to be followed at least 15-20 years to get an accurate idea of how long they last, in addition to the amount of time that elapsed while these 100 reconstructions were being performed. The problem with this is that technology is always changing, and many of the implants used 15-20 years ago are no longer being used today. Therefore, information from a prospective study initiated in 1975 may not have much useful information for surgeons in 1990.

There are several other problems involved in interpreting and comparing studies on prosthetic longevity. Surgical technique, prosthetic design, and patient selection have all been demonstrated to have an influence on prosthetic longevity [10-12,20,26,30, 35,36,43,53,61-65,80,81,85,86,98,100,112,113,115,116,121,125,128,131,132,135,139, 140,142-144,146,151,152,158-160,162,163]. In many of these studies, these parameters are not well controlled for and they are frequently different between studies, making a consensus difficult. Results for loosening published before 1985 tend to be worse than results published after that time. Loosening rates for cemented femoral components tend to be lower than for cemented acetabular components [42,49]. Femoral head size is also a factor and is different between many of the studies. There is a wide range in the literature for loosening rates, with the average currently being about 10-15 years for loosening of 10% of implanted cemented femoral components, and slightly worse results with cemented acetabular components. These results are in individuals 65 years of age or older.

Based upon these results, it can be seen that a patient who is 65 years of age will have about a 10% chance of requiring revision for loosened cemented femoral component at 80 years of age. A patient who is 45 years of age when cemented arthroplasty is performed will have at least a 10% chance of requiring revision by 60 years of age. The older patient will probably never need to have a revision performed while the younger patient will almost certainly suffer clinical aseptic loosening in his or her lifetime.

The goals of research on aseptic loosening are not directed to individuals over 65 years of age in whom reconstructive longevity is not a significant problem. These efforts are directed to the many younger individuals, as well as the many patients who suffer from diseases that impair bone quality, and are not currently considered candidates for this procedure because of the problem of aseptic loosening.

III. RETRIEVAL STUDIES

Retrieval studies focus primarily on histologic evaluation of the implant–bone interface, with some researchers examining *in vitro* properties of cells retrieved. The difficulty in analyzing the results of such studies is in the interpretation of their findings. Tissue samples have been taken from pseudocapsule, pseudomembrane, bone–cement interface, cement–metal interface, bone–metal interface, areas of focal osteolysis, acetabulum, femur, and tibial sites, depending upon the study. The variability of the findings under such different sampling conditions makes comparison difficult, as the conclusions reached based on tissue sampled in one location may be different from findings based on tissue taken from other locations. For the purpose of organization, these studies are divided according to the following six groups, based on the aspect examined:

A. Well-fixed bone–cement interface
B. Role of polymethylmethacrylate particles
C. Role of polyethylene particles
D. Focal osteolysis or aggressive granulomatous lesions
E. Role of metal particles
F. Retrieval studies that use *in vitro* methods to examine the roles of different cells/ particles in aseptic loosening

A. Well-Fixed Bone–Cement Interface

Several studies have examined well-fixed implants taken postmortem, to examine the bone–cement interface. Engh et al. [44] examined nine porous coated acetabular components, all of which had been functioning well at time of death, and all with stable radiographs. All nine specimens demonstrated growth of bone into the implant porous coating, occupying a mean of 32% of the fields examined. They also demonstrated fibrous tissue in nonossified areas that, when present, was extremely dense and well organized. No granulomas were found. Radiographs were found to underestimate gap areas and overestimate the occurrence of bone apposition.

The remaining postmortem studies were performed using tissue from cemented arthroplasties. Jasty et al. [76] examined 13 femora taken at autopsy from patients who had had cemented total-hip arthroplasty (THA), all functioning well at the time of death, with one showing radiographic loosening. Findings included host bone directly apposed to cement, with rare intervening fibrous tissue. The cement mantle was intact throughout, despite the presence of fractures in the mantle and occasional debonding at the cement–prosthesis interface. There was extensive bone remodeling, with a dense shell of new bone around and growing into the surface of the cement mantle and attached to the outer cortex. This adjacent cortex showed osteoporosis and cortical thinning.

Malcolm [102] reported on autopsy specimens from 78 total hip replacements that had been placed by Charnley between 8 and 22 years prior to examination. Histologic evaluation revealed wear particles (high-density polyethylene – HDPE – and metal) in the fibrous membranes that surrounded the prosthesis. There was an intact, viable cement-bone interface around the femoral component in 35 of the hips, and all acetabular specimens had a thick fibrous membrane between cup and bone.

Maloney et al. [103] performed biomechanical studies as well as histologic evaluation on 11 femurs (clinically and radiographically stable) retrieved at autopsy from patients who had had cemented THA. Biomechanical analysis in single limb stance and stair climbing positions using a 100-pound spinal load resulted in maximal axial micromotion of 40 μm, indicating a well-fixed prosthesis. In addition, they found marked stress shielding in the proximal medial femoral cortex, which persisted long after surgery. Histologic evaluation revealed trabecular bone intimately associated with the cement mantle on scanning electron microscopy and minimal fibrous tissue. Examination of the cement mantle revealed findings similar to that of Jasty et al. [76] with fractures of the cement mantle. These were found primarily at the prosthesis–cement interface, at sharp corners, and in association with voids in the cement.

B.   Role of Polymethylmethacrylate Particles

One of the earliest studies examining the reaction of bone to cement was that of Charnley [27], describing histologic findings of 23 human specimens between 1 month and 7 years after implantation. At 2–4 weeks, cellular damage was found to extend approximately 500 μm from the cement surface. New bone as well as fibrocartilage formation was beginning. At 1 year, transition was seen from fibrous tissue to fibrocartilage, with ossification of the fibrocartilage in direct continuity with bone. Also, necrotic bone and evidence of osteoclasis were present, as well as new osteones. The findings at 2–5 years and at 7 years resembled those seen at 1 year, but with fibrocartilage being replaced by lamellar bone. Foreign-body giant cells were seen on the surface of fibrous tissue in direct contact with cement, becoming less numerous over time.

Willert et al. [156] examined specimens taken from autopsy and at revision in 28 patients. An early postoperative change that did not persist was bone necrosis. This was followed by osseous repair. Acrylic "pearls" were noted in the tissue surrounding the implant, in association with foreign-body giant cells, some of which contained intracellular cement particles.

Willert et al. [155] sampled tissue from the capsule at reoperation for failed total-joint replacements. They reported finding a synovial-like membrane, with layers poorly defined, and a foreign-body reaction to particulate material present in the membrane. Cell types identified included histiocytes, multinucleated giant cells, and occasionally lymphocytic or plasmacytic infiltrates.

Carlsson et al. [23], in 1983, presented results of radiographic examination of 70 total hip arthroplasties exchanged for mechanical loosening of the stem. Localized bone resorption or scalloping was found in 33 of the 70 cases. In 8 of these 33, it was seen first in the proximal third of the femur. In two cases, scalloping started at the middle of the stem, and in 19 cases, it was found to start at the tip of the stem. They also graded the degree of scalloping and "mode of failure" based on stem positioning as described in Gruen et al. [59]. They found that the tip of the stem was more often in direct contact with cortical bone in cases of mechanical failure and scalloping than in failed stems without scalloping.

Johanson et al. [79] obtained 30 specimens from the bone–cement interface in hips revised for aseptic loosening. Histologic examination demonstrated histiocytosis, fibrosis, and necrosis, with particles of cement, polyethylene, and necrotic bone. Also noted were cement fractures and microfractures of bone.

To date there have been few studies that directly compared tissue taken from aseptically loose cemented, press-fit, and ingrowth prostheses. Lennox et al. [92] obtained tissue from 50 cemented, 5 press-fit, and 6 biologic ingrowth prostheses. Pseudosynovial implant-facing samples were taken from all specimens for histologic examination. Cemented implant membranes contained many macrophages and giant cells, and frequent granuloma formation. Press-fit membranes contained poorly vascularized dense fibrous tissue, with rare macrophages or giant cells. Biologic ingrowth membranes, which did contain macrophages, were the most vascular, with loosely organized connective tissue. Mast cells, when present, were associated with stainless steel and/or cobalt–chrome particles.

C. Role of Polyethylene Particles

Numerous recent studies also cite polyethylene (PE) as playing a causative role in aseptic loosening. Ohlin et al. [117] obtained tissue from 24 Christiansen total hip replacements at revision. Electron microscopy revealed an abundance of polyoxymethylene particles in the periprosthetic tissue, with associated fibrinoid necrosis and macrophage activation. Mathiesen et al. [107] also studied the Christiansen total hip implant with polyacetal socket (16 prostheses) in comparison with the Charnley–Muller ultrahigh molecular weight polyethylene (UHMWPE) hip implant (18 prostheses). Findings were similar for both groups, including the presence of necrosis, fibrosis, histiocytosis, and foreign-body giant cells, and evidence of chronic inflammation (lymphocytes, macrophages, and plasma cells). The inflammation and necrosis appeared to be more extensive in the polyacetal group. Mathieson et al. [106], in 1986, measured frictional characteristics of polyacetal compared to polyethylene and found that friction in polyacetal sockets was twice that in polyethylene sockets. In addition they found that the frictional characteristics of the polyacetal changed with age of the material *in vivo*.

Several other studies have also identified UHMWPE and high-density polyethylene (HDP) particles in the tissue surrounding loose prostheses, at sites distant from the joint in association with histiocytes and/or macrophages and/or giant cells [13,16,18,71,125, 135,137,138,157,162]. The significance of the presence of these particles is unclear at this time.

D. Focal Osteolysis and Aggressive Granulomatous Lesions

Focal osteolysis or aggressive granulomatous lesions have been reported in hip replacements [4,5,19,75,101,104,105,134,136,148] on both the acetabular and femoral side. In addition, these lesions have been noted in both cemented and uncemented arthroplasties. Many of these studies are in the form of case reports.

Santavirta et al. [134] described 6 patients (5 Lord prosthesis, 1 PCA) with aggressive granulomatous lesions after cementless hip arthroplasty, who underwent revision on average 4.8 years postoperatively for aggressive granulomatous lesion in both the femur and acetabulum (5 patients) or the femur alone (1 patient). On histologic evaluation, all granulomas contained histiocytes, giant cells, and necrotic debris, as well as particulate debris identified under polarized light as polyethylene. Santavirta et al. [136], comparing 6 patients with aggressive granulomatous lesions to 6 patients with common loosening, again demonstrated granulomas consisting of histiocytic–monocytic connective tissue at revision of cemented THA with aggressive granulomatous lesions. Immunohistologic evaluation of this tissue revealed that most cells were multinucleated giant cells and C3bi-receptor, nonspecific esterase-positive monocyte–macrophages suggestive of foreign-body reaction. This was in contrast to that found in areas around loose cemented stems (without aggressive granulomatous lesion), which consisted of dense connective tissue and a relative lack of activated fibroblasts in granulomatosis.

Jasty et al. [75] reported on 4 cases of extensive, localized bone resorption at rigidly anchored, cemented total hip replacement that demonstrated sheets of macrophages and foreign-body giant cells. Abundant methylmethacrylate particulate debris, but no polyethylene, was found. In contrast to the conclusions of Santavirta [136] above, Jasty et al. concluded that this did resemble tissue found in loosened total hip implants studied in their previous work.

Maloney et al. [105] studied 16 patients with focal femoral osteolysis after total hip replacement without cement. Two of these patients underwent revision and one underwent biopsy. Extensive ingrowth of bone was found, with dense fibrous tissue around the smooth part of the stem. There were focal aggregates of macrophages with particulate polyethylene and metallic debris. Maloney et al. [104] reviewed 25 cases of femoral endosteolysis in radiographically stable, cemented femoral implants, 3 of which were retrieved postmortem. Interval between arthroplasty and appearance of osteolysis ranged from 40 to 168 months. In 15 cases, the area of osteolysis corresponded to a defect in the cement mantle or an area of thin cement. In addition, focal cement fracture was demonstrated around implants that were otherwise rigidly fixed. Histologic exam revealed histiocytic reaction, with evidence of particulate polymethylmethacrylate.

Anthony et al. [5] described four cases of localized endosteolysis of the femur in otherwise well-fixed, cemented components. Like Maloney, they also noted areas of lysis to be related to local defects in the cement mantle, suggesting that the space between the stem and cement provided a route of entry for contents of the joint cavity to reach the endosteal surface, leading to localized bone lysis and loosening.

Maguire et al. [101] reported two cases of cemented total hip arthroplasty that had developed severe foreign-body reaction. Findings included microfragments of both polyethylene (PE) and polymethylmethacrylate (PMMA), and a foreign-body reaction. Tissue reaction consisted of foamy macrophages, giant cells, particulate debris, fibroblast proliferation, and osteoblast/osteoclast activity. Areas of necrosis were also noted.

Pazzaglia [119] reported on one case of extensive endosteolysis in the femur following total hip replacement. Fragmentation of the cement was noted, and histologic exam revealed sheets of macrophages, foreign-body giant cells, fibrin, and hemorrhagic and necrotic material. Osteoclasts and osteoblasts were also present.

Williams and McQueen [157] reported on 18 patients who presented for revision of loose, cemented total hip arthroplasty. They described a fibrous membrane consisting of three zones: a pseudosynovial lining adjacent to the cement mantle, a middle area filled with methylmethacrylate "pearls" with or without sheets of macrophages, and a third layer adjacent to trabecular bone consisting of dense connective tissue. Two populations of histiocytes were noted: foamy histiocytes with intracellular debris and vacuoles, and those with abundant granular endoplasmic reticulum and protein vacuoles. The predominant particle was PMMA, with polyethylene being much less common.

The majority of studies concerning localized osteolysis or aggressive granulomatous lesions had a histologic picture similar to that in aseptic loosening without such localized osteolysis.

E. Role of Metal Particles

Several retrieval studies have focused on the role of metal debris in aseptic loosening. Evans et al. [47] studied three aspects of the potential role of metals in prosthesis loosening. They first examined tissue taken at autopsy or revision and measured the metal concentration by neutron activation analysis in 10 specimens and by atomic absorption spectrophotometry in 3 specimens, and demonstrated elevated levels of metal in tissue adjacent to cobalt–chrome prostheses. They next performed skin sensitivity tests to cobalt, chrome, and nickel in patients with loosened prostheses. They found positive skin sensitivity to cobalt and chromium in 9 patients with loose metal-on-metal prostheses, but no sensitivity in 5 other patients with loose metal-on-metal prostheses. None of the patients with well-fixed prostheses (24) showed skin sensitivity. Histologic examination of periprosthetic tissue taken from patients with skin sensitivity was also performed. These patients were found to have a large amount of infarcted connective tissue, amorphous and cellular debris, and necrotic bone. Where there was viable tissue, sheets of macrophages and multinucleate cells with intracellular debris were present. Vascular changes included fibrous intimal proliferation, fibrinoid necrosis, and arteriolar thrombosis.

Winter [159] performed histopathologic examination of tissues taken from 44 patients with cobalt–chromium alloy implants. This study also demonstrated presence of foreign-body particles and abnormal number of macrophages in 27 of the 44 tissue samples. The tissue reaction depended on the number of particles present, with some foreign-body fragments phagocytosed by macrophages.

Agins et al. [1] examined tissue adjacent to 9 titanium–UHMWPE prostheses, 8 of which had been cemented. They found an intense histiocytic and plasma cell reaction in pseudocapsuler tissue, and metallic staining of lining cells. Evaluation of the tissue for metals using atomic absorption spectrophotometry revealed elevated levels of titanium, aluminum, and vanadium, with relative concentrations similar to those in the parent metal. This supported wear of the metal as the source rather than corrosion, which would be expected to produce concentrations different from the parent alloy.

Lombardi et al. [99] also examined aseptic loosening in the presence of a titanium alloy prosthesis, reporting two cases of early loosening. At revision in the first case, black-stained hypertrophic synovium was found with a grossly loose prosthesis. Histologic exam revealed metallic fragments in a fine dust-like pattern in histiocytes and fibrofatty tissue. Titanium tissue concentration was 280 μg per gram of tissue. At revision in the second case, again a large amount of black-stained fibrous tissue was found. Histologic exam revealed histiocytes and metallic debris. Tissue contained 14 μg of cobalt, 0.49 μg of chromium, and 10 μg of titanium. In both cases, there was burnishing of the femoral head, indicating wear.

Betts et al. [15] measured metal concentrations in periarticular tissue from 22 patients at revision surgery. They found microscopic metal particles only in failures due to infection, and the highest concentrations of metals in tissue came from infected specimens as well. Tissue metal contents, which varied widely (range 2.7–250 μg of metal per gram of dried tissue), did not correlate with histologic findings. Most frequent histologic findings were fibrosis, histiocytic reaction, hemorrhage, and necrosis. Ratios of the elemental metals reflected the parent alloy composition, suggesting wear particles rather than corrosion as the major source of metal in the tissues. They also noted the presence of cement and polyethylene particles.

Lewis et al. [94] examined tissue levels of cobalt in conjunction with serum levels in 7 control patients undergoing primary hip arthroplasty and 6 cobalt-exposed patients who had developed aseptic loosening after hip arthroplasty. Serum cobalt concentrations were not elevated in cobalt-exposed patients over control; however, cobalt concentrations were greatly increased in periprosthetic tissue in 5 of the 6 cobalt-exposed patients, compared with controls.

Huo et al. [74] examined metallic debris in 12 patients with femoral endosteolysis and aseptic loosening after cemented total hip arthroplasties. Tissue was retrieved from the area of femoral endosteolysis (FE), femoral bone–cement pseudomembrane, and pseudocapsule. Metal levels were 2.5 times higher in FE than in femoral pseudomembrane and 4.2 times higher than in pseudocapsule. Barium levels were 1.7 and 42.4 times higher in FE than in pseudomembrane or pseudocapsule, respectively. Histiocytic reaction was present in all specimens, as was particulate cement debris. Polyethylene debris was present in 11 of 12 specimens. Metallic wear debris was present within histiocytes.

F. Retrieval/*In Vitro* Studies

Goldring et al. [51] obtained tissue from the bone–cement interface in 20 patients with loose, nonseptic failed total hip replacement, remote from the pseudocapsule. Histologically, the membrane was divided into three zones: the synovial-like layer of cells at the cement surface, the midportion that contained sheets of histiocytes and giant cells, and a fibrous layer that blended into the bone. Tissue fragments were found to release prostaglandin E_2 (PGE_2) and collagenase into culture into medium. In a second study, Goldring et al. [52] further studied the bone–cement interface. Tissue was obtained from the membrane at the bone–cement interface of acetabular and/or femoral side of 41 failed total-hip replacements. All patients had had a diagnosis of osteoarthritis prior to their initial surgery, and presence of infection was excluded at the time of revision. Histologic description was similar to that in their earlier study, that is, a synovial-like lining with deeper layers containing abundant foreign particulate material (both PMMA and polyethylene) associated with a giant-cell/histiocyte reaction. Culture of cells taken from this tissue with ^{14}C-arachidonic acid resulted in a PGE_2 peak on radiochromatography, which was abolished on incubation with indomethacin. They also studied the capacity of the tissue to induce bone resorption in murine bone resorption assay, using conditioned medium. The conditioned medium from all but 1 of the 11 cultures of bone–cement interface membranes showed significantly increased calcium release above control. These results, however, had poor correlation with PGE_2 levels. Addition of indomethacin to the culture medium in this experiment did suppress PGE_2 levels and did somewhat reduce calcium release in comparison to controls.

Linder et al. [96] studied the membrane surrounding loose prostheses in 21 total hip arthroplasties revised for aseptic loosening, using histology and enzyme histochemistry. A soft tissue membrane infiltrated with macrophages was identified, which had a high acid phosphatase activity and a negative alkaline phosphatase activity. The surrounding bone was lamellar and showed evidence of remodeling, with areas of bone formation and resorption. Osteocytes were strongly positive for NADH–diaphorase, indicating metabolic activity.

Sedel et al. [140] examined production of inflammatory mediators around 29 total-hip arthroplasties with loose prostheses at revision. They compared alumina–alumina cemented, alumina–alumina cementless, metal–PE cemented, and metal–PE cementless prostheses; and demonstrated that tissue surrounding alumina–alumina prostheses produced less PGE_2 than tissue surrounding metal–polyethylene prostheses.

Kossovsky et al. [89] examined the function of macrophages obtained from periprosthetic tissue (identified by acid phosphatase activity), measuring superoxide anion production. They found a chronic moderate level of activity and a lack of responsiveness to a potent stimulator (phorbol myristate acetate), which suggested down-regulation of the periprosthetic synovium.

Santavirta et al. [135] obtained 7 tissue samples at revision for failed total hips using immunohistopathologic studies. In cases of simple loosening, they found dense connective tissue with fibroblasts, and aggressive granulomatous lesions contained fibroblasts and histiocytic–monocytic reactive zones. T-lymphocytes were few and lacked IL-2 receptors (not activated). The most frequent cell stainable for antibodies was the CD11b-positive, peroxidase-negative tissue macrophage. These cells were thought to have been recruited by polyethylene and titanium to migrate, adhere, and phagocytose particles in the tissue.

Ohlin et al. [116] obtained tissue from 6 patients at revision and used organ culture of periprosthetic and capsular tissue to study bone resorbing capacity. Conditioned culture medium from organ culture of these tissues placed in mouse calvaria culture induced significantly increased bone resorption. This effect was reduced by calcitonin (osteoclast inhibitor).

Athanasou et al. [7] also examined resorptive capacity of tissue obtained from 4 revision joint capsules. They found numerous macrophages and foreign-body macrophage polykaryons, which they distinguished from osteoclasts by antigenic phenotype and lack of response to calcitonin. They found that macrophages and macrophage polykaryons obtained from joint capsules could produce resorption pits when placed in culture on cortical bone slices.

Several studies have looked at release of various mediators from tissue retrieved from failed joint replacement. Kim et al. [86] examined 34 membranes from 20 cementless and 14 cemented prostheses, and compared them to adjacent pseudocapsular tissue as control. On histologic exam, cementless membranes contained more metal debris, while cemented membranes contained more foreign-body giant cells. Both cemented and cementless membranes produced elevated levels of collagenase, gelatinase, PGE_2, and interleukin-1 (IL-1) compared to controls, but they were not significantly different from each other.

Westacott et al. [153] examined the pseudosynovial membrane surrounding loose joint prostheses accompanied by osteolysis. They found higher numbers of IL-1B- and IL-1A-secreting cells when compared to normal controls and in comparison to synovium from rheumatoids.

Jiranek et al. [78] obtained membranous tissue from the cement–bone interface of 10 polyethylene acetabular components revised for aseptic loosening. They demonstrated macrophages to be the predominant cell type present, though fibroblasts were also present. Particulate debris—including metal, PMMA, and polyethylene—was present in all specimens and intracellular in macrophages and giant cells. IL-1B mRNA was demonstrated in macrophages by hybridization, but immunolocalization demonstrated IL-1B protein on both macrophages and fibroblasts. PDGF transcripts were present in both cell types.

Appel et al. [6] also examined the bone–cement interface for various mediators. They found explant cultures of pseudomembrane and synovium to produce IL-1, tumor necrosis factor (TNF), and PGE_2. Furthermore, they demonstrated increased ^{45}Ca release from limb bone rudiments when cultured with conditioned medium obtained from pseudomembrane cultures.

Finally, Dorr et al. [37] also examined capsule and fibrous membrane from loose titanium and cobalt–chrome stems. They found elevated levels of PGE_2, IL-1, and collagenase in these tissues. Synovial fluid and blood metal ion levels were elevated in loose cemented and cementless stems from both titanium and cobalt–chromium components, but not in fixed stems.

IV. *IN VIVO* STUDIES

There are relatively few *in vivo* models that have been developed to examine aseptic loosening. This section is organized in the following groups:

A. The rabbit tibia model (Goodman et al. [55,57]; Linder [97])
B. The intra-articular rat model (Howie et al. [70,72])
C. The rat subcutaneous air pouch model (Cuckler et al. [31,91])
D. The rat diaphysis model (Sund and Rosenquist [145])
E. Hamster cheek model (Linder and Romanus [95])
F. The guinea pig model (Stinson [144])
G. The sheep hip replacement model (Radin et al. [126])
H. The canine hip replacement model (Turner et al. [149]; Spector et al. [141]; Mendes et al. [109])

As with the retrieval studies in humans, the majority of these studies have observed response to implantation from a histologic standpoint; however, some have also done *in vitro* testing to look at biochemical factors as well.

A. Rabbit Tibia Model

Goodman et al. [56] designed an experimental model in rabbits, drilling a hole in the proximal tibia in which was placed an experimental material on one side, the opposite side serving as control. In comparing bulk versus particulate titanium and cobalt chrome alloy, they performed histologic examination of the tibias at 16 weeks postimplantation. Findings included a fibrous tissue layer surrounding both the particulate and bulk forms of these metals, with decreased cell numbers surrounding bulk material; however, they found no evidence of inflammation or foreign-body reaction. Using the same model, Goodman et al. [55] compared the effects of particulate polymethylmethacrylate and polyethylene (ultrahigh molecular weight polyethylene—UHMWPE). Histologic findings were similar for both materials and consistent with those found in human retrieval studies, that is, a foreign-body reaction with histiocytes and giant cells, though the UHMWPE interfaces were thicker, containing more histiocytes and fibrocytes. In addition, using this same model to generate tissue for *in vitro* studies [54], they demonstrated an increase in PGE_2 production from peri-implant (PMMA) tissue placed in tissue culture. Furthermore, they demonstrated that oral administration of sodium naproxen (cyclooxygenase inhibitor) was able to suppress this effect.

Linder [97] also used a rabbit tibia model to compare an implant of polymerized cement with polymerizing dough. Histologically, there was no difference between the two, suggesting that monomer trauma did not add to the acute tissue trauma of the surgery itself.

B.   Intra-Articular Rat Model

Howie et al. [70] designed a model for bone resorption using the rat distal femur, in which a non-weight-bearing plug (prehardened) of methylmethacrylate was inserted through the knee joint into the distal femur. The knee joint was then repeatedly injected with polyethylene (UHMWPE). They found a shell of bone to form around the plug, which underwent resorption after injection of polyethylene. Once again a foreign-body giant cell, macrophage reaction was seen at the interface near the joint. Howie et al. [72] also looked at the effect of intra-articular injection alone of polyethylene (HDPE, 1 μm to 200 μm, most 15 μm in greatest dimension) into the rat knee. Animals were examined 1 week after a single injection and 1 week after receiving weekly injections for 5 weeks. They found a proliferation of synoviocytes, accumulation of macrophages, and occasional multinucleated giant cells. The smaller polyethylene particles were associated with macrophages, and the larger particles with multinucleated giant cells; these findings were increased with multiple injections.

C.   Rat Subcutaneous Air Pouch Model

A third rat model, which has been used recently for study of biocompatibility of implant materials, is the rat air pouch model, initially described by Edwards et al. [41]. In this model, mechanical disruption of the subcutaneous connective tissue was created by repeated injection of air. This resulted in a cavity with a lining structure having the features of a synovial membrane. Nagase et al. [114] used this model to study the inflammatory reaction in rats to artificial ceramics. The ceramics tested (hydroxyapatite type 1, tricalcium phosphate, and apatite wollastonite glass) produced increased levels of leucocyte counts, proteinase, and PGE_2, though less than positive control (monosodium urate, MSU), and slightly later than MSU. In addition, the ceramics produced significant detectable TNF activity, while MSU did not. Cuckler et al. [31] have also used the rat subcutaneous air pouch model and found this to be superior to intramuscular injection as it produces the pseudosynovial membrane similar to that observed around loose implants [51]. On further experimentation with this model [91], Cuckler et al. found that PMMA with barium sulfate led to marked inflammatory response in comparison with PMMA without barium sulfate, based on leucocyte influx, protease activity, PGE_2 production, and TNF activity, though not on histology.

Jasty et al. [77] used subcutaneous injection of particulate polymethylmethacrylate (PMMA) powder into a wound chamber in mice (fully immunocompetent and three strains of mice with immunodeficiencies) to show a fibrous tissue reaction with foamy histiocytes and giant cells surrounding the acrylic particles, with evidence of phagocytosis. Bulk PMMA demonstrated only a fibrous reaction with fewer macrophages and giant cells. They compared these results to histologic findings in tissue retrieved from loose and well-fixed femoral components, where they had identified frequent fractures in the cement mantle and wear of the cement surfaces. They noted that the fractures were associated with sharp corners on the prosthesis, defects in the cement mantle, thin mantles, and separation at the cement–mantle interface. The histologic findings were in agreement with those found in the animal study, that is, a macrophage, foreign-body giant cell granulomatous reaction in response to particulate but not bulk PMMA.

D.   Rat Femur Diaphysis Model

One final rat model (Sund and Rosenquist [145]) used the diaphysis of the femur to compare intramedullary implantation of methylmethacrylate to periosteal elevation and removal of bone marrow by suction. They demonstrated that implantation of PMMA caused the greatest vascular disturbance and attributed it to blockage of the normal medullary blood supply.

E.   Hamster Cheek Model

Linder and Romanus [95] used a hamster model to study the effects of polymerizing bone cement on living tissue. The hamster cheek pouch was everted and stretched over a glass plate, and a superficial defect made, exposing connective tissue arterioles, capillaries, and venules. They compared polymerizing paste to liquid monomer, observing the microcirculation over time and any associated temperature changes. They found that wherever there was direct cement–tissue contact, severe, possibly irreversible microcirculatory disturbances occurred, including circulatory standstill and intravascular hemolysis. Temperature was not found to be a factor in this study.

F.   Guinea Pig Model

Stinson [144] inserted particulate PMMA, polythene, and nylon into the muscle and knee joint of guinea pigs to compare tissue reaction by histology. This study found essentially the same response to all three materials—macrophages and foreign-body giant cells, with a lymphocytic component in the reaction to polythene and PMMA. Stinson found no erosion or fragmentation of the polythene or PMMA over a 3-year period but did find disintegration of the nylon implants after 6 months.

G.   Sheep Hip Replacement Model

Radin et al. [126] used sheep in an *in vivo* model to study plastic-on-metal total hip replacement, with a controlled walking regimen. They found a decreased torsional rigidity between the prosthesis and femoral cortex in all animals; this paralleled calcar resorption and formation of a radiolucent line at the bone–cement interface, as well as histologic deterioration of the bone–cement interface.

H.   Canine Hip Replacement Model

Several canine models have been used for total joint prosthesis and the study of aseptic loosening [109,141,149]. Turner et al. [149] produced intentional aseptic loosening in 37 dogs followed by revision (using titanium porous coated femoral stem) with one of the following: no graft to osseous defect; hydroxyapatite/B tricalcium phosphate in the defect; or cancellous bone graft as part of a one-stage revision, or cancellous bone graft followed 4 months later with implantation of component in a two-stage procedure. They found that autologous bone graft led to the greatest and most consistent bone ingrowth, especially when performed in two stages. A second canine study (Mendes et al. [109]) looked at a surface replacement type prosthesis, using HDPE cup and socket in dogs. This was associated with failure in 5 of 8 by 6.5 months. Histologic exam revealed foreign material (wear particles—both methylmethacrylate and polyethylene) scattered in the synovium and capsule. They found no tissue reaction around the methylmethacrylate particles but did find such a reaction with histiocyte and giant cells around polyethylene particles, many having been phagocytosed. This is in contrast to the results of most retrieval studies from humans or animals. Spector et al. [141] also used a canine model to produce aseptic loosening for investigating *in vivo* and *in vitro* activity of cells associated with loosening. They found that the biologic response as determined by IL-1 and PGE_2 activity paralleled radiographic appearance of loosening and observations made intraoperatively as well as histologically. Radiographically, there was a radiolucent seam. On histologic exam, interface tissue displayed synovial characteristics as well as macrophages and multinucleated foreign-body giant cells, often adherent to large PMMA particles. Levels of IL-1 and PGE_2 were elevated, and the increase in PGE_2 could be suppressed by *in vitro* naproxen.

As demonstrated by this review, the findings of the *in vivo* studies are largely consistent with the findings of the retrieval studies reviewed above.

V. *IN VITRO* MODELS

The purpose of developing *in vitro* models of the loosening process is twofold. The first is to improve our understanding of the biologic mechanism of aseptic loosening by separating the individual components of this process and studying their interaction in a way that is not possible with *in vivo* models. The second major purpose is to develop a system that can eventually be used to develop strategies to improve implant longevity. These potential strategies include using this model to test different materials for their biologic response, testing of different pharmacologic agents to see if they can modify the biologic response, and testing of cell types from patients to determine if a predisposition to loosening exists—to give the orthopedic surgeon a basis for preoperative selection.

The development of *in vitro* models of the loosening process is based upon bringing the cellular elements of the interface into contact with the material elements in a controlled environment. Early models of this process centered upon exposing cells to polymethylmethacrylate (PMMA) monomer in tissue culture and then studying the degree to which this monomer was toxic [122]. This evolved from the early theories on loosening in which it was felt that a toxic response to implantation of the PMMA was a major factor in later loosening [95]. This toxicity was felt to arise from the heat generated by polymerization of the cement in the medullary canal, and also from release of monomer [45]. These theories became less popular when retrieval studies of well-fixed implants from cadavers demonstrated little if any evidence of necrotic bone. In addition, further studies on the kinetics of polymethylmethacrylate monomer dissolution demonstrated that within a few hours to at most a few days, no monomer could be detected at the site of polymerization even by the most sensitive methods. Aseptic loosening usually takes many years to occur, and so it is unlikely that any detectable monomer is present when the interface is converting from a well-fixed to a loose histologic appearance.

We began working on this model in the early 1980s. At that time, a clearer picture of the loose and well-fixed bone cement interfaces was emerging from the retrieval studies that formed the basis of this model. The well-fixed interface was found to have cement adjacent to healthy bone, with little or no inflammatory response, no cement particles, and no macrophages. In contrast, the loose interface consisted of large numbers of cement particles, with a very extensive collection of macrophages in association with these particles. This response was also shown to be associated with fibrous tissue accumulation and bone resorption. From these studies it was proposed that the mechanism of loosening may not be a toxic response to cement implantation, but instead an inflammatory response to the production of cement particulates. To study this response more accurately in tissue culture, it was decided to study the response of cells to polymethylmethacrylate particles rather than to polymethylmethacrylate monomer.

Macrophages in close contact with polymethylmethacrylate particles is a consistent feature of the aseptically loose interface that is not present in the well-fixed interface. In the tissue culture model, macrophages were exposed to these particles and then the response was analyzed. The first parameters of interest were particle toxicity. This developed because of the earlier studies on monomer toxicity [45,58] and because particle toxicity was felt to be a significant factor in granulomatous diseases such as gout and silicosis of the lung [2]. It seemed likely that, since the monomer was so toxic, the particles would also be toxic, and that this response may be the reason why a small amount of particles could exert a biologic effect over a prolonged period of time [67].

To better evaluate the potential toxicity of PMMA particles, several controls were used [67]. To control for the presence of soluble toxic substances such as residual monomer, we developed a filtrate control in which the particles were suspended in media and then filtered using a $0.2-\mu m$ filter. The filtrate is examined to be certain it is free of particles and then exposed to the cells as an additional control. If the toxic response to the particles is secondary to soluble contaminants and not the particles themselves, then it would be expected that the cells exposed to the filtrate control will also demonstrate this toxic response. In our initial study (1988), PMMA and polystyrene particles (purchased from Polysciences Co.) were used in diameters ranging from 0.3 to 0.5 μm [67]. Polystyrene of the same size was chosen as a control because these particles are considered to be inert [8,40,123,124]. By using a control particle that was nontoxic, we were able to establish whether the response was secondary to the composition of the particle or simply a dose response to the number of particles. The biologic parameters of toxicity studied were macrophage DNA synthesis and cytotoxic ability [38,39]. It was found that exposure to PMMA particles significantly inhibited both DNA synthesis and cytotoxic function with respect to controls. This response did not appear to be secondary to any soluble contaminants such as monomer, nor was it simply a dose response to the physical presence of particles.

The finding that exposure to PMMA particles was toxic to macrophages has several implications regarding the mechanism of loosening. It reveals that macrophages that migrate to the interface in the presence of these particles may undergo a cycle of phagocytosis, cell death, and then release of the particles for phagocytosis by additional macrophages [22]. This repetitive cycle of phagocytosis and death is characteristic of a granulomatous response. It is significant because it implies that a small amount of particles may have a very potent effect because they are continuously being released for interaction with other cells.

In our initial studies it was demonstrated that exposure of macrophages to bone cement particles is toxic. If this is the case *in vivo*, then it seemed very unlikely that macrophages could be directly involved in bone resorption. Macrophages are known to be capable of releasing a variety of inflammatory mediators capable of stimulating bone resorption, so it was hypothesized that the response to the particles involved phagocytosis, early mediator release, and then later cell death. The problem with this hypothesis is that it proposes that the phagocytosis of cement particles could lead to a stimulation of one aspect of macrophage function, that being mediator release, while at the same time being toxic and inhibiting other cell functions such as macrophage cytotoxic capability.

To better study the coexistence of the toxic effects of the cement particles and their ability to stimulate mediator release, we studied the effects of particle exposure upon release of the intracellular enzyme lactate dehydrogenase, as well as the release of arachidonic acid products [33,68]. Release of intracellular lactate dehydrogenase is a reflection of cell injury [3]. Arachidonic acid and its various metabolites are inflammatory mediators released by macrophages in response to a variety of stimuli [9,88]. This is considered to be a nonspecific but sensitive assay for inflammatory mediator release since any mediator in the arachidonic acid family will be detected. In this study, exposure to varying concentrations of polymethylmethacrylate particles consistently led to lactate dehydrogenase release while at the same time also stimulating release of arachidonic acid metabolites. In contrast, exposure to the styrene control particles did not lead to significant lactate dehydrogenase release but did lead to release of the inflammatory mediators. This study demonstrates the coexistence of both toxic and stimulatory effects upon macrophage physiology following particle phagocytosis.

In the previous studies it was demonstrated that exposure of macrophages to bone cement particles led to phagocytosis, mediator production, and then cell death. To understand more specifically the response of the macrophages to cement particles, we designed a study to compare the response of macrophages at the bone–cement interface in loose prostheses, with the response of macrophages to cement particles in tissue culture [69]. It was proposed that the response of macrophages to the fragmentation of the cement mantle could be thought of as a response to particles of different sizes. As the mantle fatigues, it breaks into smaller particles. The presence of the small particles is the link between the mechanical and biologic components of this process because these particles stimulate macrophages to produce mediators that ultimately result in bone resorption and aseptic loosening. To study this, electron microscopy was used to determine if the macrophages in tissue culture appeared morphologically similar to, and responded to polymethylmethacrylate particles in the same way as macrophages at the bone–cement interface. The abilities of three cement preparations—crushed simplex, crushed palacos, and prepolymerized simplex powder—to stimulate release of the bone-resorbing mediators prostaglandin E_2 and tumor necrosis factor were studied [14,17,24,25,28,29,34, 46,48,90,93,120,130,148,150]. The toxic effects of these three preparations were studied as performed previously by evaluation of their effects upon DNA synthesis (^{3}H-thymidine incorporation). Finally, the effects of changing the particle sizes from ones that were small enough to be phagocytosed to ones that were too large to be phagocytosed were evaluated with respect to these different parameters.

At the bone–cement interface, in the presence of large particles or without particles, the macrophages adhered to the surface of the cement and no phagocytosis was evident. When particles were present, only those less then 12 μm in size were phagocytosed by the cell. This size characteristic was also present when macrophages were exposed to different size particles in tissue culture. All three cement preparations consistently stimulated the cells to produce the bone-resorbing mediator tumor necrosis factor; however, none of the three preparations led to production of prostaglandin E_2. As in the previous studies, all three preparations inhibited ^{3}H-thymidine incorporation (DNA synthesis) by the cells.

On the basis of these studies, we proposed that the mechanism of aseptic loosening was a macrophage-mediated response with two components [69]. The first involves recognition of the mechanical failure of the cement mantle, which results from the production of particles small enough to be phagocytosed by macrophages (less than 12 μm). This initiates a biological response that is characterized by a repetitive cycle of particle phagocytosis and cell death with release of certain bone-resorbing mediators, one of which is tumor necrosis factor. The production of these mediators leads to bone resorption at the bone–cement interface, which destroys the bond that was formed between the cement and bone at implantation and ultimately results in aseptic loosening.

Considering the number of retrieval studies dealing with aseptic loosening that have been published in the last 20 years, there have been relatively few *in vitro* studies. There are slight differences between all the *in vitro* studies. Peripheral blood monocytes have been used in several. These cells have advantages over immortalized macrophages in that they are human, but disadvantages in that significant variability exists between monocytes obtained from different individuals in their responsiveness to inflammatory stimuli [118]. Each time an experiment is performed, new cells have to be obtained from another donor, making it difficult to compare results. In one study by Herman et al. [66], polymethylmethacrylate particles obtained by drill press stimulated monocytes to produce interleukin-1, tumor necrosis factor, and prostaglandin E_2. Davis et al. [32] performed a similar study using monocytes, but with prepolymerized simplex powder, and could not demonstrate increased levels of prostaglandin E_2 or interleukin-1. Several authors have demonstrated the capacity of this conditioned mediator to stimulate bone resorption as reflected by the release of ^{45}Ca from radiolabeled calvaria [50,66,127]. In our laboratory we have also worked with this calvarial model and have found a similar release. It should be noted that in most instances, although the release of ^{45}Ca was significantly greater than unexposed calvaria, the magnitude of this release was not great, usually less than 50% over unexposed controls. It seems likely that in the *in vivo* situation, the release of mediators by any particular macrophage is significant but not of great magnitude following cement particle phagocytosis. However, loosening is a process that takes years to develop, and so even if the biologic response is not of great magnitude, it is speculated that with time, enough bone resorption will occur to disrupt the bond between cement and bone. In addition, the toxic nature of the particles probably leads to a slow but continual influx of new macrophages to phagocytose particles and release mediators. In this way, a small amount of particles can exert a continued effect over a long period of time.

VI. CONCLUSIONS

Prosthetic joint replacement has been one of the most significant medical contributions of the last 30 years. Unfortunately, aseptic loosening continues to be the major factor limiting the use of this technology. The development of *in vivo* and *in vitro* models, as well as the continued retrieval studies, holds promise for improving our understanding of this process and ultimately leading to the development of strategies that can avoid or delay the onset of clinical loosening. These strategies may include the development of improved materials for fixation, methods to detect a biologic predisposition to loosening, or the use of pharmacologic agents to improve implant longevity. Even if effective in delaying the onset of loosening for only 5–10 years, the implementation of these strategies would have a profound influence in improving and increasing the application of joint replacement technology to society.

REFERENCES

1. Agins, H. J., Alcock, N. W., Bansal, M., Salvati, E. A., Wilson, P. D., Pellicci, P. M., and Bullough, P. G., Metallic wear in failed titanium-alloy total hip replacements, *J. Bone Joint Surg.*, *70A*, 347–356 (1988).

2. Alison, A. C., Harrington, J. S., and Birbeck, M., An examination of the cytotoxic effects of silica on macrophages, *J. Exp. Med.*, *124*, 141–154 (1966).

3. Amador, E., Dorfman, L., and Walker, W., Serum lactate dehydrogenase activity: An analytical assessment of current assays, *Clin. Chem.*, *9*, 391–399 (1963).

4. Amstutz, H. C., Campbell, P., Kossovsky, N., and Clarke, I. C., Mechanism and clinical significance of wear debris-induced osteolysis, *Clin. Orthop.*, *276*, 7–18 (1992).

5. Anthony, P. P., Gie, G. A., Howie, C. R., and Ling, R. S. M., Localised endosteal bone lysis in relation to the femoral components of cemented total hip arthroplasties, *J. Bone Joint Surg.*, *72B*, 971–979 (1990).

6. Appel, A. M., Sowder, W. G., Siverhus, S. W., Hopson, C. N., and Herman, J. H., Prosthesis-associated pseudomembrane-induced bone resorption, *Br. J. Rheum.*, *29*, 32–36 (1990).

7. Athanasou, N. A., Quinn, J., and Bulstrode, C. J. K., Resorption of bone by inflammatory cells derived from the joint capsule of hip arthroplasties, *J. Bone Joint Surg.*, *74B*, 57–62 (1992).

8. Atik, S. S., and Thomas, J. K., Polymerized microemulsions, *J. Am. Chem. Soc.*, *103*, 4279 (1981).

9. Aussel, C., and Fehlman, M., Effect of alpha-fetoprotein and indomethacin on arachidonic acid metabolism in P388D macrophages: Role of leukotrienes, *Prostaglandins Leukot. Med.*, *28*(3), 325–336 (1987).

10. Bargar, W. L., Shape the implant to the patient. A rationale for the use of custom-fit cementless total hip implants, *Clin. Orthop.*, *249*, 73–78 (1989).

11. Barrack, R. L., Mulroy, R. D., and Harris, W. H., Improved cementing techniques and femoral component loosening in young patients with hip arthroplasty. A 12-year radiographic review, *J. Bone Joint Surg.*, *74B*, 385–389 (1992).

12. Beckenbaugh, R. D., and Ilstrup, D. M., Total hip arthroplasty. A review of three hundred and thirty three cases with long follow-up, *J. Bone Joint Surg.*, *60A*, 306–313 (1978).

13. Bell, R. S., Schatzker, J., Fornasier, V. L., and Goodman, S. B., A study of implant failure in the Wagner resurfacing arthroplasty, *J. Bone and Joint Surg.*, *67A*, 1165–1175 (Oct. 1985).

14. Bertolini, D. R., Nedwin, G. E., Bringman, T. S., Smith, D. S., and Mundy, G. R., Stimulation of bone resorption and inhibition of bone formation *in vitro* by human tumour necrosis factors, *Nature*, *319*, 516–518 (1986).

15. Betts, F., Wright, T., Salvati, E. A., Boskey, A., and Bansal, M., Cobalt-alloy metal debris in periarticular tissues from total hip revision arthroplasties, *Clin. Orthop.*, *276*, 75–82 (1992).

16. Bobyn, J. D., Polyethylene wear debris, *Can. J. Surg.*, *34*, 530–531 (1991).

17. Bockman, R. S., Prostaglandin production by human blood monocytes and mouse peritoneal macrophages: Synthesis dependent on *in vitro* culture conditions, *Pop. Rep.* (*Ser. G, Prostaglandins*), *21*, 9–31 (1981).

18. Boynton, E., Waddell, J. P., Morton, J., and Gardiner, G. W., Aseptic loosening in total hip implants: The role of polyethylene wear debris, *Can. J. Surg.*, *34*, 599–605 (1991).

19. Brown, I. W., and Ring, P. A., Osteolytic changes in the upper femoral shaft following porous-coated hip replacement, *J. Bone Joint Surg., 67B*, 218–221 (1985).

20. Buchholz, H. W., and Heinert, K., Long-term results of cemented arthroplasty, *Orthop. Clin. N. Am., 19*, 531–540 (1988).

21. Bullough, P. G., DiCarlo, E. F., Hansraj, K. K., and Neves, M. C., Pathologic studies of total joint replacement, *Orthop. Clin. N. Am., 19*, 611–625 (1988).

22. Cannon, G. J., and Swanson, J. A., The macrophage capacity for phagocytosis, *J. Cell Sci., 101*, 907–913 (1992).

23. Carlsson, A. S., Gentz, C.-F., and Linder, L., Localized bone resorption in the femur in mechanical failure of cemented total hip arthroplasties, *Acta Orthop. Scand., 54*, 396–402 (1983).

24. Chambers, T. J., McSheehy, P. M. J., Thomas, B. M., and Fuller, K., The effect of prostaglandins I_2, E_1, E_2 and dibutyryl cyclic AMP on the cytoplasmic spreading of rat osteoclasts, *Br. J. Exp. Pathol., 65*, 557 (1984).

25. Chambers, T. J., McSheehy, P. M. J., Thomas, B. M., and Fuller, K., The effect of calcium-regulation hormones and prostaglandins on bone resorption by osteoclasts disaggregated from neonatal bones, *Endocrinology, 116*, 234 (1985).

26. Charnley, J., and Cupic, Z., The nine and ten year results of the low-friction arthroplasty of the hip, *Clin. Orthop., 95*, 9–25 (1973).

27. Charnley, J., The reaction of bone to self-curing cement. A long-term histology study in man, *J. Bone Joint Surg., 52B*(2), 340–353 (1970).

28. Collins, D. A., and Chambers, T. J., Effect of prostaglandin E_1, E_2, and F_2 on osteoclast formation in mouse bone marrow cultures, *J. Bone Mineral Res., 6*(2), 157–164 (1991).

29. Collins, D. A., and Chambers, T. J., Prostaglandin E_2 promotes osteoclast formation in murine hematopoietic cultures through an action on hematopoietic cells, *J. Bone Miner. Res., 7*(5), 555–561 (1992).

30. Cornell, C. N., and Ranawat, C. S., Survivorship analysis of total hip replacements. Results in a series of active patients who were less than fifty-five years old, *J. Bone Joint Surg., 68A*, 1430–1434 (1986).

31. Cuckler, J. M., Mitchell, J., Baker, D. G., Ducheyne, P., Imonitie, V., and Schumacher, H. R., A comparison of the biocompatibility of polymethylmethacrylate debris with and without titanium debris: A comparison of two *in vivo* models, *ASTM, 12*, 118–126 (1991).

32. Davis, R. G., Goodman, S. B., Smith, R. L., Lerman, J. A., and Williams, R. J., The effects of bone cement powder on human adherent monocytes/macrophages *in vitro, J. Biomed. Mater. Res., 27*, 1039–1046 (1993).

33. Decker, T., and Lohman-Mattes, M. L., A quick and simple method for the quantification of lactate dehydrogenase release in measurements of cellular cytotoxicity and tumor necrosis factor (TNF) activity, *J. Immunol. Meth., 15*, 61–69 (1988).

34. Dietrich, J. W., Goodson, J. M., and Ralsz, L. G., Stimulation of bone resorption by various prostaglandins, *Prostaglandins, 10*, 231 (1975).

35. Dercy, F., and Amstutz, H. C., Survivorship analysis in the evaluation of joint replacement, *J. Arthroplasty, 1*, 63–69 (1986).

36. Dorey, F., and Amstutz, H. C., The validity of survivorship analysis in total joint arthroplasty, *J. Bone Joint Surg., 71A*, 544–548 (1989).

37. Dorr, L. D., Bloebaum, R., Emmanuel, J., and Meldrum, R., Histologic, biochemical, and ion analysis of tissue and fluids retrieved during total hip arthroplasty, *Clin. Orthop., 261*, 82–95 (1990).

38. Drysdale, B. E., and Shin, H. S., Activation of macrophages for tumor cell cytotoxicity: Identification of indomethacin sensitive and insensitive pathways, *J. Immunol., 127*, 760 (1981).

39. Drysdale, B. E., Zarchuk, C., and Shin, H., Mechanism of macrophage-mediated cytotoxicity: Production of a soluble cytotoxic factor, *J. Immunol., 131*, 2362 (1983).

40. Edman, P., Sjoholm, I., and Brunk, U., Ultrastructural alterations in macrophages after phagocytosis of acrylic microspheres, *J. Pharm. Sci., 73*, 153 (1984).

41. Edwards, J. C. W., Sedgewick, A. D., and Willoughby, D. A., The formation of a structure with the features of synovial lining by subcutaneous injection of air: An *in vivo* tissue culture system, *J. Pathol., 134*, 147–156 (1981).

42. Eftekhar, N. S., and Nercessian, O., Incidence and mechanism of failure of cemented acetabular component in total hip arthroplasty, *Orthop. Clin. N. Am., 19*, 557–566 (1988).

43. Engh, C. A., and Bobyn, J. D., Principles, techniques, results, and complications with a porous-coated sintered metal system, *Instr. Course Lect., 35*, 169–183 (1986).

44. Engh, C. A., Zettl-Schaffer, F., Kukita, Y., Sweet, D., Jasty, M., and Bragdon, C., Histological and radiographic assessment of well functioning porous-coated acetabular components. A human postmortem retrieval study, *J. Bone Joint Surg., 75A*, 814–823 (1993).

45. Enis, J. E., Sarmiento, A., and Linker, G., Toxicity of methylmethacrylate to cells in tissue culture, *J. Bone Joint Surg., 55A*, 661 (1973).

46. Espevik, T., and Nissen-Meyer, J., A highly sensitive cell line, WEHI 164 clone 13, for measuring cytotoxic factor/tumor necrosis factor from human monocytes, *J. Immunol. Meth., 95*, 99–105 (1986).

47. Evans, E. M., Freeman, M. A. R., Miller, A. J., and Vernon-Roberts, B., Metal-sensitivity as a cause of bone necrosis and loosening of the prosthesis in total joint replacement, *J. Bone Joint Surg., 56B*, 626–642 (1974).

48. Flick, D. A., and Gifford, G. E., Comparison of *in vitro* cell cytotoxic assays for tumor necrosis factor, *J. Immunol. Meth., 68*, 167–175 (1984).

49. Garcia-Cimbrelo, E., and Munuera, L., Early and late loosening of the acetabular cup after low-friction arthroplasty, *J. Bone Joint Surg., 74A*, 1119–1129 (1992).

50. Glant, T. T., Jacobs, J. J., Moinar, G., Shanbhag, A. S., Valyon, M., and Galante, J. O., Bone resorption activity of particulate-stimulated macrophages, *J. Bone Miner. Res., 8*(9), 1071–1079 (1993).

51. Goldring, S. R., Schiller, A. L., Roelke, M., Rourke, C. M., O'Neill, D. A., and Harris, W. H., The synovial-like membrane at the bone–cement interface in loose total hip replacements and its proposed role in bone lysis, *J. Bone Joint Surg., 65A*, 575–584 (June 1983).

52. Goldring, S. R., Jasty, M., Roelke, M. S., Rourke, C. M., Bringhurst, F. R., and Harris, W. H., Formation of a synovial-like membrane at the bone–cement interface. Its role in bone resorption and implant loosening after total hip replacement, *Arthr. Rheum., 29*, 836–842 (1986).

53. Goldring, S. R., Clark, C. R., and Wright, T. M., The problem in total joint arthroplasty: Aseptic loosening [Editorial], *J. Bone Joint Surg., 75A*, 799–801 (1993).

54. Goodman, S. B., Chin, R.-C., Chiou, S. S., and Sung Lee, J., Suppression of prostaglandin E_2 synthesis in the membrane surrounding particulate polymethylmethacrylate in the rabbit tibia, *Clin. Orthop., 271*, 300–304 (1991).

55. Goodman, S. B., Fornasier, V. L., and Kei, J., Quantitative comparison of the histologic effects of particulate polymethylmethacrylate versus polyethylene in the rabbit tibia, *Arch. Orthop. Trauma Surg., 110*, 123–126 (1991).

56. Goodman, S. B., Fornasier, V. L., and Kei, J., The effect of bulk versus particulate polymethylmethacrylate on bone, *Clin. Orthop., 232*, 255 (1988).

57. Goodman, S. B., Fornasier, V. L., Lee, J., and Kei, J., The effect of bulk versus particulate titanium and cobalt–chrome alloy implanted into the rabbit tibia, *J. Biomed. Mater. Res., 24*, 1539–1549 (1990).

58. Cireen, A. S., The effect of methylmethacrylate on phagocytosis, *J. Bone Joint Surg., 57A*, 583 (1975).

59. Gruen, T. A., McNeice, G. M., and Amstutz, H. C., "Modes of failure" of cemented stem-type femoral components. A radiographic analysis of loosening, *Clin. Orthop., 141*, 17–27 (1979).

60. Harris, W. H., Schiller, A. L., Scholler, J. M., Frieburg, R. A., and Scott, R., Extensive localized bone resorption in the femur following total hip replacement, *J. Bone Joint Surg., 58A*, 612–618 (July 1976).

61. Harris, W. H., and McGann, W. A., Loosening of the femoral component after use of the medullary-plug cementing technique. Follow-up note with a minimum five-year follow-up, *J. Bone Joint Surg., 68A*, 1064–1066 (1986).

62. Harris, W. H., and Penenberg, B. L., Further follow-up on socket fixation using a metal-backed acetabular component for total hip replacement. A minimum ten-year follow-up study, *J. Bone Joint Surg., 69A*, 1140–1143 (1987).

63. Harris, W. H., and Davies, J. P., Modern use of modern cement for total hip replacement, *Orthop. Clin. N. Am., 19*, 581–589 (1988).

64. Harris, W. H., McCarthy, J. C., Jr., and O'Neill, D. A., Femoral component loosening using contemporary techniques of femoral cement fixation, *J. Bone Joint Surg., 64A*, 1063–1067 (1982).

65. Herberts, P., Ahnfelt, L., Malchau, H., Stromberg, C., and Andersson, B. J., Multicenter clinical trials and their value in assessing total joint arthroplasty, *Clin. Orthop., 249*, 4855 (1989).

66. Herman, J. H., Sowder, W. G., Anderson, D., Appel, A. M., and Hopson, C. N., Poly-methylmethacrylate-induced release of bone resorbing factors, *J. Bone Joint Surg., 71A*, 1530–1541 (Dec. 1989).

67. Horowitz, S. M., Frondoza, C. G., and Lennox, D. W., Effects of polymethylmethacrylate exposure upon macrophages, *J. Orthop. Res., 6*, 827–832 (1988).

68. Horowitz, S. M., Gautsch, T. L., Frondoza, C. G., and Riley, L., Jr., Macrophage exposure to polymethylmethacrylate leads to mediator release and injury, *J. Orthop. Res., 9*, 406–413 (1991).

69. Horowitz, S. M., Doty, S. B., Lane, J. M., and Burstein, A. H., Studies of the mechanism by which mechanical failure of polymethylmethacrylate leads to bone resorption, *J. Bone Joint Surg., 75A*, 802–813 (1993).

70. Howie, D. W., Vernon-Roberts, B., Oakeshott, R., and Manthey, B., A rat model of resorption of bone at the cement–bone interface in the presence of polyethylene wear particles, *J. Bone Joint Surg., 70A*, 257–263 (1988).

71. Howie, D. W., Cornish, B. L., and Vernon-Roberts, B., Resurfacing hip arthroplasty: Classification of loosening and the role of prosthesis wear particles, *Clin. Orthop., 255*, 144–159 (1990).

72. Howie, D. W., Manthey, B., Hay, S., and Vernon-Roberts, B., The synovial response to intraarticular injection in rats of polyethylene wear particles, *Clin. Orthop., 292*, 352–357 (1993).

73. Humes, J. L., Bonney, R. J., Pelus, L., Dahlgren, M. C., Sadowski, S. J., Kuehl, F. A., Jr., and Davies, P., Macrophages synthesize and release prostaglandins in response to inflammatory stimuli, *Nature, 269*, 149 (1977).

74. Huo, M. H., Salvati, E. A., Lieberman, J. R., Betts, F., and Bansal, M., Metallic debris in femoral endosteolysis in failed cemented total hip arthroplasties, *Clin. Orthop., 276*, 157–168 (1992).

75. Jasty, M. J., Floyd, W. E., III, Schiller, A. L., Goldring, S. R., and Harris, W. H., Localised osteolysis in stable, non-septic total hip replacement, *J. Bone Joint Surg., 68A*, 912 (1986).

76. Jasty, M., Maloney, W. J., Bragdon, C. R., Haire, T., and Harris, W. H., Histomorphological studies of the long-term skeletal responses to well fixed cemented femoral components, *J. Bone Joint Surg., 72A*, 1220–1229 (1990).

77. Jasty, M., Jiranek, W., and Harris, W. H., Acrylic fragmentation in total hip replacements and its biologic consequences, *Clin. Orthop., 285*, 116–128 (1992).

78. Jiranek, W. A., Machado, M., Jasty, M., Jevsevar, D., Wolfe, H. J., Goldring, S. R.,

Goldberg, M. J., and Harris, W. H., Production of cytokines around loosened cemented acetabular components, *J. Bone Joint Surg., 75A*, 863–879 (1993).

79. Johanson, N. A., Bullough, P. G., Wilson, P. D., Salvati, E. A., and Ranawat, C. S., The microscopic anatomy of the bone–cement interface in failed total hip arthroplasties, *Clin. Orthop., 218*, 123–135 (1987).

80. Johnston, R. C., and Crowningshield, R. D., Roentgenologic results of total hip arthroplasty. A ten year follow-up study, *Clin. Orthop., 181*, 92–98 (1983).

81. Johnston, R. C., Fitzgerald, R. H., Jr., Harris, W. H., Poss, R., Muller, M. E., and Sledge, C. B., Clinical and radiographic evaluation of total hip replacement. A standard system of terminology for reporting results, *J. Bone Joint Surg., 72A*, 161–168 (1990).

82. Kahn, A. J., Stewart, C. C., and Teitelbaum, S. L., Contact-mediated bone resorption by human monocytes *in vitro*, *Science, 199*, 988 (1978).

83. Kavanagh, B. F., Ilstrup, D. M., and Fitzgerald, R. H., Revision total hip arthroplasty, *J. Bone Joint Surg., 67A*, 517 (1985).

84. Kavanaugh, B. F., Dewitz, M. A., Ilstrup, M., Stauffer, R. N., and Coventry, M. B., Charnley total hip arthroplasty with cement. Fifteen year results, *J. Bone Joint Surg., 71A*, 1496–1503 (1989).

85. Kim, Y.-H., and Kini, V. E. M., Uncemented porous-coated anatomic total hip replacement. Results at six years in a consecutive series, *J. Bone Joint Surg., 75B*, 6–14 (1993).

86. Kim, K. J., Rubagh, H. E., Wilson, S. C., D'Antonio, J. A., and McClain, E. J., A histologic and biochemical comparison of the interface tissues in cementless and cemented hip prostheses, *Clin. Orthop., 287*, 142–152 (1993).

87. Kimura, H., Immunoassay with stable polystyrene latex particles, *J. Immun. Meth., 38*, 353 (1980).

88. Klein, D. C., and Ralsz, L. G., Prostaglandins: Stimulation of bone resorption in tissue culture, *Endocrinology, 86*, 1436–1440 (1970).

89. Kossovsky, N., Liao, K., Millett, D., Feng, D., Campbell, P. A., Amstutz, H. C., Finerman, G. A. M., Thomas, B. J., Kilgus, D. J., Cracchiolo, A., and Allameh, V., Periprosthetic chronic inflammation characterized through the measurement of superoxide anion production by synovial-derived macrophages, *Clin. Orthop., 263*, 263–271 (1991).

90. Kurland, J. L., and Beckman, R., Prostaglandin E production by human blood monocytes and mouse peritoneal macrophages, *J. Exp. Med., 147*, 952–957 (1978).

91. Lazarus, M. D., Cuckler, J. M., Mitchell, J., Schumacher, H. R., Baker, D. G., Ducheyne, P., and Imonitie, V., Biocompatibility of polymethylmethacrylate with and without barium sulfate in the rat subcutaneous air pouch model, *ASTM, 13*, 127–134 (1991).

92. Lennox, D. W., Schofield, B. H., McDonald, D. F., and Riley, L. H., Jr., A histologic comparison of aseptic loosening of cemented, press-fit, and biologic ingrowth prostheses, *Clin. Orthop., 225*, 171–191 (1987).

93. Lerner, U. H., and Ohlin, A., Tumor necrosis factors alpha and beta can stimulate bone resorption in cultured mouse calvaria by a prostaglandin-independent mechanism, *J. Bone Miner. Res., 8(2)*, 147–155 (1993).

94. Lewis, C. G., Belniak, R. M., Hopfer, S. M., and Sunderman, F. W., Jr., Cobalt in periprosthetic soft tissue. Observations in 6 revision cases, *Acta Orthop. Scand., 62(5)*, 447–450 (1991).

95. Linder, L., and Romanus, M., Acute local tissue effects of polymerizing acrylic bone cement, *Clin. Orthop., 115*, 303 (1976).

96. Linder, L., Lindberg, L., and Carlsson, A., Aseptic loosening of hip prostheses. A histologic and enzyme histochemical study, *Clin. Orthop., 175*, 93–104 (1983).

97. Linder, L., Reaction of bone to the acute chemical trauma of bone cement, *J. Bone Joint Surg., 59A*, 82–87 (1977).

98. Livermore, J., Ilstrup, D., and Morrey, B., Effect of femoral head size on wear of the polyethylene acetabular component, *J. Bone Joint Surg., 72A*, 518–528 (1990).

99. Lombardi, A. V., Mallory, T. H., Vaughn, B. K., and Drouillard, P., Aseptic loosening in total hip arthroplasty secondary to osteolysis induced by wear debris from titanium-alloy modular femoral heads, *J. Bone Joint Surg., 71A*, 1337–1342 (1989).

100. Loudon, J. R., and Charnley, J., Subsidence of the femoral prosthesis in total hip replacement in relation to the design of the stem, *J. Bone Joint Surg., 62B*(4), 450–453 (1980).

101. Maguire, J. K., Coscia, M. F., and Lynch, M. H., Foreign body reaction to polymeric debris following total hip arthroplasty, *Clin. Orthop., 216*, 213 (1987).

102. Malcolm, A. J., Pathology of longstanding cemented total hip replacements in Charnley's cases, *J. Bone Joint Surg., 70B*, 153 (1988).

103. Maloney, W. J., Jasty, M., Burke, D. W., O'Connor, D. O., Zalenski, E. B., Bragdon, C., and Harris, W. H., Biomechanical and histologic investigation of cemented total hip arthroplasties. A study of autopsy-retrieved femurs after *in vivo* cycling, *Clin. Orthop., 249*, 129–140 (1989).

104. Maloney, W. J., Jasty, M., Rosenberg, A., and Harris, W. H., Bone lysis in well-fixed cemented femoral components, *J. Bone Joint Surg., 72B*, 966–970 (1990).

105. Maloney, W. J., Jasty, M., Harris, W. H., Galante, J. O., and Callaghan, J. J., Endosteal erosion in association with stable uncemented femoral components, *J. Bone Joint Surg., 72A*, 1025–1034 (1990).

106. Mathiesen, E. B., Lindgren, U., Reinholt, F. P., and Sudmann, E., Wear of the acetabular socket. Comparison of polyacetal and polyethylene, *Acta Orthop. Scand., 57*, 193–196 (1986).

107. Mathiesen, E. B., Lindgren, J. U., Reinholt, F. P., and Sudmann, E., Tissue reactions to wear products from polyacetal (Delrin) and UHMW polyethylene in total hip replacement, *J. Biomed. Mater. Res., 21*, 459–466 (1987).

108. McMillan, R. M., Hasselbacher, P., Hahn, J. L., and Harris, E. D., Jr., Interactions of murine macrophages with monosodium urate crystals: Stimulation of lysosomal enzyme release and prostaglandin synthesis, *J. Rheumat., 8*, 555–562 (1981).

109. Mendes, D. G., Walker, P. S., Figarola, F., and Bullough, P. G., Total surface hip replacement in the dog. A preliminary study of local tissue reaction, *Clin. Orthop., 100*, 256–264 (1974).

110. Mirra, J. M., Amstutz, H. L., Matos, M., and Gold, R., The pathology of the joint tissues and its clinical relevance in prosthesis failure, *Clin. Orthop., 117*, 221 (1976).

111. Mirra, J. M., Marder, R. A., and Amstutz, H. C., The pathology of failed total joint arthroplasty, *Clin. Orthop., 170*, 175–183 (1982).

112. Mulroy, R. D., and Harris, W. H., The effect of improved cementing techniques on component loosening in total hip replacement. An 11-year radiographic review, *J. Bone Joint Surg., 72B*, 757–760 (1990).

113. Murray, D. W., and Rushton, N., Macrophages stimulate bone resorption when they phagocytose particles, *J. Bone Joint Surg., 72B*, 988–992 (1990).

114. Nagase, M., Baker, D. G., and Schumacher, H. R., Prolonged inflammatory reactions induced by artificial ceramics in the rat air pouch model, *J. Rheumatol., 15*, 1334–1338 (1988).

115. Nizard, R. S., Sedel, L., Christel, P., Meunier, A., Soudry, M., and Witvoet, J., Ten-year survivorship of cemented ceramic-ceramic total hip prosthesis, *Clin. Orthop., 282*, 53–63 (1992).

116. Ohlin, A., Johnell, O., and Lerner, U. H., The pathogenesis of loosening of total hip arthroplasties, *Clin. Orthop., 253*, 287–296 (1990).

117. Ohlin, A., and Kindblom, L.-G., The ultrastructure of the tissue surrounding the Christiansen total hip, *Acta Orthop. Scand., 59*(6), 629–634 (1988).

118. Pacifici, R., Rifas, L., Teitlebaum, S., Slatopsky, E., McCracken, R., Bergfeld, M., Lee, W., Avioli, L. V., and Peck, W. A., Spontaneous release of interleukin-1 from blood

monocytes reflects bone formation in idiopathic osteoporosis, *Proc. Natl. Acad. Sci.*, *84*, 4616–4620 (1987).

119. Pazzaglia, U. E., Fragmentation of methylmethacrylate: A cause of late failure of total hip replacement, *Arch. Orthop. Trauma Surg.*, *109*, 49–52 (1989).
120. Pederson, J. G., Lund, B., and Reiman, J., Depressive effects of acrylic cement components on bone metabolism, *Acta Orthop. Scand.*, *54*, 796 (1983).
121. Petty, W., The effect of methylmethacrylate on chemotaxis of polymethylmethacrylate leukocytes, *J. Bone Joint Surg.*, *60*, 492 (1978).
122. Pollice, P. F., Kang, J., Sliverton, S., and Horowitz, S. M., A model system of rat osteoclast precursors to study bone resorption in aseptic loosening, *Trans. Soc. Biomater.*, *26*, 61 (1993).
123. Polysciences, Inc., *Embedding with methacrylate*, Data sheet No. 104, Paul Valley Industrial Park, Warrington, PA, June 1983.
124. Polysciences, Inc., *Polybead microparticles*, Data sheet No. 238, Paul Valley Industrial Park, Warrington, PA, August 1984.
125. Pryor, G. A., Villar, R. N., and Coleman, N., Tissue reaction and loosening of carbon-reinforced polyethylene arthroplasties, *J. Bone Joint Surg.*, *74B*, 156–157 (1992).
126. Radin, E. L., Rubin, C. T., Thrasher, E. L., Lanyon, L. E., Crugnola, A. M., Schiller, A. S., Paul, I. L., and Rose, R. M., Changes in the bone–cement interface after total hip replacement. An *in vivo* animal study, *J. Bone Joint Surg.*, *64A*, 1188–1200 (Oct. 1982).
127. Raisz, L. G., and Nieman, I., Effect of phosphate, calcium and magnesium on bone resorption and hormonal response in tissue culture, *Endocrinology*, *85*, 446–452 (1969).
128. Ranawat, C. S., Rawlins, B. A., and Harju, V. T., Effect of modern cement technique on acetabular fixation total hip arthroplasty. A retrospective study in matched pairs, *Orthop. Clin. N. Am.*, *19*, 599–603 (1988).
129. Rembaum, A., and Dryer, W. S., Immunomicrospheres: Reagent for cell labeling and separation, *Science*, *208*, 364 (1980).
130. Rey, R. M., Paidment, G. D., McGann, W. M., Jasty, M., Harrigan, T. P., Burke, D. W., and Harris, W. H., A study of intrusion characteristics of low viscosity cement simplex-P and Palacos cements in a bovine cancellous bone model, *Clin. Orthop.*, *215*, 272–278 (1987).
131. Ritter, M. A., and Campbell, E. D., The survival of the cemented femoral component of a total hip replacement, *Clin. Orthop.*, *243*, 143–147 (1989).
132. Rodan, G. A., and Martin, T. J., Role of osteoblasts in hormonal control of bone resorption — A hypothesis [Editorial], *Calcif. Tissue Int.*, *33*, 349–351 (1981).
133. Sakurai, A., Satomi, N., and Haranaka, K., Tumor necrosis factor and the lysosomal enzymes of macrophages or macrophage-like cell line, *Cancer Immunol. Immunother.*, *20*, 6–10 (1985).
134. Santavirta, S., Hoikka, V., Eskola, A., Konttinen, Y. T., Paavilainen, T., and Tallroth, K., Aggressive granulomatous lesions in cementless total hip arthroplasty, *J. Bone Joint Surg.*, *72B*, 980–984 (1990).
135. Santavirta, S., Konttinen, Y. T., Hoikka, V., and Eskola, A., Immunopathological response to loose cementless acetabular components, *J. Bone Joint Surg.*, *73B*, 38–42 (1991).
136. Santavirta, S., Konttinen, Y. T., Bergroth, V., Eskola, A., Tallroth, K., and Lindholm, T. S., Aggressive granulomatous lesions associated with hip arthroplasty. Immunopathologic studies, *J. Bone Joint Surg.*, *72A*, 252–257 (1990).
137. Schmalzried, T. P., Kwong, L. M., Jasty, M., Sedlacek, R. C., Haire, T. C., O'Connor, D. O., Bragdon, C. R., Kabo, J. M., Malcolm, A. J., and Harris, W. H., The mechanism of loosening of cemented acetabular components in total hip arthroplasty. Analysis of specimens retrieved at autopsy, *Clin. Orthop.*, *274*, 60–78 (1992).
138. Schmalzried, T. P., Jasty, M., and Harris, W. H., Periprosthetic bone loss in total hip arthroplasty. Polyethylene wear debris and the concept of the effective joint space, *J. Bone Joint Surg.*, *74*(6), 849–863 (1992).

139. Schulte, K. R., Callaghan, J. J., Kelley, S. S., and Johnston, R. C., The outcome of Charnley total hip arthroplasty with cement air. A minimum twenty-year follow-up. The results of one surgeon, *J. Bone Joint Surg., 75A*, 961–975 (1993).

140. Sedel, L., Simeon, J., Meunier, A., Villette, J. M., and Launey, S. M., Prostaglandin E_2 level in tissue surrounding aseptic failed total hips, *Arch. Orthop. Trauma Surg., 111*, 255–258 (1992).

141. Spector, M., Sliortkroff, S., Hsu, H.-P., Lane, N., Sledge, C. B., and Thornhill, T. S., Tissue changes around loose prostheses—A canine model to investigate the effects of an anti-inflammatory agent, *Clin. Orthop., 261*, 140–152 (1990).

142. Stauffer, R. N., Ten-year follow up study of total hip replacements. With particular reference to roentgenographic loosening of components, *J. Bone Joint Surg., 64A*, 983 (1982).

143. Stinchfield, F. E., Symposium: Statistics on total hip replacement, *Clin. Orthop., 95*, 23–262 (1973).

144. Stinson, N. E., Tissue reaction induced in guinea-pigs by particulate polymethylmethacrylate, polyethylene and nylon of the same size range, *Br. J. Exp. Pathol., 46*, 135 (1965).

145. Sund, G., and Rosenquist, J., Morphological changes in bone following intramedullary implantation of methylmethacrylate, *Acta Orthop. Scand., 54*, 148 (1983).

146. Sutherland, C. J., Wilde, A. H., Borden, L. S., and Marks, K. E., A ten year follow-up of one hundred consecutive Muller curved-stem total hip-replacement arthroplasties, *J. Bone Joint Surg., 64A*, 970–982 (1982).

147. Tallroth, K., Santavirta, S., Konttinen, Y. T., and Lindholm, T. S., Aggressive granulomatous lesions after hip arthroplasty, *J. Bone Joint Surg., 71B*, 571–575 (1989).

148. Tashjian, A. H., Jr., Voelkel, E. F., Lazzaro, M., Goad, D., Bosma, T., and Levine, L., Tumor necrosis factor-alpha (cachectin) stimulates bone resorption in mouse calvaria via a prostaglandin mediated mechanism, *Endocrinology, 120*, 2029–2036 (1987).

149. Turner, T. M., Urban, R. M., Sumner, D. R., and Galante, J. O., Revision without cement, of aseptically loose, cemented total hip prostheses. Quantitative comparison of the effects of four types of medullary treatment on bone ingrowth in a canine model, *J. Bone Joint Surg., 75A*, 845–862 (1993).

150. Vaes, G., Cellular biology and biochemical mechanism of bone resorption. A review of recent developments on the formation, activation and mode of action of osteoclasts, *Clin. Orthop., 231*, 239–271 (1988).

151. Van der Schaaf, D. B., Deutman, R., and Mulder, T. J., Stanmore total hip replacement. A nine- to ten-year follow-up, *J. Bone Joint Surg., 70B*, 45–48 (1988).

152. Wang, J., and Leung, P. C. K., Arachidonic acid as a stimulatory mediator of luteinizing hormone-releasing action in the rat ovary, *Endocrinology, 124*, 1973–1979 (1989).

153. Westacott, C. I., Taylor, G., Atkins, R., and Elson, C., Interleukin 1 alpha and beta production by cells isolated from membranes around aseptically loose total joint replacements, *Ann. Rheum. Dis., 51*, 638–642 (1992).

154. Willert, H. G., and Semlitsch, M., Reactions of the articular capsule to wear products of artificial joint prostheses, *J. Biomed. Mater. Res., 11*, 157–164 (1977).

155. Willert, H. G., Ludwig, J., and Semlitsch, M., Reaction of bone to methacrylate after hip arthroplasty, *J. Bone Joint Surg., 56A*, 1368–1382 (1974).

156. Willert, H.-G., Bertram, H., and Buchhorn, G. H., Osteolysis in alloarthroplasty of the hip. The role of ultra-high molecular weight polyethylene wear particles, *Clin. Orthop., 258*, 95–107 (1990).

157. Williams, R. P., and McQueen, D. A., A histopathologic study of late aseptic loosening of cemented total hip prostheses, *Clin. Orthop., 275*, 174–179 (1992).

158. Wilson, P. D., Jr., Amstutz, H. C., Czerniecki, A., Salvati, E. A., and Mendes, D. G., Total hip replacement with fixation by acrylic cement. A preliminary study of 100 consecutive McKee-Farrar prosthetic replacements, *J. Bone Joint Surg., 54A*, 207–236 (1972).

159. Winter, G. D., Tissue reactions to metallic wear and corrosion products in human patients, *J. Biomed. Mater. Res. Symp., 5*(1), 11–26 (1974).
160. Wroblewski, B. M., 15–21 year results of the Charnley low-friction arthroplasty, *Clin. Orthop., 211*, 30–35 (1986).
161. Wroblewski, B. M., Wear of high-density polyethylene on bone and cartilage, *J. Bone Joint Surg., 61B*, 498–500 (1979).
162. Wroblewski, B. M., Taylor, G. W., and Siney, P., Charnley low-friction arthroplasty: 19–25-year results, *Orthopedics, 15*, 421–424 (1992).
163. Ziats, N. P., Miller, K. M., and Anderson, J. M., *In vitro* and *in vivo* interactions of cells with biomaterials, *Biomaterials, 9*, 5–13 (1988).

29

Factors Affecting Bone Ingrowth

J. Marcus Hollis and Charlene M. Flahiff
University of Arkansas for Medical Sciences
Little Rock, Arkansas

I.   INTRODUCTION

Total joint replacement is a well-accepted procedure in patients with degenerative joint disease and can often restore near normal function to arthritic and painful joints. Results of hip implants fixed with bone cement are encouraging, with good results observed at 10 or more years. However, loosening of total hip components increases over time (Sutherland et al., 1982). Noncemented porous coated components have been used in an attempt to improve these long-term results, especially in young patients and those with failed cemented joints. Porous coated implants rely on bone ingrowth into the pores on the surface of the implant for fixation. Although these implants are gaining acceptance for total joint replacement, clinical results to date indicate that bone ingrowth into porous coatings is often far from complete. In implants retrieved at reoperation, the amount of porous surface ingrown with bone has been found to be less than 10% (Cook et al., 1988b; Zettl-Schafer et al., 1992). In a study looking at femoral stems and acetabular cups, Cook et al. (1988a) found that 18% of the stems had no bone ingrowth, 45% had less than 2% of the surface ingrown, 14% of the stems had 2-5%, and 23% had 5-10% of the surface ingrown with bone. Even in functioning implants retrieved postmortem, the amount of available porous coating ingrown with bone averages only 32% (Zettl-Schafer et al., 1992). Other studies have shown that fibrous tissue often fills much of the implant (Haddad et al., 1987).

Fixation by bone ingrowth and by fibrous tissue both appear to be stable in short-term follow-up, but bone ingrowth improves clinical results (Engh et al., 1987). An implant without good bone attachment can generate wear debris due to toggling and allow wear debris into the interface. This debris can cause osteolytic activity that decreases bone supporting the implant, ultimately leading to failure of the implant system (Schmalzried and Harris, 1992). Even with bone ingrowth, failure of fixation has been observed in very active patients, suggesting that the bone had penetrated the pores and later failed in fatigue (Jasty et al., 1991). A major problem with porous coated implants is subsidence of the implant and thigh pain (Maloney and Harris, 1990). Clinical studies have shown significant migration of the acetabular component and subsidence of the femoral component at 5 years of follow-up (Heekin et al., 1993). It is postulated that this could be due to incomplete bone ingrowth, leading to impending clinical failure. More complete ingrowth of the bone into the pores and stronger ingrown bone is a possible solution to many of the problems associated with porous coated total joint replacements.

There are more than ample data to support the claim that bone will grow into a porous coated implant under the right circumstances. If fact, studies have shown that bone will go out of its way to grow into porous material in well-controlled animal studies (Bobyn et al., 1981; Robertson et al., 1976). Yet clinical retrievals at our institution and others clearly show that the porous coated implants rarely achieve a high percentage of the surface ingrown with bone. The questions then become: What could be preventing most of the surface of an implant from being invaded by ingrowing bone? And what can be done to improve the amount of bone ingrowth?

Many factors have been shown to affect bone ingrowth into porous coated implants. These factors include the relative motion of the implant and bone, referred to as *micromotion*, the pore size, the interface gap, and hydroxyapatite coatings. Long-term factors include bone remodeling, metal ion release, and polyethylene wear (Engh et al., 1992; Haddad et al., 1987; Pilliar, 1983).

II. MECHANICAL FACTORS

A. Micromotion

Motion between the implant and bone is an inevitable result of load applied to the implant prior to full ingrowth of bone into the implant surface. Studies have shown that the micromotion of joint replacement implants is affected by: (1) the load applied to the implant (O'Connor et al., 1990), (2) the design of the implant (Yoshii et al., 1991), and (3) the surgical technique used to place the implant (Hadjari et al., 1991; Maloney et al., 1990). Therefore, any information on the effect of this motion could be used in the assessment of these factors controlling the micromotion. It is somewhat difficult to distinguish between motion effects and load since motion is often a result of loading. The studies are therefore divided by the emphasis the individual authors have in their reports.

Several studies have examined the relative effect of different amounts of micromotion on ingrowth. Cameron et al. (1973) reported on a motion study in which porous Co–Cr staples were placed spanning an unstable tibial osteotomy. The staples were coated with a sintered bead surface with 50–100 μm pore size. There was no speculation as to what the magnitude of motion might have been. At 4 months, there was fibrous tissue ingrowth, and the pullout load was not increased. Controls not subjected to motion (or load) showed bone ingrowth and a large increase in pullout load.

Pilliar et al. (1986), in an attempt to quantify the relationship between bone ingrowth and motion, made measurements of the amount of motion present in femoral intramedullary rods at sacrifice 1 year after implantation in dogs. Under ± 20 N-m axial load cycling the bone ingrown implants moved 28 μm. This number represents deformation at the interface and bending of the surrounding bone. The implants that were fixed with fibrous tissue deformed from 100 to 200 μm in tension and from 50 to 310 μm in compression, giving a range for total motion of 150 μm to 510 μm. These data were extrapolated to conclude that 150 μm of motion will cause fibrous tissue ingrowth. This motion, however, was measured 1 year after implantation, and not during ingrowth. In this same paper, a second study with canine endodontic implants showed bone ingrowth at 3 months of use. The teeth were stabilized by the implant and the periodontal ligament. Data from previous studies on canine tooth loading and human periodontal ligament stiffness were extrapolated to show that the teeth probably did not move more than 28 μm. The authors concluded from these data that 28 μm of motion will not inhibit bone ingrowth into alveolar bone. No direct measurement of the amount of motion that existed during the initial ingrowth phase is reported in this study.

Burke et al. (1991) examined the effect of ±20 μm and ±75 μm (40 and 150 total) of interface motion in a distal canine femur cancellous bone model. An undersize drill hole was used to obtain a press fit. At 6 weeks, the implants with 40 μm had bone ingrowth, but it was not continuous with the surrounding bone. There was no ingrowth in the implants with 150 μm of motion.

The effect of short periods of daily motion was studied by Aspenberg et al. (1992). They used a cylindrical chamber with a 1 mm wide canal for tissue ingrowth and a titanium cylindrical core with a transverse groove completing the canal. These chambers were placed transcortically in rabbit proximal tibias. They found that 0.5 mm of core motion for only 30 sec per day at 0.67 Hz significantly decreased the amount of bone ingrowth into the chamber. The canal was found to be filled mostly with vascularized fibrous tissue in specimens with the applied motion. In a study with the same model, comparing 0.5 mm of motion with 0.75 mm of motion, Goodman and Aspenberg (1992) found that 0.75 mm of motion provided less ingrowth than the 0.5 mm motion. These researchers concluded that short daily periods of motion can cause fibrous ingrowth rather than bone ingrowth.

Soballe et al. (1992b) studied the effect of hydroxyapatite (HA) coating and motion on the host response to a knee implant in dogs. The implant bone interface had a 0.75 mm gap, and an axial motion of 150 μm was allowed during gait. A fibrous membrane had formed around both HA-coated and noncoated groups at 4 weeks in the motion groups. Titanium surface implants demonstrated a thick fibrous connective tissue while the HA-coated implants had a thin fibrocartilaginous tissue membrane. The shear strength of the implants with motion was less than that of the stable implants. Bone ingrowth was demonstrated in stable implants.

An animal model for studying the effect of micromotion on cortical bone ingrowth into porous coated implants was developed by Hollis et al. (1992a). This model allows four different amounts of motion and no motion to be examined in one animal. Four cylindrical porous coated titanium plugs with percutaneous shafts were implanted transcortically into the femurs of mature canines. A plate was clamped onto external fixation pins and the percutaneous shafts to prevent uncontrolled movement of the implants and to serve as a reference for turning the implants (Fig. 1). A small motor rotated the 200-μm shaft a small angle through a lever. This shaft, in turn, rotated the other three shafts through a series of 2 : 1 ratio pulleys. Each day postsurgery, the four implants were moved 25, 50, 100, and 200 μm, respectively, in rotation for 10 min twice a day. Four implants without percutaneous shafts were placed similarly in the contralateral side to serve as controls.

The dogs were sacrificed after 3, 4, and 6 weeks. The implant–bone composites were sectioned such that the circumference could be examined by the technique of Stewart et

A-P View

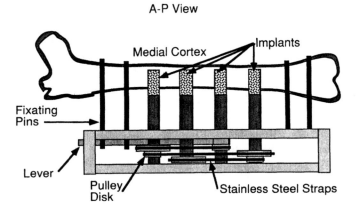

Figure 1   Implant jig to apply controlled micromotion. Rotation is supplied by the lever, which connects to a small electric motor (not shown).

al. (1993). Stained specimens were observed under a microscope at low power; the image was viewed on a computer screen and qualitative measurements were made. The percentage of the implant circumference with bone ingrowth was then calculated (Hollis et al., 1992b).

Histological results showed some bone ingrowth into all implants (Fig. 2). Almost the complete circumference in the 25, 50, and 100 μm groups had ingrowth into the surface, with bone filling the pores in some areas. The bone grew into pores smaller in width than the distance of implant motion in many cases. This implied that the bone was

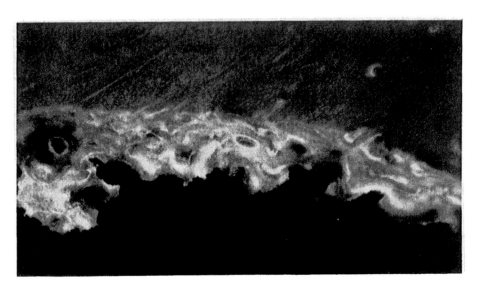

Figure 2   Histological slide of a 50 μm motion transcortical implant. New bone is seen surrounding the implant and within the pores of the porous coating. (Tetracycline, 50× magnification.)

deforming and moving with the implant. In other locations there were gaps of various widths between the bone and implant. The percentages of the circumference ingrown for the five groups are shown in Fig. 3. The different time groups were combined since no significant trend with time was seen. Implants from the control side that had no applied motion showed the least amount of ingrowth, with an average of less than 50%. The groups with 25–100 μm of motion all displayed 85–90% ingrowth. The implants with 200 μm of motion had significantly reduced ingrowth compared to the other groups with motion.

Ten minutes of motion twice a day was enough to inhibit ingrowth into the 200-μm specimens. This could be due to disruption of the growth, which could not recover before the next disruption by the application of the motion. It appears from these results that there is a range of motion that is optimal for bony ingrowth. Although it was expected that the control implants with no applied motion would have the most ingrowth, this was not the case. One possible explanation is that a limited amount of micromotion will actually induce bone formation into the pores of an implant in the early phases of ingrowth. This could be due to a shear strain being developed in the bone surrounding the implant that is enough to stimulate bone growth but not severe enough to disrupt the bone once it starts growing into the pores. Other studies have also shown that loading under controlled circumstances can increase bone ingrowth (Harris and Jasty, 1985).

In summary, the results of these studies suggest that there is a range of motion that is tolerated and allows bone ingrowth. Although these studies were conducted with different animal models and implants, they all suggest that 150–200 μm of relative motion will inhibit bone ingrowth while 25 μm of motion will allow or encourage bone ingrowth. Further work needs to be done, however, to examine the interrelation of other factors such as pore size and interface gap with the effect of micromotion.

B. Loading

The load applied to an implant can affect the interface in a few different ways. Stress is created, either a normal stress, shear stress, or a combination of the two. The load can also cause a more global stress in the bone that is not confined to the interface. In

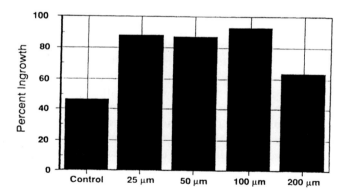

Figure 3 Percentage of implant circumference with bony ingrowth for the five motion groups. Control implants had no applied motion. Motion of 200 μm decreased the bone ingrowth, while smaller amounts of motion increased ingrowth compared to the control group.

addition, the applied load can cause motion at the interface. The studies reviewed here focus on the effect of implant load on the interface ingrowth and the effect of strain in the surrounding bone.

Ducheyne et al. (1977), in an early study of bone ingrowth, compared loaded and unloaded intramedullary rods. Stainless steel intramedullary rods with fiber metal porous coatings were implanted into both femurs of canines. On one side the femur was cut in the middle and the rods were placed with a Teflon spacer between the bone ends to prevent bone healing. The contralateral femur was left intact. Results showed that loaded rods with the Teflon spacer had a much lower interfacial strength (1/4) compared to the unloaded rods in intact femurs. The unloaded implants displayed bone ingrowth, while no calcified tissue was found in the loaded implants. They made the observation that the pore size, as it relates to ingrowth, should be different depending on the kind of loading present.

Heck et al. (1986) conducted a study on the effect of loading on ingrowth into intramedullary rods. In dogs, both femurs had implants, but one limb was suspended with an external fixator to prevent weight bearing. The other hind limb was therefore subjected to above normal weight bearing. The external fixator was used during the initial 3 weeks after surgery, and the dogs were sacrificed at 12 weeks. Radiological analysis and microradiological ingrowth assessment showed no difference between the two groups of limbs. Pushout strength, however, was 3 times higher for the unloaded as compared to the overloaded implants. The energy absorbed and stiffness were also higher for the initially unloaded implants. There was no correlation between interface strength and bone ingrowth. This was attributed to the effect of fibrous tissue fixation. Harris and Jasty (1985) implanted a group of canine acetabular implants that were denied weight bearing by dislocating the hip and compared the ingrowth to a normally loaded hip. At 6 months, ingrowth into the unloaded group (7.6%) was less than the loaded group (13.3%).

The loads in the bone surrounding the implant can also have an effect on the ingrowth. Hulbert et al. (1974) compared ingrowth into porous materials inserted into functional femurs with those inserted into amputated femurs. They found that there was good ingrowth in the functional femurs but little in the femurs without weight bearing. Rubin and McLeod (1992) found that strain at the implant site, produced by a load applied by an external fixator away from the implant, will also increase bony ingrowth. About 100 microstrain (no micromotion) was produced at the cortex of the bone at the implant site. This low strain magnitude greatly enhanced new bone formation. Unloaded implants had only 13% ingrowth, while those loaded at 1 and 20 Hz showed 21% and 74% ingrowth, respectively. Usui et al. (1989) examined the effect of vibratory bone loading on ingrowth into porous HA and on fracture healing. A 25 Hz vibration was applied for either 20 or 60 min/day to rabbit tibia into which porous HA rods had been inserted. Animals were sacrificed at 2, 3, 4, and 6 weeks. There was no significant effect of vibration on the amount or rate of new bone ingrowth. A significantly larger callus was produced by the 60 min per day vibration in the fracture model, but the strength was not significantly higher. It appears from these two reports that more research needs to be done on vibratory enhancement of bone ingrowth to determine the factors that could lead to consistent results.

It is well known that load can stimulate an increase in the mass of bones. However, the mechanisms of this effect, much less the effect of load on bone ingrowth, are not well understood. The results of some of these studies show that loading on the implant will eliminate or reduce ingrowth of bone in intramedullary models where shear forces are generated, while other studies show that some load can be beneficial. It would seem, therefore, that a specific amount of loading that can help stimulate bone formation but not create too large an interface shear might be an ideal mechanical environment for bone ingrowth.

III. GEOMETRICAL FACTORS

A. Surface Geometry and Pore Size

The surface of ingrowth fixation implants must have a geometry that accommodates the bone ingrowth. The term *surface* in this section is meant to include the entire porous layer, not just the very outer surface of this layer. Several porous surface finishes have been developed, including sintered compressed fiber metal, wire mesh, sintered beads, and plasma spray coatings. These techniques produce somewhat different surfaces, and bone ingrowth has been shown to occur successfully in all of them. Studies have shown, however, that some aspects of surface geometry are important. In a study examining the effect of porous surface depth, Bobyn et al. (1980a) constructed fracture fixation plates with a single or a multiple layer of spherical shaped metal powder particles on the surface. These plates were implanted onto the lateral aspect of canine femurs for 4, 6, 8, 12, 18, and 24 weeks. The plates were then pulled from the bone. Results of the testing indicated that implants with the multiple particle layer surface configuration developed a greater tensile strength of fixation than did implants with the single particle layer surface configuration.

Jasty et al. (1993) compared bone ingrowth into uncemented hemispherical canine acetabular components porous coated with cobalt–chrome spheres to those porous coated with titanium fiber mesh. Good bone ingrowth was noted in both types of porous coatings at 6 weeks after surgery, with no difference in the bone quality. However, quantification of bone ingrowth showed that more bone grew into the titanium fiber mesh compared to the spheres (10.5% versus 5.5% of the area, respectively). The mean area density of the ingrown bone was greater for the fiber mesh coating than for the spherical coating. The ingrown bone penetrated 66% of the depth of the porous layer with fiber mesh coatings compared to 32% for the spherical coating. The confounding variable in this study was that the surface geometry and the material were both varied, so no conclusion can be based purely on the geometry.

The size of the pores has been observed as an important factor since early studies on bone ingrowth. Lembert et al. (1972) implanted fiber metal implants with 190, 230, and 390 μm mean pore size into the intramedullary canals of dogs. The implants were not loaded. They found shear strengths of 167, 150, and 135 MPa for the three pore sizes, but the differences were not statistically significant. In results similar to Lembert et al., Cook et al. (1985) found no difference in the amount of ingrowth for pore sizes of 155–350 μm. In studies using a wider range of pore sizes, the effect is more prominent. Klawitter et al. (1976) studied the effect of pore size and time on bone growth. Porous polyethylene intramedullary rods were implanted into dog femurs for 4, 8, and 16 weeks. Histological and microradiographical results showed bone ingrowth into pores as small as 40 μm. Pore sizes in the 100 to 135 μm range provided faster rate of bone ingrowth while larger pore sizes did not increase the bone ingrowth rate. Robertson et al. (1976) studied ingrowth into Co-Cr cylinders with various surfaces. Polished, sandblasted, porous coated cylinders with 30–85, 40–106, and 50–125 μm pore sizes were placed transcortically into dog femurs. Pushout tests showed a trend of increased shear strength with increasing pore size and time after implantation.

A transcortical model was used by Bobyn et al. (1980b) to examine the effect of pore size on bone ingrowth. Pore sizes ranges of 20–50, 50–200, 200–400, and 400–800 μm were compared. Specimens were examined at 4, 8, and 12 weeks. The 20–50 μm group had the lowest strength, and the other larger pore size groups had much higher strengths. However, there was a slight trend of decreasing strength with increasing pore size in the range of 50–800 μm. Histologically, pores from 50 to 400 μm were completely ingrown with bone at 8 weeks. The 400 to 800 μm group, however, was not completely ingrown with bone even at 12 weeks. Clemow et al. (1981) found that the interfacial shear strength decreased with increasing pore size for 175, 225, and 325 μm pore sizes. In this study, titanium intramedullary rods with porous coatings of the various pore sizes were implanted in dog femurs for 6 months. The percentage of the surface with bone ingrowth was inversely proportional to the square root of the pore size. The interfacial shear strength and stiffness decreased with increasing pore diameter. The pushout strength and stiffness were proportional to the percent of bone ingrowth. Canine acetabular implants with pore sizes of 140, 200, and 450 μm were implanted by Harris and Jasty (1985). In a fourth group, a central gap was created by underreaming the bone for additional 450 μm pore size implants. A fifth group, also using 450-μm implants, was denied weight bearing by dislocating the hip. Animals were sacrificed at 6 months. Extensive bone ingrowth was observed for all three pore size groups. The percent of available area of bone ingrowth was lowest in the 140-μm group and highest in the 450-μm group. The group with the initial gap had significantly less ingrowth percent than the nongap group of the same pore size, 8.5% compared to 13.3%. Ingrowth into the unloaded group was minimal (7.6%) compared to the loaded group. The beneficial effect of larger pores in contrast to other studies was attributed to the functional loading. This is in agreement with an observation by Ducheyne et al. (1977) that the critical pore size for ingrowth is different for dynamic loading compared to static loading.

Table 1 summarizes these studies on the effect of pore size on bone ingrowth. It appears there is an optimal pore size for bone ingrowth in unloaded implants, which is in the range of 150–200 μm. The loaded implants, however, performed better with 450 μm pore size. Although the interrelationship between pore size and motion has not been studied quantitatively, it seems from these previous studies that optimum pore size has some dependence on micromotion or loading.

B. Interface Gap

It seems, intuitively, that the further the bone has to travel to grow into the implant, the less ingrowth is likely to occur. Animal studies have shown that interface gaps do affect the amount and rate of bone ingrowth. In dogs, bone ingrowth has been found to occur within 3 weeks when implants were in direct apposition with bone. With gaps up to 1.5 mm, it took 4 weeks for new bone to bridge the gap and 12 weeks for complete bone ingrowth (Cameron et al., 1976). In this excellent study, screws were porous coated (pore size from 20 to 100 μm), placed through an oversized hole of dog femurs, and screwed into the far cortex. Diameters of hole and screw were such that gaps of 1.5, 1.0, 0.5, and 0.0 mm existed between screw and near cortex. Only soft tissue was present at 2 weeks, while at 3 weeks bone was present and in contact with the surface except in 1.5-mm gaps. Ingrowth was noted in the porous coatings of all gap groups at 4 weeks. The gaps were

Table 1   Summary of Studies on the Effect of Pore Size on Bone Ingrowth

Study	Model	Pore sizes	Results
Lembert et al. (1972)	Dog, intramedullary rods	190, 230, and 390 μm	Decreasing strength with increasing pore size but not significant
Klawitter et al. (1976)	Dog, transcortical cylinders	40–206 μm	100–135 μm range optimal
Robertson et al. (1976)	Dog, transcortical cylinders	30–85, 40–106, and 50–125 μm	Increased shear strength with increasing pore size
Bobyn et al. (1980)	Dog, transcortical cylinders	20–50, 50–200, 200–400, and 400–800 μm	20–50 μm had lowest strength; slight decrease in strength with increasing pore size in the range of 50–800 μm
Clemow et al. (1981)	Dog, intramedullary rods	175, 225, and 325 μm	Shear strength decreased with increasing pore size
Harris and Jasty (1985)	Dog, acetabular cups	140, 200, and 450 μm	Increased ingrowth with increased pore size
Cook et al. (1985)	Dog, transcortical implants	155, 235, and 350 μm	No difference in the amount of ingrowth for tested pore sizes

eliminated by 8 weeks. The effect of a 1.5-mm gap was determined to be a 1-week delay in ingrowth maturation. Bobyn et al. (1981) placed porous coated intramedullary rods, with diameters of 2.5 to 5.5 mm, into femurs with average intramedullary diameters of 6.5 mm. At 12 weeks the implants had a shell of bone around the implants, but this shell was connected to the cortex with trabeculae only in areas of less than 2-mm gap. Sandborn et al. (1988) looked at intramedullary implants with varying diameters that were inserted into dog femurs. Gaps of 0.0–2.0 mm were left between implant and bone. Results after 3, 6, and 12 weeks showed bone bridging a gap as large as 2.0 mm. However, the percent of bone filling the gap was decreased for the wider gaps. Bone ingrowth was greater in the cortical region compared to the cancellous region except after 12 weeks, at which time they were similar. Soballe et al. (1991) implanted porous coated titanium alloy cylinders into femoral condyles of dogs. One condyle had an implant with a 1-mm gap, while the other condyle did not have a gap. One limb was made osteopenic. Two groups of implants were used, one with an HA coating and the other with a plain porous coating. At 4 weeks, mechanical testing showed shear strength increases of three- to fivefold in the osteopenic limb and twofold in control limb for the HA coating. The addition of a 1 mm interface gap reduced shear strength by 40–80%. The HA coating was shown to reduce the effects of the gap. Harris and Jasty (1985) showed that a central gap created by underreaming the bone in canine acetabula allows a significantly smaller ingrowth percent, 8.5% compared to 13.3%, than the nongap group of the same pore size.

From these animal studies it may be concluded that gaps as large as 2 mm are bridged by the bone ingrowth but not as completely as with smaller gaps. It appears, therefore, that the presence of gaps alone could be sufficient to cause the lack of ingrowth over large areas as has been reported in retrievals. In clinical studies the effect of the gap cannot be differentiated from the effect of increased motion on ingrowth since a poor fit would normally produce greater motion. A no-gap interface is considered ideal by most surgeons. In practice, however, this is difficult to achieve. Studies have shown that even with hemispherical acetabular implants and matched reamers, significant gaps between the implant and bone occur (Schwarts et al., 1991). The need for a perfect fit has also not been demonstrated in clinical studies. The question of the interrelation of gap size and micromotion has not been addressed previously. The effect of the gap with controlled interface motion remains to be determined.

IV. MATERIAL FACTORS

In addition to the mechanical environment of the implant and the geometrical surface characteristics, another important factor in determining bony ingrowth is the material of the surface layer. Various potential implant materials and surface coatings have been examined.

A. Implant Materials

Titanium and cobalt–chrome alloys are the most commonly used materials for porous coated implants. Jasty et al. (1993) compared bone ingrowth into uncemented hemispherical canine acetabular components porous coated with cobalt–chrome spheres to those porous coated with titanium fiber mesh. Good bone ingrowth was noted in both types of porous coatings at 6 weeks after surgery, with no difference in the bone quality. However, quantitation of bone ingrowth showed that more bone grew into the titanium fiber mesh compared to the cobalt–chrome spheres (10.5% versus 5.5% of the area, respectively). The mean area density of the ingrown bone was greater in the titanium fiber mesh coating than for the cobalt–chrome spherical coating. The ingrown bone penetrated 66% of the depth of the porous layer with titanium fiber mesh coatings, compared to 32% for the cobalt–chrome spherical coating. In this study the surface geometry and the material were both varied so the effect could be due to the material or the geometry, but it is most likely due to material differences.

Ceramics have many properties that might make them suitable for porous ingrowth implants. Robertson et al. (1976) placed 200- to 290-μm glass beads into a drilled hole to produce a porous, although not rigid, structure. They found that the inclusion of the glass beads into the drilled hole increased the rate and amount of bone formation over an empty drilled hole.

Several investigators have evaluated hydroxyapatite (HA) for enhancing bone ingrowth. Holmes et al. (1986) implanted porous HA into dog tibias and found that bone was in apposition with the ceramic, with 66.5% of the surface of the implant covered with bone ingrowth at 12 months. Porous ceramic hydroxyapatite blocks were implanted into surgically created defects in dog femora by Hoogendoorn et al. (1984). At retrieval

3.5 years after implantation, the implants were firmly attached to the bone. In order to determine the most appropriate properties for hydroxyapatite, four kinds of sintered hydroxyapatite were implanted in animals and studied histologically by Wang (1990). In addition, the responses at different implantation sites were compared. Hydroxyapatite with a 300–600 μm pore size demonstrated osteogenic activity superior to HA with a 50–250 μm pore size. Implantation at the epiphysis produced higher osteogenic activity in the early period, compared to implantations at the metaphysis or diaphysis. This difference in bone ingrowth had disappeared at 26 weeks. Parsons et al. (1988) developed a composite of HA particulate and calcium sulfate hemihydrate, which resulted in a material with better properties than HA alone. The resorption of the calcium sulfate left porosity for bone ingrowth and attachment to the nonresorbable HA particulate. They found that bone ingrowth occurred rapidly, with bone conduction from particle to particle.

In addition to HA, other ceramics such as tricalcium phosphate (TCP) and calcium aluminate have been investigated for bone-inducing properties. Graves et al. (1975) examined calcium aluminate ceramic specimens that consisted of different amounts of phosphorous pentoxide (P_2O_5). An increase in mesenchymal cell proliferation, and in fibrous and bone tissue formation at the ceramic–tissue interface and within the implant was seen with increasing concentrations of P_2O_5. Uchida et al. (1984) examined three different porous ceramics (calcium aluminate, hydroxyapatite, and tricalcium phosphate) with two pore size ranges (150–210 μm and 210–300 μm) for bone ingrowth in the absence of bone marrow. At 6 months after implantation in the skulls of rats and rabbits, tissue ingrowth into pores was seen in all three types of ceramics and in both pore sizes, but bone ingrowth was usually not seen within the pores of any of the ceramics. The density of the tissue was far less in the calcium aluminate than in the calcium hydroxyapatite or tricalcium phosphate. For each type of ceramic, the soft tissue ingrowth was denser with the larger pore size. In a subsequent study using the same animal models, Uchida et al. (1985) examined these ceramics after implantation in tibias, where bone marrow was present. They found that new bone consistently formed within the bone marrow surrounding and adjacent to all three kinds of ceramics. Bone ingrowth was seen in the pores of the calcium hydroxyapatite and tricalcium phosphate ceramics, but no bone was seen within the pores of the calcium aluminate implants.

Shimazki and Moony (1985) compared HA of two pore sizes (190–230 μm and 260–600 μm) with porous tricalcium phosphate (100–300 μm pore size) for bone ingrowth in rabbit tibias. The HA implants had almost twice as much bone infiltration as the TCP at 3 weeks and slightly more at 24 weeks. The HA with larger pores had more ingrowth than that with smaller pores. Degradation of the TCP was higher than that of the HA. Tencer et al. (1988) evaluated two kinds of coralline HA and TCP after 3 and 24 weeks in rabbit tibias. At 3 weeks, the two kinds of HA implants had 17% and 11% bone regeneration compared to the TCP, which had 7%. At 24 weeks, the HA implants were 56% and 52% filled with bone, compared to 44% for the TCP.

Anderson et al. (1984) implanted porous titanium and low-temperature isotropic (LTI) pyrolytic carbon transcortical implants into canine femurs. Bone formed in direct apposition with the LTI carbon implants, but the attachment shear strength was an order of magnitude lower than for the porous titanium implants. Tarvainen (1985) evaluated bone ingrowth into porous glassy porous carbon cylinders in rabbits. After 3 weeks, new bone formation occurred in the pores, and with time the bone became more dense. The amount of bone tissue in the pores reached a maximum at 12 weeks, when 45% of the pore volume was incorporated with bone tissue. Maistrelli et al. (1992) found that shear strength was higher and the amount of bone remodeling greater with titanium stems as compared to carbon composites. This was attributed to the larger surface area of the titanium porous coating. Other materials, mostly ceramics, have been examined for their potential to enhance bone ingrowth.

To improve the compressive properties of porous HA, Tencer et al. (1987) coated HA plugs with polylactic acid (PLA). These plugs were implanted in rabbits for 3, 12, and 24 weeks and were then compared to uncoated controls. Mechanical tests showed higher compressive strength, stiffness, and energy absorption values for coated specimens compared to uncoated specimens. At 12 weeks, the uncoated plugs had higher ultimate interfacial shear stress, but at 24 weeks there was no difference. Uncoated plugs also had higher volume fractions of new bone. Histology showed direct apposition of new bone to the PLA coating and degradation of the coating. We have examined a degradable PLA–calcium carbonate composite, which was made of interconnecting phases to slow the degradation rate (Flahiff et al., 1993). Samples were incubated in buffered saline or implanted in the backs of rats for 0, 1, or 4 weeks. Failure load, tensile strength, and elastic modulus significantly decreased for both groups during the first week, probably a result of the decreased PLA fraction, as determined by scanning electron microscopy (SEM). Continued decreases were seen at 4 weeks for the *in vitro* samples but not for *in vivo*. The stabilization and even slight increase in tensile strength and failure strain in the *in vivo* samples was thought to be due to tissue ingrowth (seen at 4 weeks) forming a tissue–implant composite.

Porous polymers have been recommended as coatings for femoral stems based on their low modulus, which allows uniform stress distribution to the surrounding bone. Application of the porous polymer coating to the metallic substrate also reduces metal ion release, and the polymer coating does not affect the mechanical properties of the device. Animal studies have shown bone ingrowth into porous polyethylene and porous polysulfone implants in cortical and cancellous bone. Pullout testing of porous polysulfone implants has shown that the strength of this material was higher than that of the surrounding bone. Less cortical bone loss was found around porous polysulfone coated stems in dogs than was reported for fully coated porous metallic prostheses, presumably because of the lower stiffness (Spector et al., 1988).

Albrektsson (1984) found that significantly more bone formed in titanium controls than in pipes made of bone cement. Poor biocompatibility of the cement compared to titanium was suggested to be one factor responsible for the reduced bone formation and was thought to be one reason for the fibrous tissue capsule generally seen around cemented implants.

Bone ingrowth into porous polyethylene rods has been investigated. Klawitter et al. (1976) implanted porous polyethylene rods into femurs of dogs, which were sacrificed 4, 8, and 16 weeks postoperatively. Results showed that porous polyethylene was capable of accepting bone growth into pores as small as 40 μm. The optimum rate of bone ingrowth was observed in pore sizes approximately 100–135 μm, with no increase in the rate of bone ingrowth in samples with larger pore sizes.

In summary, several materials that have been shown to be conducive to bone ingrowth are available. Titanium and Co–Cr are used routinely for porous coated implants with success. This can be attributed primarily to their high mechanical strength. The other materials that were shown to allow bone ingrowth are used in plastic surgery applications where graft strength is not required, but they have not been used for load-bearing implants due to strength concerns.

B. Coatings

In order to develop an implant system that has the strength of the titanium alloy or Co–Cr but the surface characteristics of some other implant materials, coatings have been developed. The most popular coating at the present time is hydroxyapatite (HA). Hydroxyapatite is a biocompatible ceramic with osteoinductive properties. Benefits include accelerated response of bone to implant, increased interfacial strength, enhanced filling of the gap, and lack of a fibrous tissue membrane.

The presence of an HA coating has been found to increase bone ingrowth and attachment strength for gaps up to 2 mm, although it is most effective in enhancing ingrowth for gaps of 1 mm or less (Cook et al., 1991). Without gaps, HA coatings have been found to increase the amount of ingrowth and interfacial shear strength in dogs for up to 4 weeks after implantation (Ducheyne et al., 1980). HA-coated plugs were implanted for 2, 4, and 12 weeks and were compared to the uncoated porous metal fiber material. At a few weeks postop, the rate of bone ingrowth and the strength of the interfacial bond was greater in the HA-coated implants. Stimulation of bone into the surface pores was cited as the reason for the increased rate of bond formation. Spivak et al. (1990) compared titanium specimens sputter coated with HA to those without HA for smooth surface and rough surface samples at 6 and 12 weeks in dogs. Significant increases in early bone ingrowth were seen for both types of surfaces. Cook et al. (1992) found that plasma-sprayed HA enhanced the amount of ingrowth and strength of interface attachment in porous coated Co–Cr–Mo transcortical implants from 2 to 52 weeks. Interface strength developed much more quickly with the HA coating, with the strength obtained at 2–4 weeks equal to that at 6–8 weeks in uncoated implants.

Maistrelli et al. (1992) examined the effect of HA coatings on femoral stems made of either carbon composite or titanium alloy. Osseointegration was greater in the HA-coated stems. Pushout tests showed a sixfold increase in interfacial shear strength and a twelvefold increase in shear stiffness with the HA-coated group. In the HA-coated group, shear strength was greatest proximally and progressively decreased distally, while the uncoated groups had the opposite trend. The bonding strength of HA-coated Ti–6Al–4V implants with bone was examined in rabbits and goats by Oonishi et al. (1989). The bonding strength of the HA-coated implants was approximately four times greater than the uncoated implants at 2 weeks and twice as strong at 6 weeks. Strengths were similar after 12 weeks of implantation. In contrast to the above-mentioned studies, earlier studies by Cook et al. (1988c) showed no significant improvement in interfacial shear strength in HA-coated implants in canine femurs.

Soballe et al. (1992a) studied the effect of HA coating on titanium alloy implants with micromotion. Fibrocartilaginous tissue was seen around the HA-coated implants with motion, while fibrous connective tissue surrounded the uncoated implants. The shear strength of the HA-coated implants exceeded that of the uncoated, for implants with and without micromotion. Without micromotion, the HA-coated implants had a tenfold increase in shear strength and fivefold increase in bone ingrowth as compared to the uncoated implants. HA also increased the gap healing capacity.

Other ceramic coatings have been shown to induce bone ingrowth. With HA–tricalcium phosphate coatings on titanium fiber mesh implants, bone formation was increased for 14 weeks in rabbit tibias in a study by Burr et al. (1991). This was attributed to early production of woven bone and the subsequent rapid formation of lamellar bone. Rivero et al. (1988) treated porous titanium fiber implants with a calcium phosphate coating and inserted them in dogs for 1, 2, 4, and 6 weeks. The mean shear strength at 4 weeks was 24% greater for the calcium-phosphate-coated implants than for paired controls. No difference in fixation strength was seen at the other time periods. Osteoconductive properties of the ceramic coating were concluded by bone forming in direct contact with the calcium phosphate. No increase in bone ingrowth volume was found for the coated implants at any time period. Anderson et al. (1984) examined carbon coating for its effect on bone ingrowth. Porous titanium implants, carbon coated and uncoated, were placed in dog femurs. At 6 months, both types of implants showed a high degree of mineralized bone ingrowth. The carbon-coated implants had a 4% increase in bone volume compared to the uncoated, and the attachment shear strength was higher.

As clearly demonstrated by these studies, hydroxyapatite coating appears to increase the rate of bone ingrowth into porous coated implants and the early interfacial strength. In addition, it appears to improve bone ingrowth in the presence of gaps. Clinically, its use could minimize the time that the patient would need to have reduced weight bearing. Since the HA- and non-HA-coated implants tend to converge in terms of percent ingrowth over time, a reduction in time to weight bearing may be the only certain benefit of the HA coatings. As HA coatings become more popular, clinical follow-ups will reveal their long-term effects. If the primary benefit is early weight bearing, an alteration in postoperative management may be a final test of this hypothesis.

V. ELECTRICAL STIMULATION

Electrical stimulation of bone is well known to increase the rate of fracture healing. Since the ingrowth of bone into an implant after reaming and insertion is similar to the process of bone healing, it is not unlikely that electrical stimulation would have an effect on bone ingrowth. Several studies have been performed to test this hypothesis.

Colella et al. (1981) used a femur transcortical model to study the effect of electrical stimulation on ingrowth into porous titanium implants. A constant current of 50 μA was applied for up to 8 days using the implant as a cathode. The animals were sacrificed at 1, 2, or 3 weeks and the interfacial shear strength was measured. The shear strength of the stimulated implants was about twice the unstimulated controls and was higher for every animal. The stiffness was similar between experimentals and controls.

The effect of current magnitude was examined by Buch et al. (1986) using titanium chamber implants inserted in the tibial metaphysis of rabbits. Constant current of either 5 μA, 20 μA, or 50 μA was passed through the implant, which was used as cathode. A platinum–iridium screw placed in the cortex served as the anode. The 5-μA and 20-μA groups, respectively, showed a 2.4-fold, and 2.6-fold increase in bone in the test chambers. The 50-μA group had a 48% decrease in bone volume compared to controls. The results suggest that a range of currents for maximum bone formation exits and is apparently a function of the implant geometry and animal model. Schutzer et al. (1990) examined bone ingrowth into porous titanium canine hip implants with and without capacitively coupled electrical field and found no significant difference in bone ingrowth after 6 weeks of stimulation. Shimizu et al. (1988) studied the effect of pulsing electromagnetic field (PEMF) on bone ingrowth into porous hydroxyapatite (HA) and porous tricalcium phosphate (TCP). The implants were placed into rabbit tibias and examined at 3 to 4 weeks. The HA implants had greater amounts of bone with the PEMF compared to control and in contrast to the TCP implants, which were not affected.

These studies show that the effect of different kinds of electrical stimulation on bone ingrowth parallels that of fracture healing. Direct current electrical stimulation provides a significant improvement in bone ingrowth, while the AC capacitive coupled and PEMF electrical stimulation do not help ingrowth enough to be noticed.

VI. BIOLOGICAL FACTORS

The vascular supply to the bone and tissue is a critical factor in determining the success of joint replacement arthroplasty, especially in the case of porous coated implants, which rely upon bony ingrowth. It is postulated that motion prevents bony ingrowth by shearing small vessels and preventing them from entering into the porous coated material, thus eliminating the essential vessels that provide the cellular and physiological factors and nutrients required to produce bone.

Studies on the insertion of acrylic bone cement and a metal implant have shown that the rate of vascular ingrowth is directly related to the type of bone and to the degree of reaming and secondary destruction of vessels (Rhinelander et al., 1979). A model has been developed by Hollis and coworkers (1994) to examine the influence of vascular changes on the speed and degree of bony ingrowth into porous coated implants. Using a canine model, both femurs were reamed at the time of surgery. In one femur a titanium plasma sprayed rod was inserted, while the other femur served as a control.

On the day of sacrifice, the hind limbs were perfused with a solution of micropaque and saline, so that only functional components of the afferent vascular system were filled, down to and including the smallest capillaries (Rhinelander, 1974). The dogs were then sacrificed and their femurs retrieved. After fixation, the femurs were cut to produce 1 cm, 1 mm, and 1.5 mm thick cross sections through the proximal, midshaft, and distal metaphyseal regions for pushout testing, microangiography, histology, and tetracycline fluorescence.

Although bony ingrowth could not be demonstrated on x ray, it was clear from histological and angiographic slides that there was adequate blood supply in all dogs by 4 weeks (Fig. 4). Bone ingrowth into pores of the implant was directly related to the amount of vascularization, and these areas were filled with new bone. Almost all of the implant pores in the metaphysis were occupied with bone, which was in intimate contact with the titanium. The percent of the implant in contact with vascularity decreased from 60% at the trochanter to 35% 4 cm distally. The diaphyseal area, where the nutrient artery was eradicated by the reaming, was different from the metaphyseal. The diaphyseal cortex that was in intimate contact with the porous coated rod was totally devoid of blood supply and necrotic with the exception of a small area in the region of linea aspera. Periosteal new bone formation was most prominent in this region, and vessels from the periosteum were seen to penetrate the outer portion of the cortex (Fig. 5). On histological examination, these areas were associated with osteoclastic replacement of the avascular cortex, accompanied by new bone formation. In some areas within the devascularized cortex there was space between the cortical bone and the porous coated surface that did not contain vessels nor any evidence of bony ingrowth. Biomechanical testing showed that the porous coated rods in these areas were not as rigidly fixed as those in the metaphyseal area, where there was abundant blood supply and new bone formation in the pores. Biomechanical results showed that interface strength correlates with the vascularity, since the strength was greater in the proximal region as compared to the distal region. Pushout strength decreased from 300 to 130 N, proximal to distal. In contrast to

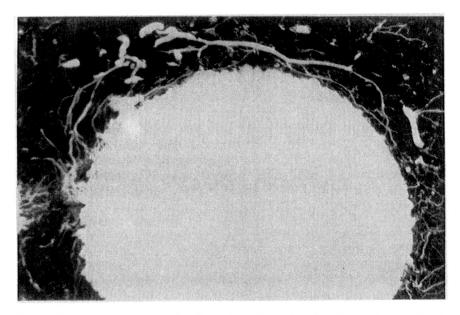

Figure 4   Microangiogram of a slice taken 15 μm distal to the trochanter. Implants in this area showed good vascularity (white) surrounding most of the implant.

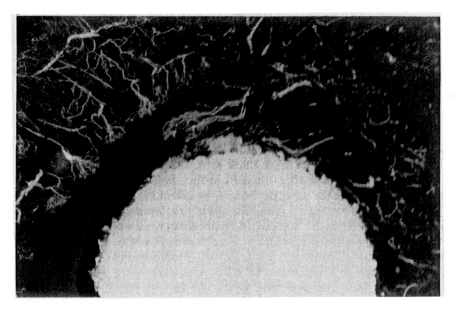

Figure 5   Microangiogram of a slice 32 μm below the trochanter. The featureless gray crescent on the left is devascularized old cortex. In contrast, the cortex on the right has been revascularized.

the above findings, Clemow et al. (1981) had previously shown a higher interface strength in cortical bone as compared to cancellous bone.

In conclusion, it appears that the reaming of the diaphyseal cortex followed by implantation of a porous coated rod devascularizes much of the cortex other than in the area of the linea aspera. The devascularized cortex becomes an impediment to revascularization, and bony ingrowth is much less than where cancellous bone is in immediate contact with the implant. The clinical implications of these findings are delayed bony ingrowth in the diaphyseal region as compared to the metaphysis and thus the emphasis on delayed weight bearing. Precise surgical technique and prevention of excessive devascularization is also important. To utilize the diaphyseal cortex for porous fixation, porous coating in the region of linea aspera might improve ingrowth of bone.

Growth factors such as bone morphogenetic protein (BMP) and transforming growth factor-beta (TGF-β) have been shown to stimulate bone formation. Several studies have looked at the use of growth factors to stimulate bone ingrowth. Urist et al. (1984) found that TCP/BMP implants had much more bone ingrowth than TCP or BMP alone at 21 days in mice. Gombotz et al. (1994) implanted calcium sulfate discs with and without TGF-β1 into rat defects. At 6 weeks discs containing TGF-β1 showed a greater amount of bone ingrowth than untreated controls. Lind et al. (1995) studied the effect of incorporating rhTGF-β into TCP and HA coatings. After 6 weeks implantation in canines, mechanical testing showed increased shear strength, stiffness and energy absorption for TCP coated implants treated with rhTGF-β compared to untreated controls. No significant increase in properties was seen for treated HA-coated implants. Incorporation of rhTGF-β also increased gap healing for the TCP-coated implants. Summer et al. (1995) found that the amount of bone ingrowth in a canine model was up to 300% greater in HA/TCP-coated intramedullary rods treated with TGF-β1 compared to untreated controls at 28 days.

Bone grafts have been used to enhance fixation of porous ingrowth implants. McLaughlin et al. (1984) used a demineralized bone matrix with porous coated rods to enhance bone ingrowth. These rods were inserted bilaterally into canine femoral medullary canals. Pullout testing and gross and roentgenographic examination confirmed that the demineralized bone matrix enhanced fixation. Ronningen et al. (1986) compared the bone-forming potential of isogenic bone marrow combined with allogenic bone matrix to that of bone marrow alone. The materials were packed into tubes of porous fiber titanium and placed in the back musculature of rats. At 12 days the combination of bone marrow and matrix had produced more bone than marrow only, but at 25 days there was no difference. It was concluded that the combination of bone matrix and marrow might enhance fixation at an early postoperative stage. A way to enhance bone ingrowth may be to use cancellous bone chips. Kienapfel et al. (1992) placed autogenous and freeze-dried allogenic cancellous bone into gaps created in a canine model. In each humerus, an implant was placed in an overreamed cavity so that a uniform 3-mm gap was present. Graft material was placed in the gap of one humerus while the gap of the other humerus was left empty and served as a control. Histologically, both autograft and allograft appeared to aid repair of the defect, but quantitatively only autograft enhanced new bone formation. While the enhancing effect was recognizable as early as 2 weeks, treatment with autograft increased the amount of bone ingrowth nearly threefold at 4 weeks and eightfold at 8 weeks. Strength of fixation was increased nearly sevenfold at 4 weeks and twofold at 8 weeks in the autograft group. These studies show that the use of bone material such as autogenous bone graft or demineralized bone improves ingrowth. This would be especially helpful where interface gaps are present.

VII. DISCUSSION

Retrieved implants often show bone ingrowth in some preferential locations such as the medial proximal area of hip stems and around pegs and spikes in acetabular and tibial tray components. Mechanical phenomena such as rigid fixation providing less motion, higher compressive stress, decreased shear stress, or perhaps smaller motion due to higher friction from increased normal compressive stress could be involved in this trend. The challenge is to control the mechanical environment of the interface in such a way as to enhance bone ingrowth. Typically, the state of stress at an interface is hard to estimate and varies within the gait cycle. Data are available on the loads experienced on limbs during various activities including non-weight-bearing motion. This is of little use, however, without some guidelines as to the appropriate range of loads for the implants. Studies show that overloading of the implant–bone interface in shear can reduce bone ingrowth. One approach to this problem would be to keep the loads as small as possible, but this could limit the activity of the patients unnecessarily and delay rehabilitation and cause disuse atrophy. In addition, some studies have suggested that zero load on the limb or implant might reduce bone ingrowth. A preferred approach would be to determine the optimum range of load for a particular implant. This would be difficult to do with accuracy due to variations in bone quality, surgical technique, and resulting fit. Also, the motion or load tolerance for different implant interfaces is not known. Clearly, more data in this area would be helpful.

A critical factor affected by surgery is the initial fit of the implant. As an example, in the preparation of the acetabula, due to the variation in bone quality and the unconfined action of the reamers, the hole is rarely prepared to the shape of the mating implant (Schwarts et al., 1991). In addition, clinicians often ream to a size 1–2 mm smaller than the implant or use an implant intentionally shaped incongruent with the reamer to achieve close fit around the rim. Difficulty in getting bony apposition in the dome is a consequence. Obtaining a precise fit is also difficult in other areas. Carefully designed instrumentation could provide a maximum fit. Bone grafting is helpful in filling gaps and eliminating defects in addition to encouraging ingrowth and improving fixation. In addition, hydroxyapatite coating is an improvement that increases the rate of bone ingrowth and minimizes the period of the patient's reduced weight bearing. The cost versus benefit justification of this addition remains to be proven.

VIII. SUMMARY

Porous coated implants rarely achieve a high percent of the surface ingrown with bone. Factors that have been shown to affect bone ingrowth into porous coated implants include the relative motion of the implant and bone, the pore size, interface gaps, and hydroxyapatite coatings. There is a range of motion that is tolerated and allows bone ingrowth. Bone ingrowth has been shown to be inhibited by 150–200 μm of relative motion while 25 μm of motion will allow or encourage bone ingrowth. The optimal pore size range for bone ingrowth in unloaded implants is 150–200 μm, while this range for loaded implants is larger, at least 450 μm. A relationship may be seen between pore size and loading. Stress in the surrounding bone will increase ingrowth; however, large shear forces on the bone–implant interface will reduce or eliminate bone ingrowth. Gaps as large as 2 mm have been shown to be bridged by bone ingrowth but not as completely as smaller gaps. Larger gaps may not be bridged. Bone graft however, has been demonstrated to improve bone ingrowth in interfaces with gaps. Hydroxyapatite coatings increase the rate of bone ingrowth into porous coated implants and the early interfacial strength. These coatings also increase the amount of bone ingrowth in the presence of gaps. Although direct current electrical stimulation provides a significant improvement in bone ingrowth, AC capacitive coupled and PEMF electrical stimulation do not appear to have the same effect.

REFERENCES

Albrektsson, T. (1984). Osseous penetration rate into implants pretreated with bone cement, *Arch. Orthop. Traum. Surg., 102*, 141–147.

Anderson, R. C., Cook, S. D., Weinstein, A. M., and Haddad, R. J., Jr. (1984). An evaluation of skeletal attachment to LTI pyrolytic carbon, porous titanium, and carbon-coated porous titanium implants, *Clin. Orthop., 182*, 242–257.

Aspenberg, P., Goodman, S., Toksvig-Larsen, S., Ryd, L., and Albrektsson, T. (1992). Intermittent micromotion inhibits bone ingrowth. Titanium implants in rabbits, *Acta Orthop. Scand., 63*, 141–145.

Bobyn, J. D., Pilliar, R. M., Cameron, H. U., Weatherly, G. C., and Kent, G. M. (1980a). The effect of porous surface configuration on the tensile strength of fixation of implants by bone ingrowth, *Clin. Orthop., 149*, 291–298.

Bobyn, J. D., Pilliar, R. M., Cameron, H. U., and Weatherly, G. C. (1980b). The optimum pore size for fixation of porous-surfaced metal implants by the ingrowth of bone, *Clin. Orthop., 150*, 263–270.

Bobyn, J. D., Pilliar, R. M., Cameron, H. U., and Weatherly, G. C. (1981). Osteogenic phenomena across endosteal bone–implant spaces with porous surfaced intramedullary implants, *Acta Orthop. Scand., 52*, 145–153.

Buch, F., Albrektsson, T., and Herbst, E. (1986). The bone growth chamber for quantification of electrically induced osteogenesis, *J. Orthop. Res., 4*(2), 194–203, 1986.

Burke, D. W., Bragdon, C. R., O'Connor, D. O., Jasty, M., Haire, T., and Harris, W. H. (1991). Dynamic measurements of interface mechanics *in vivo* and the effect of micromotion on bone ingrowth into a porous surface device under controlled loads *in vivo*, *Trans. Orthop. Res. Soc., 16*, 103.

Burr, D. B., Mori, S., Boyd, R. D., Sun, T. C., Lane, L., Blaha, J. D., and Parr, J. (1991). HA/TCP coatings induce rapid ingrowth by combination of woven bone and elevated lamellar bone formation, *Trans. Orthop. Res. Soc., USA, Japan, and Canada*, p. 86.

Cameron, H. U., Pilliar, R. M., and Macnab, I. (1973). The effect of movement on the bonding of porous metal into bone, *J. Biomed. Mater. Res., 7*, 301–311.

Cameron, H. U., Pilliar, R. M., and Macnab, I. (1976). The rate of bone ingrowth into porous metal, *J. Biomed. Mater. Res., 10*, 295–302.

Carlsson, L., Rostlund, T., Albrektsson, B., and Albrektsson, T. (1988). Implant fixation improved by close fit: Cylindrical implant–bone interface studied in rabbits, *Acta Orthop. Scand., 59*, 272–275.

Clemow, A. J., Weinstein, A. M., Klawitter, J. J., Koeneman, J., and Anderson, J. (1981). Interface mechanics of porous titanium implants, *J. Biomed. Mater. Res., 15*, 73–82.

Colella, S. M., Miller, A. G., Stang, R. G., Stoebe, T. G., and Spengler, D. M. (1981). Fixation of porous titanium implants in cortical bone enhanced by electrical stimulation, *J. Biomed. Mater. Res., 15*, 37–46.

Cook, S. D., Walsh, K. A., and Haddad, R. J. (1985). Interface mechanics and bone ingrowth into porous Co–Cr–Mo alloy implants, *Clin. Orthop., 193,* 271–280.

Cook, S. D., Barrack, R. L., Thomas, K. A., and Haddad, Jr., R. J. (1988a). Quantitative analysis of tissue growth into human porous total hip components, *J. Arthroplasty, 3*(3), 249–262.

Cook, S. D., Thomas, K. A., and Haddad, Jr., R. J. (1988b). Histologic analysis of retrieved human porous-coated total joint components, *Clin. Orthop., 234,* 90–101.

Cook, S. D., Thomas, K. A., Kay, J. F., and Jarcho, M. (1988c). Hydroxyapatite-coated porous titanium for use as an orthopedic biologic attachment system, *Clin. Orthop., 230,* 303–312.

Cook, S. D., Thomas, K. A., Dalton, J. E., and Whitecloud, T. S. (1991). Increased gap filling, bone ingrowth and fixation strength with HA-coated porous implants, *Trans. Orthop. Res. Soc., USA, Japan, and Canada,* p. 85.

Cook, S. D., Thomas, K. A., Dalton, J. E., Volkman, T. K., Whitecloud, T. S., III, and Kay, J. F. (1992). Hydroxylapatite coating of porous implants improves bone ingrowth and interface attachment strength, *J. Biomed. Mater. Res., 26,* 898–1001.

Ducheyne, P., De Meester, P., Aernoudt, E., Martens, M., and Mulier, J. C. (1977). Influence of a functional dynamic loading on bone ingrowth into surface pores of orthopedic implants, *J. Biomed. Mater. Res., 11,* 811–838.

Ducheyne, P., Hench, L. L., Kagan, A., Martens, M., Bursens, A., and Mulier, J. C. (1980). Effect of hydroxyapatite impregnation on skeletal bonding of porous coated implants, *J. Biomed. Mater. Res., 14*(3), 225–237.

Engh, C. A., Bobyn, J. D., and Glassman, A. H. (1987). Porous-coated hip replacement: The factors governing bone ingrowth, stress shielding, and clinical results, *J. Bone Joint Surg., 69B*(1), 45–55.

Engh, C. A., O'Connor, D., Jasty, M., McGovern, T. F., Bobyn, J. D., and Harris, W. H. (1992). Quantification of implant micromotion, strain shielding, and bone resorption with porous-coated anatomic medullary locking femoral prostheses, *Clin. Orthop., 285,* 13–29.

Flahiff, C. M., Blackwell, A. S., Feldman, D. S., and Hollis, J. M. (1993). A degradable hierarchical composite for bone healing, *Trans. Soc. Biomater., 16,* 129.

Gombotz, W. R., Pankey, S. C., Bouchard, L. S., Phan, D. H., and Puolakkainen, P. A. (1994). Stimulation of bone healing by transforming growth factor-beta 1 released from polymeric or ceramic implants, *J. Applied Biomat., 5,* 141.

Goodman, S., and Aspenberg, P. (1992). Effect of amplitude of micromotion on bone ingrowth into titanium chambers implanted in the rabbit tibia, *Biomaterials, 13*(13), 944–948.

Graves, G. A., Noyes, F. R., and Villanueva, A. R. (1975). The influence of compositional variations on bone ingrowth of implanted porous calcium aluminate ceramics, *J. Biomed. Mater. Res., 9*(4), 17–22.

Haddad, R. J., Cook, S. D., and Thomas, K. A. (1987). Biological fixation of porous-coated implants, current concepts review, *J. Bone Joint Surg., 69A*(9), 1459–1466.

Hadjari, M. H., Hollis, J. M., and Nelson, C. L. (1991). A biomechanical study of initial acetabular cup fixation: the effect of screw placement and screw tightness, and correlation with bone density, *Trans. Orthop. Res. Soc., 16,* 271.

Harris, W. H. (1986). Factors controlling optimal bone ingrowth of total hip replacement components, *Instructional Course Lectures, 35,* 184–187.

Harris, W. H., and Jasty, M. (1985). Bone ingrowth into porous coated canine acetabular replacements: The effect of pore size, apposition, and dislocation, in *Hip: Proceedings of the Thirteenth Open Scientific Meeting of the Hip Society,* pp. 214–234.

Heck, D. A., Nakajima, I., Kelly, P. J., and Chao, E. Y. (1986). The effect of load alteration on the biological and biomechanical performance of a titanium fiber–metal segmental prosthesis, *J. Bone Joint Surg., 68A,* 118–126.

Heekin, D. R., Callaghen, J. J., Hopkinson, W. J., Savory, C. G., and Xenos, J. S. (1993). The porous-coated anatomic total hip prosthesis, inserted without cement, *J. Bone Joint Surg., 75A*(1), 77–91.

Hollis, J. M., Hofmann, O. E., Flahiff, C. M., and Stewart, C. L. (1992a). Development of a transcortical model for quantification of the effect of micromotion on ingrowth into porous coated implants, *Trans. Orthop. Res. Soc.*, *17*, 564.

Hollis, J. M., Hofmann, O. E., Flahiff, C. M., and Stewart, C. L. (1992b). Effect of micromotion on ingrowth into porous coated implants using a transcortical model, *Trans. Fourth World Biomaterials Congress*, p. 258.

Hollis, J. M., Stewart, C. L., Griffin, F. M., and Nelson, C. L. (1994). A model for vascular, physiological, and biomechanical effects of porous implants, in *Trans. Soc. Biomater.*, Boston.

Holmes, R. E., Bucholz, R. W., and Moony, V. (1986). Porous hydroxyapatite as a bone-graft substitute in metaphyseal defects: A histometric study, *J. Bone Joint Surg.*, *68A*, 904–911.

Holmes, R., and Hagler, H. (1988). Porous hydroxyapatite as a bone graft substitute in maxillary augmentation: An histometric study, *J. Cranio-Maxillo-Facial Surg.*, *16*, 199–205.

Hoogendoorn, H. A., Renooij, W., Akkermans, L. M., Visser, W., and Wittebol, P. (1984). Long-term study of large ceramic implants (porous hydroxyapatite) in dog femur, *Clin. Orthop.*, *187*, 281–288.

Hulbert, S. F., Mathews, J. R., Klawitter, J. J., Sauer, B. W., and Leonard, R. B. (1974). Effect of stress on tissue ingrowth into porous aluminum oxide, *J. Biomed. Mater. Res. Symp.*, *5*, 85.

Jasty, M., Bragdon, C. R., Maloney, W. J., Haire, T., and Harris, W. H. (1991). Ingrowth of bone in failed fixation of porous coated femoral components, *J. Bone Joint Surg.*, *73A(9)*, 1331–1337.

Jasty, M., Bragdon, C. R., Haire, T., Mulroy, R. D., Jr., and Harris, W. H. (1993). Comparison of bone ingrowth into cobalt–chrome sphere and titanium fiber mesh porous coated cementless canine acetabular components, *J. Biomed. Mater. Res.*, *27(5)*, 639–644.

Kienapfel, H., Sumner, D. R., Turner, T. M., Urban, R. M., and Galante, J. O. (1992). Efficacy of autograft and freeze-dried allograft to enhance fixation of porous coated implants in the presence of interface gaps, *J. Orthop. Res.*, *10(3)*, 423–433.

Klawitter, J. J., Bagwell, J. G., Weinstein, A. M., and Sauer, B. W. (1976). An evaluation of bone growth into porous high density polyethylene, *J. Biomed. Mater. Res.*, *10(2)*, 311–323.

Lange, T. A., Zerwekh, J. E., Peek, R. D., Moony, V., and Harrision, B. H. (1986). Granular tricalcium phosphate in large cancellous defects, *Ann. Clin. Lab. Sci.*, *16*, 467–472.

Lembert, E., Galante, J., and Rostoker, W. (1972). Fixation of skeletal replacement by fiber metal composites, *Clin. Orthop.*, *87*, 303–310.

Lind, M., Overgaard, S., Soballe, K., Beck, S. L., Nguyen, T., Ongpipatanakul, B., and Bunger, C. (1995). Transforming growth factor-β enhances fixation of ceramic coated implants, *Trans. Orthop. Res. Soc.*, *20*, 192.

Maistrelli, G. L., Mahomed, N., Garbuz, D., Fornasier, V., Harrington, I. J., and Binnington, A. (1992). Hydroxyapatite coating on carbon composite hip implants in dogs, *J. Bone Joint Surg.*, *74B*, 452–456.

Maloney, W. J., and Harris, W. H. (1990). Comparison of a hybrid with an uncemented total hip replacement, *J. Bone Joint Surg.*, *75A(9)*, 1349–1352.

Maloney, W. J., O'Connor, D. O., Burke, D. W., Zalenski, E. B., and Harris, W. H. (1990). Micromotion of cementless hemispherical acetabular components fixed with screws: Quantification and the effect of the number of the screws on stability, *Trans. Soc. Biomater.*, *13*, 173.

Martens, M., Ducheyne, P., De Meester, P., and Mulier, J. C. (1980). Skeletal fixation of implants by bone ingrowth into surface pores, *Arch. Orthop. Traum. Surg.*, *97(2)*, 111–116.

McLaughlin, R. E., Reger, S. I., Bolander, M., and Eschenroeder, H. C. (1984). Enhancement of bone ingrowth by the use of bone matrix as a biologic cement, *Clin. Orthop.*, *183*, 255–261.

O'Connor, D. O., Burke, D. W., Sedlacek, R. C., Zalenski, E. B., and Harris, W. H. (1990). Bone–implant micromotion with the PCA mid-stem, *Trans. Soc. Biomater.*, *13*, 149.

Oonishi, H., Yamamoto, M., Ishimaru, H., Tsuji, E., Kushitani, S., Aono, M., and Ukon, Y. (1989). The effect of hydroxyapatite coating on bone growth into porous titanium alloy implants, *J. Bone Joint Surg., 71B*, 213–216.

Parsons, J. R., Ricci, J. L., Alexander, H., and Bajpai, P. K. (1988). Osteoconductive composite grouts for orthopedic use, *Ann. NY Acad. Sci., 523*, 190–207.

Pilliar, R. M. (1983). Bone micropore ingrowth, *J. Orthop. Res., 1*(2), 226.

Pilliar, R. M., Lee, J. M., and Maniatopoulos, C. (1986). Observations on the effect of movement on bone ingrowth into porous-surfaced implants, *Clin. Orthop., 208*, 108–113.

Rhinelander, F. W. (1973). Effects of medullary nailing on the normal blood supply of diaphyseal cortex, in *A.A.O.S. Instructional Course Lectures*, C.V. Mosby, St. Louis, pp. 161–187.

Rhinelander, F. W. (1974). Tibial blood supply in relation to the fracture healing, *Clin. Orthop., 105*, 34.

Rhinelander, F. W., Nelson, C. L., Stewart, R. D., and Stewart, C. L. (1979). Experimental reaming of the proximal femur and acrylic cement implantation vascular and histologic effects, *Clin. Orthop., 141*, 74–89.

Rivero, D. P., Fox, J., Skipor, A. K., Urban, R. M., and Galante, J. O. (1988). Calcium phosphate-coated porous titanium implants for enhanced skeletal fixation, *J. Biomed. Mater. Res., 22*, 191–201.

Robertson, D. M., Pierre, L., and Chahal, R. (1976). Preliminary observations of bone ingrowth into porous materials, *J. Biomed. Mater. Res., 10*(3), 335–344.

Ronningen, H., Solheim, L. F., Barth, E., and Langeland, N. (1986). Osteogenesis promoted by bone matrix combined with marrow. Titanium implants studied in rats, *Acta Orthop. Scand., 57*, 15–18.

Rubin, C. T., and McLeod, K. J. (1992). Promotion of bony ingrowth by frequency specific, low amplitude mechanical strain, *Trans. Orthop. Res. Soc., 17*, 69.

Sandborn, P. M., Cook, S. D., Spires, W. P., and Kester, M. A. (1988). Tissue response to porous-coated implants lacking initial bone apposition, *J. Arthroplasty, 3*(4), 337–346.

Schmalzried, T. P., and Harris, W. H. (1992). Periprosthetic bone loss in total hip replacement: The role of high density polyethylene (HDP) wear debris and the concept of the effective joint space, *Trans. Orthop. Res. Soc., 17*, 243.

Schutzer, S. F., Jasty, M., Bragdon, C. R., Harrigan, T. P., and Harris, W. H. (1990). A double-blind study on the effects of a capacitively coupled electrical field on bone ingrowth into porous-surfaced canine total hip prostheses, *Clin. Orthop., 260*, 297–304.

Schwarts, J. T., Engh, C. A., Forte, M. R., Kukita, Y., Arias, M., and Gualiteri, G. (1991). Evaluation of initial surface apposition in porous coated acetabular components, *Trans. Orthop. Res. Soc., 16*, 243.

Shimazki, K., and Moony, V. (1985). Comparative study of porous hydroxyapatite and tricalcium phosphate as bone substitute, *J. Orthop. Res., 3*, 301–310.

Shimizu, T., Zerwekh, J. E., Videman, T., Gill, K., Mooney, V., Holmes, R. E., and Hagler, H. K. (1988). Bone ingrowth into porous calcium phosphate ceramics: Influence of pulsing electromagnetic field, *J. Orthop. Res., 6*(2), 248–258.

Soballe, K., Hansen, E. S., Brockstedt-Rasmussen, H., Hjortdal, V. E., Juhl, G. I., Pedersen, C. M., Hvid, I., and Bunger, C. (1991). Gap healing enhanced by hydroxyapatite coating in dogs, *Clin. Orthop., 272*, 300–307.

Soballe, K., Brockstedt-Rasmussen, H., Hansen, E. S., and Bunger, C. (1992a). Hydroxyapatite coating modifies implant membrane formation. Controlled micromotion studied in dogs, *Acta Orthop. Scand., 63*(2), 128–140.

Soballe, K., Hansen, E. S., Rasmussen, H. B., and Bunger, C. (1992b). Hydroxyapatite coating converts fibrous anchorage to bony fixation during continuous implant loading, *Trans. Orthop. Res. Soc., 17*, 292.

Spector, M., Heyligers, I., and Roberson, J. R. (1988). Porous polymers for biological fixation, *Clin. Orthop., 235*, 207–219.

Spivak, J. M., Ricci, J. L., Blumenthal, N. C., and Alexander, H. (1990). A new canine model to evaluate the biological response of intramedullary bone to implant materials and surfaces, *J. Biomed. Mater. Res., 24*, 1121–1149.

Stewart, C. L., Skinner, R., and Hollis, J. M. (1993). Plexiglas modified Spurr low viscosity embedding medium composite mold system for study of the effect of micromotion on bone ingrowth, *J. Histotech., 16*, 145–149.

Sumner, D. R., Turner, T. M., Purchio, A. F., Gombotz, W. R., Urban, R. M., and Galante, J. O. (1995). Transforming growth factor beta enhances gap healing and bone ingrowth, *Trans. Orthop. Res. Soc., 20*, 191.

Sutherland, C. J., Wilde, A. H., Borden, L. S., and Marks, K. E. (1982). A ten-year follow-up of one hundred consecutive Muller curved-stem total hip-replacement arthroplasties, *J. Bone Joint Surg., 64A*(7), 970–982.

Tarvainen, T., Patiala, H., Tunturi, T., Paronen, I., Lauslahti, K., and Rokkanen, P. (1985). Bone growth into glassy carbon implants. A rabbit experiment, *Acta Orthop. Scand., 56*(1), 63–66.

Tencer, A. F., Woodard, P. L., Swenson, J., and Brown, K. L. (1987). Bone ingrowth into polymer coated porous synthetic coralline hydroxyapatite, *J. Orthop. Res., 5*, 275–282.

Tencer, A. F., Woodard, P. L., Swenson, J., and Brown, K. L. (1988). Mechanical and bone ingrowth properties of a polymer-coated, porous, synthetic, coralline hydroxyapatite bone-graft material, *Ann. NY Acad. Sci., 523*, 157–172.

Uchida, A., Nade, S. M., McCartney, E. R., and Ching, W. (1984). The use of ceramics for bone replacement. A comparative study of three different porous ceramics, *J. Bone Joint Surg., 66B*, 269–275.

Uchida, A., Nade, S., McCartney, E., and Ching, W. (1985). Bone ingrowth into three different porous ceramics implanted into the tibia of rats and rabbits, *J. Orthop. Res., 3*, 65–77.

Urist, M. R., Lietze, A., and Dawson, E. (1984). β-tricalcium phosphate delivery system for bone morphogenetic growth, *Clin. Orthop., 187*, 277.

Usui, Y., Zerwekh, J. E., Vanharanta, H., Ashman, R. B., and Mooney, V. (1989). Different effects of mechanical vibration on bone ingrowth into porous hydroxyapatite and fracture healing in a rabbit model, *J. Orthop. Res., 7*(4), 559–567.

Wang, F. R. (1990). Experimental study of osteogenic activity of sintered hydroxyapatite — On the relationship of sintering temperature and pore size, *Nippon Seikeigeka Gakkai Zasshi, J. Jpn. Orthop. Assoc., 64*(9), 847–859.

Yoshii, I., Whiteside, L. A., and White, S. E. (1991). The effect of material properties of the tibial tray on micromovement — CoCr vs. Ti6Al4V, *Trans. Orthop. Res. Soc., 16*, 167.

Zetti-Schafer, K. E., Engh, C. A., Sweet, D., and Bragdon, C. (1992). Histologic and roentgenographic assessment of well functioning porous coated acetabular components: A human postmortem retrieval analysis, *Trans. Implant Retrieval Symp. Soc. Biomater., 15*, 43.

30
Intravital Microscopy-Based *In Vivo* Observation of Polymer Erosion in Bone

Howard Winet
Orthopaedic Hospital and University of Southern California, Los Angeles, California
Jeffrey O. Hollinger
Oregon Health Sciences University, Portland, Oregon
Tomas Albrektsson
Göteborgs Universität, Göteborg, Sweden

I. INTRODUCTION

Erodible polymers are becoming increasingly attractive as modalities for bone fixation and reconstructive surgery. They offer advantages of eliminating revision surgery for removal of metal and delivery of osteoinductive molecules. In the rush to develop the ideal polymer, however, technology has outdistanced its basic science foundation. For example, 8% of polylactic acid (PLA) plated ankle fractures have been beset by aseptic foreign-body reactions after 12 weeks of implantation [14]. Acidosis has been postulated as the probable mechanism [26] and the lactic acid monomer generated by its hydrolysis cited as the agent. Neither *in vitro* [60–62] nor *in vivo* [86] studies have confirmed this conclusion. Yet so little of the basic science of the PLA erosion process is known that a reasonable hypothesis for an alternative mechanism has been elusive.

Investigations of polymer erosion usually include two approaches: (1) *in vitro* studies in which a baseline degradation pattern is determined under well-defined conditions and (2) *in vivo* studies intended to clarify the particular effects of the host tissue bed. For bone, *in vivo* studies are typically indirect. Histological assessment is performed on harvested polymer samples from sacrificed host animals to determine tissue reactions. Unfortunately, embedding and staining solutions tend to dissolve erodible polymers such as PLA. Consequently, it is difficult to assess relationships of polymer and tissue bed. Polarized light microscopy is a promising tool for locating birefringent erosion remnants [13], and one can alternate stained and unstained sections to reconstruct a "snapshot" of the implant environment. Nevertheless, harvesting techniques miss the interaction of eroding polymer with its surroundings, the fluid matrix and cells of host tissue. Direct observation of these events *in situ* in an intact living animal will solve this problem. It requires, however, the specialized optics of intravital microscopy (IVM).

When IVM is performed periodically on the same subject, that implanted animal

823

serves as its own comparison standard. Accordingly, data obtained can be normalized to adjust for subject variations unrelated to experimental conditions. This review describes how bone chamber IVM is being applied to study bioerodible implant incorporation, that is, the replacement of poly(α-hydroxy acid) copolymer with regenerated bone tissue.

II. BONE CHAMBER IVM

A. Development

Albrektsson [3] has reviewed extensively the history and development of the bone chamber. With the exception of a sketchy summary and some reference to vascular studies, this section is an update. The modern era of bone chamber IVM began with Sandison's [77] development of the rabbit ear chamber window in 1924. By mounting the rabbit with its ear on an intravital microscope stage, investigators could view the healing of tissue between two glass slips that formed the upper and lower window surfaces. The device has contributed significantly to understanding wound healing (e.g., Ref. 52). Without ear chambers or their variants, intravital microscopic studies would be restricted to acute procedures on *ex vivem* specimens. The majority of *in vivo* microcirculation studies have indeed been acute [70].

In 1958 Brånemark [16] performed the first intravital microscopic observations of bone blood flow after grinding a rabbit's fibula to a sheet thin enough to view medullary and endosteal microcirculation with transillumination. By 1964 he had replaced this procedure with an implantable tibial window that allowed chronic viewing of the microcirculation in femurs, vertebrae, and joints [17]. After replacing its metal rings and glass slips with a titanium screw and glass rods, these investigators were able to utilize the material characteristics of bone to maintain a constant field of view without the risk of fracture. The glass rods were glued into the titanium shell to maintain an interwindow separation space into which bone could heal. A critical requirement for stability of the bone chamber was osseointegration of the titanium screw threads. Without osseointegration the chamber would loosen and no bone would regenerate. IVM of bone healing also was carried out in ear chambers [35]. But these ectopic preparations resembled "graft" incorporation more than normal healing and offered limited insight.

McCuskey et al. [65–67] and Albrektsson [4], a student of Brånemark, refined the bone chamber implant (BCI) and investigated the effect of various agents and conditions on osteogenesis and angiogenesis, which for the BCI are more appropriately termed *neoosteogenesis* and *neoangiogenesis* (see below). By the late 1970s, Albrektsson and his students were the only investigators utilizing this optical BCI. Their IVM studies included the effects of irradiation [6], curing bone cement [7], fibrin [5], heat [33], and compression-induced ischemia [3] on mature and healing bone.

B. Baseline Gap Healing in the BCI: The Historical Control

Any model developed to evaluate the mutual influence of tissue and erodible implant must have a definitive baseline state that, for a quantitative control, will provide valid reference values. The current BCI model was developed from Albrektsson's [3] adaptation. Its *in situ* positioning is shown in Fig. 1. Implantation is similar to that of any bicortical screw with the exception that alignment is more critical and thermal necrosis is significantly reduced by saline-cooled low-velocity (1500 rpm) burring [33]. The 100-μm separation between its two quartz elements (the "slit") must align with cortex exposed by

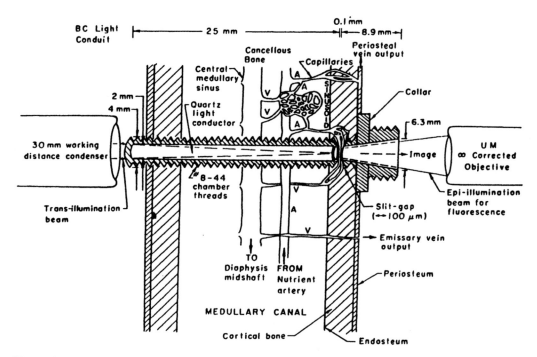

Figure 1 Implanted bone chamber *in situ*. Not to scale and without musculature. Chamber "head" is at right. Note positioning of slit-gap in cortex, which requires that collar be flush with proximal tibia medial surface. (From Ref. 90.)

surgical burring that created the bone gap/defect. Cortical (Haversian) bone regenerates into this slit-gap, the observation of which via IVM is the modus operandi of data gathering. Healing into the slit-gap is by creeping substitution through necrotic bone at the defect boundary, followed by apposition that eventually appears in the field of view.

1. Implantation and Exposure Surgeries

In the historical control [93,94], blood from the medullary canal exposed by burring is injected into the slit-gap. Accordingly, the initial healing tissue is a hematoma matrix bordered by necrotic cortical bone, quartz, and titanium. The bone chamber carrying this tissue is screwed into threaded bicortical burr holes through the medial surface, and the sides of the slit-gap not bounded by titanium face the same two directions as the bone long axis. Surgery is completed by closing the wound and allowing screw threads to osseointegrate for 20 days.

At 20 days (D20), both the medial (head) and lateral (tail) ends of the bone screw are exposed and fitted with delrin skin reflection buttons. The exposed implant ends are long enough to lift the buttons from underlying skin to prevent pressure necrosis. As long as the BCI ends remain exposed, the wound site is treated with daily H_2O_2 lavage and coating with gentamicin ointment. Infections (usually from *Pseudomonas* sp.) resulting from failure to maintain this antibacterial protocol and misalignment of the BCI are probably the two most frequent causes of failure in this model.

2. *Observation and Recording*

Observations commence 3 weeks postimplantation (W3) when the chamber's titanium shell has osseointegrated. They continue weekly until the ends are closed over (without buttons) or the BCI is explanted (for harvesting of slit-gap tissue or use as a transplant). Each observation begins 20 min after an injection of 5 mg/ml morphine sulfate (or Demerol). No ketamine (the anesthetic of choice) is utilized, in order to minimize artificial stimulation of cardiac output [30]. The rabbit, enclosed in a torso sling and held in sitting position by a supporting rail, is placed on the stage of a horizontal intravital microscope (hIVM). The BCI-carrying leg is carefully lifted into a yoke that clamps the BCI head and tail, aligning its optical axis with that of the microscope. Relative positioning is shown in Fig. 2, where it will be noted that the animal is in dorsal recumbency. A catch spring on the yoke's tightening screw allows quick release of the leg if the rabbit jumps. Also, BCI holders on the yoke compress the implant, minimizing pressure on leg musculature, which would affect circulation [90].

The hIVM is similar to other intravital microscopes in having the long focal lengths and working distances associated with telescopes [89]. It is designed for photomicro-

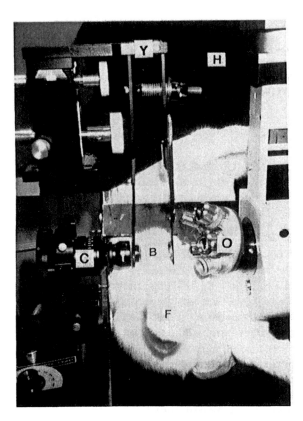

Figure 2 Rabbit with BCI mounted in hIVM. H = head and F = foot of animal. Y = top of spring-loaded yoke. O = microscope objectives and C = condenser. B marks location of BCI held by yoke.

graphy and videomicrography of bright-field, polarized-light and epifluorescent images, and has the optical flexibility to accommodate a variety of recording devices. Observations characteristically require 30–40 min utilizing the sequence

1. Bright-field images of nonvascular tissues; video recorded.
   a. Simple transmitted light to detect trabeculae.
   b. Polarized light to indicate collagen orientation.
2. Epi-illuminated fluorescence images; video recorded.
   a. 420-nm excitation filter for tetracycline uptake by trabeculae (oxytetracycline, demeclocycline, or calcein blue is injected at least 3 days prior to observation).
   b. Injection and observation of fluorescent microspheres (1.75 μm) under 490 μm excitation filter.
   c. Injection and observation of dextran 70 kDa conjugated with either fluorescein isothiocyanate (FITC-D70) under 490-nm excitation filter or rhodamine isothiocyanate (RITC-D70) under 540-nm excitation filter. Videorecording covers at least 2.5 min following this injection.
3. Four photographs are then taken, including images under:
   a. Simple transmitted light.
   b. Polarized transmitted light.
   c. Tetracycline epifluorescence.
   d. Epifluorescence appropriate for FITC-D70 or RITC-D70.
4. Epi-illuminated fluorescence images for permeability analysis; video recorded. Either FITC-D20 or RITC-D20 is injected and observed for at least 1 min.

Typical examples of transmitted/bright-field and epi-illuminated fluorescence images of the slit-gap field of view are presented in Fig. 3. The magnifications shown are greater than those used for analysis. The latter include the entire circle of the field of view.

3. Image Processing and Analysis

Images must be converted from analog to digital mode before quantitative analysis can be performed. The parameters processed are:

1. Trabecular area.
2. Vessel length and caliber, which must be obtained individually from each vessel segment to detect variations in static caliber. (Vasomotion cannot be resolved by the present optics.)
3. Velocity of microspheres.
4. Fluorescence intensity as a function of radial distance from the nearest vessel.

While assessment of the progress of bone apposition may be followed by both bright-field illumination and tetracycline fluorescence histomorphometry, slit thickness and long focal lengths limit resolution so that isolated single cells (except blood cells or osteocytes in lacunae) cannot be discriminated. No other technique, however, has been able to resolve perfused microvasculature, microcirculation, and nutrient exchange in bone as well as BCI IVM. Accordingly, by allowing simultaneous observation of trabecular healing, angiogenesis, and transport, this model forms a cell–tissue bridge in the total picture of local physiological relationships under relatively defined conditions.

Analysis of each parameter can be longitudinal or latitudinal. Latitudinal analyses group data from all subjects at a particular week into the same pool, from which statistics may be calculated. Graphing of data pools from each week yields a pattern indistinguish-

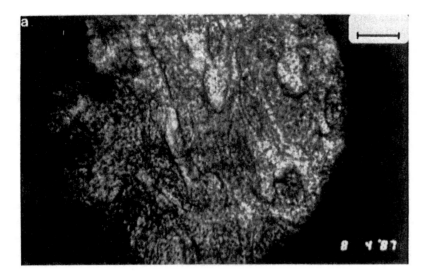

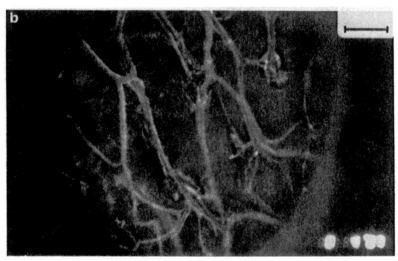

Figure 3 Examples of control images obtained in W8. Slit-gap is filled with remodeled bone (Haversian canals/secondary osteons), which is apparent in (a), the bright-field image. Note how vasculature in (b), the epifluorescence image, matches the Haversian canals visible in (a). Scale bar is 200 μm. (From Ref. 90.)

able from acute studies, where a different set of animals is observed each week and each animal is sacrificed following its observation. Longitudinal analysis can be performed via two statistical models: family of curves and normalization. The family of curves, or "flexifit," model, developed by Guardabasso and his colleagues [45], creates time-dependent data graphs for each subject in a chronic study and determines if they belong to the same family, for which a "family representative" plot is derived.

The normalization model also separates each animal, allowing its history to be accounted for in the analysis. It also allows each animal to serve as its own frame of reference by designating one of its measurements (e.g., maximum or minimum bone area) as the baseline, of which all others are fractions. The advantage of such normalization over the family of curves approach is that it reduces distortions due to scale that arise when comparing a rabbit that may have a better circulation, for example, than the least-perfused subject. Thus, experimental differences are preserved. Once normalization has linked all measures from each subject, the gains of a chronic study are sustained during subsequent statistical pooling, for example, grouping values from all subjects at each given week.

4. Norms

Neoosteogenesis Norms.   In designating bone regeneration in this model, the term *neoosteogenesis* is preferable to *osteogenesis* or *reosteogenesis* because, in the BCI, bone is regenerating into a slit-gap filled with hematoma (the blood injected into the BCI during implantation) and not into a simple defect or necrotic bone. The term is a necessary reminder that the model is not equal to a normal healing state.

Another limitation of the model arises from the fact that trabeculae formed by neoosteogenesis are most detectable via transillumination. The visible projection that results outlines an area that is the basis for neoosteogenesis calculations. Such "bone mass" measures mask remodeling to the extent that osteoclast activity is insufficient to produce a net reduction in projected area. Hence, it is understood that the values obtained are literally net neoosteogenesis. Volume calculations to obtain dimensionally correct bone measures do not add error because trabeculae thickness usually matches that of the slit [94].

Bone growth is traditionally measured in two techniques: (1) grossly by increase in bone volume using stained tissue sections or x-radiographs and (2) fluorescent detection of mineralization. One of the simplest forms of the first technique is to follow porous ingrowth into a prosthetic implant. As in the BCI, these implants allow "fingers"/trabeculae of bone to penetrate their pores (in the case of the BCI, the "pore" traverses the implant). Linear apposition rate is the distance penetrated divided by time. It could be expressed in terms of area, volume, or percentage of pore space occupied, but these measures are usually reserved for complex pore geometries (e.g., penetration into ceramic implants).

Projected trabecular area is the basic bone measure in the BCI model. A variety of video image analysis programs have been utilized for measuring this parameter. Each utilizes the same procedure of allowing the user to trace an outline of the bone image with a mouse/trackball-controlled cursor and computing an area in pixels. The pixels are converted to square micrometers with a measured scale factor and to cubic centimeters after multiplying this result by the average slit thickness. The latter is rarely exactly 100 μm or the same at both ends of the slit. It is computed by measuring and averaging the two openings. Apposing fronts have been sampled and viewed in sagittal histological sections to determine their pointedness. Characteristically, they were parabolic but blunt and it is assumed that the error in approximating a constant trabecular thickness is not significant [94].

For BCI data, change in trabecular area is expressed as change in percentage of slit-gap filled by the projected bone area ($\Delta\%B$). Trabecular neoosteogenesis into the slit-gap ($\Delta\%B/t$) followed a sigmoid regression characteristic of growth curves [94].

Linear apposition rate values were obtained by approximating the advancing front as an arc of a circle whose change in radius was equivalent to net apposition. Thus calculated, advance of trabeculae averaged 60 μm/day between W3 and W6, which agreed well with linear apposition rate values from other models as shown in Table 1. Woven bone formation followed by remodeling and lamellar bone formation were detectable with polarized light in the model. Evidence of remodeling, decrease in bone area, was seen as early as W5 [94].

Fluorescent labeling of mineralization fronts was also tried so that comparisons could be made with parallel data from other models. Certain fluorescent dyes (e.g., tetracycline) label osteoid as it is being mineralized. By injecting into a subject two dyes of different emission spectra at different time points and measuring the shortest distance between their labels, a measure of apposing front advancement can be obtained that is essentially equivalent to mineral apposition rate (MAR). In one measure, the MAR was 13 μm/day, an order of magnitude higher than published reports for mature cortical bone from other models using this technique [72]. Nevertheless, it is well below the MAR range for growing bones [9], a result that supports viewing the advancing fronts as apposing bone (growing bone is more embryonic and increases size faster) trabeculae. Note also that the BCI MAR value is also below that for linear apposition cited earlier. This difference is simply explained by the observation that linear apposition includes a number of osteons, each of which adds its own new mineralization to overall trabecular length.

The choice between the two techniques depends upon how their results are to be interpreted. If one is concerned with evaluating metabolic rates of the basic multicellular unit (BMU/osteon), MAR would be the measure of choice. If total trabecular regeneration is the focus, as has been the case for the BCI model, some form of apposition rate would be more appropriate.

Neoangiogenesis Norms. Traditionally, in orthopedics, the necessity for measuring neo-osteogenesis is obvious. The same cannot always be said for its parallel, "neoangiogenesis" [93]. While it is generally recognized that angiogenesis is a critical component of wound healing and that tissue reaction to implantation is a form of wound healing, the number of vessel regeneration studies in healing bone is small in comparison to the number addressing bone regeneration. Given that vasculature delivers inflammatory cells

Table 1 Osteogenesis Following Implant Surgery

Model	Device	<21 days	W3–W6[a]	W6–W8[a]	Ref.
Rabbit femur	4.76-mm Ti mesh	110	55	?	40
Dog femur	4.76-mm Ti mesh	90	60	?	40
Dog mandible	Ti mesh	150	65	?	34
Rabbit tibia	1-mm harvest chamber	175	?	?	2
Rabbit tibia	100-μm bone chamber	?	50	?	1
Rabbit tibia	100-μm bone chamber	?	60	34	94

Ingrowth/apposition (μm/day)

[a]W: week

and nutrients, maintains chemical homeostasis, and may provide osteoprogenitors [18] for the healing process, the lack of interest is hard to understand, although difficulty in visualizing bone vasculature *in situ* is a major cause. The unfortunate result, in any case, is that less is probably known about vascular physiology in bone than in any other organ, a state of affairs that has restricted our understanding of other facets of bone physiology.

To the obvious parallels with neoosteogenesis analysis, the study of neoangiogenesis adds some complications that must be understood for valid interpretation of results. Similar to the trabeculae, vessels may disappear from week to week [14], so the modifier "net" is implicit in this parameter as well. Typically, the vessels become occluded and are phagocytosed by macrophages. Many occluded vessels are visible with transmitted light illumination because they are filled with red blood cells. Thus, they are not providing a microcirculatory function and their inclusion in "vascularity" is misleading. Only perfused vasculature as revealed by intravascular FITC-D70/RITC-D70 is measured in the BCI. It provides the sole basis for calculating neoangiogenesis. *Neovascularization* denotes the consequence of neoangiogenesis.

Video images of epi-illuminated fluorescent vasculature were measured with the same image processing utilities as were the trabeculae. Two measures were obtained: internodal (between branch points) vessel length (l) and caliber (c) at the vessel midpoint. It was assumed that a vessel with varying c would have the shape of a truncated cone. From these two measures, surface area ($s_i = \pi c_i l_i$) and volume ($v_i = \pi c_i^2 l_i/4$) were calculated. (The subscript i is an index meaning each measurement). Microvasculature was characterized by:

1. Total vessel length, $L = \Sigma l_i$ and vascularity (L/V), where V is the volume of tissue containing the vessels. Separate calculations for vascularity of trabecular versus nontrabecular tissue were also obtained.
2. Average caliber, $\bar{c} = (\Sigma l_i c_i)/L$.
3. Total vascular surface area, $S = \Sigma s_i$; from which the total surface area of vessels within a specific range of c values—for example those associated with permeable vessels—could be extracted.
4. Total vascular volume (= blood volume), $V_b = \Sigma v_i$; with which the blood volume fraction for the slit-gap tissue (of volume V_c), $\phi = V_b/V_c$ could be calculated. If the average hematocrit of the slit-gap tissue were known, an estimate of O_2 delivery could be attempted, using ϕ values.

Net angiogenic rates for the BCI and other healing models are presented in Table 2. As is the case with healing bone, two forms of data representation dominate the literature. Where single vessels are identifiable over the observation period, micrometer/day values can be obtained. Although far less often used, L/V measures are the alternative. In sum, angiogenesis in bone is comparable to that in other tissues, although a little low with respect to cerebral cortex.

During the W3–W8 healing period in the BCI, vasculature was either labile or mobile, as it was difficult to find the same vessel at a given location from week to week. As a result, single-vessel values were difficult to obtain, and L/V became the exclusive measure of vascularity. Values of L/V tended to increase, due primarily to the high vascularity of ingrowing trabeculae. Average c ($\bar{c}$) tended to decrease during the same period, suggesting a corresponding increase in perfused new and/or previously plugged narrow vessels. It was predicted from these observations that because more vasculature was in the permeable size range, filtration would increase with time during this period.

Table 2   Angiogenesis

Model	Device	Net angiogenic rate	Ref.
Rabbit tibia	Bone chamber		
	Cortical bone	$\leq 300 \ \mu m/day$	
	Cancellous bone	$\leq 400 \ \mu m/day$	3
Rabbit ear	Ear chamber	$\leq 170 \ \mu m/day$	24
Rabbit ear	Ear chamber	$220 \ \mu m/day$	23
Rabbit eye	Cornea	$320 \ \mu m/day$	82
Rat brain	Cerebral cortex	$7 \times 10^7 \ \mu m/cm^3/day$	29
Rabbit tibia	100-μm bone chamber	$2 \times 10^5 \ \mu m/cm^3/day$ (W3–W6)[a]	
		$2 \times 10^6 \ \mu m/cm^3/day$ (W6–W8)	b

[a]W: week
[b]Calculated from Winet, Ref. 96 and unpublished data

Microcirculation Norms.   Microcirculation analysis [99] yields measures of local blood supply (Q), which is an indirect indicator Of oxygen delivery, since RBCs are confined to the vessels and the partition coefficient for O_2 is 1.0 in all venular capillaries. Molecular oxygen is important to the wound healing environment for its effect on cell viability and its effect on the composition of cellular products released to the interstitium. Lack of O_2 increases glycolysis by decreasing oxidative phosphorylation in mitochondria. As a result there is an increase in lactic acid, which attracts macrophages and induces them to produce angiogenins [54]. This sequence of events is only one example of how blood supply can influence neoangiogenesis.

Specific P_{O_2} values for given vessel segments cannot be calculated directly from Q, however, because hematocrit is not uniformly distributed over the microvasculature and venular capillaries cannot be identified. For the BCI studies, Q was computed from velocity u of 1.75-μm fluorescent microspheres viewed with epifluorescence illumination. Blood supply is calculated from $Q = \Sigma q_i$, where q_i is the blood supply of each influx (to the slit-gap tissue) vessel and is calculated from $q_i = \pi c_i^2 u_i / 8$, which assumes microspheres are in the flow centerline.

Representative values for Q are compared with those from other models and tissues in Table 3. It is evident that the locally obtained BCI values were higher than those from global procedures performed on other controls. The difference appears to result from relative purity of tissue. In the BCI, healing tissue only is observed and it is limited to vessels, their fibrous/collagen matrix, and newly formed bone. No necrotic or poorly vascularized tissues are present to average-out highly perfused regions.

Three relationships indicated by these studies are particularly relevant for the current review:

1. Trabeculae entered the slit-gap when P_{O_2} was relatively low (low Q_{in}). This observation was consistent with osteogenesis taking place under relatively anaerobic conditions.
2. $\Delta \% B$ decreased when Q_{in} increased, until the latter achieved its minimum, whereupon the relationship reversed. These observations were consistent with a lowering of osteogenesis under relatively aerobic conditions.
3. Q_{in} decreased from a pre-W3 value but rose after W4. These observations conflicted

Table 3 Blood Supply

Model	Device	Q (ml/min/100 g)	Ref.
Canine inguinal adipose tissue	Bleeding through cannula	8.0	76
Canine cerebrum	Entrapped micro-spheres	170 (during hypercapnia)	64
Canine tibia	Entrapped 15-μm microspheres	Mature cortical = 2.5 Immature cortical = 7.0 Mature cancell. = 38.3 Immature cancell. = 15.4	56
Canine tibia fracture	Isotope washout	36.2	71
Rabbit tibia	1.75-μm micro-spheres in BCI	Min. avg. 68 (W4) Max. avg. 227 (W7)	a

[a]Winet, unpublished data

directly with those in global fracture models [71]. As noted above, they may be explained by observation that vascularity was higher in the trabeculae than the surrounding fibrovascular tissue.

In general, however, these observations agreed with the more global ones of Brighton et al. [19], in which matrix formation is favored by high P_{O_2} (high Q_{in}) and osteogenesis by low P_{O_2} (low Q_{in}). The new insight provided by BCI observations is the localization of low versus high P_{O_2} regions in the healing tissue. Since bone carries more perfused vasculature, it has a higher internal P_{O_2}. Outside the apposing bone, conditions are relatively anaerobic. Thus, there is an oxygen gradient from bone to fibrovascular tissue that may play a critical role in triggering osteogenesis at the interface between the two tissues. The relative impacts of O_2 gradients versus absolute values on a given physiological process are important considerations in microcirculatory physiology of all other organs. So it would not be surprising to find a similar pattern in bone.

Nutrient Exchange Norms. Circulation's primary function is to exchange materials with tissues in microvascular beds [91]. An understanding of which solutes are being delivered (by extravasation) to the tissue interstitium, when and how much, and a corresponding understanding of the same variables for vessel uptake of interstitial solutes, is crucial for comprehending vessel–cell (and cell–cell) interactions during wound healing. Transmural transport across vessel endothelium occurs through pore-like structures, located primarily in venular capillaries, which come in two pore caliber ranges, 40–70 Å and 250–300 Å [75]. The basement membrane acts as a primary filter only when endothelial cells are separated, which may occur early in wound healing, when separations of up to 1 μm have been observed [73].

FITC-D70 (D70 = 70-kDa dextran), with a hydrodynamic diameter of 140 Å [78], can permeate only the large pores, which occur at a ratio to small pores of 1 : 30,000 [75]. Incidence of large pores increases under stress conditions, such as venous occlusion [100]. Little extravasation of this 70-kDa dextran is expected in mature bone [69], so the dye serves to outline the vessel lumen with fluorescence. In normal microcirculation, large molecules such as albumin (hydrodynamic diameter 140 Å) enhance the buffering capacity of interstitial fluid.

A measure of the incidence of such pores would reflect the degree to which large buffering molecules were available to the interstitium. To evaluate the incidence of such pores, an investigation of sites of FITC-D70 extravasation, called "leak points" (LP), was conducted. It was found that:

1. LP incidence (LP per unit tissue volume = LP/V) increased as Q_{in} decreased.
2. Rate of trabecular apposition ($\Delta\%B$) increased as LP/V in bone increased.

Averaged out over the entire slit-gap tissue, however, there was no significant relationship between $\Delta\%B$ and LP/V [92]. The change of extravasation with Q_{in} indicated that extravasation of this solute in bone was not a diffusion-limited process, an important consideration when attempting to relate Q to implant erosion rates of biodegradable polymers.

FITC-D20 (D20 = 20-kDa dextran), in contrast, has a hydrodynamic diameter of 56 Å (extrapolated from Schaeffer et al., Ref. 78). It was easily extravasated, yielding fluorescence that diffused away from each vessel. Measurements of this diffusion were used to obtain some preliminary estimates of vessel permeability. First, two video frames 10 sec apart were grabbed and digitized. Each frame showed a change in extravascular fluorescence, starting with 3 sec following its appearance in perfused vessels. The fluorescence intensity profile was determined. This is a measure of the concentration distribution in space of fluorescent molecules, and it changed as a function of time and vessel permeability. For a given solute, concentration at a given distance (x) from the vessel surface (C_x) will change at a known rate ($\Delta C_x/\Delta t$), if diffusion is the sole determinant of its transport. It has been shown by Wayland and Fox [88] that, by using the mathematical form of the intensity profiles of a given solute, and comparing the rate of change of its concentration (C_x^*) at x over the same time period ($\Delta C_x^*/\Delta t$), one would obtain a measure of the exclusivity of diffusion in this system ($[\Delta C_x^*/\Delta t]/[\Delta C_x/\Delta t] = \Delta C_x^*/\Delta C_x$), with a result of 1.0 indicating "free" diffusion.

Two BCI samples were measured for exclusivity of diffusion. Each rabbit received injections of FITC-D70 and -D20 only if the larger molecule did not extravasate. An example of the time-separated intensity profiles is presented in Fig. 4. Samples were

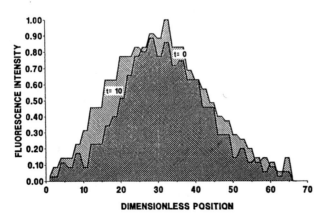

Figure 4 Fluorescence intensity profile showing extravasation of FITC–dextran 40 over a 10-second interval. Vessel centerline is at position 30.

obtained at D13 (13 days postimplantation) and D27. It was found that large pores were present at D13 and that FITC-D70 extravasated faster than the free diffusion rate. In contrast, FITC-D20 was the only molecule that leaked at D27, and at a rate slower than free diffusion. Clearly, diffusion was not acting alone at D13 and it was inhibited (by pore wall interference?) by D27. If these preliminary results are confirmed by larger-sample studies, a more complete permeability pattern for stages of acute bone healing will emerge. (One may then address the question of how an eroding polymer interacts with vessel small pore permeability. A parallel study with large pore permeability would also be logical.). The pattern suggested by preliminary data is that by D13 a number of large- and small-vessel pores, presumably associated with posttraumatic hyperemia, were still present. By W3, large-pore incidence was reduced, as bone was being laid down outside the field of view. With the entrance of trabeculae from W4 on, the incidence of large pores and mineralization of the matrix in the slit-gap tissue increased.

III. BCIs AS CARRIERS OF TRANSPLANTS

A. Incorporation of Homotopic (Implanted in Bone) Autogenous Bone

The "platinum standard" for bone grafting is vascularized autograft, which is the only true graft because both donor and host bone remain alive postimplantation [83]. In the absence of vessel anastomoses, the donated tissue "survives" as a necrotic sequestrum or is decomposed via a process termed "incorporation" [21]. The "gold standard" for incorporation is autogenic bone, a totally histocompatible tissue. Some of its donor cells may survive [68], but the fate of the autogenic implant usually depends upon its porosity, the degree of hypoxia-induced necrosis, the effectiveness of invading host cells [21], and the size of the host bed [79].

Autogenous bone incorporation has been studied extensively by Albrektsson and his collaborators [3]. Their procedure was to allow a BCI to fill with bone and transplant it to the contralateral tibia or rotate it in place. Any osteogenic effect [31] (stimulation of osteoblast activity at a site distant from trauma) presumably was discounted. Bone apposition, microcirculation, and angiogenesis were all semiquantitatively evaluated in Albrektsson's studies. It was found that early revascularization of the donor bone was associated with its successful incorporation. Host vessels penetrated donor bone by 4 days postimplantation (D4) and completely revascularized the 100 μm thick, 3×10^{-4} cm^3 tissue by D21. Generally, revascularization networks did not match those present in the donor fragment at implantation. In fact, the resulting arborization was so "irregular" that it prohibited identification of ingrowing microvasculature on a basis other than caliber [2] (venules, arteries, and capillaries were assigned size ranges).

Remodeling of the donor bone was not evident until it had been almost completely revascularized. Thus, one is faced with the question of how canals for the new networks were "carved out." Perhaps answers can be derived from those unusual cases where host and donor vessels appeared to anastomose spontaneously, an event called "recirculation" by Albrektsson [1]. In these cases, remodeling of the donor bone was evident by the end of W1. Histoincompatibility cannot be invoked as a mechanism for this difference in remodeling in an autogenic model. However, the release of oxygen radicals and other products of tissue necrosis during the inflammatory response to surgery can influence remodeling by stimulating osteoclasts to resorb necrotic bone [10] and thereby release "stormones" (matrix-bound cytokines [38]) such as bFGF (and other angiogenins),

TGF-βs (which probably mobilize mesenchymal cells [43]) and BMPs (bone morphogenetic proteins, which influence osteoinduction) [101].

Among the other functions of the extracellular matrix in the wound focus are mechanical bridging of the wound edges and providing a suitable surface for migrating cells. The fibrin clot entraps platelets that secrete cytokines and is coated with fibronectin (from plasma and platelets [44]). Macrophages have no difficulty navigating such a structure, particularly since they can "remodel" it with the aid of the plasminogen activator they secrete and phagocytosis. Migrating fibroblasts [85] and endothelial cells [32] "see" a fibronectin matrix that is haptotropic (stimulates haptotaxis: directed cell movement due to cellular adhesion gradients to substratum-attached components [39]). Upon reaching the awaiting macrophages, the fibrovascular tissue organizes in response to their secreted cytokines and the orientation of fibronectin fibers [53]. All three of these cell types are capable of secreting fibronectin, but the implied interactions have not been designated [44].

Macrophages may also be induced to secrete fibrinogens that attract collagenase-secreting fibroblasts [74], which will digest collagen remnants from trauma or strands aligned in conflict with the prevailing mechanical stresses [53]. Thus, one has the impression that the state of the matrix following fibrin digestion by plasmin during normal healing is not permanent, and that the presence of an implant: would further complicate its behavior. Consider the fibronectin layer that undoubtedly coats any implant following clot digestion. It should be haptotropic for fibroblasts and endothelial cells. If the implant degrades, macrophages penetrating its fractures would be in an ideal location to lay down fibronectin, which would attract the other two cell types. To the degree that degradation products and implant geometry determine penetrating macrophage itinerary, they could have considerable influence on healing direction.

The studies of Albrektsson and his colleagues utilized lamellar bone of cortical and endochondral origin. While the anatomical origin of the donor bone is of merely tangential interest to the present review, the structure of its matrix, with respect to its mechanical strength, is of direct concern. Intramembranous bone typically develops by a process that results in a shell [46], where the distance from its cellular components and external vascular nourishment are relatively small. Thus, it tends to be relatively compact and unporous. Vascular penetration of a transplanted block of such bone is a major challenge for host bed giant cells or osteoclasts, because of its small surface-to-volume ratio. This situation contrasts with that for endochondral bone, which provides ample porosity, that is, surface for resorbing cells and migrating endothelial cells [21,47]. Accordingly, Smith and Abramson [80] found little volume change of onlayed membranous as compared to endochondral implants at the same host site. Nevertheless, Kusiak et al. [57] found better vascular penetration of intramembranous than endochondral onlay implants.

Another geometric consideration is the differences between trabecular and cortical bone (e.g., the cancellous bone in the metaphysis vs. the compact bone in the diaphysis). These become germane to bone transplant bone chamber studies, however, only when the implant site is inconsistent (i.e., varies between being too proximal and too distal from its standard location at the diaphysis–metaphysis junction). The host bone growing into the slit-gap would be forced by geometry in either case to assume the form of a trabeculum advancing at first by creeping substitution and at last by apposition, but the mechanical support for the chamber would differ.

B. Incorporation of Homotopic Allogeneic Bone

Unless extraordinary genetic matching between host and donor has occurred, histoincompatibility responses of the former will range from prolonged local inflammatory nonspecific foreign-body reaction to full systemic immune reaction against the Class I and II donor cell surface antigens. The latter reaction would result in implant rejection [81]. Once T-lymphocytes have been alerted by sufficient antigen, they can, via secreted cytokines—interleukins (ILs) and/or interferons—alert helper T-cells and/or macrophages; and either of these can, via secretion of cytokines (tumor necrosis factor), stimulate osteoblasts to secrete colony-stimulating factors and IL-6, activating osteoclast precursors to differentiate into osteoclasts to resorb donor bone [81]. The few donor surface osteoblasts that survive implantation are gone by the end of 2 weeks, due to host foreign-body reaction [42].

By the time resorption commences, host vessels have penetrated the implant along preexisting Haversian and Volkmann canals. In large implants this revascularization is reversed as a function of histoincompatibility by inflammatory cells that occlude the vessels, initiating their degeneration [42]. Resorption penetrates only enough to allow deposition of new bone to a thickness of 20–80 μm around the implant [21]. Incorporation ends with both host bone and soft tissue occupying resorbed space [21]. The mechanical success of the incorporation is linked to minimizing this space.

Bone chamber allogeneic bone studies utilized a sufficiently small implant volume to allow complete revascularization of the donor bone disk without the inflammatory response triggering vessel degeneration. Thus, the disk was often well vascularized when the first signs of its resorption were detected. Histoincompatibility was not completely masked in this implant, however, as a space of at least 50 μm persisted between resorbing implant and apposing (would this pattern fit the definition of "creeping substitution"?) host trabeculae [95]. Moreover, revascularization is delayed by at least 2 weeks [96] as compared with the bone chamber autogeneic bone studied by Albrektsson et al. [1].

IV. BIOERODIBLE POLYESTERS IN BONE GRAFTING AND BONE FIXATION

Of the synthetic polymers currently available for human implantation, the aliphatic poly (α-hydroxy acids), such as polylactic acid (PLA) and polyglycolic acid (PGA) have the longest clinical history. PLA has been used as a surgical implant material for at least 25 years [11]. It depolymerizes to form pyruvic and lactic acid, which are eventually metabolized to CO_2 and H_2O if sufficient O_2 is present. PGA depolymerizes to form glycolic acid, which may be excreted or transformed to pyruvic acid. The molecular weights commonly utilized range from 40 to 100 kDa. Depolymerization in both is by hydrolytic scission and is accelerated *in vitro* by increasing pH [22]. The rate of depolymerization varies with the molecular configuration of the polymer. In general, PLA, with a half-life of 195 days, degrades slower than PGA, with a half-life of 90 days [22]. But the latter has a greater tensile strength [50]. There are other sources of polyester implant variation such as crystalline-to-amorphous ratio that relate to isomer ratios. As an example of the latter, poly(L-lactic acid) is mostly crystalline and resistant to hydrolysis while poly(DL-lactic acid) is mostly amorphous [25]. At present it is not possible to control the structure of a given batch of either homopolymer so that the distribution of various molecular configurations is known [58,63]. Thus, erosion rates of two batches of the "same" polymer are not the same in identical environments [50] and data from well-controlled *in vitro* tests show significant dispersion [59,63]. These sources of variation in polymer samples of the same molecular weight must be considered when interpreting observations.

Orthopedic application of erodible polymers for internal fixation has been explored for over 10 years [36]. Notwithstanding the challenges to synthesis reproducibility, attempts to combine the mechanical advantages of PGA with the erosion advantages of PLA have led to the development of PLGs (copolymers of PLA and PGA). Common, commercial PLG formulations have molar ratios of 50 : 50 and 85 : 15 (PLA : PGA), with the former preferred for maxillofacial bone reconstruction [50]. The half-life for dissolution of 50 : 50 PLG can be as rapid as 7 days, but a shift of the molar ratio in either direction increases this value [50]. Fixation with PLG has been reviewed by Böstman et al. [11] and maxillofacial grafting by Hollinger and Battistone [50]. Johnson et al. [55] loaded PLG strips with human BMP and applied them to femoral nonunions for up to 6 months with no reported foreign-body reactions. However, Böstman et al. [14] found that 5% of ankle fractures fixed with rods and sutures made of 90 : 10 PLG developed sterile draining sinuses after 12–16 weeks and 7% developed malunions, the latter suggesting mechanical failure. In response to this result, these workers developed PGA fiber reinforced PGA plates and screws. While mechanical results appeared to be promising, the tendency for both PGA and PLA fixators to stimulate a late (12 weeks to almost 3 years) foreign-body reaction in almost 8% of the cases [11], as noted above, is cause for concern.

In a majority of the applications by the Böstman group, the polymer was essentially a composite, even though its component monomers were the same species. This synthetic anisotropy and the natural tendency toward variability of isomer and form (crystalline vs. amorphous) within any polymer batch make it difficult to maintain precision for comparison studies. Intermediate breakdown products will retain these heterogeneities to varying degrees. Nevertheless, breakdown products (e.g., lactic acid) probably dominate the chemical interaction of tissue with implant. Since these fragments are too small to transmit loads, the results of studies that concentrate on the chemistry of the interaction should be equivalent. Accordingly, it is not necessary to duplicate load regimes to gain insight into the physiological events during incorporation of a given polymer. Sufficiently basic information from the study of these events is applicable to both fixation and grafting. Indeed, given that erodible polymeric screws must be replaced by bone and that eroding plates may form part of a callus, one may view fixation with erodible implants as a form of grafting. There are limitations to such extrapolation, of course. Also, since the presence of chondrocytes is the essential difference between membranous and endochondral bone healing, care should be taken in predicting membranous maxillofacial healing from callus-forming long bone models.

The shape of a polymer implant acting as an osteoconductive support matrix (OSM) has an important influence on both its physiologic effects and mechanical stability. The rate of imbibition is strongly related to OSM surface-to-volume ratio ($S : V$) and surface contour. As the surface area of the OSM increases relative to its total volume more surface is exposed to the interstitial fluid, thereby enhancing imbibition and erosion rate. Furthermore, density and surface-to-density ratio ($S : \rho$) are inversely related to imbibition and subsequent hydrolysis [84]. Törmälä et al. [84] found, for fiber-reinforced PGA rod implants, a strong correlation between $S : \rho$ and retention of high elastic modulus with time. In general, as $S:V$ increases and/or $S:\rho$ decreases, the rate of erosion will be more rapid.

The initial tissue response to a PLG OSM is probably due to mechanical perturbation of the host tissue bed. Because PLG is relatively biocompatible, the few reports of early foreign-body reactions describe a mild transient response [49]. However, release of monomers and acidic oligomers may be sudden enough to evoke the chronic late foreign-body inflammatory response reported by Böstman et al. [11]. Between these two tissue responses there is undoubtedly an evolving reaction of the microvasculature to the biodegrading copolymer that slowly undermines the latter's tertiary (chain-based, not just group-based) structure.

The PLG–OSM reaction to the initial tissue edema is probably also mechanical, due to changing pressure environment (osmotic and hydrostatic). Chu has postulated that *in vivo*, the amorphous regions of PLG thread are hydrolyzed first [22]. Crystalline zones are protected by a "cage effect." When the crystalline domains depolymerize, cracks develop and paths open for penetration by hydrolyzing agents, causing an accelerated release of monomers [22]. In sutures, the transition from amorphous to crystalline phase hydrolysis takes place at about W3 *in vitro* [22]. It is likely that the process is slower for the dense (low $S:V$) bone screws observed by Böstman et al. [11] than for the suture threads described by Chu [22]. However, one cannot assume a predictable transition pattern, since amorphous-to-crystalline transitions may occur spontaneously [8].

Investigations of responses of bone to polymer implants have been conducted primarily through histomorphometry and histology. The methods employed parallel those used in evaluating so-called incorporation of porous ceramic implants [51]. Accordingly, Hollinger [49] implanted a 2 mm diameter, 1.25 mm thick disk of 80-kDa 50:50 PLG into rat tibia and found osteoblasts in the space between the recipient bed boundary and a dissolving implant by 7 days. Trabeculae had formed by 21 days, when the implant was reduced to small "islands." No inflammatory response was observed. Observation of capillaries was restricted, however, to beyond the first 28 days postimplantation.

V. THE ROLE OF THE VASCULAR SYSTEM IN INCORPORATION OF POLYMER IMPLANTS

Implantation adds a complication to normal wound healing of any tissue that is reflected in vascular responses. With data from autogeneic and allogeneic bone implants providing arbitrary boundaries for the range of biocompatibility responses, it is expected that the reactions of bone microvasculature to nonantigenic yet histoincompatible (as opposed to "inert") polymers would fall between the extremes describe above. Formulating predictions of expected vascular behavior for bone is, however, problematic. The lack of quantitative studies on this subject for bone healing was noted above, and Glowacki [47,57] has pointed out a similar lack of vascular information for the process by which implant is replaced with regenerated host tissue (incorporation).

Accordingly, in previous investigations of poly(α-hydroxy acid) erosion in bone, there apparently have been no reports quantitating vascular events during the incorporation process. It is generally accepted that poly(α-hydroxy acid) dissolution in bone is more rapid in a highly vascular host bed [50], but this prediction has not been tested. Reference has been made by a number of investigators to the presence of vessels and there has been considerable interest in inflammatory responses. Accordingly, Hollinger and

Battistone [50] found a transient inflammatory reaction to PLG at 72 h in a rat or mouse muscle pouch and Böstman et al. [12] report the appearance of edema in orthopedic patients at the implant site about 12 weeks postimplantation. Bouet et al. [15], using laser doppler velocimetry in rabbit muscle, have tried to correlate blood flow and biocompatibility of a number of nonaliphatic polymers to develop a standardized *in vivo* biocompatibility test. They concluded their technique had promise, particularly for detecting incompatibilities based on "interface" toxicity, as opposed to leached-product toxicity.

Inducing a pattern of incorporation from these observations is not trivial. One can, however, build reasonable hypotheses by inducing how implant decomposition will interact with normal wound healing from what is known about each process. In response to trauma, a cascade of healing events is initiated that brings macrophages to the wound focus where they elaborate fibrogenins and angiogenins. Lactic acid, which is normally present in the anaerobic environment, stimulates macrophages to secrete angiogenic factors, but pyruvate and low pH per se do not [54]. Low pH increases blood supply [27], bringing in more O_2 to allow oxidation of metabolites. Oxidation and the release of buffering macromolecules from the numerous large pores, at this stage of healing [73], will raise the pH. As pH rises, macrophages depart, lowering free angiogenin concentration and, consequently, the number of vessels. A decrease in O_2 and blood supply ensues. Osteoblasts/osteoprogenitors attracted to the wound site by the release of "stormones" from damaged matrix or fellow osteoblasts, secrete collagen I [19]. Where O_2 concentration and pH fall below a critical level, osteogenesis commences [19], accompanied by angiogenesis and mineralization. Angiogenesis at this juncture may be stimulated by the release of stormone angiogenins, such as basic FGF from subendothelial extracellular matrix [37] during vessel absorption. Both the low O_2 concentration and low pH at the start of trabecular regeneration stimulate microcirculatory autoregulatory mechanisms to increase blood flow in bone [28]. Vascularity and bone apposition rate are positively correlated in the BCI model as they are in other models [48].

Vessel permeability selects which buffers or polymer-degrading agents diffuse to the implant environment. It, together with the lymphatics, also selects the metabolites and monomer products of erosion that are removed. Observations of *LP/V* reported earlier [92] suggest large-pore incidence was greatest in healing bone trabeculae during maximum apposition, which occurred between W4 and W6 (after deposition of the collagen I matrix). During this period of maximum osteogenesis, angiogenesis brought in more new (small caliber) vessels [93], which, in bone, exhibited more large, buffer-extravasating pores [92]. This raised local pH [20], as mature remodeling bone was becoming established. Small pores, which occupy at least 3 orders of magnitude more of the vascular surface, appeared, from preliminary data, to be less permeable at W4. However, the fact that the vessel yielding these data was in fibrovascular tissue must be kept in mind for their interpretation.

The reported effects of lactic acid on macrophages suggest a greater angiogenic response to PLA or high-PLA fraction PLG than to PGA, but no such comparison has been reported. The high incidence of large pores during inflammation [73] suggests an increase in pH following an initial drop due to hypoxia and cell death [20]. As pH increases, there should be an acceleration of polymer erosion, as has been reported for PLG threads [22]. As long as buffering is maintained there will be a diffusion gradient for transport of monomers from the polymer. To the extent that macromolecular buffering agents from the microvasculature accelerate polymer erosion, the existence of two large pore incidence peaks suggests two periods of attack on the implant, independent of any effect polymer erosion may have on the host.

Missing from the above account are macrophages, giant cells, and PMNLs, which attack implants, and local edema from increased microvascular permeability, which dilutes the interstitium, enhancing the exchange pool for degradation products.

VI. BCIs AS CARRIERS OF BIOERODIBLE POLYMERS

Traditional studies of PLG incorporation have been histological. Few have applied quantitative methods to study bone defects filled with PLG plugs and harvested at various time intervals to assess the changes in cell and tissue populations [49]. Bone apposition was quantitatively, and vascularity qualitatively evaluated in these studies. Results indicated a PLG-generated enhancement of bone healing [49].

The BCI appeared to be an ideal tool for studying incorporation of erodible polymers in bone. The BCI houses a slit-gap, essentially a culture cell with culture medium supplied by the organism. Its location in bone guaranteed that the same site was being sampled each week. Direct comparisons could be made with chronic *in vitro* studies of degradation of the same polymer. Before a valid interpretation of observations is possible, however, limitations of the BCI model for revealing implant–tissue interactions must be understood.

Materials placed in the slit-gap are not, initially, in contact with bone. They are merely imbedded in the fibrin–platelet matrix of a hematoma. This is not to say that bone growing into the slit-gap is significantly stress shielded. While the titanium screw obviously distorts the distribution of stresses exhibited during normal gap healing, it does not affect osteogenesis sufficiently to prevent ingrown bone from persisting for up to 2 years [98]. During incorporation, however, mechanical interactions of any material in the slit-gap with surrounding bone are delayed until apposing trabeculae contact the device. Thus, the BCI model essentially isolates chemical from mechanochemical interactions between implant material and host tissue, at least in the early stages of healing. BCI data, consequently, give insight into the purely chemical interaction of eroding implant with host tissue during incorporation.

To date only PLG has been subjected to BCI IVM. Samples were obtained from extruded 100 μm thick threads of 40-kDa, 50 : 50 (PLLA : PGA) molar ratio material prepared by the Ethicon division of Johnson & Johnson, Inc. The thread was not reprocessed to control nonuniformities. Thus, microscopic examination revealed regions of slubbing (i.e., bulges).

It was hypothesized for this study that bone apposition rate ($\Delta\%B/t$) would not be altered by PLG erosion. It was reasoned that in the Hollinger studies [49], healing rat bone tissue was able to use the PLG plug as a scaffolding. Moreover, the intimate contact between bone and plug shortened the distance invading vessels had to traverse with their acid-buffering plasma. In the BCI, there was a space of about 1 mm between the perimeter of the burr hole and the PLG—the total defect diameter was 4 mm—which would probably serve as a reservoir for the accumulation of lactic and glycolic acid until blood vessels could cross into the slit-gap field of view. The PLG used was a 100 μm diameter thread, a poor scaffolding candidate in a 2 mm wide tissue, even when penetrated by advancing vessels. The interaction of PLG with tissue was postulated, consequently, to be more chemical than mechanical. Accordingly, it was predicted that the acidic monomers of PLG degradation could accumulate in the reservoir sufficiently to inhibit neoosteogenesis from the cortex. At this point, the report by Vasenius et al. [86] showing that, except for a point well after incorporation, blood pH changed insignificantly around polylactide intramedullary rods, had not appeared.

The two conflicting predictions suggested a balance between agents that favor and those that inhibit neoosteogenesis. Consequently, it was hypothesized that their effects would offset each other, and that neoosteogenesis into a BCI would occur at the same rate in controls (i.e., unloaded BCIs) as in experimentals (i.e., BCIs loaded with PLG); which is, in effect, the null hypothesis. There appear to be no studies of the direct effect of PLG bioerosion on cytokine physiology, so predictions about this effect were not formulated.

For the *in vitro* standard study, segments of the thread were placed in Tyrode's solution at 37°C and microphotographed daily the first week, and weekly from then on. The first apparent changes occurred by 8 days. They were: (1) an apparent thickening of the thread, which may have been accompanied by shortening; and (2) increase in optical density. It took 6 weeks for significant fracturing to appear and at least 18 weeks for the remnants to be reduced to shards.

For the *in vivo* studies, segments about 4 mm long were cut off with iridectomy scissors and placed between the two quartz windows of each chamber as it was assembled. Care was taken to compress each segment only enough to keep it from slipping out of the slit-gap. The loaded BCIs were sterilized with ethylene oxide gas at room temperature for 12 h and degassed for 24 h using laminar-flow filter-sterilized air. Implantation, exposure, and animal maintenance was the same as for the controls described above. The one variable changed was time. Whereas the control studies were completed in 8 weeks, these required 10 and included some samples at 12 weeks.

Observations commenced at W3 and two experimental groups were immediately identified. In the first group the PLG appeared to have unravelled. Some vessels were present but characteristically were limited to the periphery. This result was attributed to the existence of highly amorphous sections of the copolymer and served as an indicator of variability in the syntheses of PLG. No trabeculae appeared and vasculature was markedly reduced in these slit-gaps over the course of the study.

In the second group, erosion, neoosteogenesis, and neoangiogenesis appeared to progress in an ordered fashion. Both results have been reported [97]. Observations from a more typical specimen are depicted in Fig. 5. Data from the second group are summarized in Fig. 6. Trabeculae usually appeared at W5, occasionally being delayed to W6 or W7. Osseous filling of the slit-gap was rarely achieved before W10, and the maximum neoosteogenic rate occurred between W7 and W8. The delay in comparison with the controls was statistically significant between W5 and W9. After this delay, however, osteogenesis, as indicated by the curve slope, proceeded at the same rate as the controls. An apparent "recovery" of osteogenesis after W5 produced apposition rates as high as 4.3%, a value 20% higher than the fastest control rate. Such accelerations were not, however, sufficiently characteristic to generate a steeper regression curve (Fig. 6).

There was no evidence of incompatibility between trabeculae and polymer. It appeared that the regenerating bone interfaced directly with the polymer (Fig. 5). Confirmation of this observation at the cellular level awaits further histological study.

Neoangiogenesis analysis showed that L/V versus time was delayed in the presence of PLG [99]. Maximum perfused vascularity occurred between W10 and W11, 3 weeks after the control peak. Neoangiogenesis was depressed, with the minimum L/V value almost

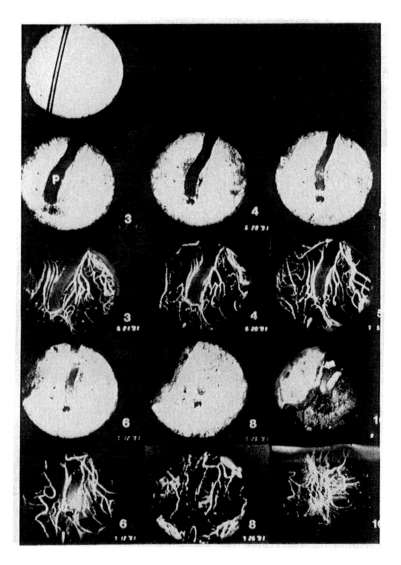

Figure 5 Neo-osteogenesis, neo-angiogenesis, and PLG erosion in a representative bone chamber. All panels are at the same magnification with slit-gap circles 2 mm in diameter. Times (W3, etc.) are in weeks post-implantation. Polymer (P) and trabeculae (B) are identified in first two panels only. Fibrovascular tissue (F) shows orientation of perfused vessels (PV) parallel with the bone long axis. W10 is represented by two photographs, the last panel showing its oxytetracycline deposition at mineralization sites (arrow) and regions from which it has not yet diffused (photograph taken less than 4 days after injection).

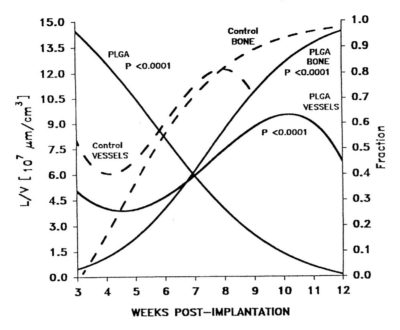

Figure 6 Summary of measurements of neo-osteogenesis and neo-angiogenesis in control and experimental subjects, and PLG erosion in the latter. Vascularity is defined as perfused vessel length per unit tissue volume. Ossification is fraction of slit-gap field-of-view filled with trabeculum. Error bars are omitted for clarity but may be found in original reports. The control bone regression curve has been continued well beyond W9 (the final observation point if beyond W8) for symmetry. Note that neo-osteogenesis is delayed and neo-angiogenesis is both delayed and inhibited around the eroding PLG. (From Ref. 98.)

halved (Fig. 6). Nevertheless, the pattern of neoangiogenesis persisted, including a projected maximum L/V prior to W3. Thus, the agreement of these results with control observations of Brighton et al. [19], that osteogenesis is enhanced by low P_{O_2} and collagen synthesis by high P_{O_2}, indicates that PLG incorporation does not alter basic physiological relationships. Separate evaluation of trabecular and fibrovascular L/V has not been performed. It appears, however, that while the delay in neoangiogenesis can be explained as an effect of trabecular apposition delay, the cause of its inhibition is more elusive. Further analysis will be necessary to determine if vascularity in the trabeculae has significantly changed in the presence of eroding PLG.

No correlation could be found between the disappearance of PLG and rate of neoosteogenesis or neoangiogenesis. The plots in Fig. 6 suggest a negative correlation between bone apposition and polymer erosion. If the study had been performed using acute observations, calculation would have given a statistically significant linkage. The advantage of a chronic model like the BCI, is that each rabbit serves as its own reference. Resulting correlations were, accordingly, animal specific and, consequently, more accurate reflections of cause and effect.

Biocompatibility appeared to be supported by neoangiogenesis patterns. There was often evidence of vessel penetration of polymer fractures (Fig. 5). Nevertheless, neoosteogenic and neoangiogenic delay during PLG erosion was significant. There is an apparent paradox between this circumstantial relationship and the lack of correlation between the disappearance of PLG and rates of the two regeneration processes cited above. The paradox may be resolved by postulating that one of the two apparently time-dependent processes is not truly time dependent. Since tissue regeneration is demonstrably time dependent [93,94], the candidate must be the PLG. A scenario in which the visible erosion of polymer is not representative of the actual loss of mass is not difficult to fashion for bulk eroders such as PLG. Visible erosion readings are based on changes in the polymer's profile. Bulk eroders degrade internally before degradation affects their outer boundary, which apparently acts like a semipermeable membrane [87]. Accordingly, monomer efflux through the "membrane" results in polymer weight loss and may influence tissue regeneration, but is not visible as area changes. This shortcoming of the BCI model may be surmounted by incorporating a covalently bound fluorescent dye in the polymer that would be released during depolymerization.

The retardation of bone and vessel regeneration did not appear to be caused by geometry of the PLG in the slit-gap field, because there was sufficient room for both vessels and bone before either contacted the polymer surface. Moreover, a persistent effect would have diminished, rather than delayed, the two regenerations. The fact that neoosteogenic rates "recovered" following their delay, and that neoangiogenic plots retained their two-peaked pattern, supports the conclusion that normal homeostatic wound healing mechanisms were intact in the slit-gap tissue. Although the PLG strands were too small to exert pressure on the surrounding tissue when expanding, they could have deposited particles during erosion that are analogous to "wear" particles from prostheses. Accordingly, there remain mechanical effects that cannot be ruled out.

Of the possible chemical effects, acidosis is not supported by recent observations on PLA *in vivo* [86] and PLG *in vitro* [62]. However, pH in the PLA study was measured in nearby blood vessels rather than near the eroding surface. Thus, there is as yet no accounting for relatively unbuffered, local effects. In the present study, the expected stimulation by lactic acid monomers of neoangiogenesis did not materialize. A reduction of macrophages by W3, which typically occurs following the clearance phase (removal of necrotic tissue and clot) of healing, may have been the reason. In any case, bioincompatibility—much less toxicity—did not appear to be a significant factor in these studies. This concurs with other rabbit studies [86]. Specific chemical interactions yet to be investigated include the role of blood-borne agents and their rate of delivery in the erosion process. Accordingly, analyses of permeability and blood supply in the BCI–PLG model are currently in progress to obtain insight into the transport aspects of the incorporation of this copolymer.

VII.   CONCLUSION

Given that degradation mechanisms for erodible implants are dominated by macrophage/giant cell and bathing fluid, it is clear that the role of microcirculatory responses to, and effects on, the synthetic guest must be understood. Biocompatibility can be assessed in terms of speed and degree of perfused vascularization of the implant, and incorporation can be described in terms of the state of the microcirculation at the time of implant disappearance. In order to achieve these assessments one must either sacrifice a large number of subjects over short intervals to obtain large sample sizes at many time points, or chronically sample a relatively small number of subjects.

BCI–IVM provides the latter approach with its inherent advantage of normalization. In addition to providing a defined group of subjects, it provides a defined tissue. The same 2 mm is being observed each time. In essence, one has simultaneously a closed system in terms of location and an open system in terms of exposure to the integrated organism — a culture cell with natural medium, as it were. The slit-gap provides a compartment into which any implant material may be placed for evaluation. On the down side, a bone screw does not allow truly "normal" healing and a gap/defect is not a fracture. The distortions, however, are almost exclusively mechanical.

Accordingly, chemical and carefully delineated mechanical conclusions may be drawn about the physiology of implant incorporation from BCI–IVM analysis. In the case of PLG, it is evident that the recipient host bed recognizes the implant as foreign. It does not, however, undertake a defensive response. There is, instead, a "cautious" healing. What remains to be determined is:

1. The specific vascular permeability changes associated with the state of the polymer
2. The degree to which the observed responses can be generalized to other preparations of PLG

Future directions for application of BCIs to the study of implant–host interaction are suggested by the nature of the model. Any material that can be formed to fit the BCI slit-gap, including nonerodables such as titanium, can be tested for biocompatibility. The data produced from these observations can provide clinically relevant and basic knowledge about physiological responses to implant materials.

REFERENCES

1. Albrektsson, T., *In vivo* studies of bone grafts: The possibility of vascular anastomoses in healing bone, *Acta Orthop. Scand., 51*, 9–17 (1980).
2. Albrektsson, T., Repair of bone grafts, *Scand. J. Plast. Reconstr. Surg., 14*, 1–12 (1980).
3. Albrektsson, T., Implantable devices for long-term vital microscopy of bone tissue, in *CRC Critical Reviews of Biocompatibility*, CRC Press, Boca Raton, FL, 1987, pp. 25–51.
4. Albrektsson, T., and B. Albrektsson, Microcirculation in grafted bone, *Acta Orthop. Scand., 49*, 1–7 (1978).
5. Albrektsson, T., A. Bach, S. Edshage, and A. Jönsson, Fibrin adhesive system (FAS) influence on bone healing rate, *Acta Orthop. Scand., 53*, 757–763 (1982).
6. Albrektsson, T., M. Jacobsson, and I. Turesson, Irradiation injury of bone tissue, *Acta Radiol. Oncol., 19*, 235–239 (1980).
7. Albrektsson, T., and L. Linder, Bone injury caused by curing bone cement. A vital microscope study in the rabbit tibia, *Clin. Orthop. Rel. Res., 183*, 280–287 (1984).
8. Anderson, J. M., Perspectives on *in vitro* interactions with biodegradable polymers, in *Portland Bone Symposium* (J. O. Hollinger and A. Seyfer, eds.), University of Oregon Health Sciences, Portland, 1993, pp. 435–448.
9. Aronson, J., B. Harrison, C. M. Boyd, D. J. Cannon, H. J. Lubansky, and C. Stewart, Mechanical induction of osteogenesis. Preliminary studies, *Ann. Clin. Lab. Sci., 18*, 195–203 (1988).
10. Ashhurst, D. E., The influence of mechanical conditions on the healing of experimental fractures in the rabbit: A microscopic study, *Phil. Trans. R. Soc. Lond. B, 313*, 271–302 (1986).
11. Böstman, O. M., Absorbable implants for the fixation of fractures, *J. Bone Joint Surg. A, 73A*, 148–153 (1991).
12. Böstman, O. M., E. Hirvensalo, J. Mäkinen, and P. Rokkanen, Foreign-body reactions to

fracture fixation implants of biodegradable synthetic polymers, *J. Bone Joint Surg. B, 72B*, 592–596 (1990).

13. Böstman, O. M., U. Päivärinta, E. Partio, M. Manninen, J. Vasenius, A. Majola, and P. Rokkanen, The tissue–implant interface during degradation of absorbable polyglycolide fracture fixation screws in the rabbit femur, *Clin. Orthop. Rel. Res., 285*, 263–272 (1992).

14. Böstman, O. M., S. Vainionpää, E. Hirvensalo, A. Mäkela, K. Vihtoner, P. Törmälä, and P. Rokkanen, Biodegradable internal fixation of malleolar fractures. A prospective randomized trial, *J. Bone Joint Surg. B, 69B*, 615–619 (1987).

15. Bouet, T., K. Toyoda, T. Ikarashi, T. Uchima, A. Nakamura, T. Tsuchiya, M. Takahashi, and R. Eloy, Evaluation of biocompatibility, based on quantitative determination of the vascular response induced by material implantation, *J. Biomed. Mater. Res., 25*, 1507–1521 (1991).

16. Brånemark, P.-I., A method for vital microscopy of mammalian bone marrow *in situ*, *Lunds Univ. Arsskrift, 54*, 1–41 (1958).

17. Brånemark P.-I., U. Breine, B. Johansson, P. J. Roylance, H. Rokert, and J. M. Yoffey, Regeneration of bone marrow, *Acta Anat. (Basel), 59*, 1–46 (1964).

18. Brighton, C. T., D. G. Lorich, R. Kupcha, T. M. Reilly, R. Rose, and R. A. I. Woodbury, The pericyte as a possible osteoblast progenitor cell, *Clin. Orthop. Rel. Res., 275*, 287–299 (1992).

19. Brighton, C. T., J. L. Schaffer, D. B. Shapiro, J. J. S. Tana, and C. C. Clark, Proliferation and macromolecular synthesis by rat calvarial bone cells grown in various oxygen tensions, *J. Orthop. Res., 9*, 847–854 (1991).

20. Brueton, R. N., W. J. Revell, and M. Brookes, Haemodynamics of bone healing in a model stable fracture, in *Bone Circulation and Vascularization in Normal and Pathological Conditions* (A. Schoutens, J. Arlet, J. W. M. Gardeniers, and S. P. F. Hughes, eds.), Plenum Press, New York, 1993, pp. 121–128.

21. Burchardt, H., The biology of bone graft repair, *Clin. Orthop. Rel. Res., 174*, 28–42 (1983).

22. Chu, C. C., The degradation and biocompatibility of suture materials, in *CRC Critical Reviews of Biocompatibility*, CRC Press, Boca Raton, FL, 1985, pp. 261–322.

23. Clark, E. R., and E. L. Clark, Microscopic observations on new bone formation of cartilage and bone in the living mammal, *Am. J. Anat., 70*, 167–200 (1942).

24. Cliff, W. J., Kinetics of wound healing in rabbit ear chambers, a time lapse cine microscopic study, *Q. J. Exp. Physiol. Cog. Med. Sci., 50*, 79–89 (1965).

25. Daniels, A. U., M. K. O. Chang, and K. P. Andriano, Mechanical properties of biodegradable polymers and composites proposed for internal fixation of bone, *J. Appl. Biomater., 1*, 57–78 (1990).

26. Daniels, A. U., M. S. Taylor, K. P. Andriano, and J. Heller, Toxicity of absorbable polymers proposed for fracture fixation devices, *Trans. Orthop. Res. Soc. 38th Mtg., 17*, 88 (1992).

27. Davis, T. R. C., and M. B. Wood, The direct effects of hydrogen ion concentration on long bone vascular resistance, *Trans. Orthop. Res. Soc. 37th Mtg., 16*, 674 (1991).

28. Davis, T. R. C., and M. B. Wood, Endothelial control of long bone vascular resistance, *J. Orthop. Res., 10*, 344–349 (1992).

29. de Paermentier, F., P. Heuschling, B. Knoops, P. Janssens de Varebeke, and P. van den Bosch de Aguilar, A new model for quantification of microvascular regeneration after a lesion of the rat cerebral cortex, *Brain Res., 398*, 419–424 (1986).

30. Duffy, M. (ed.), *Physicians Desk Reference*, 46th ed., Medical Economics Data, Montvale, NJ, 1992.

31. Einhorn, T. A., G. Simon, V. J. Devlin, J. Warman, S. P. S. Sidhu, and V. J. Vigorita, The osteogenic response to distant skeletal injury, *J. Bone Jt. Surg., 72A*, 1374–1378 (1990).

32. Ejim, O. S., G. W. Blunn, and R. A. Brown, Production of artificial-oriented mats and strands from plasma fibronectin: A morphological study, *Biomaterials, 14*, 743–748 (1993).

33. Eriksson, A. R., T. Albrektsson, B. Grane, and D. McQueen, Thermal injury to bone. A vital-microscopic description of heat effects, *Int. J. Oral Surg., 11*, 115–121 (1982).

34. Evaskus, D. S., W. Restocker, and D. M. Laskin, Evaluation of sintered titanium fiber composite as a subperiosteal implant, *J. Oral Surg., 38*, 490 (1980).

35. Ezra-Cohn, H. E., P. G. Bullough, and J. Trueta, The growth of bone autografts in rabbit ear chambers, *J. Bone Jt. Surg., 51B*, 372–379 (1969).

36. Finnegan, M., The tissue response to internal fixation devices, in *Critical Reviews in Biocompatibility*, CRC Press, Boca Raton, FL, 1989, pp. 1–11.

37. Folkman, J., Angiogenesis, in *Thrombosis and Haemostasis* (M. Verstraete, J. Vermylen, H. R. Lijnen, and J. Arnout, eds.), Leuven University Press, 1987, pp. 583–596.

38. Folkman, J., M. Klagsbrun, J. Sasse, M. Wadzinski, D. Ingber, and I. Vlodavsky, A heparin-binding angiogenic protein—basic fibroblast growth factor—is stored within basement membrane, *Am. J. Pathol., 130*, 393–400 (1988).

39. Furcht, L. T., Critical factors controlling angiogenesis: Cell products, cell matrix and growth factors, *Lab. Invest., 55*, 505–509 (1986).

40. Galante, J., W. Rostocker, R. Lueck, and R. Ray, Sintered fiber metal composites as a basis for attachment of implant to bone, *J. Bone Jt. Surg., 53A*, 101–114 (1971).

41. Glowacki, J., Tissue response to bone-derived implants, in *Bone Grafts and Bone Substitutes* (M. B. Habal and A. H. Reddi, eds.), W. B. Saunders, Philadelphia, 1992, pp. 84–92.

42. Goldberg, V. M., and S. Stevenson, Natural history of autografts and allografts, *Clin. Orthop. Rel. Res., 225*, 7–16 (1987).

43. Goldring, M. B., and S. R. Goldring, Skeletal tissue response to cytokines, in *Portland Bone Symposium*, Oregon Health Sciences University, Portland, 1993, 61–132.

44. Grinnell, F., Fibronectin and wound healing, *J. Cell. Biochem., 26*, 107–116 (1984).

45. Guardabasso, V., P. J. Munson, and D. Rodbard, A versatile method for simultaneous analysis of families of curves, *FASEB J., 2*, 209–215 (1988).

46. Ham, A. W., and D. H. Cormack, *Histology*, J. B. Lippincott, Philadelphia, 1979.

47. Hardesty, R. A., and J. L. Marsh, Craniofacial onlay bone grafting: A prospective evaluation of graft morphology, orientation and embryonic origin, *Plast. Reconstr. Surg., 85*, 5–15 (1990).

48. Heppenstall, R. B., Fracture healing, in *Fracture Treatment and Healing* (R. B. Heppenstall, ed.), W. B. Saunders, Philadelphia, 1980, pp. 35–64.

49. Hollinger, J. O., Preliminary report on the osteogenic potential of a biodegradable copolymer of polylactide (PLA) and polyglycolide (PGA), *J. Biomed. Mater. Res., 17*, 71–82 (1983).

50. Hollinger, J. O., and G. C. Battistone, Biodegradable bone repair materials. Synthetic polymers and ceramics, *Clin. Orthop. Rel. Res., 207*, 290–305 (1986).

51. Holmes, R. E., R. W. Bucholz, and V. Mooney, Porous hydroxyapatite as a bone-graft substitute in metaphyseal defects, *J. Bone Joint Surgery A, 68A*, 904–911 (1986).

52. Hunt, T. K., and W. J. Van Winkle, Wound healing, in *Fracture Treatment and Healing* (R. Heppenstall, ed.), W. B. Saunders, Philadelphia, 1980, pp. 1–34.

53. Ingber, D. E., and J. Folkman, How does extracellular matrix control capillary morphogenesis? *Cell, 58*, 803–805 (1989).

54. Jensen, J. A., T. K. Hunt, H. Scheuenstuhl, and M. J. Banda, Effect of lactate, pyruvate, and pH on secretion of angiogenesis and mitogenesis factors by macrophages, *Lab. Invest., 54*, 574–578 (1986).

55. Johnson, E. E., M. R. Urist, and F. A. M. Finerman, Bone morphogenetic protein augmentation grafting of resistant femoral nonunions, *Clin. Orthop. Rel. Res., 230*, 257–265 (1988).

56. Kelly, P. J., Pathways of transport in bone, in *Handbook of Physiology. The Cardiovascular System. Part 1: Peripheral Circulation and Organ Blood Flow* (S. R. Geiger, ed.), American Physiological Society, Bethesda, 1983, pp. 371–396.

57. Kusiak, J. F., J. E. Zins, and L. A. Whitaker, The early revascularization of membranous bone, *Plast. Reconstr. Surg., 76*, 510–516 (1985).

58. Lane, J. M., and H. S. Sandhu, Current approaches to experimental bone grafting, *Orthop. Clin. N. Am., 18*, 213–225 (1987).

59. Lewis, D. H., Controlled release of bioactive agents from lactide/glycolide polymers, in *Biodegradable Polymers as Drug Delivery Systems* (M. Chasin and R. Langer, eds.), Dekker, New York, 1990, pp. 1–41.

60. Li, S. M., H. Garreau, and M. Vert, Structure–property relationships in the case of the degradation of massive aliphatic poly-(α-hydroxy acids) in aqueous media. Part 1. Poly(DL-lactic acid), *J. Mater. Sci.: Mater. Med., 1*, 123–130 (1990).

61. Li, S. M., H. Garreau, and M. Vert, Structure–property relationships in the case of the degradation of massive aliphatic poly-(α-hydroxy acids) in aqueous media. Part 2. Degradation of lactide–glycolide polymers: PLA37.5GA25 and PLA75GA25, *J. Mater. Sci.: Mater. Med., 1*, 131–139 (1990).

62. Li, S. M., H. Garreau, and M. Vert, Structure–property relationships in the case of the degradation of massive aliphatic poly-(α-hydroxy acids) in aqueous media. Part 3, *J. Mater. Sci.: Mater. Med., 1*, 198–206 (1990).

63. Logan, W. T., personal communication (1991).

64. Marcus, M. L., D. D. Heistad, J. C. Ehrhardt, and F. M. Abboud, Total and regional cerebral blood flow measurement with 7-, 10-, 15-, 25- and 50-μ microspheres, *J. Appl. Physiol., 40*, 501–507 (1976).

65. McClugage, S. G., and R. S. McCuskey, Relationship of the microvascular system to bone resorption and growth *in situ*, *Microvasc. Res., 6*, 132–134 (1973).

66. McClugage, S. G., R. S. McCuskey, and H. A. Meineke, Microscopy of living bone marrow *in situ*. II. Influence of the microenvironment on hemopoiesis, *Blood, 38*, 96–107 (1971).

67. McCuskey, R. S., S. G. McClugage, and W. J. Younker, Microscopy of living bone marrow *in situ*, *Blood, 38*, 87–95 (1971).

68. Motoki, D. S., and J. B. Mulliken, The healing of bone and cartilage, *Clin. Plast. Surg., 17*, 527 (1990).

69. Owen, M., and J. T. Triffitt. Extravascular albumin in bone tissue, *J. Physiol., 257*, 293–307 (1976).

70. Paaske, W. P., and P. Sejrsen, Permeability of continuous capillaries, *Dan. Med. Bull., 36*, 570–590 (1989).

71. Paradis, G. R., and P. J. Kelly, Blood flow and mineral deposition in canine tibial fractures, *J. Bone Jt. Surg., 57A*, 220–226 (1975).

72. Parfitt, M. A., M. K. Drezner, F. H. Glorieux, J. A. Kanis, H. Malluche, P. J. Meunier, S. M. Ott, and R. R. Recker, Bone histomorphometry: Standardization of nomenclature, symbols and units, *J. Bone Miner. Res., 2*, 595–610 (1987).

73. Renkin, E. M., Transport pathways and processes, in *Endothelial Cell Biology* (N. Simionescu and M. Simionescu, eds.), Plenum Press, New York, 1988, pp. 51–67.

74. Riches, D. W. H., The multiple roles of macrophages in wound healing, in *The Molecular and Cellular Biology of Wound Repair* (R. A. Clark and P. M. Hensen, eds.), Plenum Press, New York, 1988, pp. 213–239.

75. Rippe, B., and B. Haraldsson, How are macromolecules transported across the capillary wall? *NIPS, 2*, 135–138 (1987).

76. Rosell, S., Tissue–blood transport and metabolism in canine adipose tissue during hemorrhage and shock, in *Microcirculation: Transport Mechanisms. Disease States* (J. Grayson and W. Zingg, eds.), Plenum Press, New York, 1975, pp. 152–162.

77. Sandison, J. C., A new method for the microscopic study of living growing tissues by the introduction of a transparent chamber in the rabbit's ear, *Anat. Rec., 27*, 281–287 (1924).

78. Schaeffer, R. C. J., R. R. Renkiewicz, S.-M. Chilton, D. Marsh, and R. W. Carlson, Preparation and high-performance size-exclusion chromatographic (HPSEC) analysis of fluorescein isothiocyanate-hydroxyethyl starch: Macromolecular probes of the blood–lymph barrier, *Microvasc. Res., 32*, 230–243 (1986).

79. Schmitz, J. P., and J. O. Hollinger, The critical size defect as an experimental model for craniomadibulofacial non-unions, *Clin. Orthop. Rel. Res., 205*, 299–308 (1986).

80. Smith, J. C., and M. Abramson, Membranous vs. endochondral bone autografts, *Arch. Otolaryngol., 99*, 203 (1974).

81. Stevenson, S., and M. Horowitz, The response to bone allografts, *J. Bone Jt. Surg., 74A*, 939–950 (1992).

82. Taylor, S., and J. Folkman, Protamine as an inhibitor of angiogenesis, *Nature, 297*, 307–312 (1982).

83. Thorogood, P. V., and J. C. Gray, The cellular changes during osteogenesis in bone and bone marrow composite autografts, *J. Anat., 120*, 27 (1975).

84. Törmälä, P., J. Vasenius, S. Vanionpää, J. Laiho, T. Pohjonen, and P. Rokkanen, Ultrahigh strength absorbable self-reinforced polyglycolide (SR-PGA) composite rods for internal fixation of bone fractures, *J. Biomed. Mater. Res., 25*, 1–22 (1991).

85. Tsukamoto, Y., W. E. Helsel, and S. M. Wahl, Macrophage production of fibronectin, a chemoattractant for fibroblasts, *J. Immunol., 127*, 673 (1981).

86. Vasenius, J., A. Majola, E.-L. Miettinen, P. Törmälä, and P. Rokkanen, Do intramedullary rods of self-reinforced poly-*L*-lactide or poly-*DL/L*-lactide cause clactic acid acidosis in rabbits? *Clin. Mater., 10*, 213–218 (1992).

87. Vert, M., S. M. Li, G. Spenlehauer, and P. Guerin, Bioresorbability and biocompatibility of aliphatic polyesters, *J. Mater. Sci.: Mater. Med., 3*, 432–446 (1992).

88. Wayland, H. J., and J. R. Fox, Quantitative measurement of macromolecular transport in the mesentery, in *Cardiovascular Dynamics* (J. Baan, A. Noordergraat, and J. Raines, eds.), MIT Press, Cambridge, 1978, pp. 215–223.

89. Wayland, J., Intravital microscopy, in *Advances in Optical and Electron Microscopy* (R. Barer and V. Cosslett, eds.), Academic Press, New York, 1975, pp. 1–47.

90. Winet, H., A horizontal intravital microscope bone chamber system for observing microcirculation, *Microvasc. Res., 37*, 105–114 (1989).

91. Winet, H., and J. Y. Bao, Relationship between volumetric flow and blood vessel dimensions in healing cortical bone, in *Engineering Science, Fluid Mechanics* (G. T. Yates, ed.), World Scientific, New York, 1990, pp. 161–169.

92. Winet, H., and J. Y. Bao, Microvascular leakage in apposing trabeculae of a healing cortical defect: A bone chamber study in the rabbit tibia, *Trans. Orthop. Res. Soc. 37th Mtg., 16*, 673 (1991).

93. Winet, H., J. Y. Bao, and R. Moffat, A control model for tibial cortex neovascularization in the bone chamber, *J. Bone Miner. Res., 5*, 19–30 (1990).

94. Winet, H., J. Y. Bao, and R. Moffat, Neo-osteogenesis of haversian trabeculae through a bone chamber implanted in a rabbit tibial cortex: A control model, *Calcif. Tiss. Int., 47*, 24–34 (1990).

95. Winet, H., P. Dossick, J. Y. Bao, W. Stetson, S. Anderson, T. M. Moore, and L. Menendez, Neo-osteogenesis at the interface between allograft and host bone as viewed in the bone chamber, *Trans. Orthop. Res. Soc. 34th Mtg., 13*, 395 (1988).

96. Winet, H., P. Dossick, J. Y. Bao, W. Stetson, S. Anderson, T. M. Moore, and L. Menendez, Neovascularization of 2 mm allograft discs: A preliminary intravital microscope bone chamber study in the rabbit, in *Bone Circulation and Bone Necrosis* (J. Arlet and B. Maziéres, eds.), Springer-Verlag, New York, 1988, pp. 369–373.

97. Winet, H., and J. O. Hollinger, Incorporation polylactide–polyglycolide in a cortical defect: Neo-osteogenesis in a bone chamber, *J. Biomed. Mater. Res., 27*, 667–676 (1993).

98. Winet, H., and J. O. Hollinger, Intravital microscopic evidence that polylactide–polyglycolide (PLGA) delays neo-osteogenesis and neo-angiogenesis in healing bone, *Cells Mater., 3*, 273–281 (1993).

99. Winet, H., and J. O. Hollinger, Incorporation of polylactide–polyglycolide in a cortical defect: Neo-angiogenesis and blood supply in a bone chamber, *J. Orthop. Res.* (1995, in press).

100. Wolf, M. B., L. P. Porter, and P. D. Watson, Effects of elevated venous pressure on capillary permeability in cat hindlimbs, *Am. J. Physiol., 257*, H2025–H2032 (1989).

101. Yasko, A. W., J. M. Lane, E. J. Fellinger, V. Rosen, J. M. Wozney, and E. A. Wang, The healing of segmental bone defects, induced by recombinant human bone morphogenetic protein (rhBMP-2). A radiological, histological, and biochemical study in rats, *J. Bone Jt. Surg., 74A*, 659–670 (1992).

DATE DUE
